Detection of Optical Signals

Series in Optics and Optoelectronics

For more information about this series, please visit:
https://www.crcpress.com/Series-in-Optics-and-Optoelectronics/book-series/TFOPTICSOPT

Detection of Optical Signals

Antoni Rogalski
Zbigniew Bielecki

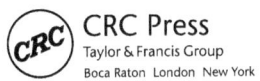

CRC Press
Taylor & Francis Group
Boca Raton London New York

CRC Press is an imprint of the
Taylor & Francis Group, an **informa** business

First edition published 2022
by CRC Press
6000 Broken Sound Parkway NW, Suite 300, Boca Raton, FL 33487-2742

and by CRC Press
2 Park Square, Milton Park, Abingdon, Oxon, OX14 4RN

CRC Press is an imprint of Taylor & Francis Group, LLC

Library of Congress Cataloging-in-Publication Data
Names: Rogalski, Antoni, author. | Bielecki, Zbigniew, author.
Title: Detection of optical signals / Antoni Rogalski and Zbigniew Bielecki.
Description: First edition. |
Boca Raton: CRC Press, [2022] |
Series: Series in optics and optoelectronics | Includes bibliographical references and index.
Identifiers: LCCN 2021045715 | ISBN 9781032059488 (hbk) |
ISBN 9781032069227 (pbk) | ISBN 9781003263098 (ebk)
Subjects: LCSH: Image converters. | Optical detectors. | Charge coupled devices.
Classification: LCC TK8316 .R64 2022 |
DDC 621.36/7–dc23/eng/20211110
LC record available at https://lccn.loc.gov/2021045715

ISBN: 978-1-032-05948-8 (hbk)
ISBN: 978-1-032-06922-7 (pbk)
ISBN: 978-1-003-26309-8 (ebk)

DOI: 10.1201/9781003263098

Typeset in Times
by Newgen Publishing UK

Access the Support Material: www.routledge.com/9781032059488

Contents

Preface

This book provides a comprehensive overview of the important technologies for photon detection, from the X-ray through ultraviolet, visible, infrared to far-infrared spectral regions. It unique feature relays on combining subject matter from many disciplines, especially physics and electronics – which usually have little interaction – into a comprehensive treatment of a unified topic. In textbooks, we frequented at least a dozen distinct areas in the global literature. While excellent textbooks exist in many of those fields, there was a need to have a single publication that adopts the perspective of linking the specific mechanisms in the context of optical receivers.

The receiver of optical radiation consists of a photodetector, preamplifier and signal-processing circuit. In a photodetector, the optical signal is converted into an electrical one, which is amplified before further processing. *Detection of Optical Signals* treats optical receivers and system components and considers various readout electronics in fabrication of detector arrays. It is expected that the reader will gain a good understanding of the similarities and contrasts, the strengths and weaknesses, of the multitude of approaches that have been developed over a century of effort to improve our ability for photon detection. In the past, the emphasis was always on the methods of operation and physical limits to detector performance.

The specific goals of this textbook are to

- Provide a bridge from physical mechanisms into the methods used for photon detection in a wide spectral range;
- Guide readers into more detailed and technical treatments of readout optical signals;
- Give a broad overview of the optical signal detection, including the terahertz region and two-dimensional material;
- Make the book accessible to the widest possible audience;
- Each chapter ends with recommended problems to help readers in further studies.

The level of presentation is suitable for graduate students in physics and engineering who have received standard preparation in modern solid-state physics and electronic circuits. This book is also of interest to individuals working with aerospace sensors and systems, remote sensing, thermal imaging, military imaging, optical telecommunications, infrared spectroscopy and light detection and ranging. To satisfy the needs of the first group, many chapters discuss the principles underlying each topic before bringing the reader the most recent information available. The book could especially be used as a reference for participants in relevant workshops and short courses.

Detection of Optical Signals is divided into twelve chapters. The first four chapters give general information about optical detectors and systems. In fact, this part is a source of fundamental information needed in understanding the other parts of book. Chapter 1 establishes the formalism and definitions used in signal imaging. General detector characteristics and their merits are discussed in Chapter 2. Chapter 3 is devoted to the fundamentals of detector noise, which limits the performance of detectors. The detection mechanisms in most widely used thermal and photon detectors and in analysis of the fundamental performance limits common to all of detectors, are provided in Chapter 4. The objective of the next six chapters (5 to 10) is to present the status of different types of thermal (Chapter 5), photoemissive (Chapter 6) and a wide class of photon detectors operated in spectral regions from X-rays to far-infrared (Chapter 7), quantum well, superlattice and quantum dot photodetectors (Chapter 8), a new generation of 2D material photodetectors (Chapter 9), and terahertz detectors (Chapter 10). Since the output signal from any of the detector must be processed by external electronics, Chapter 11 describes direct and same advanced detection systems. Several types of discrete devices or integrated circuits suitable for the active element in preamplifiers, bipolar (BJT) and field-effect transistor (FET), or an integrated circuit with an input bipolar transistor FET or MOSFET transistor, are described. Chapter 12 describes the progress in focal plane array techniques – in their fabrication and in integrated circuit design. Particular attention is put on monolithic arrays in the visible region (CCD and CMOS) and hybrid arrays in infrared.

Detection of Optical Signals gives, we hope, a comprehensive analysis of the latest developments in optical light detector technology and basic insight into the fundamental processes important to evolving detection techniques. The book covers a broad spectrum of detectors, including theory, types of materials and their fundamental physical properties, and detector fabrication.

We are confident that you will enjoy using this textbook covering the fundamentals of optical signal detection, that you will derive fascination and pleasure from the extremely fast-growing sub-discipline of optoelectronics and photonics, and that you will use your knowledge in the development of your own scientific research.

Acknowledgements

In the course of writing this book, many people have assisted us and offered their support. We would like to express appreciation to the managements of the Institute of Applied Physics and the Institute of Optoelectronics, Military University of Technology, Warsaw, Poland for providing the environment in which we worked on the book. The writing of the book has been partially done under financial support of both institutes. We also sincerely thank Stuart Murray of CRC Press for providing assistance and accommodating our schedule.

Author Bios

Antoni Rogalski is a professor at the Institute of Applied Physics, Military University of Technology in Warsaw. He is one of the world's leading researchers in the field of infrared (IR) optoelectronics. He has made pioneering contributions in the areas of theory, design, and technology of different types of IR detectors. In 1997, Professor Rogalski received an award from the Foundation for Polish Science, the most prestigious scientific award in Poland, for his achievements in the study of ternary alloy systems for infrared detectors. His monumental monograph, *Infrared and Terahertz Detectors* (published in three editions by Taylor and Francis), has been translated into Russian and Chinese. In 2013, Professor Rogalski was elected as an Ordinary Member of the Polish Academy of Sciences and as a member of the Central Commission for Academic Degrees and Titles. Since early 2015, he has been the Dean of the Faculty of Technical Sciences of the Polish Academy of Sciences, and, from 2016, he has been a member of the group for affairs of scientific awards of the Prime Minister of Poland.

Professor Rogalski is a fellow of the International Society for Optical Engineering (SPIE), vice-president of the Polish Optoelectronic Committee, editor-in-chief of the journal *Opto-Electronics Review* (1997–2015), deputy editor-in-chief of the *Bulletin of the Polish Academy of Sciences: Technical Sciences* (2003–present), and a member of the editorial boards of several international journals. He is an active member of the international technical community – as chair and co-chair, organizer, and member of scientific committees of many national and international conferences on optoelectronic devices and materials sciences.

Zbigniew Bielecki, PhD, D.Sc., Eng. is a graduate of the Faculty of Electronics of the Military University of Technology in Warsaw. Since 1983 he has been working at the Institute of Optoelectronics of the Military University of Technology. He received a PhD degree in 1992, obtained his post-doctoral degree in 2002 and received the title of professor in 2008.

Professor Bielecki has held many managerial positions at his alma mater. Currently, he is a full professor at the Military University of Technology. His scientific achievements include over 450 publications in the field of optical detection signals (including 4 monographs, 2 academic scripts, 11 chapters in foreign monographs, 7 chapters in domestic monographs, and over 70 publications in indexed journals). Since he received the title of professor, the subjects of his scientific activity have been highly sensitive sensors of hazardous gases, optoelectronic sensors of disease markers contained in exhaled air, and optical communication in open space.

In 2017, Professor Bielecki received the Award of the Minister of National Defense for his lifetime achievements.

1 Radiometry and Photometry

In this chapter we will introduce definitions and parameters characterising electromagnetic radiation. In practice, the term *radiometry* is usually limited to the measurement of infrared, visible and ultraviolet light using optical instruments. The radiometric calculations are an essential part in the characterisation of detectors and in determining the signal-to-noise ratio. Radiometry not only means detecting and measuring the energy of electromagnetic radiation, but it is also used to determine the power of radiation transferred from one object to another.

The term radiometry has a meaning similar to *photometry*, related to the visible range of radiation, where the notion of radiation photons is used. Photometry is the measurement of light, which is defined as radiation detectable by the human eye. It is restricted to the visible region, and all quantities are weighted by the spectral response of the eye. It is a quantitative science based on a statistical model of the human visual response to light – that is, our perception of light – under carefully controlled conditions.

Radiometry deals with radiant energy of any wavelength. Photometry is restricted to radiation in the visible region of spectrum. The basic unit of power in radiometry is the watt (W). Typical photometric units include lumen (luminous flux), candela (luminous intensity), lux (illuminance), and candela per square meter (luminance). The lumen is simply radiant power modified by the relative spectral sensitivity of the eye.

In this chapter we will review the radiometric measurements that form the basis of the detector performance analysis. We are not able to design a correct construction of devices without specifying the spectrum and the value of the radiation power emitted by the object (target) and falling on the detector. We will try to answer the basic question: what energy value is collected and transferred to the detector surface if we know the geometric configuration of the radiation source, detector and system optics? The answer to this question makes it possible to clearly determine the signal-to-noise ratio of the system.

In order to simplify our theoretical considerations, we will limit ourselves to non-coherent sources, which are perfectly black bodies. We will exclude lasers and other sources that are partially or completely coherent. Then, the calculation of the energy distribution on the surface is the result of a simple scalar summation and not the result of a vector sum of amplitudes, as in the case of a coherent interference. In addition, we ignore the influence of diffraction effects and assume the approximation of small angles (this is a significant limitation, as it does not include cases where the object is close to the measuring equipment). Under such conditions, the sine of a given angle can be approximated by the value of the angle expressed in radians.

This chapter provides some guidance in radiometry. For further details, see References [1–8].

DOI: 10.1201/9781003263098-1

1.1   INTRODUCTION

Electromagnetic radiation is divided into sub-bands depending on the wavelength: gamma radiation, X, ultraviolet, visible, infrared, microwave and radio waves. This division is determined by the nature of the sources and the detector technologies used for individual spectrum ranges. The present book is dedicated to the detection of optical signals, so it is necessary to define this spectral range. Optical radiation is a part of electromagnetic radiation in the frequency range between 3×10^{13} and 3×10^{16} Hz. This range corresponds to wavelengths between 10 nm and 10 μm and includes the regions commonly called the ultraviolet, the visible, and the infrared [9, 10]. The most important spectral range determined by the sensitivity of the human eye is the visible range, corresponding to a wavelength between 0.38 μm and 0.78 μm. These values should be treated as approximate as they depend on the value of the energy flux of radiation acting on the retina and on the sensitivity of the observer. Figure 1.1 shows the electromagnetic radiation spectrum, while Figure 1.2 shows the spectrum of optical radiation.

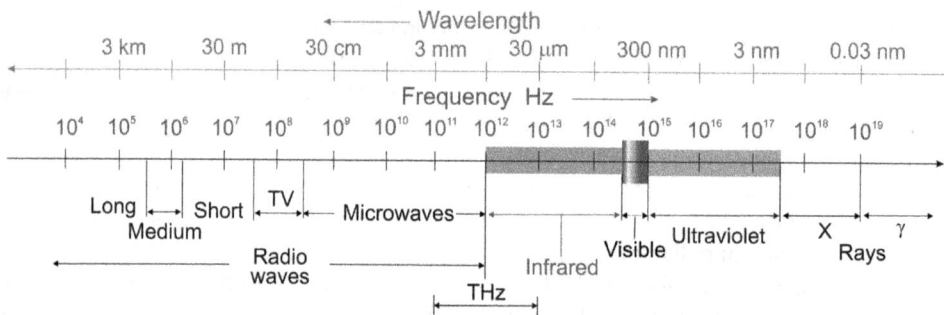

FIGURE 1.1   The electromagnetic wave spectrum.

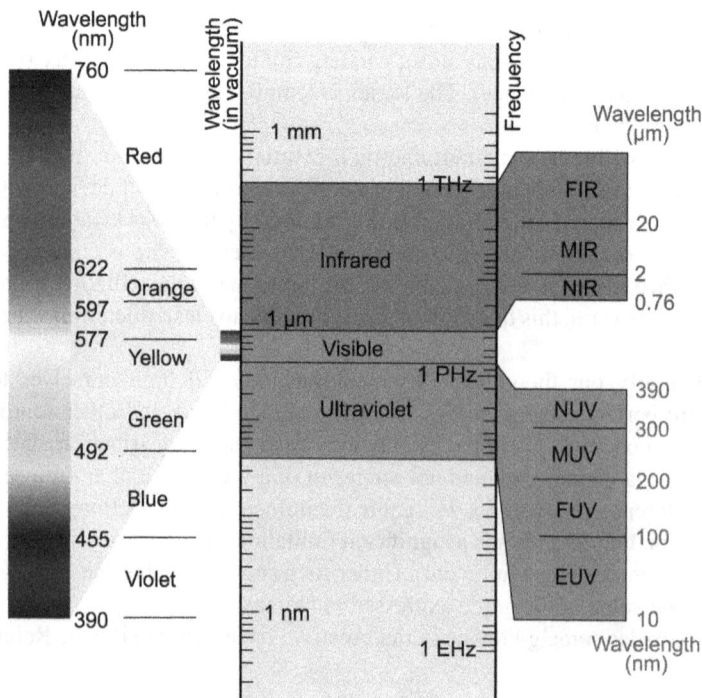

FIGURE 1.2   The optical wave spectrum.

The electromagnetic wavelength is related to two other parameters, the frequency v and the photon energy E, by the following equations:

$$v = \frac{c}{\lambda}, \tag{1.1}$$

$$E = h v [J] = \frac{hc}{\lambda q} [eV], \tag{1.2}$$

where $c = 3 \times 10^8$ m/s is the speed of light in a vacuum, λ is the wavelength, and $h = 6,626 \times 10^{-34}$ Js is the Planck constant. The electromagnetic waves propagate at different speeds depending on the type of medium in such a way that their frequency remains constant. For infrared radiation of a wavelength of 1 μm, from dependence (1.1) and (1.2), we obtain a frequency of about 3×10^{14} Hz and a photon energy of 2×10^{-19} J. For a wavelength of 10 μm, the frequency and energy values are by an order of magnitude smaller and are of 3×10^{13} Hz and 2×10^{-20} J (0.124 eV), respectively.

1.2 RADIOMETRIC AND PHOTOMETRIC QUANTITIES AND UNITS

Historically, the power of a light source was obtained by observing brightness of the source. It turns out that brightness perceived by the human eye depends upon wavelength – that is, colour of the light – and differs from the actual energy contained in the light. The eye is sensitive to radiation over a range of approximately 11 orders of magnitude from bright sunlight to a flash of light containing only a few photons.

The retina of the human eye contains two different types of photoreceptors called rods and cones that produce nerve impulses that are passed on to subsequent stages of the human visual system for processing (see Figure 1.3). The cones are spread over the entire retina, together with a large concentration within a small central area of our vision, called the fovea, which results in our high visual acuity at the centre of the field of view of the eye. The cones are responsible for our daytime colour

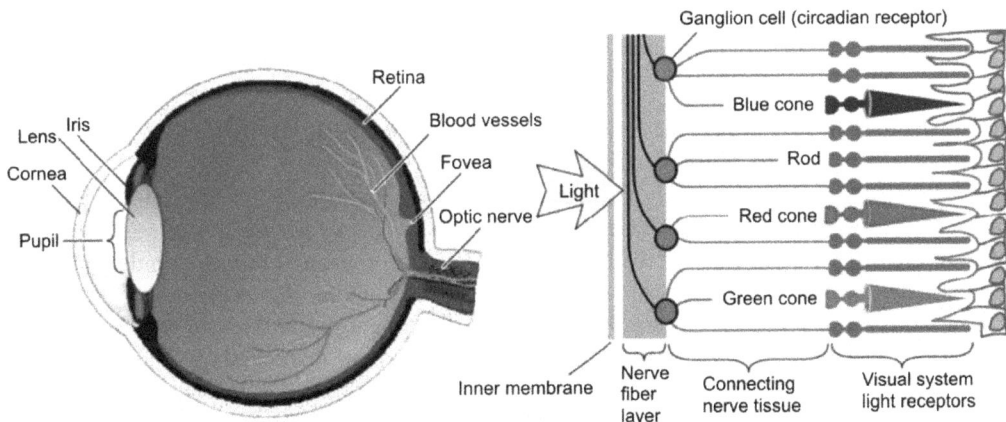

FIGURE 1.3 Schematic illustration of the human eye. The illustration shows the fovea, a cone-rich central region of the retina which affords the high acuteness of central vision. The cell structure of the retina includes the light-sensitive rod cells and cone cells. The ganglion cells and nerve fibres transmit the visual information to the brain. Rod cells are more abundant and more light-sensitive than cone cells. Rods are sensitive over the entire visible spectrum.

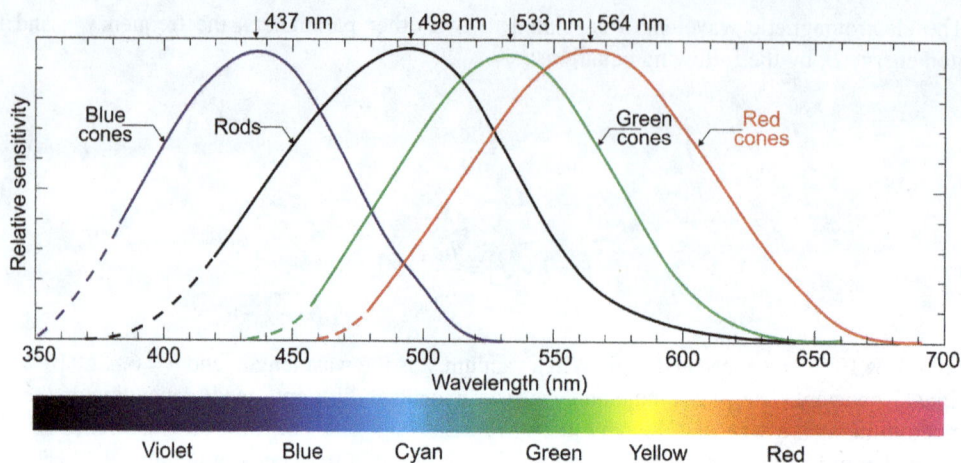

FIGURE 1.4   The spectral sensitivity functions of the rods and three types of cones sensitive in blue, green and red spectral range.

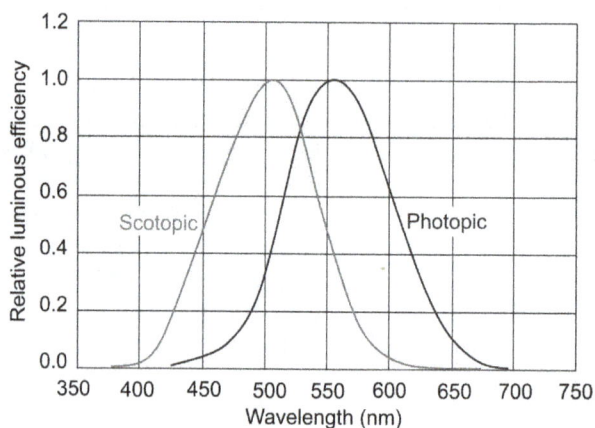

FIGURE 1.5   CIE spectral luminous efficiency functions.

vision. The rods are spread over the entire retina except the fovea and are responsible for our night, basically black-and-white, vision.

The approximate spectral sensitivity functions of the rods and three types of cones are shown in Figure 1.4. Inspection of the figure reveals that night vision (scotopic vision) is weaker in the red spectral range and thus stronger in the blue spectral range as compared to vision in daytime (photopic vision). The following discussion mostly relates to the photopic vision regime.

The eye is most sensitive to yellow-green light ($\lambda \approx 555$ nm) and less sensitive to red and blue lights of the spectrum. This means that a monochromatic wave of this length gives the impression of being much brighter than monochromatic waves of other lengths carrying the same energy. To take the difference into account, a new set of physical measures of light is defined for the visible light that parallels the quantities of radiometry, where the power is weighted according to the human response by multiplying the corresponding quantity by a spectral function, called the $V(\lambda)$ function or the spectral luminous efficiency for photopic vision, defined in the domain from 360 to 830 nm, and is normalised to one at its peak, 555 nm (Figure 1.5). The $V(\lambda)$ function tells us the appropriate response of the human eye to various wavelengths. This function was first defined by

TABLE 1.1
Radiometric and Photometric Quantities and Units

Photometric quantity	Unit	Radiometric quantity	Symbol	Unit	Unit conversion
Luminous flux	lm (lumen)	Radiant flux	Φ	W (Watt)	1 W = 683 lm
Luminous intensity	cd (candela) = lm/sr	Radiant intensity	I	W/sr	1 W/sr = 683 cd
Illuminance	lx (lux) = lm/m^2	Irradiance	E	W/m^2	1 W/m^2 = 683 lx
Luminance	cd/m^2 = lm/(sr m^2)	Radiance	L	W/(sr m^2)	1 W/(sr m^2) = 683 cd/m^2
Luminous exitance	lm/m^2	Radiant exitance	M	W/m^2	
Luminous exposure	lx s	Radiant exposure		W/(m^2 s)	
Luminous energy	lm s	Radiant energy	Q	J (Joule)	1 J = 683 lm s

the Commission Internationale de l'Éclairage (CIE) in 1924 [11] and is an average response of a population in a wide range of ages. It should be noted that the $V(\lambda)$ function was defined assuming additivity of sensation and a 2° field of view at relatively high luminance levels (>1 cd/m^2): the high radiation range is mediated by the cones. The spectral responsivity of human eyes deviates significantly at very low levels of luminescence (<10^{-3} cd/m^2) when the rods in the eyes are the dominant receptors. This type of vision is called scotopic vision.

There is a relationship between a photometric quantity X_v and a radiometric quantity $X_{e,\lambda}$ [6]:

$$X_v = K_m \int_{360\,nm}^{830\,nm} X_{e,\lambda} V(\lambda) d\lambda, \tag{1.3}$$

where K_m is the photometric radiation equivalent. It is defined as the ratio of the luminous flux to the corresponding energy flux, for the wavelength corresponding to the highest eye sensitivity, V (λ = 555 nm) = 1.

The units as well as the names of similar properties in photometry differ from those in radiometry. For instance, power is simply called power in radiometry or radiant flux, but it is called the luminous flux in photometry. While the unit of power in radiometry is the watt, in photometry it is the lumen. A lumen is defined in terms of a fundamental unit, called candela, which is one of the seven independent quantities of the SI system of units (meter, kilogram, second, ampere, Kelvin, mole and candela). Candela is the SI unit of the photometric quantity called luminous intensity, or luminosity that corresponds to the radiant intensity in radiometry. Table 1.1 lists the radiometric and photometric quantities and units along with translation between both groups of units.

Quantitative characterisation of radiation sources requires a precise definition of units. There are three types of radiometric quantities: energetic, light (photometric), and photon. The basic symbols are the same, but each of these quantities is identified, where necessary, by an appropriate index: e (energetic), v (luminous), p (photonic). Luminous quantities are used only to determine the properties of visible radiation. Tables 1.2, 1.3 and 1.4 collect the names of these quantities, their symbols and units.

In the case of infrared radiation, the energy and photon quantities are used. The basic unit of energy is the Joule (J); Table 1.2 gives the values based on it. Similar units can be introduced based on photon quantities. Such quantities and the units assigned to them marked with index p are presented in Table 1.3. The conversions of units between two systems can be done on the basis of the relation defining the amount of energy per photon: $E = hc/\lambda$. For example:

$$\Phi_e (J/s) = \Phi_p (photon/s) \times E (J/photon). \tag{1.4}$$

TABLE 1.2
Energetic Quantity

Symbol	Energetic quantity	Unit	Definition
Q_e	Radiant energy	J	Energy emitted, transferred or incident to the surface
Φ_e	Radiant flux	W	Power emitted, transmitted or incident to the surface
I_e	Radiant intensity	W/sr	Radiant flux emitted per unit solid angle
E_e	Irradiance	W/m^2	Radiant flux per unit area
M_e	Radiant exitance	W/m^2	Density radiant flux leaving a surface
L_e	Radiance	W/(m^2 sr)	Radiant flux per unit solid angle emitted from a unit surface element

TABLE 1.3
Photon Quantity

Symbol	Photon quantity	Unit	Definition
Q_p	Number of photons	photons	
Φ_p	Photon flux	photons/s	Number of photons per time unit emitted, transferred or incident
I_p	Photon flux density	photons/(s sr)	Photon flux emitted per unit solid angle
E_p	Photon irradiance	photons/(s m^2)	Photon flux incident per unit area
M_p	Photon exitance	photons/(s m^2)	Photon flux emitted by the unit area of the source
L_p	Photon luminance	photons/(s m^2 sr)	Photon flux density emitted from a unit surface element

TABLE 1.4
Photometric Quantity

Symbol	Photometric quantity	Unit	Definition
Q_v	Luminous energy	lm s	
Φ_v	Luminous flux	lm	Luminous energy per unit time
I_v	Luminous intensity	lm/sr	Luminous flux per unit solid angle
E_v	Illuminance	lm/m^2 (lx)	Luminous flux incident on a surface
M_v	Luminous exitance	lm/m^2	Luminous flux emitted from a surface
L_v	Luminance	lm/(m^2 sr)	Luminous flux per unit solid angle per unit projected source area

As we will see later, photon-based units are more convenient for describing photon detectors, whose sensitivity is proportional to the number of incident photons, while energy-based units are more useful for describing thermal detectors, sensitive to absorbed radiation energy.

Radiometry is plagued by a confusion of terminology, symbols, definitions, and units. The origin of this confusion is largely because of the parallel or duplicate development of the fundamental radiometric practices by researchers in different disciplines. Consequently, considerable care should be exercised when reading publications. The terminology used in this chapter follows international standards and recommendations [7,12].

1.3   RADIOMETRIC QUANTITIES

Radiant flux, also called radiant power, is the energy Q (in joules) radiated by a source per unit of time and is defined by

$$\Phi = \frac{dQ}{dt}. \tag{1.5}$$

The unit of radiant flux is the Watt (W = J/s).

Radiant exitance and irradiance have identical units (W/cm²) but have different interpretations. The irradiance is characterised by the spatial power density associated with the surface absorbing or emitting the incident radiation, while the exitance refers to the surface emitting the radiation. For example, exitance is characterised by energy-emitting sources, and irradiance may be characterised by passive areas of the receiver. Radiant exitance can be described as follows:

$$M = \frac{\partial \Phi}{\partial A}, \tag{1.6}$$

and can be approximated for small areas as $M = \Phi/A$, where A is the area. Figure 1.6 shows an illustration of radiant exitance (a) and irradiance (b).

Radiant intensity is the radiant flux from a point source emitted per unit solid angle in a given direction, and is expressed as

$$I = \frac{\partial \Phi}{\partial \Omega} = \frac{\partial^2 Q}{\partial t \partial \Omega}, \tag{1.7}$$

where $d\Phi$ is the radiant flux leaving the source and propagating in an element of solid angle $d\Omega$ containing the given direction (see Figure 1.7). The unit of radiant intensity is W/sr.

The solid angle may be expressed in differential form as

$$d\Omega = \frac{dA}{r^2}. \tag{1.8}$$

The unit of solid angle is steradian (sr).

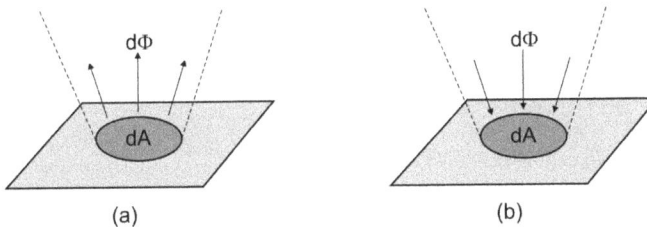

FIGURE 1.6 Radiation exitance (a) and irradiance (b).

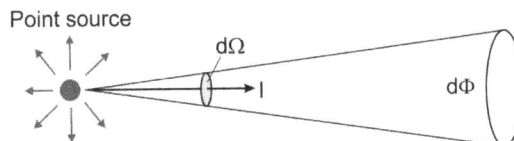

FIGURE 1.7 Radiant intensity.

If we use the spherical coordinate system seen in Figure 1.8, and use $dA = r^2 \sin\theta d\theta d\varphi$, we can write as

$$d\Omega = \sin\theta d\theta d\varphi. \tag{1.9}$$

Given this relationship, we can derive the expression for the solid angle of a flat disk with a half angle θ_{max} in the form of

$$\Omega = \int d\Omega = \int_0^{2\pi} d\varphi \int_0^{\theta_{max}} \sin\theta d\theta = 2\pi(1 - \cos\theta_{max}). \tag{1.10}$$

If a disc is small enough in relation to its distance from the beginning of the coordinate system, the solid angle of a flat disc is the ratio of the disc area divided by the square of the distance. In this case, the difference between the disk surface and the part of the spherical surface can be ignored.

Usually, we do not calculate the total power radiated by the source, because the optical system or detector takes only part of the power emitted in a limited solid angle. The radiant intensity from a point source decreases in an inverse proportion to the square of the distance from the source (see Figure 1.9).

We consider the receiver of the area A, which is placed at various distances from the point source having a uniform radiant intensity I (Figure 1.9). Using Eq. (1.7), we get

$$\Phi = I\frac{A}{r^2}, \tag{1.11}$$

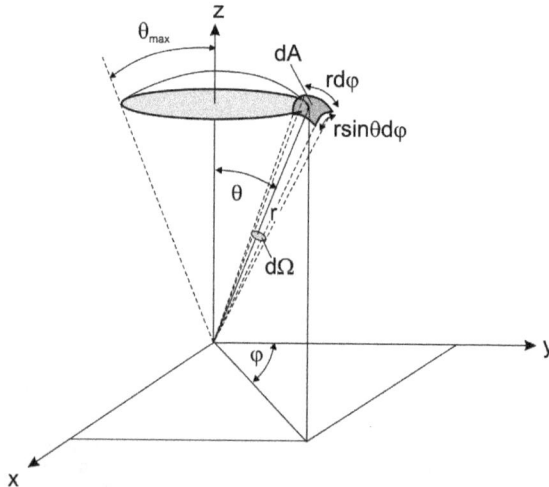

FIGURE 1.8 Relationship of solid angle to planar angle.

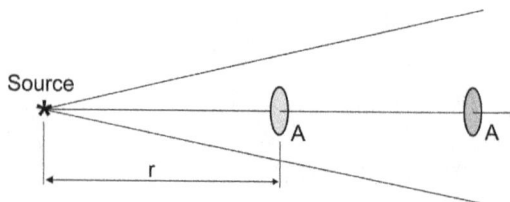

FIGURE 1.9 Irradiance falloff as a function of r from source.

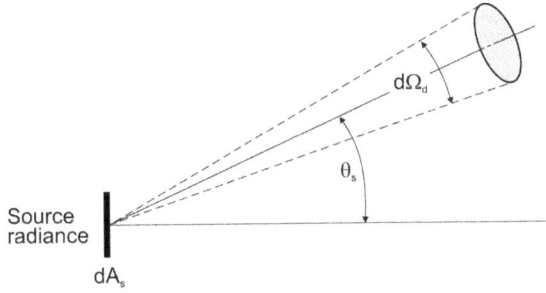

FIGURE 1.10 Radiance of an extended source.

and next:

$$E = \frac{\Phi}{A} = \frac{I}{r^2}. \tag{1.12}$$

Because the solid angle subtended by the detector falls off as $1/r^2$, the collected flux and the irradiance also decrease proportionally.

1.4 LUMINANCE

Luminance, or radiance, is used in the case of an extended source (see Figure 1.10) where its surface area is comparable to the square of the distance between the source and receiver. It defines the radiant flux or luminous flux emitted by a unit surface of the source in a unit solid angle. In a differential notation, luminance takes the form of:

$$L = \frac{\partial^2 \Phi}{\partial A_s \cos \theta_s \, \partial \Omega_d}, \tag{1.13}$$

where $\partial \Phi$ is the radiant flux emitted from the surface element and propagating in the solid angle $\partial \Omega$ containing the given direction, ∂A_s is the area of the surface element, and θ_s is the angle between the normal to the surface element and the direction of the beam. The term $\partial A_s \cos \theta$ gives the projected area of the surface element perpendicular to the measurement direction. Eq. (1.13) indicates that the power received by the detector is differential with regard to both the incremental projected area of the source and the incremental solid angle of the detector. By rearranging this equation, we obtain:

$$\partial^2 \Phi = L \partial A_s \cos \theta_s \, \partial \Omega_d, \tag{1.14}$$

and integrating one with regard to the source surface, we obtain the intensity:

$$I = \frac{\partial \Phi}{\partial \Omega_d} = \int_{A_s} L \partial A_s \cos \theta_s. \tag{1.15}$$

Similarly, by integrating over a solid angle, we obtain the expression for the existence:

$$M = \frac{\partial \Phi}{\partial A_s} = \int_{\Omega_d} L \cos \theta_s \, \partial \Omega_d. \qquad (1.16)$$

A Lambertian source (radiator) has a constant radiance that is independent of a viewing direction. This type of reflector is also referred to as an ideal diffuse radiator (emitter or reflector); see Figure 1.11. In practice, there are no true Lambertian surfaces. Most matte surfaces approximate an ideal diffuse reflector, but typically exhibit semi-specular reflection characteristics at oblique viewing angles. An ideal thermal source (blackbody) is perfectly Lambertian, while certain special diffusers also closely approximate the condition. An actual source is typically approximately Lambertian within the range of view of the angle θ_s that is less than 20°.

Even for a Lambertian source, the intensity depends on θ_s. Assuming that L is independent of the source position, we can exclude the term $L \cos \theta_s$ from the integral sign, from Eq. (1.15) as follows:

$$I = LA_s \cos \theta_s = I_n \cos \theta_s. \qquad (1.17)$$

It is Lambert's Cosine Law, where I_n is the intensity of the ray leaving in a direction perpendicular to the surface. For non-Lambertian surfaces, the radiance L is a function of the angle itself, and the falloff of I with θ_s is faster than $\cos \theta_s$.

To receive a relationship between the radiation exitance and the radiance for a planar Lambertian source, we return to Eq. (1.16) and integrate

$$M = \frac{\partial \Phi}{\partial A_s} = \int_{\Omega_d} L \cos \theta_s \, d\Omega_d = \int_0^{2\pi} d\varphi \int^{\pi/2} L \cos \theta_s \sin \theta d\theta = 2\pi L \frac{1}{2} = \pi L, \qquad (1.18)$$

where the Lambertian-source assumption has been used to pull L outside of the angular integrals. For a non-Lambertian source, the integration yields the proportionality constant different from π.

Let us simplify further considerations assuming $\theta_s = 0$. Then, for the geometrical configuration shown in Figure 1.12, the detector solid angle is given by:

$$\Omega_d = \frac{A_d}{r^2}. \qquad (1.19)$$

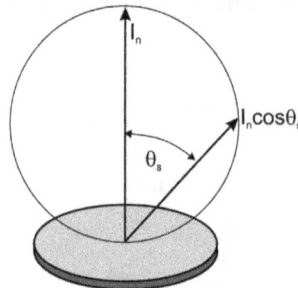

FIGURE 1.11   Radiant intensity as a function of θ_s for a Lambertian source.

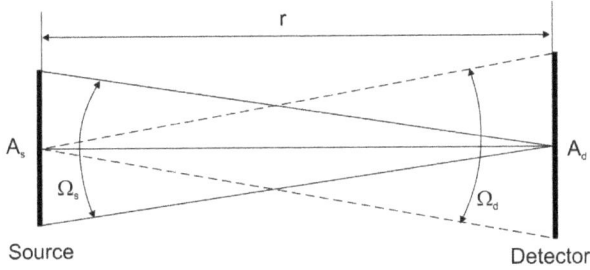

FIGURE 1.12 Radiant power transfer from source to detector.

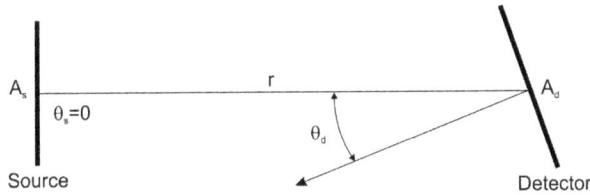

FIGURE 1.13 Radiant power transfer from source to a titled detector.

The radiant power on the detector can be obtained by multiplying the detector solid angle by the area of the source and the radiance of the source:

$$\Phi_d = LA_s\Omega_d = \frac{LA_sA_d}{r^2} = L\Omega_sA_d. \tag{1.20}$$

From this equation we can see that the flux on the detector is expressed as the radiance of the source multiplied by an area×solid angle ($A_d\Omega_s$) product. To fulfil Eq. (1.20), two limitations are required: a small angle assumption for the approximation of the solid angle of a flat surface by A/r^2 and the flux transfer is unaffected by absorption losses in the system.

Another situation occurs for a tilted receiver shown in Figure 1.13. The source normal is along the line of centres, so $\theta_s = 0$ in this case. The angle θ_d is the angle between the line of centres and the normal to the detector surface. In this situation,

$$\Phi_d = LA_s\Omega_d, \tag{1.21}$$

and since $\Omega_d = A_d\cos\theta_d / r^2$, thus

$$\Phi_d = LA_s\frac{A_d\cos\theta_d}{r^2}. \tag{1.22}$$

Thus, the flux collected and the irradiance (Φ/A_d) are decreased by a factor of $\cos\theta_d$.

We now proceed to calculate the flux on the detector when both θ_s and θ_d are nonzero, assuming a flat Lambertian source (Figure 1.14). A cosine falloff factor arises at both the source and the receiver. In this case:

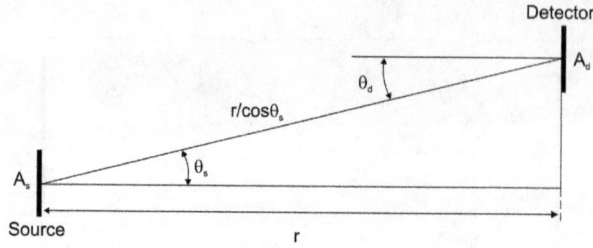

FIGURE 1.14　Radiation emitted from a source where θ_s and θ_d are non-zero.

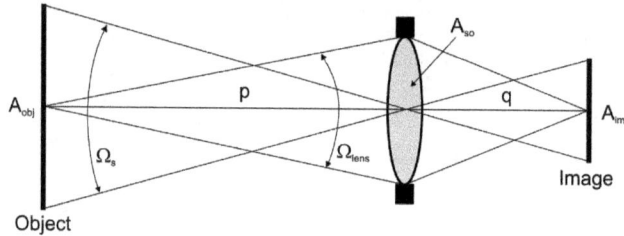

FIGURE 1.15　Radiant power collected by an optical system.

$$\Phi_d = LA_s \cos\theta_s \frac{A_d \cos\theta_d}{\left(r/\cos\theta_s\right)^2}. \tag{1.23}$$

Assuming that the surfaces of source and detector are parallel and $\theta_s = \theta_d = \theta$, the radiant intensity is proportional to $\cos^4\theta$. On account of this Eq. (1.23) is the so-called cosine to the fourth law.

Finally, we consider the flux transfer in the image-forming systems, assuming the limitations of paraxial optics (small angles) as shown in Figure 1.15. Only a certain amount of the flux Φ is collected by the optical system, an amount that can be calculated letting the lens aperture (A_{lens}) act as an intermediate receiver:

$$\Phi = LA_{obj}\Omega_{lens} = LA_{lens}\Omega_{obj}. \tag{1.24}$$

It should be noted that in a more complex system, the entrance pupil is the intermediate receiver and the $A_{lens}\Omega_{obj}$ product is the area–solid angle product of the optical system. At these conditions, the collected radiant flux equals and is reformatted by the lens and forms an image of the original object at an appropriate magnification.

The image irradiance can be found simply by dividing the flux collected in Eq. (1.24) by the image area:

$$\Phi = LA_{lens}\Omega_{lens} = LA_{lens}\Omega_{obj} = L\frac{A_{lens}A_{obj}}{p^2} = L\frac{A_{lens}A_{img}}{q^2}, \tag{1.25}$$

where p is the distance of the object from the lens, q is the distance of the image from the lens, and the last equality was obtained by using $A_{img} = A_{obj}(q/p)^2$. From Eq. (1.25), the image irradiance is equal to:

$$E_{img} = \frac{\Phi}{A_{img}} = L\frac{A_{lens}}{q^2}.$$ (1.26)

1.5 BLACKBODY RADIATION

Thermal radiation is the most common form of radiation emission. All bodies at a temperature above absolute zero emit radiation in all directions over a wide range of wavelengths. The amount of radiation energy emitted from a surface at a given wavelength depends on the material of the body and the surface temperature. Therefore, different bodies may emit different amounts of radiation at the same temperature per unit surface area. The maximum amount of radiation can be emitted and absorbed by an idealised body, called a blackbody. A blackbody is defined as a perfect absorber and emitter of radiation. It emits the radiation energy uniformly in all directions per unit area normal to the emission direction (Figure 1.16), and absorbs all incident radiation, regardless of its direction and wavelength. Its unique feature is that the spectral distribution of the emitted radiation depends solely on temperature.

The concept of the blackbody is an idealisation, as perfect black bodies do not exist in nature; however, they are good approximations to a black material. Its good approximations are: a hollow sphere or a cone (Figure 1.17) with a hole (a tiny one compared to the cavity dimensions, but a large one compared to the wavelength, so that marginal diffraction effects can be omitted), or radiant heaters covered with substances of high and non-selective emissivity (blacks, e.g., carbon black,

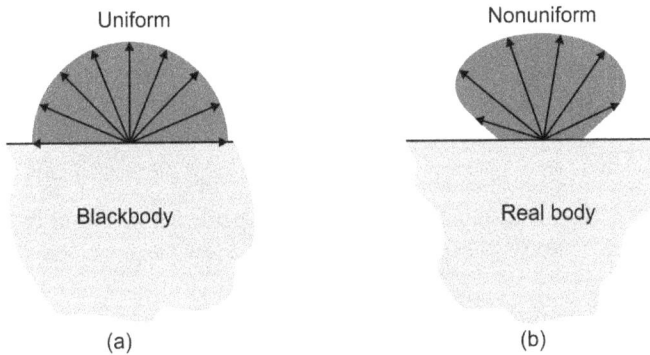

FIGURE 1.16 Radiation: (a) a blackbody, (b) a real body.

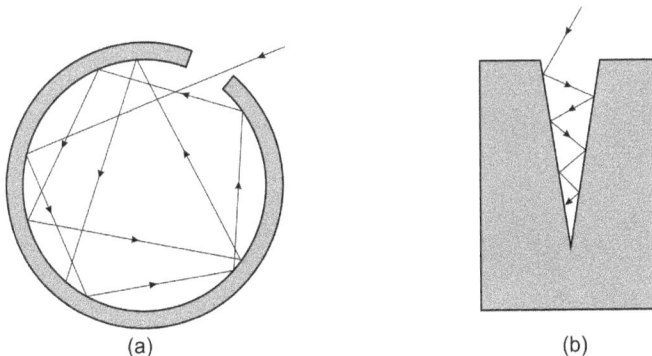

FIGURE 1.17 Model of blackbody: (a) a hollow sphere, (b) a cone.

gold black, and others). It should also be noted that knowledge of blackbody radiation laws is helpful in learning about the radiation laws of real bodies.

All objects are composed of continually vibrating atoms, with higher energy atoms vibrating more frequently. The vibration of all charged particles, including these atoms, generates electromagnetic waves. The higher the temperature of an object, the faster the vibration and, thus, the higher the spectral radiant energy. As a result, all objects are continually emitting radiation at a rate with a wavelength distribution that depends upon the temperature of the object and its spectral emissivity, $\varepsilon(\lambda)$.

Radiant emission is usually treated in terms of the concept of a blackbody [4]. A blackbody is an object that absorbs all incident radiation and, conversely, according to Kirchhoff's Law, is a perfect radiator. The energy emitted by a blackbody is the maximum theoretically possible for a given temperature. A device of this type is a very useful standard source for the calibration and testing of radiometric instruments. Further, most sources of thermal radiation radiate energy in a manner that can be readily described in terms of a blackbody emitting through a filter, making it possible to use the blackbody radiation laws as a starting point for many radiometric calculations.

1.5.1 PLANCK'S LAW

At the end of the nineteenth century very careful measurements of a perfect blackbody thermal radiation were carried out. It turned out, however, that attempts to derive a law describing this spectrum, based on the principles of classical physics, led to absurd results. For example, Rayleigh and Jeans, applying the laws of classical electrodynamics for balanced radiation (in which the radiation emitted by vibrating atomic electrons, which are oscillators, is absorbed by other atoms), obtained the following formula determining the spectral flux of the radiation emitted by a unit surface:

$$M(v,T) = \frac{2\pi v^2}{c^2} kT. \qquad (1.27)$$

Note that from this formula it results that the flux is proportional to v^2 and at $v \to \infty$ it is heading towards infinity. This is contrary to experience. Only in the low frequency range does it agree well with experience.

Trying to remove the discrepancies between theory and experience, Planck in 1900 put forward a hypothesis that an electric harmonic oscillator, which is a model of an elementary source of radiation, in the process of radiation emission can lose energy only in discrete packets, that is, quantum ΔE, of a value proportional to the frequency v of its own vibrations. That is,

$$\Delta E = hv, \qquad (1.28)$$

where $h = 6.626 \times 10^{-34}$ Js is the Planck's constant. The dimension h is action = energy × time = length × linear momentum = angular momentum. Generalising his deliberations, Planck suggested that the oscillator energy can take the values of

$$E_n = nhv \quad n = 0,1,2\ldots, \qquad (1.29)$$

where n is the quantum number.

The blackbody, or Planck equation, was one of the milestones of physics. Planck's Law describes the spectral radiance (spectral radiant exitance) of a perfect blackbody as a function of its temperature and the wavelength of the emitted radiation, in the form

$$M_{e,v}(v,T) = \frac{2\pi h v^3}{c^2} \frac{1}{\exp(h v / kT) - 1} \quad [\text{W} / (\text{cm}^2 \text{Hz})]. \tag{1.30}$$

This formula determines the spectral distribution of a body radiation which is very well in line with experience. In the low frequency range, it takes a form of the Reyleigh-Jeans formula (1.27).

Equation (1.30) can also be expressed according to the wavelength as

$$M_{e,\lambda}(\lambda,T) = \frac{2\pi h c^2}{\lambda^5} \frac{1}{\exp(hc / \lambda kT) - 1} \quad [\text{W} / (\text{cm}^2 \mu\text{m})]. \tag{1.31}$$

The analogous equation in photon units is as follows:

$$M_{p,\lambda}(\lambda,T) = \frac{2\pi c}{\lambda^4} \frac{1}{\exp(hc / \lambda kT) - 1} \quad [\text{photons} / (\text{scm}^2 \mu\text{m})]. \tag{1.32}$$

Similarly, dependencies determining energy and photon spectral luminance can be obtained from

$$L_{e,\lambda}(\lambda,T) = \frac{2h c^2}{\lambda^5} \frac{1}{\exp(hc / \lambda kT) - 1} \quad [\text{W} / (\text{cm}^2 \text{sr} \mu\text{m})]. \tag{1.33}$$

$$L_{p,\lambda}(\lambda,T) = \frac{2c}{\lambda^4} \frac{1}{\exp(hc / \lambda kT) - 1} \quad [\text{photons} / (\text{s} \, \text{cm}^2 \text{sr} \, \mu\text{m})]. \tag{1.34}$$

Corresponding equations for the spectral radiant exitance, $M(\lambda,T)$, and the spectral radiance, $L(\lambda,T)$, are related by $M = \pi L$.

Figure 1.18 shows a plot of these curves for a number of blackbody temperatures. As the temperature increases, the amount of energy emitted at any wavelength increases, too, and the wavelength of peak emission decreases.

1.5.2 Wien's Displacement Law

For each blackbody temperature T, the spectral exitance of the radiation $M_{e,\lambda}$ reaches a maximum at a certain wavelength λ_m, which can be determined by differentiating formula (1.31) with respect to the wavelength and comparing the derivative to zero. This produces the wavelength of

$$\lambda_m = \frac{2898}{T} \quad [\mu\text{m}]. \tag{1.35}$$

This is called Wien's Displacement Law. The plot of λ_m versus source temperature is a hyperbola.

In a similar way, we can obtain the maximum sensitivity for the photon spectral exitance of radiation, differentiating the formula (1.32) and comparing the derivative to zero. Then, we obtain the wavelength at which this maximum occurs is

$$\lambda_m = \frac{3670}{T} \quad [\mu\text{m}], \tag{1.36}$$

and depends on the blackbody temperature.

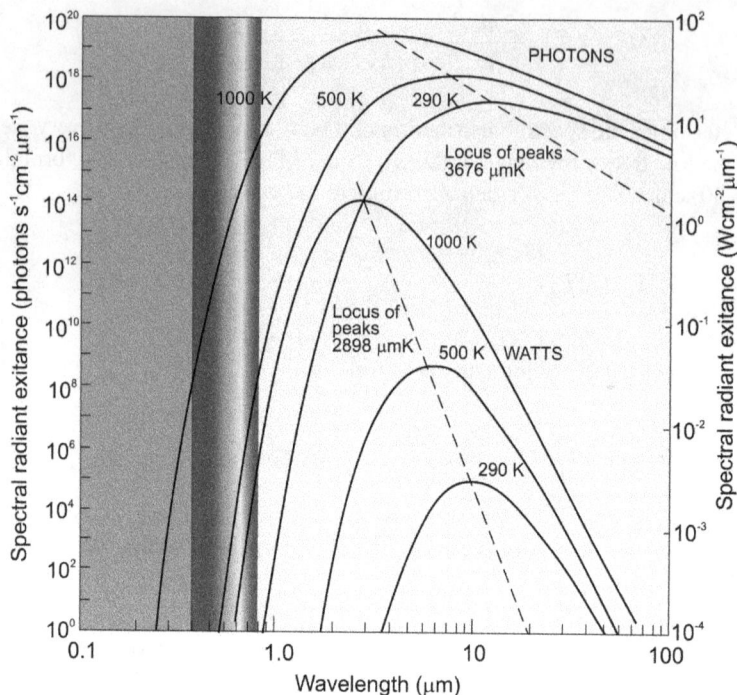

FIGURE 1.18 Planck's Law for spectral radiant exitance.

The loci of these maxima are shown in Figure 1.18 [13]. Note that for an object at an ambient temperature of 259 K, λ_m occur at 10.0 μm [Eq. (1.35) and 12.7 μm [Eq. (1.36)], respectively. We need detectors operating near 10 μm if we expect to "see" room-temperature objects such as people, trees and vehicles without the aid of reflected light. For hotter objects, such as engines, maximum emission occurs at shorter wavelengths. Thus, the waveband 2–15 μm in infrared or thermal region of the electromagnetic spectrum contains the maximum radiative emission for thermal imaging purposes. It is interesting to note that the λ_m for the Sun is near 0.5 μm, very close to the peak of sensitivity of the human eye.

1.5.3 STEFAN-BOLTZMANN'S LAW

Total radiant exitance $M_e(T)$ from a blackbody at the temperature T is the integral of the spectral exitance $M_e(\lambda, T)$ over all wavelengths:

$$M_e(T) = \int_0^\infty M_{e,\lambda}(\lambda,T) d\lambda = \int_0^\infty \frac{2\pi hc^2 d\lambda}{\lambda^5 \left[\exp(hc/\lambda kT) - 1\right]}. \tag{1.37}$$

This can be interpreted as the area under the spectra entrance curves for a given temperature, as shown in Figure 1.19. Carrying out this integral over all wavelengths we obtain

$$M_e(T) = \frac{2\pi^5 k^4}{15c^2 h^3} T^4 = \sigma_e T^4. \tag{1.38}$$

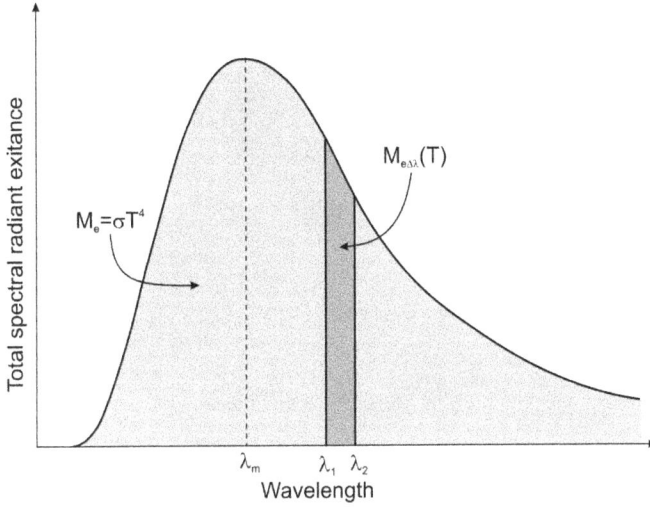

FIGURE 1.19   Total spectral radiant exitance at the temperature T and over the wavelength band from λ_1 to λ_2.

The relationship described by Eq. (1.38) is called Stefan-Boltzmann's Law, where σ_e is called the Stefan-Boltzmann constant and has an approximate value of 5.67×10^{-12} W/(cm^{2}K^4).

The radiant exitance of the blackbody between λ_1 and λ_2 is obtained by integrating Planck's Law over the integral $[\lambda_1, \lambda_2]$, as shown in Figure 1.19. The relationship between the total exitance of a blackbody over the wavelength band and its temperature is

$$M_{e,\Delta\lambda}(T) = \int_{\lambda_1}^{\lambda_2} M_{e,\lambda}(\lambda, T) d\lambda. \tag{1.39}$$

The exitance at 300 K over the interval 8–14 µm is equal to 1.22×10^2 W/m^2 and is equivalent to the exitance over the interval 3–5 µm at 410 K. The exitance over 8–14 µm is larger than exitance over 3–5 µm up to 600 K [14]. These results show the advantage of using the 8–14 µm region for low temperature targets.

1.5.4   EXITANCE CONTRAST

Consideration of how much the exitance changes with temperature is important to infrared system sensitivity. For a system operating within a finite passband ($\Delta\lambda$) it is important at what wavelength the source (target) exitance changes the most with temperature.

This consideration of the exitance contrast involves the following second partial derivative:

$$\frac{\partial}{\partial\lambda}\left[\frac{\partial M_{e,\lambda}(\lambda, T)}{\partial T}\right] = 0, \tag{1.40}$$

which produces a constraint of the similar form to Wien's Displacement Law:

$$\lambda_m = \frac{2410}{T} \quad [\mu m]. \tag{1.41}$$

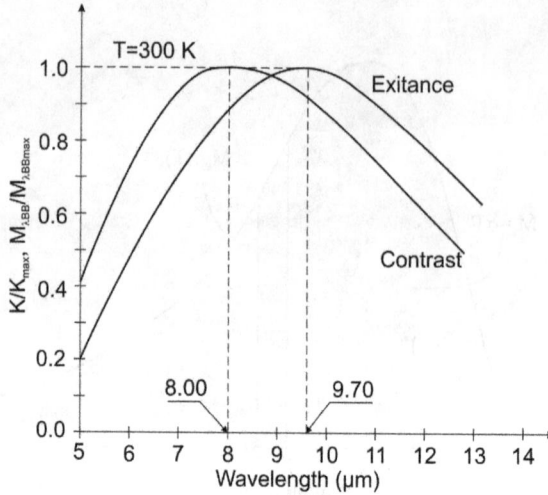

FIGURE 1.20 Comparison of contrast curve and radiant exitance of a perfect blackbody.

The function of

$$\left[\frac{\partial M_{e,\lambda}(\lambda,T)}{\partial T} \right] = K(\lambda,T), \tag{1.42}$$

is defined as the temperature contrast [8]. Dependency (1.41) determines the wavelength of blackbody radiation for which we have the maximum contrast value.

Figure 1.20 shows, according to dependencies (1.41) and (1.42), the curves of contrast and radiant exitance of a perfect blackbody as a function of a wavelength, for $T = 300$ K. Both curves are given in relative units related to the maximum function values. The maximum of contrast determined in accordance with the Wien's Law is for $\lambda \approx 8$ µm. This value does not correspond to the maximum exitance (about 9.7 µm).

There is an important proposal for a design of detection systems for use in military equipment (Eq. 1.40). If we assume that these devices should operate in the temperature range $\Delta T = -30°C$ to $+45°C$, then, the optimal conditions for detecting the minimum temperature changes of the detected object are in the band $\Delta\lambda = (7.6 - 9.9$ µm$)$.

1.6 EMISSIVITY

The questions that naturally arise are as follows:

- How does blackbody model perfectly describe real sources?
- How closely does the radiation spectrum of a real heated body correspond to that of a blackbody?

As mentioned previously, the blackbody curve provides the upper limit of the overall spectral exitance of a source for any specific temperature. Most thermal sources are not perfect blackbodies. Many are called graybodies. A graybody is one that emits radiation in the exact same spectral distribution as a blackbody at the same temperature, but with a reduced intensity. The graybody and blackbody have the same shape spectrally (see Figure 1.21).

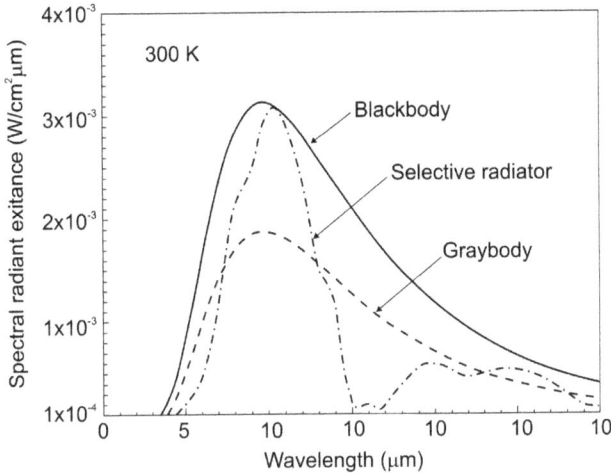

FIGURE 1.21 Spectral radiant exitance of three different radiators.

The ratio between the exitance of the actual source and the exitance of a blackbody at the same temperature is defined as emissivity. In general, emissivity depends on the wavelength λ and the temperature T:

$$\varepsilon(\lambda,T) = \frac{M_{e,\lambda}(\lambda,T)_{\text{source}}}{M_{e,\lambda}(\lambda,T)_{\text{blackbody}}}, \tag{1.43}$$

and represents a dimensionless number between zero and one ($0 \leq \varepsilon \leq 1$). This is called the spectral emissivity. Other types of emissivity are also defined (e.g., total emissivity), but we will not deal with it any further.

For a perfect blackbody, $\varepsilon = 1$ for all wavelengths. The emissivity of a graybody is independent of a wavelength. A selective source has an emissivity that depends on a wavelength. The total radiant exitance for a graybody at all wavelengths is equal to

$$M_e^{gb} = \varepsilon \sigma_e T^4. \tag{1.44}$$

For a completely transparent or fully reflective body, $\varepsilon = 0$. A more complicated situation is in the case of a selective radiator, where emissivity is a wavelength complex function (see Figure 1.21).

Emissivity provides a convenient parameter for use in the real sources modelling.

When radiation strikes a surface, part of it is reflected, Φ_r, part of it is absorbed, Φ_a, and the remaining part is transmitted, Φ_t:

$$\Phi = \Phi_r + \Phi_a + \Phi_t. \tag{1.45}$$

Figure 1.22 shows the absorption, reflection, and transmission of incident radiation by a semi-transparent material.

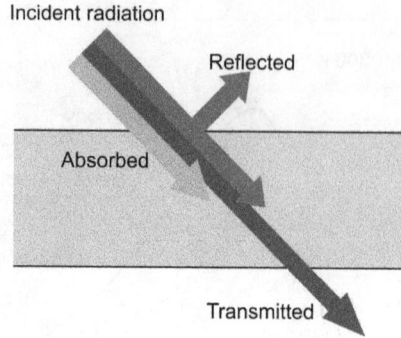

FIGURE 1.22 Processes occurring during interaction of optical radiation with matter.

By dividing both sides of the equation (1.45) by Φ, we obtain

$$a + r + t = 1. \tag{1.46}$$

The fraction of an irradiation absorber by the matter is called absorptivity, a, the fraction reflected by the surface is called reflectivity, r, and the fraction transmitted is called transmissivity, t.

For an opaque body, when there is a transmittance, $(t = 0)$, we obtain

$$a + r = 1 \quad \text{or} \quad a = 1 - r. \tag{1.47}$$

If the body does not fully absorb incident radiation, it will emit less radiation to remain in thermal equilibrium. Therefore:

$$\text{watts absorbed} = \alpha EA = \varepsilon MA = \text{watts radiated.} \tag{1.48}$$

According to Kirchhoff's Law, the integrated absorptivity equals the integrated emissivity ($a = \varepsilon$). Kirchhoff's Law also holds for spectra quantities $a(\lambda,T) = \varepsilon(\lambda,T)$, where α and ε are the functions λ and T. A blackbody has $\varepsilon = 1$ and is also perfectly black, that is, it is a perfect absorber ($a = 1$). Good absorbers are also good emitters. For example, matte black paint has a low reflectivity, so absorptivity and emissivity are high. Typically, poor emitters are good reflectors. Another example is polished brass, for which the reflectance is high, so absorptivity and emissivity are low. A body can be absorbing radiation from a high-temperature source (e.g., the Sun) and re-radiating as a lower temperature source (≈ 300 K). Recall that the peak exitance for Sun is at 0.5 μm and the peak exitance of a 300 K body is around 10 μm. However, it is not generally true that $a(\lambda = 0.5$ μm) equals $a(\lambda = 10$ μm). Since emissivity is a wavelength function, we cannot estimate it in the infrared by the visible appearance. An example of this is white paint (TiO_2). At 0.5 μm, its emissivity is 0.19, while at 10 μm, its emissivity is 0.94.

Table 1.5 lists the emissivity of a number of common materials [15]. The quality of the treated surface is very important to radiative properties. The emissivity values of various substances are usually given without taking into account the functional dependence on λ and T.

However, some general trends about emissivity as a function of temperature follow. For non-metallic substances, emissivity value is typically $\varepsilon > 0.8$ for room temperature and decreases with increasing temperature [16]. For metallic substances, the emissivity is very low at room temperature, unless the surface is oxidised. Generally, for metallic substances, the emissivity increases proportionally to temperature (Figure 1.23). The main reason for this is the surface oxidation process that occurs with increasing temperature.

TABLE 1.5
Relative Values of the Emissivity of Several Materials

Material	Temperature [K]	Emissivity
Tungsten	500	0.05
Polished silver	650	0.03
Polished aluminium	300	0.03
	1000	0,07
Polished copper		0.02–0.15
Polished iron		0.2
Polished brass	4–600	0.03
Oxidised iron		0.8
Black oxidised copper	500	0.78
Aluminum oxidised	80–500	0.75
Water	320	0.94
Ice	273	0.96–0.985
Paper	293	0.92
Glass		0.94
Lampblack	273–373	0.95
Laboratory blackbody cavity		0.98–0.99

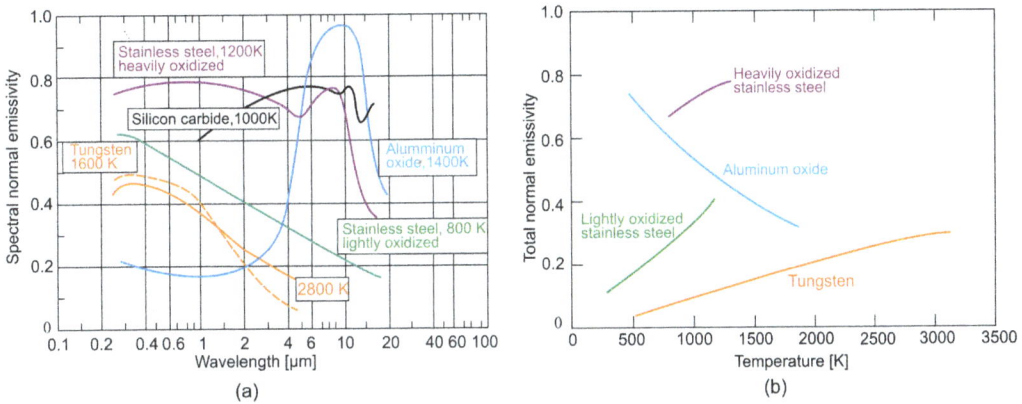

FIGURE 1.23 The dependence of the emissivity on (a) wavelength, (b) temperature for several real bodies.

1.7 PROPAGATION OF OPTICAL RADIATION

Most optoelectronic devices are designed to record optical signals that are transmitted in the Earth's atmosphere. Figure 1.24 shows a diagram of the detection system, which enables the measurement of an optical signal coming from the object under investigation. Typically, the detection system consists of an optical block (reflective or refractive), detector, detector cooler, low-noise preamplifier, signal processing system and display.

1.7.1 PROPAGATION OF OPTICAL RADIATION THROUGH THE ATMOSPHERE

Before the optical radiation is focused on the detector surface, it passes through the atmosphere and an optical system. The atmosphere interacts with the optical radiation due to some phenomena

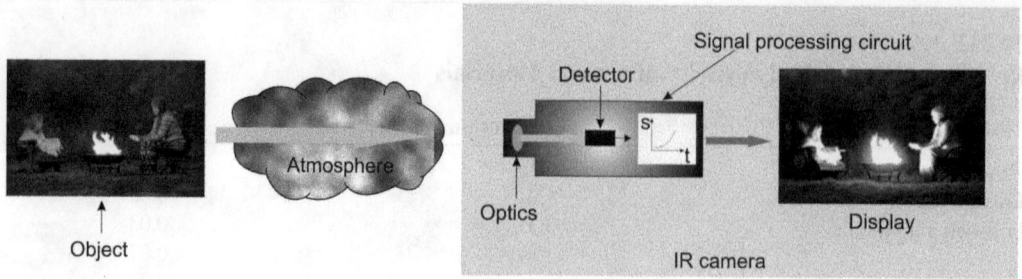

FIGURE 1.24 Diagram of the detection system enabling the measurement of an optical signal transmitted through the atmosphere.

depending on its composition. Practically, atmosphere consists of different molecular species and small particles like aerosols (fog, forest exudates, dust, sea-salt particles, soil particles, volcano debris, particulate, air pollutants, smog and smoke), ice particles and water droplets. Thus, atmosphere causes attenuation of an optical signal by absorption, scattering and scintillation.

In general, the atmospheric attenuation τ is described by Beer's Law:

$$\tau = \exp\left[-\left(\alpha_{abs} + \beta_{scat}\right)L\right],\tag{1.49}$$

where L is the distance between transmitter and receiver, α_{abs} and β_{scat} are the coefficients of atmosphere absorption and scattering, respectively.

Absorption is caused by atmospheric molecules, the energy levels of which can be excited by incident photons. The absorption coefficient depends on type, effective absorption cross section σ_{abs}, and concentration N_{abs} of gas molecules. This parameters value is expressed as follows [17]:

$$\alpha_{abs} = \sigma_{abs} N_{abs}.\tag{1.50}$$

The scattering process causes a redirected radiation beam to propagate in various directions away from the original direction [9]. There are three main types of scattering: Rayleigh, Mie and non-selective. The scattering type depends on a relationship between both scattering particles' size and the wavelength of the propagating light. Rayleigh scattering is caused by particles with a size much smaller than the light wavelength. In this case, the scattering intensity decreases with the wavelength as $\sim\lambda^{-4}$. When the particle size is comparable or as large as a radiation wavelength, Mie scattering is observed. Non-selective scattering occurs for a particle with a size larger than the beam wavelength. In this case, Mie theory is approximated by the principles of reflection, refraction and diffraction. The scattering coefficient depends on the concentration N_{scat} and the effective cross section parameters σ_{scat} of the particles and can be described by

$$\beta_{scat} = \sigma_{scat} N_{scat}.\tag{1.51}$$

The fog particles float in the air for a longer time by comparison with rain droplets. Additionally, they are characterised by smaller size comparable to a radiation wavelength. Thus, the scattering due to rainfall (non-selective scattering) is less effective than scattering due to fog (Mie scattering). The rain scattering coefficient can be determined using Stroke's Law [18]:

$$\beta_{rain\,scat} = \pi r^2 N_a Q_{scat}\left(r/\lambda\right),\tag{1.52}$$

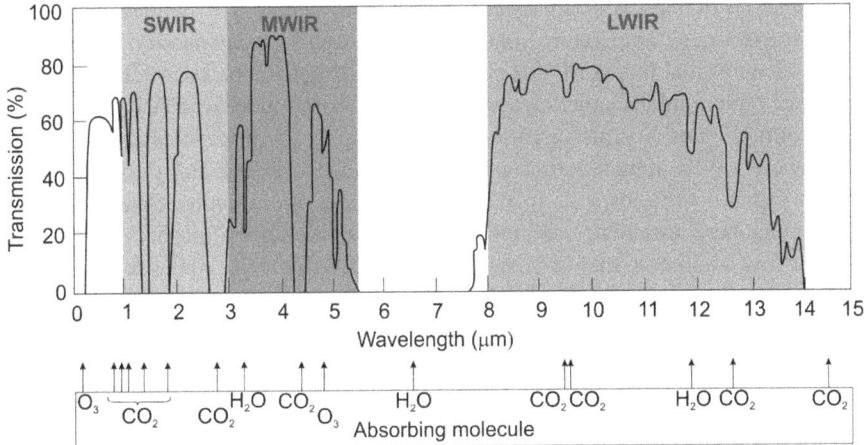

FIGURE 1.25 Transmission of the atmosphere for a 6,000-ft horizontal path at sea level containing 17 mm of precipitate water.

where r is the radius of a raindrop (from 0.001 cm to 0.1 cm), N_a is the raindrop distribution, and Q_{scat} is the scattering efficiency.

Another important atmospheric factor that limits transmission of optical radiation is turbulence. Clear-air turbulence is defined as a chaotic streams and eddies of the air masses in the absence of any clouds. Such air movements are described as turbulent because of the air masses moving at widely different speeds [19]. As a result of this phenomenon, the phase shifts of the propagating optical radiation are noticed. The distortions of a front-wave can be observed as intensity changes, referred to as scintillation. Aerosols, moisture, temperature and pressure fluctuations produce variations of the air density and, thus, its refractive index [20]. The air eddies can bend optical paths if the eddies' size is larger than the beam diameter. In the opposite situation, constructive and destructive interferences are created resulting in temporal fluctuations of light intensity (spots) at the receiver surface.

Figure 1.25 is a plot of the transmission through 6,000 feet of air as a wavelength function [21]. Specific absorption bands of water, carbon dioxide and oxygen molecules are indicated, which restricts the atmospheric transmission to three windows, at 1.4–3 μm, 3–5 μm and 8–14 μm.

The short wavelength infrared (SWIR) band (1.4–3 μm) offers unique imaging advantages over visible and thermal bands [20]. Like visible cameras, the images are primarily created by reflected broadband light sources, so SWIR images are easier for viewers to understand. Most materials used to make windows, lenses and coatings for visible cameras are readily useable for SWIR cameras, keeping costs down. Ordinary glass transmits radiation to about 2.5 μm. SWIR cameras can image many of the same light sources, such as YAG laser wavelengths. Thus, with safety concerns shifting laser operations to the "eye-safe" wavelengths where beams do not focus on the retina (beyond 1.4 μm), SWIR cameras are in a unique position to replace visible cameras for many tasks. Due to the reduced Rayleigh scattering of light at longer wavelengths by particulates in the air, such as dust or fog, SWIR cameras can see through haze better than visible cameras.

The long wavelength infrared (LWIR) band (8–14 μm) is preferred for high-performance thermal imaging because of its higher sensitivity to ambient temperature objects and its better transmission through mist and smoke. However, the middle wavelength infrared (MWIR) band (3–5-μm) may be more appropriate for hotter objects, or if sensitivity is less important than contrast. Also, additional differences occur; for example, the advantage of the MWIR band is a smaller diameter of the optics required to obtain a certain resolution, and some detectors may operate at higher temperatures (TE cooling) than is usual in the LWIR band, where cryogenic cooling is required (about 77 K).

Summarising, MWIR and LWIR µm spectral bands differ substantially with regard to background flux, scene characteristics, temperature contrast and atmospheric transmission under diverse weather conditions. Factors that favour MWIR applications are higher contrast, offer superior clear weather performance (favourable weather conditions, e.g., in most countries of Asia and Africa), higher transmittivity in high humidity, and higher resolution due to ~3 times smaller optical diffraction. Factors that favour LWIR applications are better performance in fog and dust conditions, winter haze (typical weather conditions, e.g., in Western Europe, northern United States, Canada), higher immunity to atmospheric turbulence and reduced sensitivity to solar glints and fire flares. The possibility of achieving a higher signal-to-noise (S/N) ratio due to greater radiance levels in the LWIR spectral range is not persuasive because the background photon fluxes are higher to the same extent, and, also because of readout limitation possibilities. Theoretically, in staring arrays, the charge can be integrated for a full frame time, but because of restrictions in the charge-handling capacity of the readout cells, it is much less compared to the frame time, especially for LWIR detectors for which the background photon flux exceeds the useful signals by orders of magnitude.

1.7.2 TRANSMISSION RANGE OF OPTICAL MATERIALS

An important element of any detection system is the optical block. It consists of optical elements (windows, lenses, plane mirrors, spherical and aspherical mirrors, light-splitting plates, prisms, filters, and others) that create image of observed objects in the plane of detector(s).

There are two types of optical elements: refractive elements and reflective ones. Sometimes refractive-reflective blocks are used. The role of reflective elements is to reflect the incident radiation, and the role of refractive elements is to refract and transmit the incident radiation.

Reflective elements are commonly used in IR systems (e.g., in scanners and lidars). The most important advantages of their use include the absence of chromatic aberrations. Moreover, they are lighter than refractive systems. Their disadvantage is susceptibility to assembly errors, and high requirements for surface shape tolerances [20]. Metallic coatings are usually used as reflective coatings of mirrors. They should be characterised by a large, close to unity, reflection coefficient. For this purpose, aluminium, chromium, silver, gold and others are used. Flat mirrors are widely used to fold the optical path, and reflective prisms are often used in scanning systems.

The choice of material for refractive elements in optical systems is primarily dictated by the spectral dependence of the transmittance of the material under consideration (Figure 1.26).

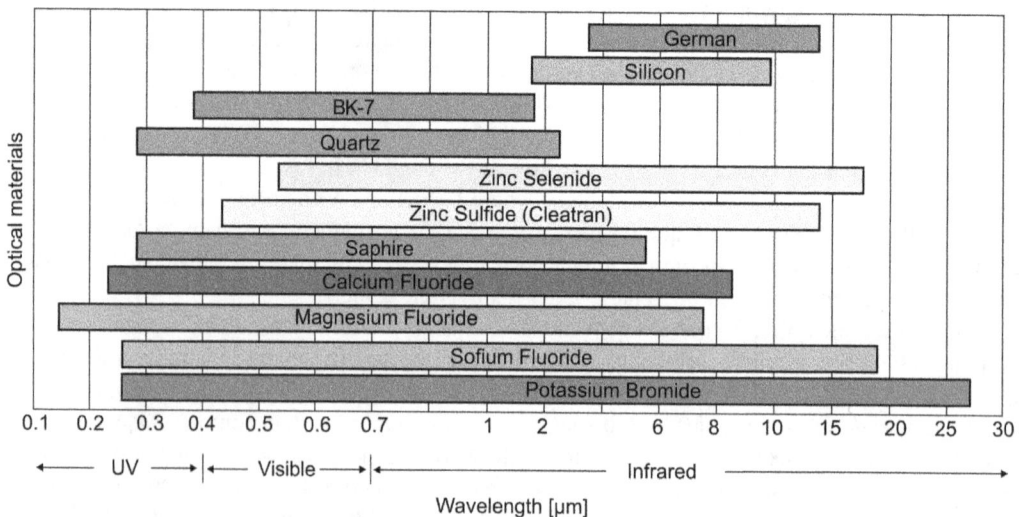

FIGURE 1.26 Spectral ranges of transmittance of selected optical materials.

Classical optical glasses (e.g., BK-7) used to manufacture optical elements for the visible and near-infrared range transmit light up to about 2.5 μm, and quartz glass up to 4.5 μm [22]. Thermal imagers use two spectral bands: 3–5 μm or 8–14 μm. Therefore, a list of materials that could be used to manufacture infrared refractive optics is quite long. The most popular materials in this spectral range include: germanium Ge, silicon Si, zinc selenide ZnSe, barium fluoride BaF_2, gallium arsenide GaAs, lithium fluoride LiF, zinc sulfide ZnS, and others. More information about optical materials can be found in the monography [23]. Plots of transmission versus wavelength for the most common optical materials used for manufacturing optical components in optical radiation detection systems, are shown in Figure 1.27.

In some applications, it is necessary to cut off unwanted spectrum bands that serve to improve the signal-to-noise ratio. There are two general categories of optical filters: absorptive and interference (dichroic) filters. Absorptive filters have a coating of different materials that absorb certain wavelengths of light, thus allowing the desired wavelengths to pass through. Interference filters consist of a series of optical coatings with precise thicknesses that are designed to reflect unwanted wavelengths and transmit the desired wavelength range. Their advantage is the ability to precisely match the characteristics to specific applications. Such filters are used, for example, in optoelectronic gas sensors (Figure 1.28).

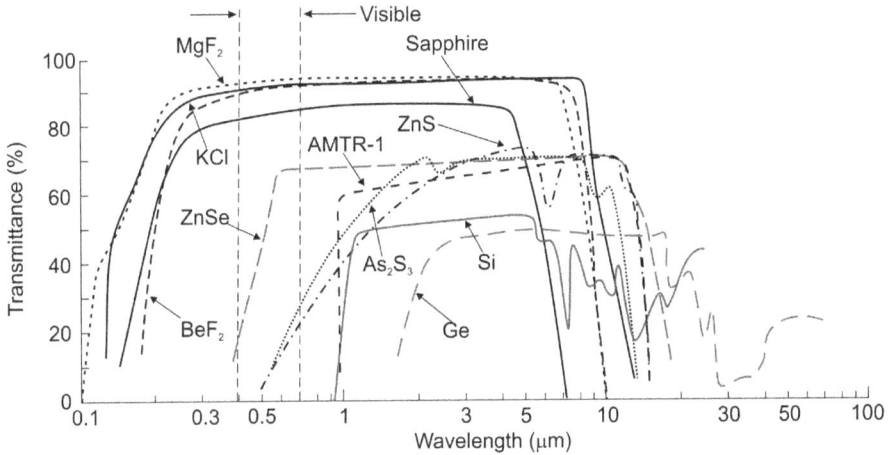

FIGURE 1.27 Transmission range of optical materials (thickness about 2 mm) (after Reference 24).

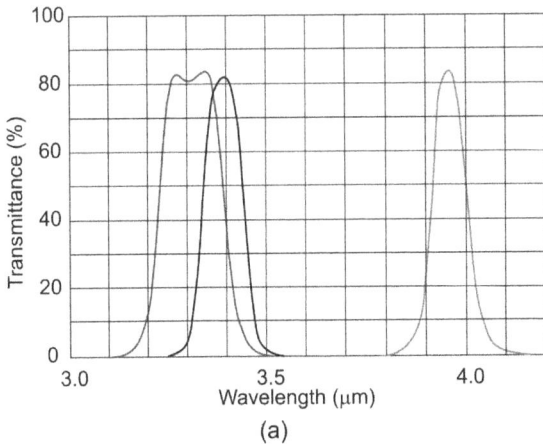

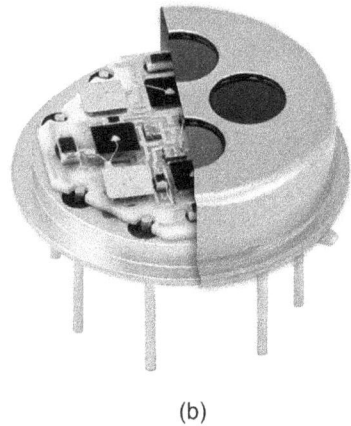

FIGURE 1.28 Optical filters: (a) examples of characteristics, (b) application in thermal detectors (after References 25 and 26).

PROBLEMS

Example 1.1

Consider a 10-cm diameter spherical ball at 500 K. Assuming that the area of the ball is a blackbody, determine (a) the total blackbody emissive power, (b) the total amount of radiation emitted by the ball in 1 min, and (c) the spectral blackbody emissive power at the wavelength of 5 μm.

Example 1.2

The temperature of a blackbody is 500 K. Determine the wavelength at which the emission of the radiation from the blackbody peaks.

Example 1.3

The distribution of solar radiation reaches its maximum at a wavelength of about 500 nm. Calculate the temperature on the surface of the Sun.

Example 1.4

Consider a radiating source has an irradiance of 2 W/cm^2 and an area of 1 mm^2. What is the total radiant flux?

Example 1.5

Consider the irradiance falling on a surface equal to 1 cm^2 is 5 W/cm^2. How much of the radian flux does 1 mm^2 of the receiving surface get?

Example 1.6

Consider the geometrical configuration shown in Figure 1.12. How much of the radian flux falls on the detector if the source area is 1 cm^2, radiance $L_e = 4$ W/cm^{2}sr, $T_s = 500$ K, detector area $A_d = 1$ mm^2, and distance $r = 5$ m?

Example 1.7

The area $A_s = 1$ cm^2 emits radiation as a blackbody at $T = 500$ K. Part of the radiation strikes the detector area A_d (see figure). Determine the solid angle subtended by the detector area $A_d = 0.1$ cm^2 when viewed from A_s and the radiant flux emitted by A_s that strikes A_d. The normal of A_d makes $\theta_d = 30°$ with the viewing direction, the normal of A_s equals $\theta_s = 60°$, and $r = 100$ cm is the distance between source and detector.

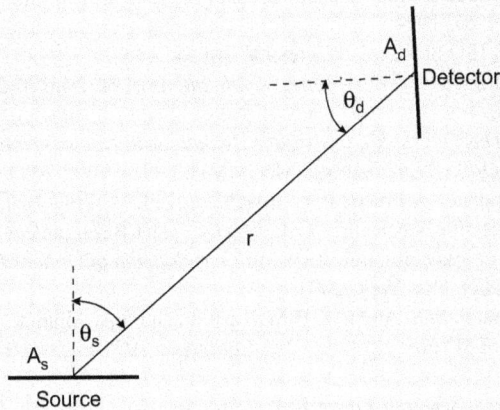

Radiant power transfer from source to a tilted detector

Example 1.8

Calculate the total power of radiation (radiant flux) emitted from the surface A_s (data from Example 1.6).

Example 1.9

Calculate the fraction of the angle subtended by A_d (data from Example 1.6).

Example 1.10

How much power is radiated through the circular hole in the screen with a radius of 1 mm, which is 2 m from the point source and which radiant intensity is 2 W/sr?

REFERENCES

1. F. Grum and R.J. Becherer, *Optical Radiation Measurements*, Vol. 1. Academic Press, San Diego, CA, 1979.
2. W.L. Wolfe and G.J. Zissis, *The Infrared Handbook*, SPIE Optical Engineering Press, Bellingham, WA, 1990.
3. W.L. Wolfe, "Radiation theory," in *The Infrared and Electro-Optical Systems Handbook*, Vol. 1, pp. 1–48, ed. G. J. Zissis, SPIE Optical Engineering Press, Bellingham, WA, 1993.
4. W.R. McCluney, *Introduction to Radiometry and Photometry*, Artech House, Boston, 1994.
5. W.L. Wolf, *Introduction to Radiometry*, SPIE Optical Engineering Press, Bellingham, WA, 1998.
6. Y. Ohno, "Basic concepts in photometry, radiometry and colorimetry," in *Handbook of Optoelectronics*, Vol. 1, pp. 265–279, eds. J.P. Dakin and R.G. W. Brown, Taylor & Francis, Boca Raton, 2018.
7. J.M. Palmer and B.G. Grant, *The Art of Radiometry*, SPIE Press, Bellingham, WA, 2010.
8. E.L. Dereniak and G.D. Boreman, *Infrared Detectors and Systems,* Wiley, New York, 1996.
9. S. Kasap, H. Ruda, and Y. Boucher, *Handbook of Optoelectronics and Photonics*, Cambridge University Press, Cambridge, 2009.

10. B.E.A. Salech and M.C. Teich M.C., *Fundamental of Photonics*, 3rd edition, Wiley, Hoboken, NJ, 2019.

11. *CIE Compte Rendu*, p. 67, 1924

12. *Quantities and Units*, ISO Standards Handbook, 3rd ed., 1993.

13. S.G. Burnay, T.L. Williams, and C.H. Jones, *Applications of Thermal Imaging*, Adam Hilger, Bristol, England, 1988.

14. G. Gaussorgues, *La Thermographie Infrarouge, Technique et Documentation*, Lavoisier, Paris, 1984.

15. W.J. Smith, *Modern Optical Engineering*, McGraw Hill, New York, 2000.

16. Y.A. Cengel. Heat Transfer. A Practical Approach. 2nd. ed. McGraw Hill, Boston, 2002. https://kntu. ac.ir/DorsaPax/userfiles/file/Mechanical/OstadFile/Sayyalat/Bazargan/cen58933_ch11.pdf.

17. S. Arnon, "Optical wireless communication," in *Encyclopedia of Optical Engineering*, edited by R.G. Driggers, Marcel Dekker, New York, 2003.

18. M.F. Talib, A.K. Rahman, M.S. Anuar, C.B.M. Rashidi, and S.A. Aljunid, "Investigation on heavy precipitation effects over FSO link", *MATEC Web Conference*, 97 01113 (2017). doi: 10.1051/matecconf/20179701113.

19. R.B. Stull, *Atmospheric Sciences Library: An Introduction to Boundary Layer Meteorology*, Kluwer Academic Publishers, Dordrecht, 1988.

20. A.G. Alkholidi and K.S. Altowij, "Free space optical communications – theory and practices", InTech, 2014, http://dx.doi.org/10.5772/58884.

21. R. Hudson, *Infrared System Engineering*, Wiley, New York, 1969.

22. Edmund Optics. The correct material for infrared applications. www.edmundoptics.com/knowledge-center/application-notes/optics/the-correct-material-for-infrared-applications/.

23. K. Potter and J. Simmons, *Optical Materials*, Elsevier, Amsterdam, 2021.

24. M.E. Couture, "Challenges in IR optics", *Proc. SPIE* 4369, 649–661 (2001).

25. *Pyroelectric & Multispectral Detectors*, Infra Tec Catalog, 2013.

26. "New four-channel detector in single supply operation with high sensitivity. Pyroelectric detector LM-274 for gas analysis now available", 07/03/2015, Infra Tec, www.infratec-infrared.com/press/press-releases/details/2014-11-20-new-four-channel-detector-in-single-supply-operation-with-high-sensitivity.

2 Characteristics of Optical Detectors

Measurement of detector parameters is a complex issue due to the large number of experimental variables involved. A variety of electrical and radiometric parameters must be taken into account and carefully controlled. With the increasing use of large, two-dimensional detector arrays, detectors characterisation has become even more complex and demanding. In this chapter we will first define the basic parameters of the detectors and then discuss the basic measuring systems for their characterisation.

2.1 INTRODUCTION

The correct work of the optical signal receiver depends mainly on the detector properties. The photodetector is the key device in the front end of an optical receiver that converts the incoming optical signal into an electrical signal. It should be characterised by high sensitivity, short response time, low power consumption, compatibility with the electronic input circuit, high durability, as well as operational reliability, high quantum efficiency, good thermal properties, low dark current, low noise, long lifetime, small size and low manufacturing costs.

In this subsection, we will define the basic parameters of the detectors.

Active area. The physical area of a photodetector, usually the active region that converts an incoming optical radiation into an electric output signal. For detectors with a circular surface, the diameter is usually given whereas, for detectors with a rectangular and square surface, its length and width are given.

Optical active area. The apparent active area of an optically immersed detector, which may differ from the physical active area due to immersion lens properties.

Detector supply voltage (bias). Many detectors require a low noise DC voltage supply. The detector output signal and noise are a function of the bias and radiation modulation frequency. The bias should provide the conditions for a maximum signal-to-noise ratio at a certain frequency.

Incident power. In order to correctly define the detector parameters, it is necessary to know the incident radiation power, its spectral and spatial distribution. For testing infrared detectors, blackbody simulators of 500 K are commonly used. A perfect blackbody has a precisely defined characteristic of the spectral distribution of the radiation power [1].

Usually, the radiant flux falling on the detector is modulated. Since the modulation can be performed in various ways (rectangular, sinusoidal, triangular modulation, etc.), the radiation flux of the fundamental component of the Fourier expansion of the modulation waveform is assumed [2]. The modulation frequency is the fundamental frequency. Rectangular modulation is commonly used in the measurements of detector parameters.

DOI: 10.1201/9781003263098-2

Detector impedance. The detector impedance Z_d is the slope of the *I-V* curve (dV/dI) evaluated at V_b (see Figure 2.1), and can be written down as

$$Z_d = \frac{dV(t)}{dI(t)}\bigg|_{V_b}.$$

(2.1)

The detector impedance depends on detector bias voltage, detector capacity and intensity of the incident radiation.

Shunt resistance of photodiode. Figure 2.1 (b) is a magnified view of the zero region of the curve shown in Figure 2.1 (a). The shunt resistance R_d is the slope of the current-voltage curve of the photodiode at the origin, that is, $V_b = 0$. In the Hamamatsu catalogues, the shunt resistance values are obtained using a dark current measured with a 10-mV voltage applied to the cathode [3, 4]. An ideal photodiode will have an infinite shunt resistance, but actual values may range from the order of 10s Ω to 1000s MΩ, and it is dependent on the photodiode material. This can significantly impact the noise current on the photodiode. For the best photodiode performance, the highest shunt resistance is desired.

Series resistance. Series resistance, R_s, of a photodiode results from contact resistance and wire bonds, as well as from non-depleted quasi-neutral material. For an ideal photodiode the value of the series resistance is equal to zero, whereas for a real photodiode, depending on the spectral range, it can be from several to several hundred ohms.

Detector signal. The detector signal is usually the value of a voltage or current that appears at the detector output by the incident radiation. The signal value depends on the detector bias voltage V_b, the modulation frequency f, the wavelength λ, the radiant flux Φ, and the detector area A:

$$V_s = V_s\left(V_b, f, \lambda, \Phi, A\right).$$

(2.2)

For most detectors, the detector signal is a linear function of the radiant flux when the power of the incident radiation to the surface is less than a certain limit value. Since only such detectors are considered in the present book, the ratio $V/\Phi A$ is fixed at certain V_b, f and λ. In many cases, the signal dependence on f and λ can be separated.

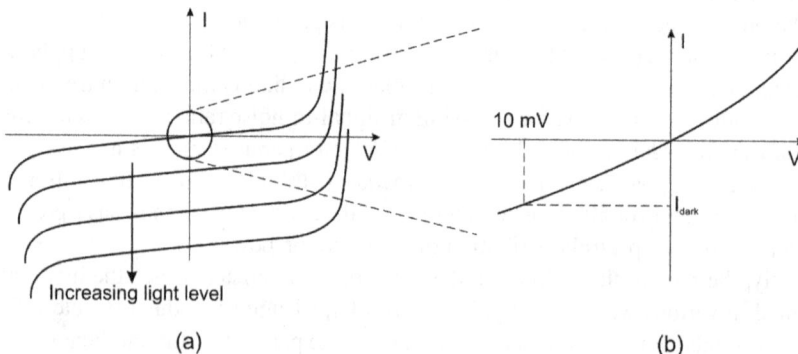

(a)   (b)

FIGURE 2.1   Current-voltage characteristics: (a) current versus voltage at different light level, (b) enlarged view of the curve zero region.

In order to determine the frequency characteristics of the detector, the relationship between the signal value and the frequency of radiation modulation is measured. These measurements are carried out at a constant radiation power and a constant bias voltage. The frequency dependence diagram of the detector signal can be used to determine the time constant (see point 2.2.5).

The spectral response is measured at a defined value of bias voltage, modulation frequency, and incident constant power. It is presented in the form of a graph of the spectral response of the signal (e.g., responsivity, detectivity, or quantum efficiency) on the wavelength.

If the radiation reaches only part of the detector surface, the signal may depend on a position of the illuminated area. For example, Si photodiodes offer an excellent sensitivity uniformity in the photosensitive area. Their nonuniformity in 80 per cent of the effective photosensitive area is less than 2 per cent [5]. Sensitivity uniformity measurements of the detector are rarely used.

2.2   DETECTOR PARAMETERS

The optical detectors can be operated under different conditions. In this book only detectors whose output signal is proportional to the radiant power are considered.

2.2.1   QUANTUM EFFICIENCY

Quantum efficiency, η, is usually defined as the number of electron-hole pairs generated in the active area of the detector divided by the number of incident photons. This is a standardised value, usually less than unity or expressed as a percentage. In this way, we limit the generation of electron-hole pairs to their creation, eliminating, for example, avalanche multiplication of the carriers. Deviations from the above definition are observed in the case of high energy of photons where quantum efficiency can reach the values beyond unity. Not all absorbed photons may generate free electron-hole pairs that can be collected. Some may disappear by recombination or become immediately trapped. If the semiconductor length is comparable with the penetration depth ($1/\alpha$, where α is the absorption coefficient), then not all photons will be absorbed. The quantum efficiency depends also on reflection from the detector surface, absorption coefficient, and device structure. It can be increased by the following: reducing the reflections at the semiconductor surface, increasing absorption, and preventing the recombination or trapping of carriers. The quantum efficiency of an ideal photodetector is a binary function – the photon energy is sufficient enough to excite the medium ($\eta = 100\%$) or is insufficient ($\eta = 0$). Figure 2.2 shows the quantum efficiency versus the wavelengths for the ideal and real detector.

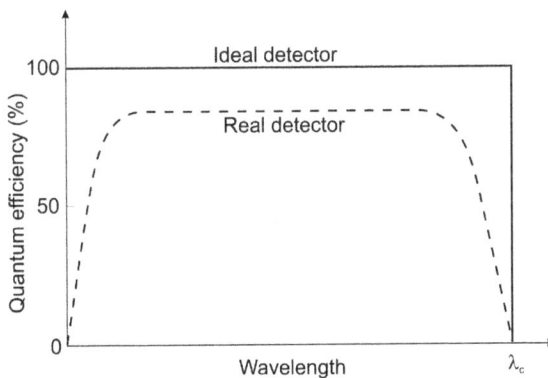

FIGURE 2.2   Quantum efficiency versus wavelengths for the ideal and real detector, where λ_c is the wavelength (cut-off wavelength) at which the responsivity decreases to half.

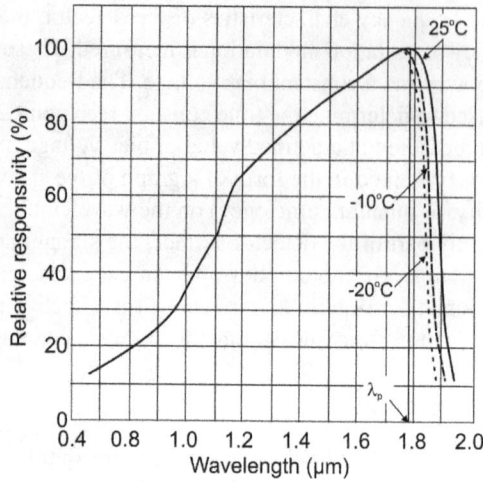

FIGURE 2.3　Relative current responsivity of the InGaAs photodiode; where λ_p is the wavelength at which responsivity reaches its maximum value (after Reference 6).

2.2.2　RESPONSIVITY

The responsivity $R(\lambda)$ of a detector is defined as the ratio of the root mean square (RMS) value of the fundamental component of the detector electrical output signal to the RMS value of the fundamental component of the input radiation power.

The voltage (or analogous current) spectral responsivity is given by

$$R_v\left(\lambda, f\right) = \frac{V_s}{\Phi_e\left(\lambda\right)}, R_I\left(\lambda, f\right) = \frac{I_s}{\Phi_e\left(\lambda\right)}, \tag{2.3}$$

where V_s and I_s are the signal voltage and signal current, respectively, and $\Phi_e(\lambda)$ is the spectra radiant incident power. The units of responsivity are either volts per watt or amperes per watt depending on whether the output is an electric voltage or a current one.

For infrared detectors, the spectral dependence of detector responsivity or the detector responsivity to blackbody radiation, at a certain temperature (usually 500 K), are given. The blackbody responsivity is defined as the ratio of the signal (voltage or current) and the total power emitted by a blackbody:

$$R_v\left(T, f\right) = \frac{V_s}{\int_0^\infty \Phi_e\left(\lambda\right) d\lambda}. \tag{2.4}$$

In catalogues of many companies there are published characteristics of current responsivity normalised to the maximum value of responsivity. It can be written in a form of $R_{relative} = R(\lambda)/R(\lambda_p) \times 100\%$ (Figure 2.3).

2.2.3　NOISE EQUIVALENT POWER

Noise-equivalent power (*NEP*) is the incident power on the detector that produces a signal-to-noise ratio of unity at the output of a given optical detector at a given data-signalling rate or modulation frequency, operating wavelength and effective noise bandwidth. Some manufacturers and authors define *NEP* as the minimum detectable power per square root bandwidth [W/Hz$^{1/2}$].

In terms of responsivity, it can be written:

$$NEP = \frac{V_n}{R_v} = \frac{I_n}{R_i}.$$ (2.5)

The unit of *NEP* is the watt.

The *NEP* is also quoted for a fixed-reference bandwidth, which is often assumed to be 1 Hz. This "*NEP* per unit bandwidth" has a unit of watts per square root Hertz (W/Hz$^{1/2}$). The *NEP* depends on the optical wavelength, as well, since the detector responsivity is wavelength dependent.

For a given detector, the lowest value of $NEP = NEP_{min}$ is obtained at the wavelength with the maximum detector responsivity. Thus,

$$NEP(\lambda) = NEP_{min} \frac{R_{max}}{R(\lambda)},$$ (2.6)

where R_{max} is the detector maximum responsivity and $R(\lambda)$ is the detector responsivity at the wavelength λ [7].

The minimum detectable power P_{min} can be calculated using the following equation:

$$P_{min} = NEP(\lambda)\Delta f^{1/2},$$ (2.7)

where Δf is the measurement bandwidth.

2.2.4 DETECTIVITY

The detectivity $D(\lambda)$ is the reciprocal of *NEP*:

$$D(\lambda) = \frac{1}{NEP}.$$ (2.8)

Many experimental and theoretical studies have shown that the detectivity is inversely proportional to the square root of the detector area and, therefore,

$$DA^{1/2} = const.$$ (2.9)

Given this, R.C. Jones has introduced the normalised detectivity D^* (or *D*-star) related to the unit detector area and the unit bandwidth [8]. This means that both *NEP* and detectivity are functions of the electrical bandwidth and detector area:

$$D^* = D\left(A_d \Delta f\right)^{1/2} = \frac{\left(A_d \Delta f\right)^{1/2}}{NEP}.$$ (2.10)

It is the most important detector parameter which allows the comparison of the same type detectors but having different areas. D^* is expressed in the unit of cmHz$^{1/2}$/W, which is more commonly called "Jones".

The normalised detectivity D^* depends on signal-to-noise ratio (SNR), voltage and current responsivity:

$$D^* = \frac{\left(A_d \Delta f\right)^{1/2}}{V_n} R_v = \frac{\left(A_d \Delta f\right)^{1/2}}{I_n} R_i = \frac{\left(A_d \Delta f\right)^{1/2}}{\Phi_e}(SNR). \quad (2.11)$$

The blackbody $D^*(T, f)$ can be determined by knowing the spectral detectivity:

$$D^*(T, f) = \frac{\int_0^\infty D^*(\lambda, f)\Phi_e(T, \lambda)d\lambda}{\int_0^\infty \Phi_e(T, \lambda)d\lambda} = \frac{\int_0^\infty D^*(\lambda, f)E_e(T, \lambda)d\lambda}{\int_0^\infty E_e(T, \lambda)d\lambda}, \quad (2.12)$$

where $\Phi_e(T, \lambda) = E_e(T, \lambda)A_d$ is the incident blackbody radiant flux (in W) and $E_e(T, \lambda)$ is the blackbody irradiance (in W/cm^2).

2.2.5 RESPONSE SPEED

In many applications where the frequency response is being measured or where a fast photoreceiver is required, the rise and fall time of the detector become very important. The rise time of the detector output signal, which is the response of the detector to a rectangular pulse extortion, is the time required for the photodetector to increase its output from 10 per cent to 90 per cent of the final output level (Figure 2.4). The fall (decay) time of the detector is defined as the time required for the signal to fall from 90 per cent to 10 per cent of the final value. This parameter can be also expressed as frequency response, which is the frequency f_c at which the photodiode output decreases by 3 dB. It can be presented by the following equation:

$$t_r = \frac{0.35}{f_c}. \quad (2.13)$$

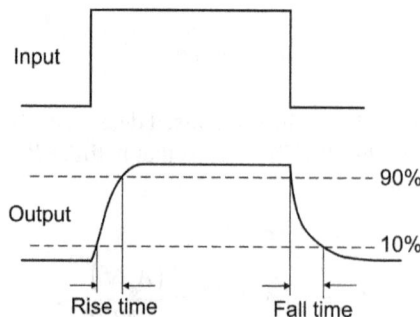

FIGURE 2.4 Examples of the response waveform.

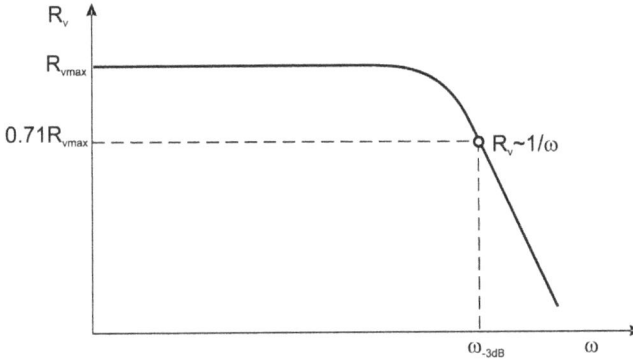

FIGURE 2.5 Detector responsivity versus angular frequency.

The frequency response characteristics of the detector can be approximated by the following equation:

$$R_v = \frac{R_{vo}}{\left(1 + \omega^2 \tau^2\right)},$$ (2.14)

where R_{vo} is the detector responsivity at zero frequency of the incident radiation modulation and τ is the time constant of the detector-preamplifier combination response:

$$\tau = \left(\omega_{-3dB}\right)^{-1},$$ (2.15)

where ω_{-3dB} is the angular frequency at which the responsivity has fallen to 0.71 of its maximum value (see Figure 2.5). In addition, the relation

$$\omega_{-3dB} = 2\pi f_c,$$ (2.16)

exists.

More complex cases are possible when the detector has different recombination mechanisms, and it can have several time constants.

2.3 DETECTOR PERFORMANCE LIMITED BY PHOTON NOISE

The ultimate performance of IR detectors is reached when the detector and amplifier noises are low compared to the photon noise. The radiation falling on the detector is a composite of components originating from the target and that from the background. Thus, the mean square value of the noise current is as follows:

$$I_n^2 = 2q^2 g^2 \left(G_{opt} + G_{th} + R\right)\Delta f,$$ (2.17)

where G_{opt} is the optical generation rate, G_{th} is the thermal generation rate, R is the radiative and nonradiative recombination rate, and Δf is the frequency band.

We can distinguish two extreme cases where it is dominant:

- signal photon noise – we are talking about the detector performance limited by signal fluctuations;
- background photon noise – we are talking about the detector performance limited by background fluctuations.

The detector operating conditions defined by the first case occur relatively rarely in the short wavelength spectrum (ultraviolet and visible range), for example, in photomultipliers. However, they do not occur in detectors made of semiconductors, the performance of which is determined by the self-noise, or the noise of the electronic system connected to the detector. Detectivity and *NEP* of detectors working in the two above-described cases are described in many monographic items [9–16].

The practical operating limit for most IR detectors is not the signal fluctuation limit (SFL) but the background fluctuation limit, also known as the BLIP (background limited infrared photodetector) limit. The photon noise is fundamental in the sense that it does not arise from any imperfection in the detector or its associated electronics, but rather from the detection process itself, as a result of a discrete nature of the radiation field.

If recombination does not contribute to the noise, then the mean square value of the noise current depends on the optical generation rate, G_{opt}, of the signal [15], which depends on the signal photon flux density ϕ_s, the detector area A_d, and the quantum efficiency η:

$$I_n^2 = 2q^2 g^2 G_{opt} \Delta f = 2\phi_s A_d \eta q^2 g^2 \Delta f. \tag{2.18}$$

Using Eq. (2.18) we obtain the expression for the detector detectivity, the performance of which is limited by the SFL:

$$D^* = \frac{\lambda}{hc} \left(\frac{\eta}{2\Phi_s} \right)^{1/2}. \tag{2.19}$$

This is the ideal situation, when the noise of the detector is determined entirely by the noise of the signal photons. The *NEP* in the SFL is given as [16]

$$NEP_{min} = \frac{9.22 hc \Delta f}{\eta \lambda}, \tag{2.20}$$

that the detector area does not enter into the expression and that NEP_{min} depends linearly upon the bandwidth Δf, which varies from the case in which the detection limit is set by the internal or background noise.

Seib and Aukerman [9] also have derived an expression for the SFL identical to Eq. (2.20) except that the multiplicative constant is not of 9.22 but $2^{3/2}$ for an ideal photoemissive or a photovoltaic detector, and $2^{5/2}$ for a photoconductor. These differences in the values of the constant coefficients result from differing assumptions in the derivation of final expressions.

In the case of infrared detectors, the practical limitation is the noise of the background radiation caused by fluctuations in the background photon flux falling on the detector. The background radiation fluctuation determines the minimum flux that must fall on the detector from the detected source in order to distinguish the signal from the background noise.

Assuming that the detector noise is determined by the noise described by the equation

$$I_n^2 = 2\phi_B A_d \eta q^2 g^2 \Delta f, \tag{2.21}$$

where ϕ_B is the background photon flux density, the detectivity is limited by the background noise:

$$D_{BLIP}^* (\lambda, f) = \frac{\lambda}{hc} \left(\frac{\eta}{2Q_B} \right)^{1/2}. \tag{2.22}$$

Here Q_B is the total background photon flux density reaching the detector. This flux can be determined by the spectral radiant exitance $M_p(\lambda, T_B)$, taking the ideal spectral characteristics of the detector (when the cut-off wavelength λ_c is equal to λ_p):

$$Q_B = \sin^2 (\theta/2) \int_0^{\lambda_c} M_p (\lambda, T_B) d\lambda, \tag{2.23}$$

where θ is the field of view (FOV) of the detector as shown in Figure 2.7. The blackbody exitance at temperature T_B is determined by the Planck Eq. (1.32) in photons/(scm²µm) units.

Figure 2.6 shows the dependence of the integral background flux density on the wavelength for different blackbody temperatures and 2π FOV [18]. The values of the integral Eq. (2.23) are given in the tables by Lowan and Blanch [17].

From Eq. (2.23), we obtain

$$\frac{Q_B (\theta)}{Q_B (2\pi)} = \sin^2 (\theta/2), \tag{2.24}$$

and the background-limited D^* relative to 2π FOV becomes

$$\frac{D_{BLIP}^* (\theta)}{D_{BLIP}^* (2\pi)} = \frac{1}{\sin(\theta/2)}. \tag{2.25}$$

The D^* varies with FOV as $[sin(\theta/2)]^{-1}$.

Figure 2.7 is a curve showing how ideal D_{BLIP}^* is improved as the cone angle θ is reduced for any given background temperature [19]. This figure also shows a different way of marking the detector viewing angle by the symbol $f/\#$. It denotes the ratio of the system focal length to the diameter of the entrance pupil D called the f-number (e.g., $f/1$ means $f/D = 1$; and $f/2$ means $f/D = 2$).

Photoconductive detectors which are generation-recombination noise-limited have a lower D_{BLIP}^* by a factor of $2^{1/2}$:

$$D_{BLIP}^* (\lambda, f) = \frac{\lambda}{2hc} \left(\frac{\eta}{Q_B} \right)^{1/2}. \tag{2.26}$$

The photon noise-limited expressions Eqs. (2.22) and (2.26) are correct only for Poisson statistics when the Bose-Einstein factor $b = [\exp(hc/\lambda kT) - 1]^{-1}$ is close to 1. If the Bose–Einstein factor is included, for example, Eq. (2.26) becomes

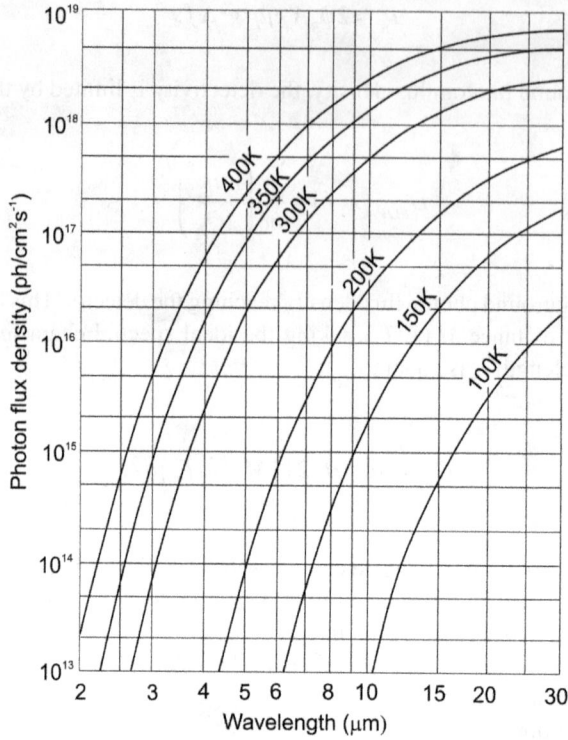

FIGURE 2.6 Dependence of the integral background flux density on a wavelength for different blackbody temperatures and 2π FOV.

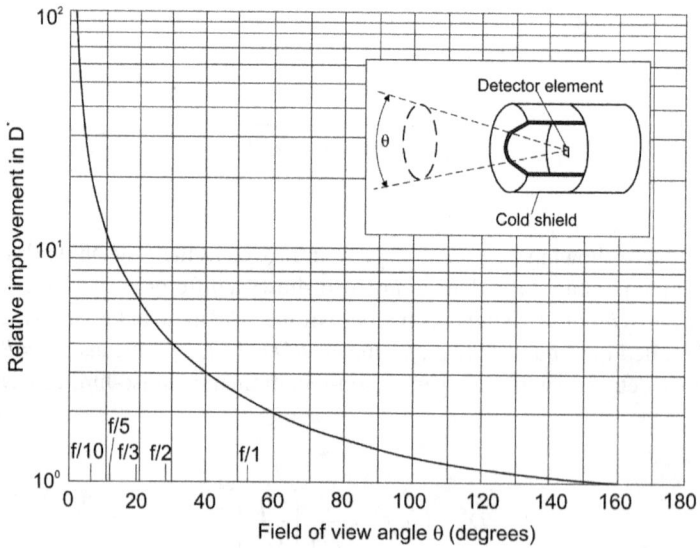

FIGURE 2.7 Relative improvement factor for detectivity with a reduction in the FOV cone angle for a BLIP detector (after Reference 19).

$$D^*_{BLIP}(\lambda,f) = \frac{\eta\lambda}{2hc\sin(\theta/2)}\left[\int_0^{\lambda_c}\eta(\lambda)Q_p(\lambda,T_B)(1+b)d\lambda\right]^{-1/2}. \qquad (2.27)$$

The highest performance possible will be obtained by the ideal detector with unity quantum efficiency and ideal spectral responsivity (where responsivity increases with the wavelength to the cutoff wavelength λ_c at which the responsivity drops to zero). This limiting performance is of interest for comparison with actual detectors. Detectivity for ideal photoconductors as the function λ_c for the background temperature T_B and for a 2π FOV is shown in Figure 2.8.

The dashed line for $T_B = 300$ K is a detectivity obtained by neglecting the Boson factor, which is considered to make a small but increasing effect as the wavelength is extended. As T_B is decreased, the Boson factor correction becomes increasingly less significant.

Figure 2.9 shows the required operating temperatures of the detectors at which they obtain detectivity limited by the influence of background radiation at a temperature of 300 K, at a viewing angle of 30° [21]. We can see that HgCdTe detectors have the highest operating temperatures; for operation close to 3 μm, thermoelectric cooling (200 K) is sufficient. Accordingly, "deeper" cooling is required for detectors operating in the 8–12 μm range (below 100 K). By the way, it is worth noting that the cooling requirements for quantum well infrared photodetectors (QWIPs) are less critical than for silicon-doped detectors.

The detectivity of BLIP detectors can be improved by reducing the background photon flux Q_B. Practically, there are two ways to do this: a cooled or reflective spectral filter to limit the spectral band or a cooled shield to limit the angular FOV of the detector. The former eliminates background radiation from spectral regions in which the detector does not need responding. The best detectors yield background-limited detectivities in a quite narrow FOV.

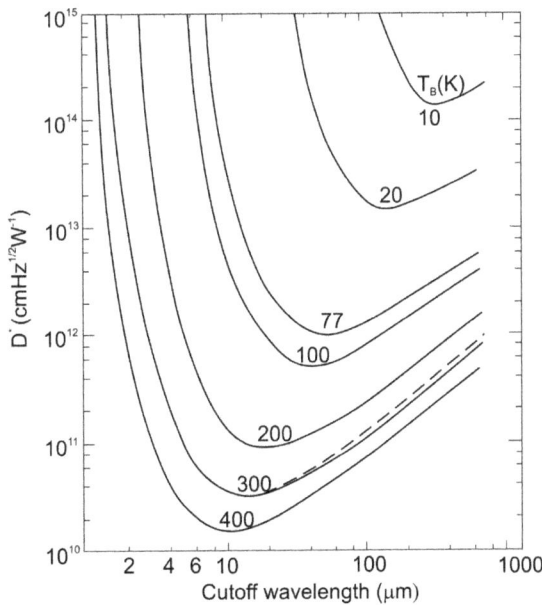

FIGURE 2.8 Detectivity at λ_c versus. λ_c for ideal photoconductive detectors operating at $T_B = 400, 300, 200, 77, 20$ and 10 K for a 2π FOV. The dashed line for 300 K neglects the Boson factor (after Reference 20).

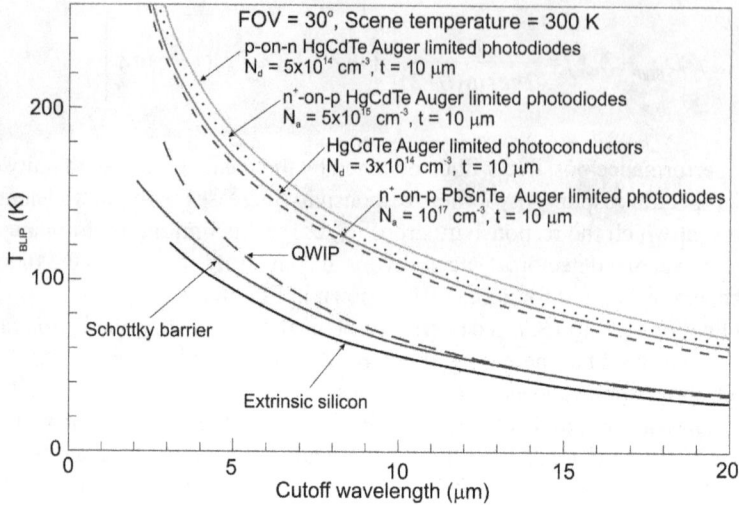

FIGURE 2.9 The required operating temperature at which infrared detectors achieve detectivity limited by the influence of background radiation, with a viewing angle of 30° and a background temperature of 300 K.

It can be shown that when the signal source is a blackbody at the temperature T_s and the radiation background is a blackbody at the temperature T_B, then the background noise-limited blackbody D^*_{BLIP} as a function of peak spectral D^*_{BLIP} is the following:

$$D^*_{BLIP}(T_s, f) = D^*_{BLIP}(\lambda_p, f) \frac{(hc/\lambda_p)}{\sigma T_s^4} \int_0^{\lambda_c} M(T_s, \lambda) d\lambda, \qquad (2.28)$$

where λ_p is the wavelength of a peak detectivity which is also the cut-off wavelength for an ideal photondetector, and σ is the Stefan–Boltzmann constant. All the D^*_{BLIP} expressions have assumed a Lambertian source subtending a half-angle of $\pi/2$ radians.

The ratio of the BLIP peak spectral D^* to the BLIP blackbody D^* is as follows:

$$K(T, \lambda) = \frac{D^*_{BLIP}(\lambda_p, f)}{D^*_{BLIP}(T_s, f)} = \frac{\sigma T_s^4}{\frac{hc}{\lambda_p} \int_0^{\lambda_c} M(T_s, \lambda) d\lambda}. \qquad (2.29)$$

Figure 2.10 is a plot of $K(\lambda)$ for $T_s = 500$ K and a 2π steradian FOV [16]. The quantity $K(T, \lambda)$ is useful because the IR detector testing yields blackbody D^* values. The peak spectral D^* is then calculated using $K(T, \lambda)$.

Jensen has made an interesting comparison between different types of infrared detectors with a long-term sensitivity limit $\lambda_c = 12.5$ μm by determining the maximum temperature at which BLIP conditions are maintained (Figure 2.11). In the calculations he assumed the independence of the refractive index from a wavelength and quantum efficiency of 100 per cent. Note that the best performance is presented by the photodiode with HgCdTe [22].

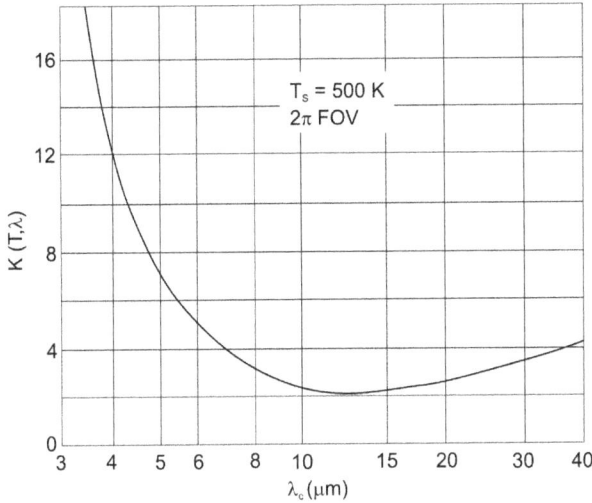

FIGURE 2.10 The ratio of the peak spectral D^* to the blackbody D^* versus the detector cut-off wavelength for T_s = 500 K and FOV = 2π FOV.

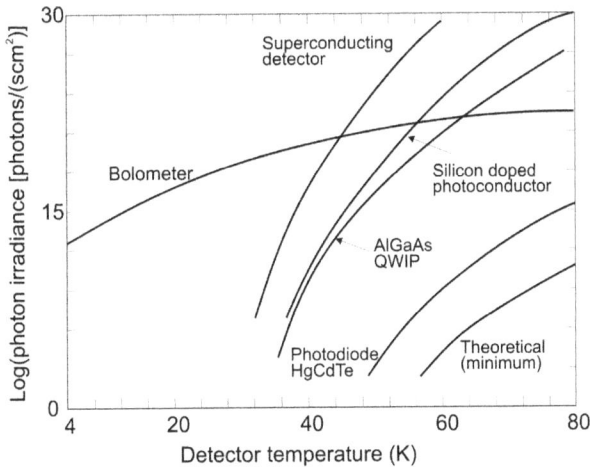

FIGURE 2.11 Dependence of the logarithm from the density of the photon flux of background radiation incident on the detector as a function of the detector operating temperature under BLIP conditions for detectors with λ_c = 12.5 μm. The individual curves are calculated for theoretical limit (minimum), HgCdTe photodiode, bolometer, AlGaAs quantum well detector, superconducting detector and Si doped photoresistor (after Reference 22).

2.4 MEASUREMENTS OF DETECTOR PARAMETERS

In order to measure the detector parameters, in addition to the electronic measuring devices, the following ones are necessary: technical model of a blackbody, modulated source of radiation with adjustable frequency, source of monochromatic radiation and reference detector. The electronic measuring devices include the following: preamplifiers, end amplifiers, Fourier spectrometers, spectrum analysers (including Fourier ones) and selective voltmeters. Auxiliary measuring devices are the following: signal generators, calibrated attenuators and detector supply systems.

2.4.1 RESPONSIVITY MEASUREMENTS

The spectral sensitivity of detectors is defined and measured differently depending on the spectral range. For detectors operating in the visible and near infrared range ($< 2.0\ \mu m$), the spectral characteristic or λ_p, at which the detector has a maximum sensitivity are given. In the latter case, wavelengths for which the sensitivity decreases to 10 per cent of the maximum value should be reported. For these detectors, the current responsivity R_i in A/W is given. This is due to the relatively high impedance of the detectors and possible errors in measuring the voltage responsivity (instruments with high Q factor of 1 GΩ/V are required). The longer wavelength infrared detectors are usually characterised by low resistance. Therefore, to measure the voltage responsivity, R_v of these detectors, it is necessary to use an instrument that measures a voltage signal with an input resistance much greater than that of the detector. There is a simple relationship between these quantities:

$$R_v = R_d R_i,\tag{2.30}$$

where R_d is the detector resistance. This condition is valid when the measured values refer to the same detector operating conditions (supply voltage and current).

For most detectors, the signal is directly proportional to the power of the incident radiation. The irradiance of a single μW/cm^2 is sufficient enough to test many types of detectors.

As indicated previously [Eq. (2.2)], the detector signal depends on the supply voltage V_b, the power of the incident radiation P_s the surface of the detector A_d, the wavelength λ, and the frequency f. In many cases the expression for the detector signal can be separated as follows:

$$V_s\left(V_b, P_s, A_d, \lambda, f\right) = u\left(V_b, P_s, A_d\right) u\left(\lambda\right) u\left(f\right).\tag{2.31}$$

Assuming, that the incident radiation power and the detector area are constant, then the above expression takes the form of

$$V_s\left(V_b, \lambda, f\right) = u\left(V_b\right) u\left(\lambda\right) u\left(f\right).\tag{2.32}$$

Thus, three independent characteristics of $u(V_b)$, $u(\lambda)$ (called spectral) and $u\left(f\right)$ (called frequency) are obtained, which can be measured independently.

Usually, the spectral dependence of the detector responsivity (for detectors in the visible and near infrared range) or the responsivity of the detector to blackbody radiation at a certain temperature, usually $T = 500$ K for thermal infrared detectors, is given.

For visible or near infrared detectors, a blackbody of 2870 K is sometimes used. Let us take a closer look at how to measure both types of responsivity.

2.4.1.1   Measurement of the Spectral Responsivity of the Detector

Figure 2.12 shows an example of the stand for measuring spectral characteristics of the detector responsivity. The measuring system consists of radiation source, optical system, modulator, monochromator, detectors (reference and tested) and signal amplification systems. Nowadays, instead of a monochromator, a Fourier spectrophotometer with a broadband source of radiation is commonly used.

The sensitivity measurement consists in measuring the voltage obtained at the output of a preamplifier connected to the detector as a function of radiation wavelength, for a specific modulation frequency and supply voltage. If the source modulation frequency changes, the analyser centre frequency is continuously tuned.

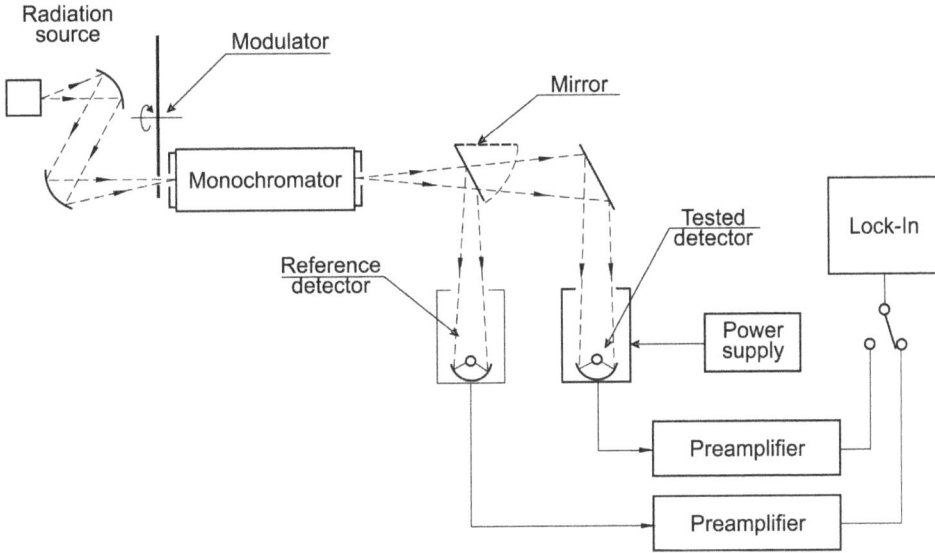

FIGURE 2.12   Diagram of the system for measuring the spectral characteristics of the detectors.

To determine the radiation power at the monochromator output, the current is measured with a reference detector with known spectral sensitivity characteristics. Pyroelectric detectors with a flat spectral responsivity characteristic, modified only by the transmission of the input window, are commonly used.

The following procedure should be followed to determine the current responsivity of the detector:

1. the radiation beam is switched to the reference detector and, then, to the tested detector using a suitable optical system;
2. if we have measured the voltage signals at the I/V preamplifiers output of the reference detector $V_r(\lambda)$ and the tested $V_s(\lambda)$, and we know the current responsivity of the reference detector, $R_{ir}(\lambda)$, then, we can calculate the current responsivity of the tested detector $R_i(\lambda)$:

$$R_i(\lambda) = R_{ir}(\lambda)\frac{V_s(\lambda)}{V_r(\lambda)} = R_{ir}(\lambda)\frac{I_s(\lambda)R_f}{I_r(\lambda)R_f} = R_{ir}(\lambda)\frac{I_s(\lambda)}{I_r(\lambda)}. \tag{2.33}$$

In practice, the relative spectral characteristics of the detector are often given. Such characteristics are obtained by dividing the responsivity of the detector $R_i(\lambda)$ by its maximum value $R_{imax}(\lambda_o)$:

$$R_{i\%}(\lambda) = \frac{R_i(\lambda)}{R_{imax}(\lambda_o)}100\%. \tag{2.34}$$

In order to measure the spectral characteristics, advanced systems offered by many companies are used, equipped with microprocessors and cooperating with microcomputers.

The spectral responsivity of IR detectors is usually measured using Fourier Transform Infrared Spectrometer (FTIR). The typical FTIR spectrometer consists of an IR light source, interferometer, sample compartment, detector, amplifier, and computer. The light source generates radiation which

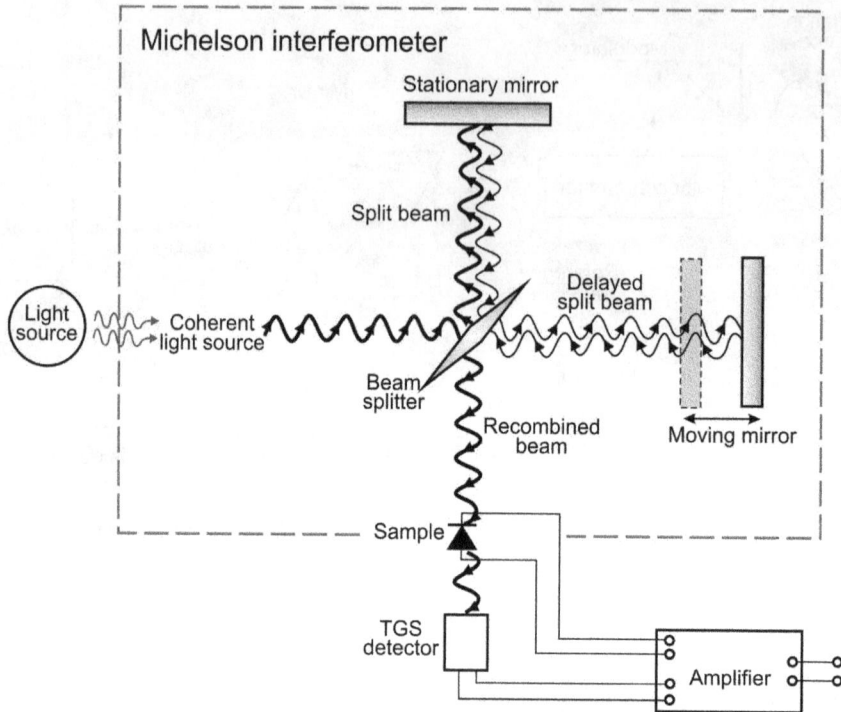

FIGURE 2.13   FTIR instrumentation.

strikes the sample (studied detector) passing through the interferometer and reaches the detector – see Figure 2.13. Then the signal is amplified and converted to digital signal (interferogram) by the amplifier and analogue-to-digital converter, respectively. In another way, the interferogram is translated to spectrum through the fast Fourier transform algorithm. The main core of FTIR spectrometer is the Michelson interferometer. It consists of a beam splitter, fixed mirror, and a moveable mirror that translates back and forth, very precisely. One beam is transmitted through the beam splitter to the fixed mirror, and the second is reflected off the beam splitter to the moving mirror. The fixed and moving mirrors reflect the radiation back to the beam splitter. Accordingly, both of these reflected radiations are recombined at the beam splitter, resulting in one beam that leaves the interferometer and interacts with the sample and strikes the detector (a typically pyroelectric TGS detector is used with flat spectral sensitivity). The detector now reports variation in energy-versus-time for all wavelengths simultaneously. A mathematical function known as a Fourier transform is used to convert the intensity-versus-time spectrum into an intensity-versus-frequency spectrum. Thus, the FTIR spectrometer collects and digitises the interferogram, performs the FT function, and displays the spectrum.

2.4.1.2   Measurement of the Detector Responsivity to Blackbody Radiation

An example of the measuring system designed to measure the responsivity of infrared detectors to blackbody radiation is shown in Figure 2.14. In this case, the monochromator with a suitable radiation source is replaced by the blackbody. This system uses a technical blackbody model with a conical cavity. The special shape of the blackbody cavity and the selected ratio of its dimensions, as well as the diameter of the iris cover, ensure high emissivity of the effective radiation source ($\varepsilon = 0.998$). The radiating cavity is heated to the required operating temperature by resistance heaters.

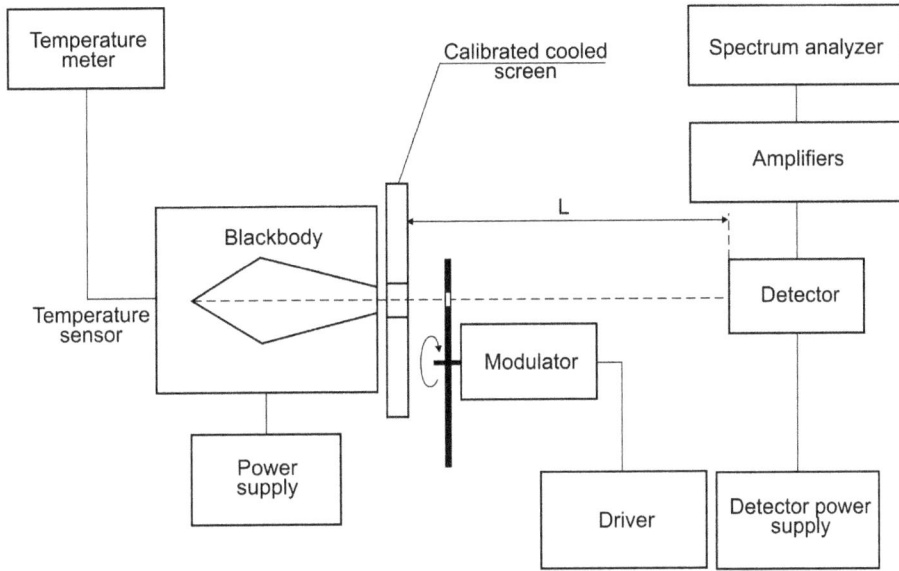

FIGURE 2.14 System for measuring the responsivity of detectors to blackbody radiation.

Many detectors require an external power supply. For this reason, the detector power supply range is determined. Efforts should be made to ensure that the detector supply current value is at a maximum value.

The excessive bias current can cause thermal instability of the detector and increased noise. On the other hand, too low value of the bias current will not provide a sufficient signal-to-noise ratio. The highest allowable power supply voltage or maximum detector current is usually specified by the manufacturer. If measurements are carried out with a supply voltage greater than that specified by the manufacturer, they shall be carried out in accordance with the safety rules. The detector bias voltage should then be changed by a small value while observing the noise level. If either the supply voltage or current is higher than the limit value, then a slight increase in the supply current and noise level will be observed. Polarisation of detectors with voltage limit values is very risky and may lead to system instability or detector destruction. The value of the radiation stream incident perpendicular to the detector area should ensure the detector linear operation.

The detector responsivity at a constant frequency modulated radiation is most often measured. In order to measure the voltage of a signal from the detector, a mechanical radiation modulator and a spectrum analyser (phase-sensitive nano-voltmeter or lock-in amplifier) are used. In the range of acoustic and sub-acoustic frequencies, mainly mechanical modulators are used. The analyser centre frequency is equal to the frequency of the mechanical modulator (chopper). Modulation frequencies higher than 50 kHz are difficult to achieve due to the need to use discs with large diameters, small slot sizes, and high spin speeds. The rectangular modulation is most often use, so it is assumed that the power of the fundamental component of the modulation waveform Fourier expansion is given (the modulation frequency is understood as the fundamental frequency). For spectral measurements, the modulator should be placed at the input slot of the monochromator. It should be able to adjust frequency.

The density of the radiation stream incident on the detector photosensitive area should be uniform. If the radiation reaches only part of the detector area, the signal may depend on the position of the illuminated field.

The power radiated through the source outlet is determined by the Stefan-Boltzmann equation:

$$P_R = \sigma\left[\left(T_R^4 - T_B^4\right)A\right], \tag{2.35}$$

where T_R is the source operating temperature, T_B is the ambient temperature, and A is the hole surface.

The radiation power falling on the detector is equal to the product of the irradiance, E_e, and the area of the detector, A:

$$P_o = AE_e,$$

(2.36)

and the power delivered to the receiver P_s, set on the optical axis at the measuring distance L from the calibrated outlet screen is determined by the equation

$$P_s = P_R \frac{A_d}{\pi L^2}.$$

(2.37)

With the measured RMS value of the voltage at the detector output $V_s(V_b, f)$, it is possible to calculate the detector voltage sensitivity to blackbody radiation:

$$R_B(V_b, f) = \frac{V_s(V_b, f)}{P_s}.$$

(2.38)

The $R_B(V_b, f)$ measurements should be made for the full range of detector bias and operating frequency.

2.4.2 Noise Measurements

When measuring the noise characteristics of detectors, a lot of experience and knowledge is required to ensure that the measurement conditions are such that the noise comes only from the detector, load resistance, and preamplifier. Due to their random nature, noises are subject to statistical description used in the analysis of stochastic processes. Therefore, the measurement of noise signals requires the use of methods and apparatus other than those used in the measurement technique of deterministic signals. In particular, it is necessary to eliminate the influence of external disturbances. Industrial interferences transmitted through the electrical network are difficult to eliminate. The detector power supply circuit can also cause additional interference if it is powered from the main power supply (Figure 2.15). An effective way to reduce the level of industrial interference is to bias the detector and the preamplifier from the battery (Figure 2.16). The detector and power supply should be placed in a common, shielded housing. A correctly designed detector power supply system should not cause additional noise. Excessive noise from the detector power supply can be detected if a low noise (metal) resistor with a resistance equal to the parallel connection of the detector and the power supply resistor is turned on instead of the detector. The resistor noise shall be independent of the flowing current. A broadband oscilloscope is often used to observe them. Schemes of measurement systems are presented in Figures 2.15 and 2.16.

Noise voltage measurements can be made with fast Fourrier transform (FFT) spectrum analyser, selective nano-voltmeter, lock-in amplifier, or selective (in the radio frequency range) micro-voltage meter. Attention shall be paid to how the indicators of these instruments are calibrated. It is particularly important in the case of spectrum analysers that have implemented procedures for displaying the signal level, usually in the following units: power (dBm – power related to 1 mW), power spectral density (dBm/Hz), linear (A or V), or square (V² or A²) scaling by multiplying a direct result by a constant of 0.02 depending on the load (analyser input resistance, which is typically 50 Ω).

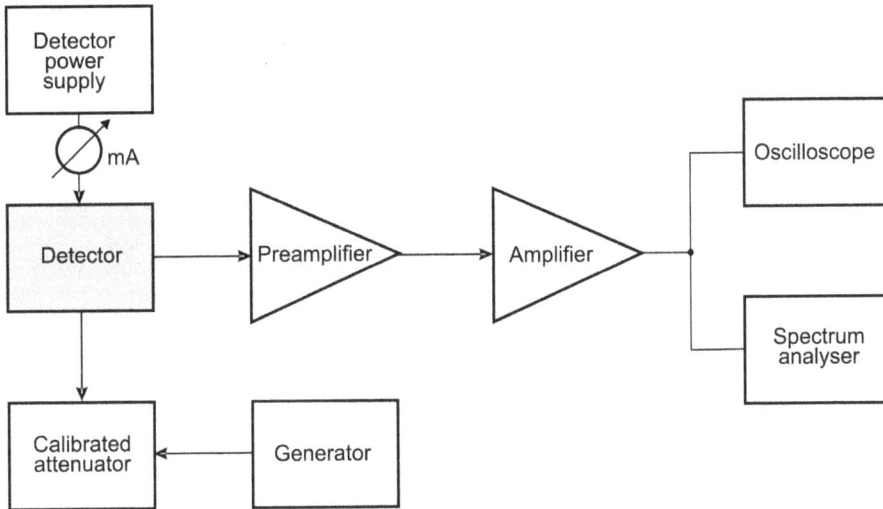

FIGURE 2.15   Block diagram of a system for measuring signal voltage and detector noise in the frequency range from 1 kHz to 1 MHz.

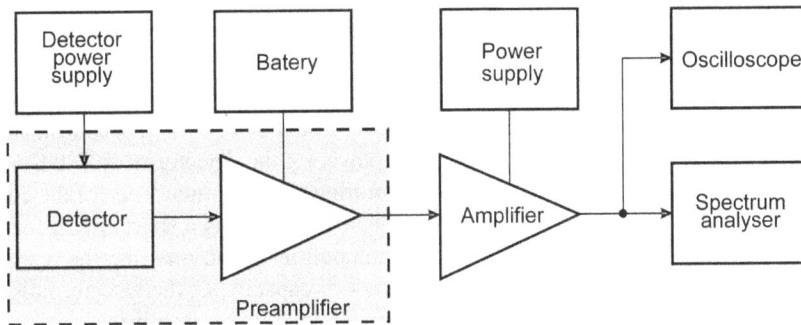

FIGURE 2.16   Block diagram of a system for measuring signal voltage and detector noise in the frequency range from 1 Hz to 100 Hz.

All these units can be referred to the RMS value of the measured voltage (noise voltage). The detector shall be shielded from all radiation sources except background radiation, before taking measurements. After turning on the power supply, the RMS noise voltage value at the preamplifier output $V_{no}(V_b, f)$ should be measured as a function of frequency. The detector shall then be exchanged for a replacement metal resistor with a resistance equal to the detector dark resistance. Again, we measure the output noise voltage as a function of frequency. The value of this voltage is marked as $V_{na}(f)$. In order to determine the voltage gain of the system, the calibration signal V_c from the generator (BFO output – beat frequency oscillator) should be given at its input. The measurement of the voltage V_c at the system input is made on a calibration resistor. To protect the system against overdrive and interference detection, a well shielded silencer should be used. The voltage value V_c should be about 100 times higher than the detector noise.

After tuning the spectrum analyser to the frequency of the calibration signal, the output voltage value V_o should be measured. The measurements are made in the same frequency range as before.

The gain of the measuring system $K_v(f)$ should be calculated as the quotient of the voltages V_o and V_c, with parametrically variable frequency.

The RMS value of the noise voltage of the detector V_{ni}, related to the input of the photodetector-preamplifier system, is determined by the equation

$$V_{ni}(V_b, f, \Delta f) = \left[\frac{V_{no}^2(V_b, f, \Delta f) - V_{na}^2(V_b, f, \Delta f)}{K_v^2(f)} + V_J^2(\Delta f) \right]^{1/2}, \qquad (2.39)$$

where R_d is the detector resistance, V_{no} is the RMS value of the noise voltage at the system output and V_J is the RMS value of the Johnson noise voltage generated by the detector in the noise band Δf.

To calculate the spectral density of the detector noise voltage, the obtained value of V_{ni} should be divided by the root of the band Δf.

$$V_{ni}(V_b, f) = \frac{V_{ni}(V_b, f, \Delta f)}{\Delta f^{1/2}}. \qquad (2.40)$$

The above equations are valid for an even distribution of the noise voltage spectral density.

Since the noise voltage depends on the detector power supply voltage, measurements should be taken for different values. Knowing the dependence of the signal-to-noise ratio on the detector supply voltage makes it possible to determine the optimal value of this voltage (e.g., for photoresistors).

Especially troublesome are the noise measurements in the lowest frequency range, where $1/f$ type noise dominates. Diagram of an example system for the measurement of this type of noise occurring in infrared detectors is shown in Figure 2.17 [23]. The tested detector is placed in a cryostat. The dividers R_1 and R_2 and the voltage source $+V$ allow powering the detector with V_b DC voltage. The R_1 resistor protects the detector against damage by limiting the maximum value of the current in the circuit. The capacitance value, C, must be so large that it introduces a short circuit for alternating signals. Then, the current i_D flows entirely to the preamplifier input, omitting the resistors R_1 and R_2. In the event of an incomplete short-circuit or a lack of capacity, C, the detector noise current is dissipated, and only a part of the preamplifier input is fed into the preamplifier.

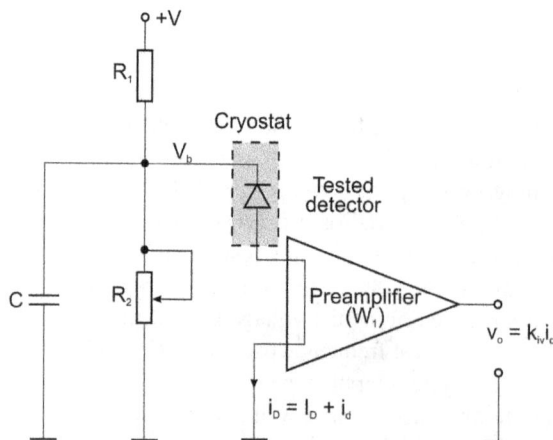

FIGURE 2.17 Scheme of a system for measuring the low-frequency noise of infrared detectors, where k_{iv} is a preamplifier transimpedance (after Reference 23).

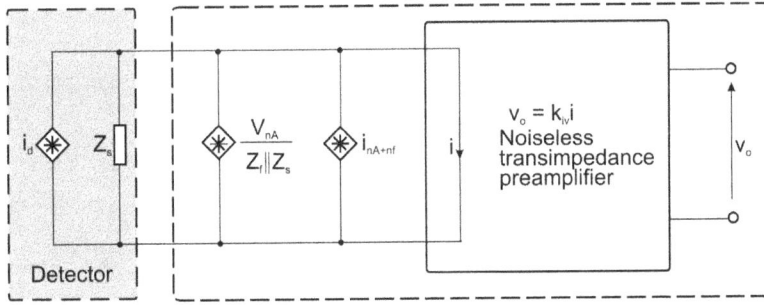

FIGURE 2.18   Simplified noise scheme of the measuring system with a transimpedance amplifier.

The average value of the detector current I_D and its fluctuation i_d are converted into a voltage using the transimpedance preamplifier W_1. At the AC output of the preamplifier, the voltage fluctuations $v_o = k_{iv} i_d$ are proportional to the fluctuation i_d of the detector current. A simplified noise equivalent scheme of the measurement system is presented in Figure 2.18. The detector noise is represented by the current source i_d. The preamplifier noise is represented by the current source i_{nA+nf} and the voltage source v_{nA}. The share of the second source in the current equivalent noise depends on the impedance Z_s loading the amplifier input and the impedance Z_f in the feedback of the operational amplifier.

The measured power spectral density S_i of the total current i flowing into the preamplifier input is given by the equation:

$$S_i = S_{in} + \frac{S_{vn}}{\left| Z_s \right| \left| Z_f \right|^2} + S_{id}. \tag{2.41}$$

It contains the spectral power density of the detector current noise S_{id} and the spectral power density of the current noise associated with the measuring system, that is, S_{in} current and S_{vn} voltage equivalent preamplifier input noise source. The share of the second component of Eq. (2.41) in the measured power spectral density of the noise current depends on the square of a module of the parallel impedance combination Z_s and Z_f. Eq. (2.41) may be used to determine the spectral density of the detector noise power, provided that the other amplifier, measurement path and detector characteristics are known.

Figure 2.19 shows a schematic diagram of the measurement system, which allows for measuring not only noise characteristics of the detectors, but also spectral characteristics and current-voltage characteristics of photodiodes. The idea of measuring the spectral and noise detector characteristics is analogous to the methods discussed above. Thanks to the use of helium cryostat, nitrogen cryostat, Peltier module and high temperature module, it is possible to measure the parameters and characteristics of the detectors in the temperature range of 10–450 K.

Keithley's 236 type precision force-measuring source was used to measure the curent-voltage characteristics of photodiodes. It enables the imposition of voltage extortion and current measurement, or current extortion and voltage measurement. The photodiode is reverse biased by an adjustable DC voltage source which is connected to a non-inverting of current-to-voltage converter.

2.4.3   MEASUREMENT OF FREQUENCY CHARACTERISTICS

The value of the detector output signal depends not only on the factors discussed in Section 2.1, but also on its frequency characteristics and the frequency of optical radiation modulation. The block diagram of the system for measuring the frequency characteristics of the detectors is shown

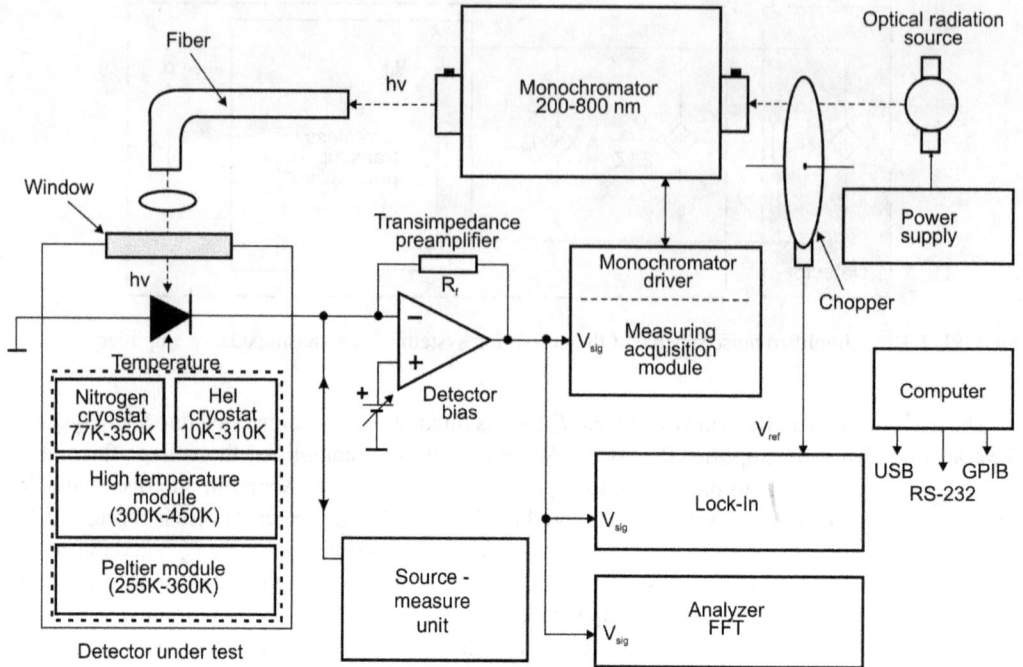

FIGURE 2.19 Scheme of the measurement system, which enables the measurement of spectral characteristics of detectors, current-voltage characteristics of photodiodes, and noise characteristics (after Reference 24).

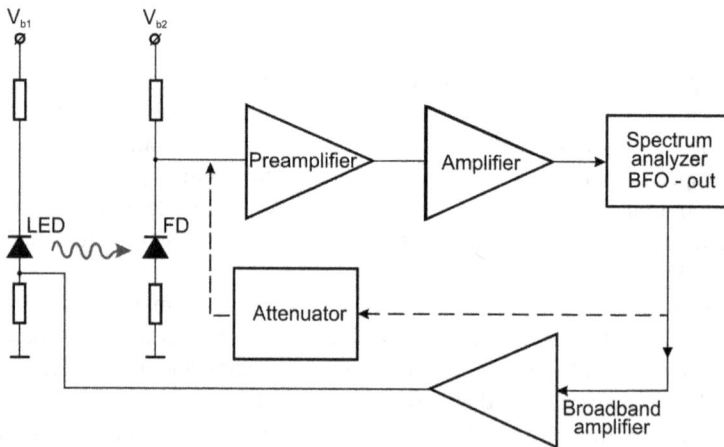

FIGURE 2.20 Block diagram of the system used to measure the frequency characteristics of the detectors.

in Figure 2.20. When measuring this characteristic, it must be ensured that the spectrum of the radiation source used is within the range of the detector spectral sensitivity. These sources may be non-modulated, such as blackbody models. However, they can be supplemented by mechanical modulators with a variable modulation frequency. Such sources are mainly used in infrared technology and low-frequency detectors. In other cases, modulated radiation sources such as LEDs and laser diodes are applied.

Measurements of the frequency characteristics should be made at constant radiation power and optimal value bias of the detector. In the system shown in Figure 2.20, the signal from the BFO output of the analyser is fed by a broadband amplifier to the radiation source. The modulated radiation emitted by the LED is focused on the detector area. The electrical signal from the detector output is amplified and then fed to the analyser input.

It follows from the spectrum analyser principle that the voltage frequency at the BFO output follows the frequency of the radiation source. This means that if the voltage frequency at the input of the analyser changes within the frequency of the detector operation, the voltage frequency at the BFO output automatically adjusts to these changes.

The advantage of the system shown in Figure 2.20 is the ease of measuring the frequency characteristics. Moreover, the narrow bandwidth of the analyser provides a high signal-to-noise ratio. Therefore, it is possible to use radiation sources with a low output power. The disadvantage of the system is the narrow spectrum of the radiation source. The use of LEDs – for example, GaAs or InAs – allows the obtaining of radiation sources with the wavelengths λ of 0.8 and 3.2 μm, respectively.

In order to determine the frequency characteristics of the detector, the dependence of the output signal voltage on the modulation frequency $V_s(f)$ must be measured. After these measurements, the radiation source should be switched off, and a generator with an attenuator connected to the preamplifier. For the same frequencies, the voltage V_c indicated by the analyser meter should be measured.

The relative frequency response $w(f)$ of the detector shall be calculated from the equation

$$w(f) = \frac{V_s(f)V_c(f_o)}{V_c(f)V_s(f_o)}, \tag{2.42}$$

where f_o is the frequency at which $w(f_o) = 1$.

Knowing the spectral characteristics (also known as frequency) of the detector voltage or noise current density, the frequency characteristics of the noise equivalent power density can be determined (Figure 2.21).

For this purpose the noise current spectral density should be divided by the maximum value of the current responsivity $R_{imax}(\lambda)$ of the detector under test (as NEP is usually given for R_{imax}):

$$NEP_{min}(f) = \frac{I_{nd}(f)}{R_{imax}}. \tag{2.43}$$

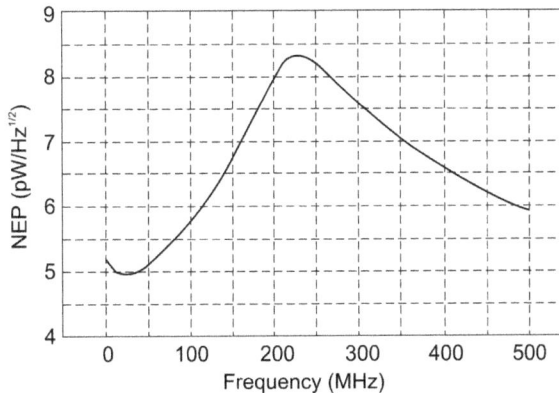

FIGURE 2.21 *NEP* spectral characteristics of *p-i-n* InGaAs photodiodes PDB460C type by Thorlabs (after Reference 7).

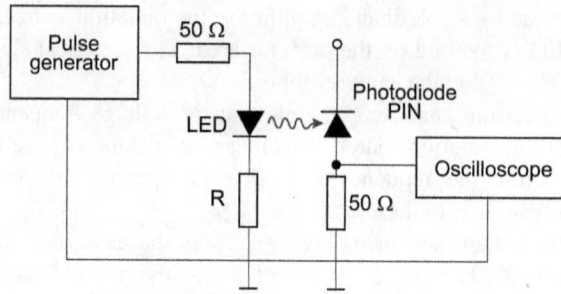

FIGURE 2.22 System for determining the rise and fall time of the photodiode output signal which is a response to a rectangular pulse extortion.

Then, using the spectral sensitivity characteristics of the detector $R_i(\lambda)$, the *NEP* frequency characteristics can be determined from the equation

$$NEP(f) = NEP_{min}(f)\frac{R_{imax}}{R_i(\lambda)}. \tag{2.44}$$

Knowing this characteristic (for any frequency range) can determine the minimum P_{min} power that can be detected by a given detector:

$$P_{min} = \int_{f_l}^{f_u} NEP(f)df. \tag{2.45}$$

2.4.4 MEASUREMENT OF THE RISE AND FALL TIME OF THE DETECTOR RESPONSE

The rise and fall times of the detector response to the rectangular pulse can be determined in the system shown in Figure 2.22. This system consists of a rectangular pulse generator and laser diode LD or LED diode, tested photodiode, as well as oscilloscope. The LED or laser diode is pulse-powered from a generator and illuminates the photodiode. The output signal from the photodiode is measured at a load resistance of 50 Ω, with a broadband oscilloscope.

PROBLEMS

Example 2.1

An InSb detector bandgap at 80 K equals 0.23 eV. Calculate the cut-off wavelength λ_c.

Example 2.2

A photoconductive detector with an area of 1 mm² is irradiated by 200 μW/cm² generating a voltage signal of 20 μV. Calculate the voltage responsivity of this detector.

Example 2.3

A PbS detector characterised by an active area of $A = 3 \times 3$ mm^2 and a voltage responsivity of $R_v = 10^5$ V/W has a noise voltage of $V_n = 40$ μV in a 10-kHz bandwidth. Calculate the detectivity of this detector.

Example 2.4

For the detector of Example 2.3 calculate the noise equivalent power *NEP*.

Example 2.5

Considering a 1-mm^2 PV detector illuminated by 10^{15} photons/cm^{2}s. Calculate a photocurrent generated in this detector if its quantum efficiency is $\eta = 0.8$.

Example 2.6

Calculate a signal-to-noise ratio registered by a photodiode with an area of $A = 1$ mm^2, a noise bandwidth of $\Delta f = 100$ kHz, and a detectivity of 10^{11} cmHz$^{1/2}$/W. Its area is irradiated $E_e = 5$ μW/cm^2.

Example 2.7

Calculate a radiant flux and a current responsivity if a photocurrent of $I_{ph} = 0.4$ μA is generated in a detector with an area of $A = 1$ mm^2 as the result of a photon irradiation $L_p = 10^{15}$ photons/cm^{2}s with a wavelength of $\lambda = 4$ μm.

Example 2.8

As can be seen from Figure 4.22, the absorption coefficient α for InGaAs at a wavelength of 1.55 μm equals 6×10^3 cm^{-1}. What is the penetration depth x of the radiation at which $P(x)/P_i = 1/e$?

Example 2.9

When 5×10^{11} photons (N_{ph}) of radiation strike a photodiode, the charge (Q) of 4.8×10^{-8} C is generated at the photodiode terminals. Determine the quantum efficiency (η) of this photodiode.

Example 2.10

For data from Example 2.9, specify the current responsivity (R_i) at a wavelength (λ) of 0.85 μm.

REFERENCES

1. W.L. Eisenman, J.D. Merriam, and R.F. Potter, "Operational characteristics of infrared photodetectors", in *Semiconductors and Semimetals*, vol. 12, pp. 1–37, edited by R.K. Willardson and A.C. Beer, Academic Press, New York, 1977.
2. M. Johnson, *Photodetection and Measurement. Maximizing Performance in Optical Systems*, McGraw-Hill, New York, 2003.
3. "Si photodiodes. Lineup of Si photodiodes for UV to near IR radiation", Selection guide 2018. www.hamamatsu.com/resources/pdf/ssd/si_pd_kspd0001e.pdf.
4. L. Orozco, "Programmable-gain transimpedance amplifiers maximise dynamic range in spectroscopy systems", *Analog Dialogue* 47–05, May, 2013.
5. www.hamamatsu-news.de/hamamatsu_optosemiconductor_handbook/14/.
6. "Compound semiconductor photosensors", Chapter 6, Hamamatsu Catalogue, 2014. www.hamamatsu.com/resources/pdf/ssd/e06_handbook_compound_semiconductor.pdf.
7. V. Mackowiak, J. Peupelman, Y. Ma, and A. Gorges, "NEP-Noise equivalent power", Thorlabs. www.thorlabs.com/images/TabImages/Noise_Equivalent_Power_White_Paper.pdf.
8. R.C. Jones, "Performance of detectors for visible and infrared radiation", in *Advances in Electronics*, Vol. 5, pp. 27–30, ed. by L. Morton, Academic Press, New York, 1952.
9. D.H. Seib and L.W. Aukerman, "Photodetectors for the 0,1 to 1,0 μm spectral region", in *Advances in Electronics and Electron Physics,* Vol. 34, pp. 95–221, ed. by L. Morton, Academic Press, New York, 1973.
10. J.D. Vincent, *Fundamentals of Infrared Detector Operation and Testing,* Wiley, New York, 1990.
11. G.H. Rieke, *Detection of Light: From the Ultraviolet to the Submillimeter,* 2nd edition, Cambridge University Press, Cambridge, 2003.
12. E.L. Dereniak and G.D. Boreman, *Infrared Detectors and Systems*, Wiley, New York, 1996.
13. M. Henini and M. Razeghi, *Handbook of Infrared Detection Technologies,* Elsevier, Amsterdam, 2002.
14. A. Rogalski, *Infrared and Terahertz Detectors*, 3rd edition, CRC Press, Boca Raton, 2019.
15. A. Rogalski, *Infrared Detectors*, 2nd edition, CRC Press, Boca Raton, 2011.
16. P.W. Kruse, "The photon process", in *Optical and Infrared Detectors*, pp. 5–69, edited by R.J. Keyes, Springer, Berlin, 1977.
17. A.N. Lowan and G. Blanch, "Tables of Planck's radiation and photon functions", *J. Opt. Soc. Amer.* 30, 70–81 (1940).
18. R.D. Hudson, *Infrared System Engineering,* Wiley, New York, 1969.
19. P.R. Bratt, "Impurity germanium and silicon infrared detectors", in *Semiconductors and Semimetals*, Vol, 12, pp. 39–141, edited by R.K. Willardson and A.C. Beer, Academic Press, 1977.
20. N. Sclar, "Properties of doped silicon and germanium in infrared detectors", *Prog. Quant. Electr.* 9, 149–257 (1984).
21. A. Rogalski, "Assessment of HgCdTe photodiodes and quantum well infrared photoconductors for long wavelength focal plane arrays", *Infrared Phys. Technol.* 40, 279–294 (1999).
22. A.S. Jensen, "Temperature limitations to infrared detectors", *Proc. SPIE* 1308, 284–292 (1990).
23. Ł. Ciura, A. Kolek, W. Gawron, A. Kowalewski, and D. Stanaszek, "Measurements of low frequency noise of infrared photodetectors with transimpedance detection system", *Metrol. Meas. Syst.* 21(3), 461–472 (2014).
24. R. Ćwirko, J. Ćwirko, and Z. Bielecki, "Measurement system testing the optical radiation detectors in a broad temperature range", *Metrol. Meas. Syst.* 16, 491–500 (2009).

3 Noise Sources

In the broadest sense of the word, noise is defined as any unwanted signal interfering with the correct reading of information contained in a useful signal [1, 2]. Noise can be caused by fluctuations in electrical quantities as the result of the discrete structure of matter. It is always present and reduces the signal quality. Noises accompanying many physical phenomena of a random nature are subject to a statistical description used in the analysis of stochastic processes. When developing their models, we use the theory of probability, theories of stochastic processes and mathematical statistics.

The performance of all detectors will be limited by random noise processes, which will determine the minimum detectable power that can be measured. The noise sources may arise in the detector, in the incident radiant energy or in the electronic circuitry associated with the detection system. The object of any system design must be to reduce the electronic noise sources below that in the output of the detector, and ideally to minimise the internal detector noise such that the overall system noise is dominated by the incident radiation noise.

Physical noise processes are inherent in any natural process or electronic component such as the detectors or transistors. Some noise processes can be derived and expressed in rigorous mathematical terminology, whereas other processes are not well understood. In detectors of light, the physical noise sources include Johnson (thermal or Nyquist) noise, shot noise, temperature-fluctuation noise and generation–recombination (g-r) noise. Johnson noise results from random charge movement due to thermal agitation in a conductor. Shot noise arises from the statistical occurrence of discrete events, such as when charges cross a bandgap potential barrier in a semiconductor. Generation-recombination noise occurs when electron-hole pairs (with finite carrier lifetime) are generated or recombined in a semiconductor. From the other side, the noise with $1/f$ (f is electrical frequency) fractal power spectrum defies physical explanation. $1/f$ noise is present in detectors, electronic circuits, flow processes such as natural rivers and traffic, biological processes and music.

A more complex situation is in the optical systems. System noise sources include interference noise, fixed-pattern noise in detector arrays and microphonic noise. Interference is caused by external events injecting spurious electrical signals by capacitive, inductive, or earth loop coupling into an electronics circuit. In the case of large detector arrays, due to statistical variations between pixels, some pixels provide a stronger signal than others. Individual pixels have different absolute responsivity values, different spectral responsivity values and/or nonlinear responses. The statistical nature of these values is modelled as so-called fixed pattern noise. Microphonic and triboelectric noise results from minute mechanical deformation of an electronic device or conductors, causing signal generation in piezoelectric or triboelectric materials, or variation in device capacitance

In this chapter only the internal noise mechanisms associated with the optical detectors presented in this book will be discussed. More detailed treatments of noise theory can be found in many reviews and books including, for example, References [1–4].

DOI: 10.1201/9781003263098-3

3.1   INTRODUCTION

Noise power can be treated as the variance σ^2 related to the standard deviation σ of the noise voltage or current. Both ways lead to a similar result. For a noise voltage source, the noise is determined as follows:

$$\sigma = \sqrt{\sigma^2} = \left[\overline{\Delta V^2}\right]^{1/2} = \left\{\overline{\left[V - \overline{V}\right]^2}\right\}^{1/2} = \left\{\frac{1}{\Delta t}\int_0^{\Delta t}\left[V(t) - \overline{V}\right]^2 dt\right\}^{1/2}, \tag{3.1}$$

where, $\overline{V}$ is the mean signal voltage and Δt is the time interval (assuming the ergodic function when the time averaged values are equal to the values averaged over the set of realisations [1]; that is the situation in the case of stationary processes). The resultant noise from multiple sources is as follows:

$$\sigma_{rms} = \left[\sum_{i=1}^{n}\sigma_i^2\right]^{1/2} = \Delta V_{rms} = \left[\sum_{i=1}^{n}\overline{\Delta V_i^2}\right]^{1/2}, \tag{3.2}$$

where, ΔV_{rms} is known as the root-mean-square (RMS) value of the resultant noise voltage:

$$\Delta V_{rms} = \left\{\frac{1}{n\Delta t}\sum_{i=1}^{n}\int_0^{\Delta t}\left[V_i(t) - \overline{V}\right]^2 dt\right\}^{1/2}. \tag{3.3}$$

Although noise is a stochastic process, its instantaneous values in general do not change in any way, and there is a certain relationship between them. The self-correlation function is used to evaluate this relationship.

If the noise can be treated as a stationary random ergodic process, we can use the Fourier transformations. Since the output signal voltage fluctuates over time as a result of an un-periodic generation process (generation rate), we will consider these fluctuations in the noise power spectrum or in the spectral power density $S(f)$.

To determine the noise content in a frequency band unit, the notion of spectral density (of the current S_i or the voltage S_v) and the function of noise power spectral density are introduced [5]. This function is defined by the following equation:

$$\left\langle\overline{V^2}\right\rangle = \int_0^{\infty}S_v(f)df, \tag{3.4}$$

and it relates the voltage mean square value to the noise power spectral density.

Let us assume that the voltage as a function of time runs as shown in Figure 3.1(a). To simplify the considerations, we will assume that the average voltage value is zero (coupling through capacity). Then, the autocorrelation function R_{vv} for such a voltage waveform has the form

$$R_{vv}(\Delta t) = \int_{-\infty}^{\infty}V(t)V(t + \Delta t)dt, \tag{3.5}$$

and is presented in Figure 3.1(b).

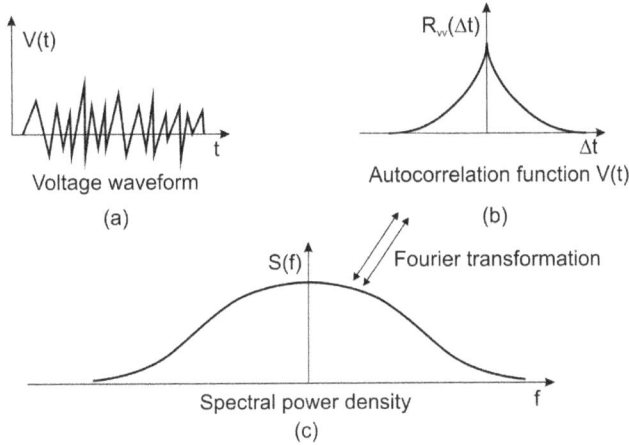

FIGURE 3.1 Noise: (a) stochastic process of voltage fluctuation, (b) autocorrelation function, (c) spectral power density.

The Fourier transform of the autocorrelation $R_{vv}(\Delta t)$ is the spectral power density $S(f)$ shown in Figure 3.1(c). The Fourier transform for $\Delta t = 0$ takes the value [6] of

$$R_{vv}\left(\Delta t = 0\right) = \int\limits_{-\infty}^{\infty} S\left(f\right) df, \tag{3.6}$$

and it is also the total power in the case of no time shift ($\Delta t = 0$). Also,

$$R_{vv}\left(\Delta t = 0\right) = \int\limits_{-\infty}^{\infty} V\left(t\right)V\left(t\right) dt = \int\limits_{-\infty}^{\infty} V^2\left(t\right) dt, \tag{3.7}$$

which means that the autocorrelation function is equal to the value of the voltage fluctuation mean square.

Because the noise power for each frequency component adds up, thus the noise voltage adds up in a square. By adding or integrating the spectral density of power (by adding powers at different frequencies), we obtain the total (resultant) noise power. If the noise power is constant (independent of the frequency f), then this noise is called a white noise. The noise power or variance is proportional to the bandwidth Δf:

$$\overline{\left(\Delta V\right)^2} \propto \Delta f, \tag{3.8}$$

and the RMS of the noise voltage is proportional to the root of the bandwidth

$$\sqrt{\overline{\left(\Delta V\right)^2}} \propto \sqrt{\Delta f}. \tag{3.9}$$

Proceeding similarly, the sum of the independent randomly changing noise power components equals

$$(\Delta V)^2 = \overline{(\Delta V)_1^2} + \overline{(\Delta V)_2^2} + \overline{(\Delta V)_3^2}, \tag{3.10}$$

where, the mean square value of the voltage fluctuation is proportional to the power. The square root of $\overline{(\Delta V)^2}$ is the RMS value:

$$\Delta V_{rms} = \sqrt{\overline{(\Delta V)^2}} = \sqrt{\overline{(\Delta V)_1^2} + \overline{(\Delta V)_2^2} + \overline{(\Delta V)_3^2}}. \tag{3.11}$$

It follows from the above considerations that the noise power sums up (noise voltages add up as their squares) and that in the case of a white noise the noise voltage is proportional to the square root of the bandwidth [see Eq. (3.9)].

Considering the noise research, it is necessary to introduce the concept of a noise band. This bandwidth is different from that of a 3-decibel amplifier. The amplifier bandwidth (3-dB) is defined as a difference in frequencies for which the power gain $K_p(f)$ decreases to half. The points on the frequency axis where the power amplification decreases to half are at the same time the points where the voltage gain $K_v(f)$ decreases by 3 dB in relation to the gain in the middle of the transmission bandwidth [Figure 3.2(a)]. Thus, the 3-dB bandwidth of the amplifier is equal to the difference between the upper f_u and the lower f_l of the limiting frequency and equals $\Delta f_{3dB} = f_u - f_l$.

In the analysis of noise detection models, the energy bandwidth Δf (also called the effective noise band or the effective band) is used that corresponds to the base of a hypothetical rectangle with a height equal to the maximum value of the power spectrum density $K_{P\,max} = K_{v\,max}^2$ and to a field equal to the area under the curve $K_v^2(f)$ [see Figure 3.2(b)]. Thus,

$$\Delta f = \frac{1}{K_{v\,max}^2} \int_0^\infty K_v^2(f)\,df, \tag{3.12}$$

where, $K_v(f)$ is the voltage gain as a frequency function.

Figure 3.2(a) shows that the noise bandwidth is wider than the detection circuit 3-dB bandwidth. If the steepness of frequency characteristic is 20 dB/dec, then the noise bandwidth equals $\Delta f = (\pi/2)f_{-3dB}$. When the steepness of the $K_v(f)$ characteristic increases and provides a faster decrease of the gain, then Δf tends to f_{-3dB}.

The detector performance is limited by statistical noise processes determining the minimum power that can be measured. There may be many sources of noise; these sources include detector,

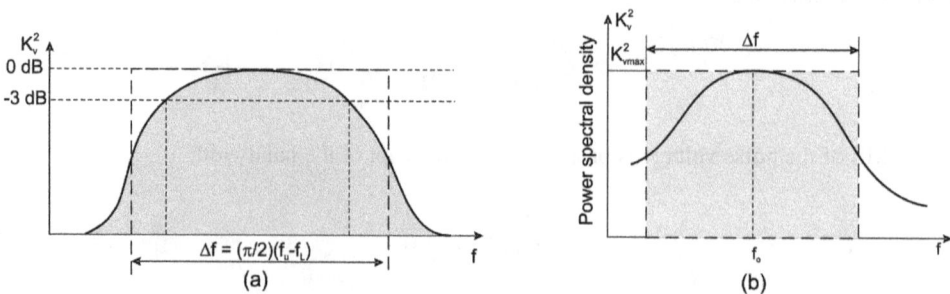

FIGURE 3.2 Determination of: (a) relationship between the noise bandwidth and the detection circuit passband, (b) illustration of a noise bandwidth, where f_o is the centre frequency of the bandwidth Δf.

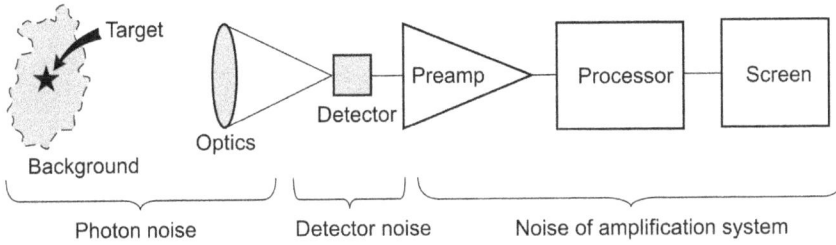

FIGURE 3.3   Detector noise classification.

incident radiation and electrical system related to the detection system (see Figure 3.3). An important challenge for detector manufacturers is to design the detector in such a way so as to reduce an internal detector noise below the noise level caused by incident radiation.

Noises related to the detection system can be divided into three groups [4,7–10]:

    I. photon noise
- signal fluctuations noise; and
- background radiation fluctuations noise.

    II. detector noise
- Johnson noise;
- shot noise;
- generation-recombination noise;
- $1/f$ noise;
- temperature noise; and
- microphone noise.

    III. amplification systems noise
- Johnson noise;
- shot noise;
- generation-recombination noise;
- $1/f$ noise;
- temperature noise;
- microphone noise; and
- popcorn noise.

3.2   PHOTON NOISE

Photon noise results from the radiation nature and is present in every detector. It is a fundamental noise in the sense that it is not due to imperfections in the detector or the electronics associated with it, but it is due to the nature of radiation. The radiation incident on the detector is a flux of photons created in individual and independent energy radiation processes. The photon flux will therefore show fluctuations around the average value. Photon noise can be considered either as the result of a statistical process of individual photons colliding with the detector or as a stochastic result during photoelectron emission acts. The first point of view requires treating radiation as a quantum system and considering some aspects of the process included in Bose-Einstein statistics. Both ways of description are presented, for example, in Boyd's monograph [4].

By photon noise we mean uncertainty in the amount of electromagnetic radiation emitted by a given source over a certain time period. For example, the variability of the radiation emission is shown in Figure 3.4. The most probable value of exitance is also shown as M_p, and the mean square deviation, σ, which is a measure of the uncertainty of its determination, that is the noise.

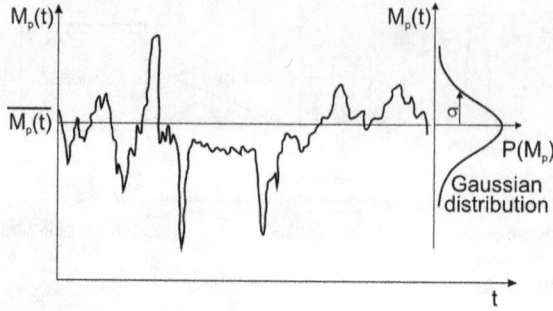

FIGURE 3.4 Instantaneous photon existence variability.

It can be shown that the variance of the photon noise has the following form:

$$\sigma^2 = \bar{n}\left(\frac{e^{hv/kT}}{e^{hv/kT}-1}\right), \tag{3.13}$$

where, $\bar{n}$ is the average number of photons emitted over the period Δt. The variance of the photon noise is equal to the variance for the Poisson distribution $\bar{n}$ multiplied by the Bose factor.

For most optical applications in the wavelength range from 0.3 μm to 30 μm and for temperatures below 500 K, the energy per photon is much higher than the thermal energy ($hv >> kT$), and then

$$\frac{e^{hv/kT}}{e^{hv/kT}-1} \approx 1, \tag{3.14}$$

and Poisson statistics can be used to determine the photon noise. If we have high energy sources or sources emitting in the millimetre range, the correction factor in Eq. (3.14) must be taken into account.

If we omit the Bose correction, then the noise of the incident photon flux Φ_p (for which $\bar{n}$ photons are expected to be emitted at the time Δt) is given by the equation

$$\sigma = \sqrt{\bar{n}} = \sqrt{\Phi_p \Delta t}. \tag{3.15}$$

The signal-to-noise power ratio takes the form of:

$$\frac{S}{N} = \frac{\overline{n^2}}{\sigma^2} = \bar{n}, \tag{3.16}$$

thus, the minimum detectable number of photons $\bar{n}$ = 1 photon [11].

Figure 3.5 shows the signal and background waveforms [12]. As can be seen from this figure, the photon noise is conditioned by the fluctuations of an optical signal and a background radiation.

3.2.1 SIGNAL FLUX FLUCTUATION NOISE

Optical flux generation is a Poisson process, which carries with the average value an inherent noise variance equal to the mean flux level. The shot noise fluctuation is smaller at long wavelengths

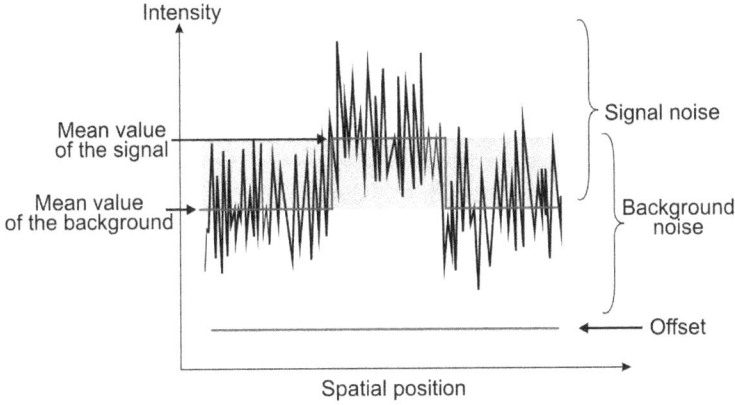

FIGURE 3.5   Illustration of the photon noise from a signal and background sources.

(infrared region) but becomes significant at very low flux levels for ultraviolet and visual light since the photons have higher energy per photon at shorter wavelengths. The noise inherent in the signal sets a minimum detectable signal level. The following derivation determines this minimum signal level under the assumption that there are no other signal or noise sources.

The optical generation rate signal (photons/s) is as follows:

$$G_{ph} = \Phi_{ph} A_d \eta, \tag{3.17}$$

where, Φ_{ph} is the photon flux density, A_d is the detector area and η – the quantum efficiency. Then, the magnitude of photocurrent is $I_{ph} = \eta q A_d \Phi_{ph}$, and the mean square value of a noise current density coming from signal fluctuation is directly proportional to the optical generation rate [13].

$$i_{nph}^2 = 2q^2 \Phi_{ph} \Delta f, \tag{3.18}$$

where q is the electron charge and Δf is the noise bandwidth. Since the radiant flux density $\Phi_e = hc\Phi_{ph}/\lambda$, then signal-to-noise ratio (SNR) becomes

$$SNR = \sqrt{\frac{\eta \lambda \Phi_e}{2hc\Delta f}}, \tag{3.19}$$

and the noise equivalent power is equal

$$NEP = \frac{2hc\Delta f}{\eta \lambda}. \tag{3.20}$$

The last equation states that for a given wavelength λ and noise bandwidth Δf, the noise equivalent power due to the signal fluctuation is determined by the detector quantum efficiency η. In the infrared region, the noise caused by fluctuations in the optical signal is negligible in relation to the background noise and the thermal generation noise (see Figure 3.6).

3.2.2   BACKGROUND FLUX FLUCTUATION NOISE

If the detector performance is limited by the noise caused by the background, the detector is operated in BLIP (background limited infrared photodetectors). Figure 3.6 indicates that the intersections of curves for signal fluctuation (SFL) and background fluctuation (BLIP) limits lie about 1.2 μm. Below about 1.2 μm, the wavelength dependence is small. Above 1.2 μm, it is a very large steep dependence of detectivity upon wavelength of the short wavelength end of the room-temperature background spectral distribution.

The principle used to determine the BLIP limit is the same as was used for SFL, except that in this case the limit is set by the noise caused by the background. For a monochromatic source at frequency v, the minimum detectable power of an open detector against a thermal background radiation is [10]:

$$NEP = \frac{hv}{\eta(v)}\sqrt{2\Delta f \int_{v_o}^{\infty} \frac{\eta(v)2\pi v^2 \exp\left(hv/kT_b\right)dv}{c^2\left[\exp\left(hv/kT_b\right)-1\right]^2}}.$$

(3.21)

At the end of this point, let us compare the contribution of the photonic noise of the signal and the photon background noise on *NEP* depending on the spectral range. Figure 3.6 illustrates the spectral *NEP* in the wavelength range from 0.1 to 20 μm assuming a background temperature of 290 K, detector areas of 1 cm^2 and 1 mm^2 (applicable only to the background fluctuation limit), a 2π steradian FOV, and bandwidths of 1 and 10^4 Hz [10]. These additional values of parameters are specified due to different dependencies of *NEP* (upon area and bandwidth) for signal fluctuation and background fluctuation limits. Note that the intersections of three pairs of curves for which the bandwidths of the signal and background fluctuation limits are equal, lie between 1.0 and 1.5 μm. A similar intersection of the curves for both operating conditions takes place for detectivity (see Figure 4.6).

Figure 2.8 shows the spectral detectivity plotted as a function of wavelength for selected values of background temperature assuming unit quantum efficiency. Although this figure assumes rather specialised conditions (i.e., background radiation due to blackbody source), it provides a useful standard against which to compare the performance of actual detectors fabricated by commercial manufactures.

3.3   JOHNSON NOISE

Thermal noise was observed for the first time by J.B. Johnson in 1927, and a theoretical analysis was performed by H. Nyquist in 1928 [11]. For this reason, this noise is also called Johnson-Nyquist noise and is associated with thermal fluctuations in the speed of free carriers. It is only generated in the dissipative real component of complex impedances. Johnson-Nyquist noise is the basic type of noise; it occurs even when there is no current passing through the element and represents the minimum noise level in the element and unambiguously limits the resolution of each measurement path.

Johnson noise can be considered as a one-dimensional form of blackbody radiation because its derivation is based on the density of states [11]. Its spectral density is given by

$$v_n^2 = 4kTR\left(\frac{x}{e^x+1}\right),$$

(3.22)

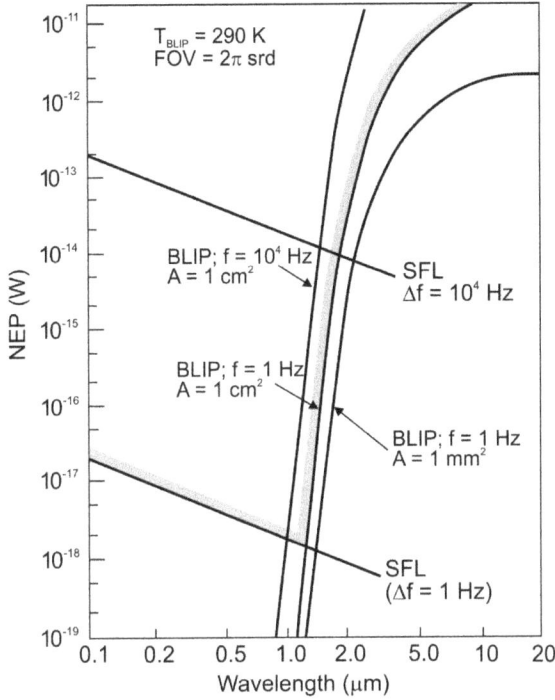

FIGURE 3.6 Minimum detectable monochromatic power as a function of the wavelength for a composite of SFL and BLIP limit for two detector areas and electrical bandwidths. Background temperature is 290 K and FOV is 2π steradians. Detector long wavelength limit is equal to the source wavelength (after Reference 10).

and

$$i_n^2 = \frac{4kT}{R}\left(\frac{x}{e^x+1}\right), \tag{3.23}$$

where R is the resistive element in Ω, v_n and i_n are the RMS noise voltage and current power spectral densities in V^2/Hz and A^2/Hz, respectively; $x = hf/kT$, where f is the electrical frequency. Because $e^x = 1 + x + x^2/2! + x^3/3! + \ldots$, thus, for small x the term $x/(e^x + 1)$ has unity value.

The Johnson-Nyquist noise has a flat power spectral density up to the frequency of 10^{12}–10^{14} Hz (the inverse of electrical relaxation time). This means that the noise power with frequencies contained in the 1 Hz bandwidth is the same for each frequency. Figure 3.7(a) shows the time course of a thermal noise that can be observed on the oscilloscope screen, while Figure 3.7(b) shows its power spectral density distribution. Thermal noise determines the lower limit of the noise voltage or the noise current in each detector, or the real part impedance of any element.

Fluctuations of the random Brownian motion of free charge carriers mean that at the terminals of the resistor with the value of R there will be an electromotive force with a non-zero mean square value determined by the equation

$$V_{nJ}^2 = 4kTR\Delta f, \tag{3.24}$$

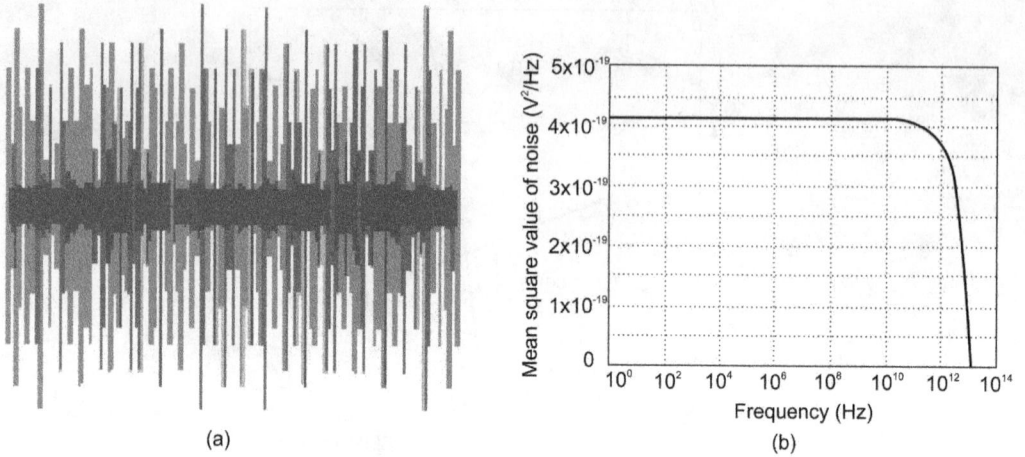

FIGURE 3.7 Thermal noise: (a) illustration of time course, (b) power spectral density distribution.

where Δf is the noise bandwidth of the system. Thus, the RMS value of the thermal noise voltage is the following:

$$V_{nJ} = \sqrt{4kTR\Delta f}. \tag{3.25}$$

When the noise source is loaded with a matching resistor, we will get the available noise power

$$P_t = \left(\frac{V_{nJ}}{2}\right)^2 \frac{1}{R} = kT\Delta f. \tag{3.26}$$

Eq. (3.26) shows that noise power does not depend on the noise generator resistance, but is directly proportional to the temperature on the absolute scale and the band of the measuring system.

Thermal noises are also described by means of a current source. According to Norton's claim, the RMS value of the current source efficiency is the following:

$$I_{nJ} = \sqrt{\frac{4kT\Delta f}{R}}. \tag{3.27}$$

To obtain the noise voltage spectral density S_{vJ}, the RMS value of the voltage is divided by the square root of the band:

$$S_{vJ} = \sqrt{4kTR}. \tag{3.28}$$

In the same way, we obtain the noise current spectral density S_{iJ}:

$$S_{iJ} = \sqrt{\frac{4kT}{R}}. \tag{3.29}$$

Equation (3.25) is very important in noise theory. Several important conclusions can be drawn from this equation. The noise voltage is proportional to the bandwidth square root, regardless of the frequency range covering the bandwidth. To minimise the thermal noise effect, one should narrow the bandwidth as much as possible when carrying a useful signal.

3.4 SHOT NOISE

Another type of noise that occurs in photodetectors and signal-processing systems is the shot noise. This noise is related to the current passing through the potential barrier and is conditioned by a discrete nature of the passing charge as a series of independent events. Current passing through the barrier is the sum of many elementary pulses and, therefore, the flow of discrete charges (note that the current passing through the resistor cannot have such a noise component). Although all these pulses are identical, their position on the timeline is random. Deviations from the ideal flow caused by an accidental generation of discontinuous portions of the electric charge are the shot noise (Figure 3.8).

Shot noise is generated in photovoltaic and photoemissive detectors. It is not found in photoconductive detectors. The importance of the shot noise increases when the number of particles carrying the charge is relatively small. This is due to Poisson distribution describing the fluctuations of the charge carrier passing through the potential barrier. With the large number of carriers, Poisson distribution changes to normal distribution.

It turns out that the current of the p-n junction shot noise current is defined as follows [1]:

$$I_n = \left[\left(2qI + 4qI_s \right) \Delta f \right]^{1/2},$$ (3.30)

where I is the total junction current and I_s is the saturation current. The second component of Eq. (3.30) is caused by the statistical process of carrier diffusion through the junction. In the case of zero bias, $I = 0$, whereas in the case of a sufficiently high diode polarisation in the reverse direction, $I = I_s$, therefore:

$$I_n = \left(2qI_s \Delta f \right)^{1/2}.$$ (3.31)

In the photoemission vacuum photocathodes the current pulse starts from the moment when an electron is emitted from the cathode and ends with the electron hitting the anode where it recombines

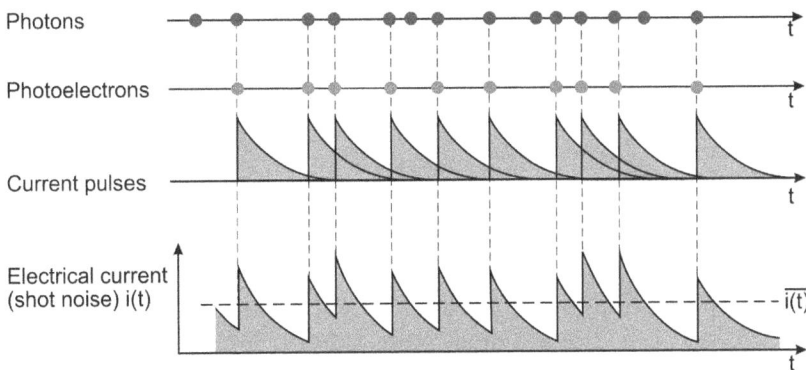

FIGURE 3.8 Shot noise. The induced photocurrent comprises a superposition of current pulses, each associated with a detected photon. The superposition of the individual current pulses constitutes shot noise.

with a positive charge. The shot noise expression for photocathodes is similar to Eq. (3.31), but in this case of I_s it becomes a photocathode dark current due to photoemission, field emission or anode-cathode leakage current.

Note that the photon noise spectrum is flat, and the shot noise current is directly proportional to the root of the bandwidth, not to the position of that bandwidth. This means that we are dealing with a white noise, with a Gaussian probability distribution carrying a constant amount of power in each bandwidth unit.

According to Eq. (3.31), the shot noise increases with the increase of the detector current intensity and, thus, also with the increase of a received signal level. This is what distinguishes it from the thermal noise, which is independent of the optical power level. Equation (3.31) is true if there is no interaction between charges forming the electric current, for example, for the current passing through the junction of a semiconductor diode. In this case, the charges are moving thanks to diffusion cross, and independently of each other, the potential barrier.

For large numbers of events, the Poisson distribution approximates a Gaussian distribution and shot noise has a Gaussian distribution. However, when small event numbers are considered (e.g., low light level at visual or ultraviolet wavelengths), the distribution is not Gaussian.

Let us pay attention to one more difference between a photoresistor and a photodiode. The share of photons in the generation and recombination noise of the photoresistors is $\sqrt{2}$ times greater than given by Eq. (3.30). Since the recombination does not occur in an ideal diode (a strong electric field of the junction eliminates the possibility of recombination), it is reasonable to distinguish between detectors showing shot noise (i.e., photovoltaic detectors) and those showing generation-recombination noise (i.e., photoresistors).

3.5 GENERATION-RECOMBINATION NOISE

Statistical fluctuations of thermal and optical speed of generation and recombination of free carriers in a semiconductor are the source of generation-recombination (g-r) noise. In an imperfect semiconductor material, there are structural imperfections (vacancies, unplanned admixtures, dislocations, etc.) creating energy levels located in a forbidden band. They can act as traps and intercept or generate current carriers. As a result, there are fluctuations in their number in a conductor or valence band. On the other hand, fluctuations in the average concentration of carriers cause fluctuations in current, voltage and electrical resistance. Very often, the analysis of a generation-recombination noise (g-r) is limited only to noise caused by fluctuations of thermal speed of generation and recombination of free carriers in a semiconductor (Figure 3.9). The free electrons can find empty donor levels where they randomly recombine in time because the carrier lifetime is short compared to the transit time between electrodes.

In photoconductive detectors, the primary noise contributor at medium-to-high frequencies is the g-r noise. The generation-recombination noise is not found in most photovoltaic detectors because

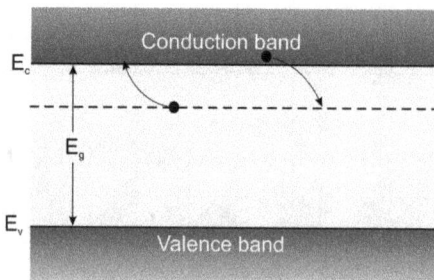

FIGURE 3.9   Generation-recombination noise idea.

the carriers are quickly swept out of the junction before recombination. However, some materials do have g-r noise in photovoltaic devices.

The generation of free carriers can be caused by two processes: thermally excited carriers or optically excited carriers. Thermally excited carriers are created by virtue of the energy levels in the material due to its operating temperature. At higher temperatures, more thermally excited carriers are generated (due to increasing kT value).

The g-r noise power density has the general form

$$S_{gr} \propto \frac{\tau^2}{1 + \omega^2 \tau^2}, \tag{3.32}$$

where τ is the carrier lifetime and ω is the electrical frequency. Note that the carrier introduce a pool in the transfer function, which results in a roll-off at higher frequencies. The statistical fluctuation in the carrier concentration produces the white noise (constant), which has electrical frequencies less than the inverse of carrier lifetime. In other words, the generation-recombination noise spectrum is flat up to a frequency value approximately equal to the inverse of the free carrier lifetime. The high-frequency roll-off is not as high as for shot noise or thermal noise because the carrier lifetimes are much longer than the brief events associated with shot noise and thermal noise.

In the literature there are many analytical expressions for the generational-recombination noise. They depend on a temperature and a mechanism of the generation-recombination process – whether there are interband processes or doped band-level-type processes.

Generally, the RMS current expression for generation-recombination noise is given by

$$I_{ngr} = 2qg\sqrt{\eta E_p A_d \Delta f + g_{th} A_d \Delta f t}, \tag{3.33}$$

where g is the photoconductive gain, E_p is the photon flux (photon irradiance) on the detector, and g_{th} is the rate of thermal generation, and t is the detector thickness in the optical propagation direction.

In the case of an n-type doped photoconductor, the current noise is determined by the following equation [12]:

$$I_{ngr}^2 = \frac{4qI_b g\Delta f}{1 + \omega^2 \tau^2}, \tag{3.34}$$

where, I_b is the bias current of the detector, τ is the free carrier lifetime, g is the photoconductive amplification, and ω is the angular frequency.

For an almost intrinsic semiconductor, the RMS value of the noise voltage is as follows [13]:

$$V_{ngr} = \frac{2V_b}{\sqrt{A_d t}} \frac{1+b}{bn+p} \left(\frac{np}{n+p} \right)^{1/2} \left(\frac{\tau \Delta f}{1+\omega^2 \tau^2} \right)^{1/2}, \tag{3.35}$$

where, $A_d t$ is the detector volume, $b = \mu_e / \mu_h$ is the ratio of electron mobility to holes mobility, n and p are the concentration of electrons and holes, respectively, and τ is the lifetime of free carriers, assuming that this time is the same for electrons and holes.

The above equation is valid for simple band transitions and also for recombination through Schockley-Read-Hall centres, if the recombination centres density is sufficiently low.

In the case of a compensated doped semiconductor, where the concentration of n carriers is much lower than the concentration of a compensating dopant, the correct equation is [14]:

$$I_{ngr} = 2I_b \left[\frac{\tau \, \Delta f}{A_d t \, n \left(1 + \omega^2 \tau^2\right)} \right]^{1/2}.$$

(3.36)

When the sample is uncompensated, the right-hand side of Eq. (3.36) should be multiplied by $(N_d - n)/(2N_d - n)$, where N_d is the concentration of donors.

Generation-recombination noise can be used to test defects of semiconductor devices. The method of defects characterisation based on the knowledge of g-r noise is called noise spectroscopy.

3.6 1/F NOISE

This type of noise is probably the most studied. It is called $1/f$ noise because its spectral power decreases with the increasing frequency. It is believed that the source of this noise is the non-ohmic of electrode electrical contacts, fluctuations of leakage current and the presence of potential barriers at the contacts, inside or on the surface of a semiconductor [15]. Reduction of $1/f$ noise to an acceptable level is an art that depends greatly on the processes employed in preparing the contacts and surfaces. Up until now, no fully satisfactory general theory has been formulated.

The empirical expression defining the RMS value of the low-frequency noise current is as follows:

$$I_{1/f} = \left(\frac{K I_b^\alpha \Delta f}{f^\beta} \right)^{1/2},$$

(3.37)

where, K is the proportionality factor, I_b is the bias current, α, β are the constants characterising the detector material. In most cases, it takes values close to 2, and β changes in the range from 0.8 to 1.5.

There are several models of this kind of noise [16]. The best-known include the McWhorter and Hooge models [12,17]. The McWhorter model assumes the presence of traps in a semiconductor with an appropriate distribution of time constants of trapping processes. On the other hand, in the Hooge model the noise intensity is inversely proportional to the number of free carriers and the frequency.

The frequency f_c, at which the noise intensity of the $1/f$ type equals the intensity of the white noise, is called the corner frequency. Its value is very different from single Hz to several tens of MHz and depends on a semiconductor device type.

$1/f$ noise always occurs in photoconductors and bolometers that require a bias current. A typical noise spectrum of a photoconductive detector is shown in Figure 3.10.

The best performance is achieved when the photoconductor operates in the frequency range where the generation-recombination noise dominates. This is achieved by an appropriate modulation of the source signal and using a filter in the signal readout circuits allowing the required frequency spectrum. The bandwidth depends on the type of application.

The next figure presents experimentally measured noise in two narrow gap semiconductor photodiodes. Measurements of $1/f$ noise taken at DRS for CdTe passivated vertically integrated n$^+$-n$^-$-p HgCdTe photodiodes indicate a dependence of noise on device dark current density, as shown in Figure 3.11(a), for material with dislocation density below 2×10^5 cm^{-2} [18]. The noise depends on the absolute value of dark current (as $I_d^{0.926}$, where I_d is the dark diode current), regardless of the mole HgCdTe composition or operating temperature. Figure 3.11(b) shows the share of $1/f$ noise, thermal noise, shot noise, and preamplifier depending on the frequency and bias voltage of the p-i-n MWIR

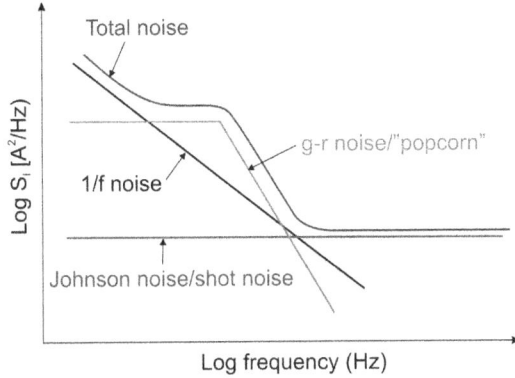

FIGURE 3.10 Typical noise power spectrum for a photoconductor versus frequency.

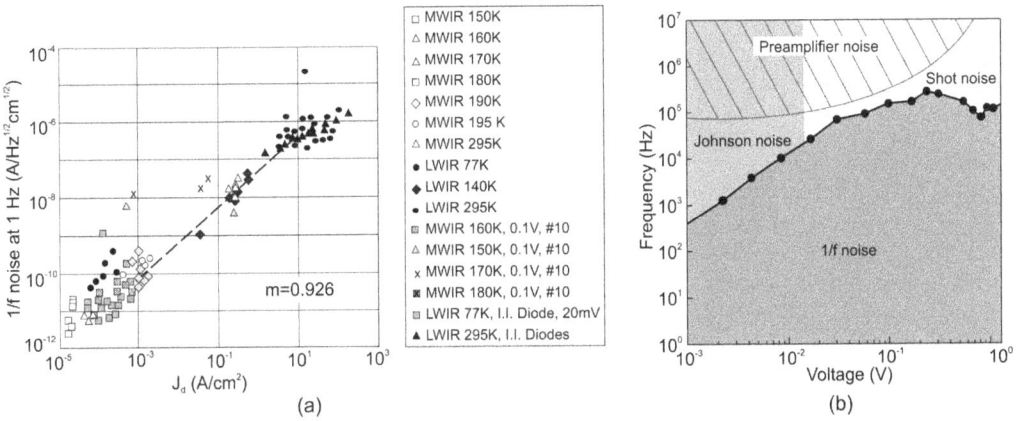

FIGURE 3.11 Experimentally measured noise in two narrow-gap semiconductor photodiodes: measurements $1/f$ noise figure versus dark current density for various HgCdTe photodiodes (after Reference 18); (b) share of different types of noise for p-i-n MWIR InAs/GaSb superlattice photodiode (after Reference 19).

InAs/GaSb superlattice photodiode. Let us note that the share of the $1/f$ type noise is dominant in the range of the lowest frequencies and increases with an increase of the detector bias voltage.

3.7 TEMPERATURE NOISE

Temperature noise is only observed in thermal detectors and is caused by a change in the detector temperature, which in turn is conditioned by fluctuations in the heat flow between the detector and the environment. The heat exchange can take place either through a radiation exchange or through a thermal conductivity with detector support elements. This type of noise is introduced to distinguish it from Johnson noise. Among the sources of the thermal detector noise are ambient temperature fluctuations. Changes in the ambient (background) temperature are transmitted by thermal resistance of the detector and cause a change in its temperature. The noise resulting from these fluctuations is called the temperature noise.

The temperature distribution is white noise Gaussian with a mean value of T and variance [20]:

$$\overline{(\Delta T)^2} = \frac{kT^2}{C},\tag{3.38}$$

where C is the heat capacity of the object.

The detector temperature variance is determined by the following equation [20, 21]:

$$\overline{\Delta T^2} = \frac{4kTR_{th}}{1 + \omega^2 \tau_{th}^2} \Delta f, \tag{3.39}$$

where, R_{th} is the thermal resistance and τ_{th} is the thermal time constant. It can be shown that the temperature-fluctuation noise of the power spectral density is

$$\left(\Delta T\right)_n^2 = \frac{4kT^2}{\sqrt{G^2 + \left(\omega C\right)^2}}, \tag{3.40}$$

where G is the thermal conductance.

Fluctuations in the detector temperature cause changes at voltage contacts. The average square value of a noise voltage caused by temperature fluctuations is the following [20,21]:

$$V_{th}^2 = K^2 \overline{\Delta T}^2 = \frac{4kTK^2R_{th}}{1 + \omega^2 \tau_{th}^2} \Delta f, \tag{3.41}$$

where the K coefficient is defined by Eq. (4.7).

The temperature noise proportion is the highest in the lowest frequency range. Minimising this noise is particularly important in cooled bolometers.

3.8   MICROPHONIC NOISE

Microphonic noise is caused by a mechanical displacement. This noise is the result of changes in the inter-electrode wire capacity, caused by its displacement relative to the housing (ground).

The capacity of the wire-housing system is equal to [see Figure (3.12)]

$$C = \frac{\varepsilon A}{d}, \tag{3.42}$$

where, ε is the medium dielectric constant and A is the capacitor effective area.

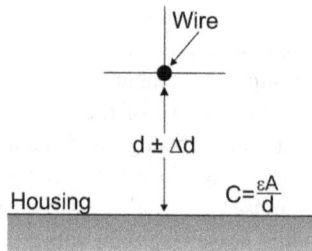

FIGURE 3.12   Microphone noise model.

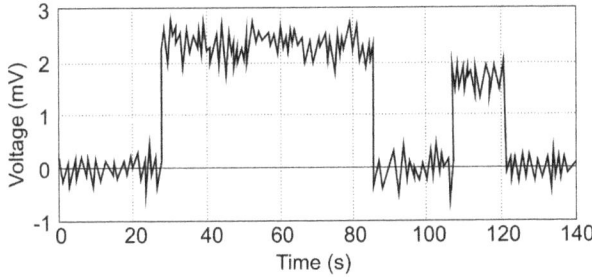

FIGURE 3.13   Illustration of the explosive noise time course.

If the wire moves by Δd, causing a change in capacity, the voltage caused by the charge will change due to wire vibrations. The basic principle of avoiding the microphone noise is the construction of mechanically stable instruments.

3.9   POPCORN NOISE

Manifestations of this noise, called popcorn noise, appear in the form of sudden or explosive voltage increases at the detector output [22]. It is found in the low-frequency mode – see Figure 3.10. The name of this noise comes from the fact that its sound is similar to bursts of corn kernels heard from a loudspeaker. You can imagine this noise as pulses on the oscilloscope screen similarly to those shown in Figure 3.13. Their amplitude may be an order of magnitude greater than the amplitude of a white noise, and the spectral density of the noise current is described by the following equation:

$$I_n = \frac{KI\Delta f}{1 + \left(f/f_c\right)^2},\tag{3.43}$$

where, K is the constant depending on the electronic element type, f_c is the corner frequency, and I is the DC current [23].

Explosive noise is caused by defects in the network, usually metal impurities, or by the incorrect detector electrical contact technology. Emerging pulses are attributed to an impact ionisation of neutral admixtures caused by high-energy electrons. The electric field value in the detector with optimal performance is smaller than the impact ionisation critical field. Improved technology minimises this effect. Usually, the explosive noise depends on the bias direction.

The influence of these noises on the detection system output signal can be reduced by using appropriate signal processing circuits and algorithms. Detailed information on this subject can be found in works [24, 25].

PROBLEMS

Example 3.1

If a photodiode bandwidth is of 1 MHz, what should be the bandwidth so that the noise is reduced 10 times?

Example 3.2

If a noise of 2 μV is observed in a bandwidth of 1 MHz, calculate the average noise voltage spectral density.

Example 3.3

Calculate the RMS value of the thermal (Johnson) noise voltage and the thermal noise current of a 100-kΩ resistor at 300 K in a bandwidth of 1 MHz.

Example 3.4

Determine the output noise voltage density produced by the load resistance $R_L = R_d = 1$ kΩ (see Figure). Assume, that the detector is noiseless.

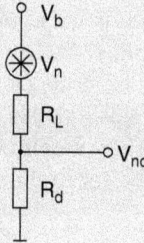

Example 3.5

If a detector has a noise voltage density of 10 μV and a responsivity of 10^7 V/W, calculate *NEP*.

Example 3.6

A detector with an area of $A = 100 \times 10^{-6}$ cm² and a detectivity of $D^* = 5 \times 10^{10}$ Jones is illuminated with an irradiance of $E_e = 0.25$ mW/cm². Calculate the signal-to-noise ratio at the output of the detector that has a 250-kHz bandwidth.

Example 3.7

An InGaAs p-i-n photodiode (G10899-02 type) has the following parameters: responsivity R_v = 0.80 A/W at λ_p = 1550 nm, dark current I_d = 1 nA, and a bandwidth of 20 MHz. Radiation with a power of 300 nW falls on the detector surface. Calculate the mean-square shot noise current and the mean-square dark noise current.

Example 3.8

Consider an ideal Si photodiode ($\eta = 1$, $R_d = \infty$, $I_d = 0$). Calculate the minimum optical power required for $SNR = 1$ at 900 nm with a bandwidth of 1 MHz. What is the corresponding photocurrent?

Example 3.9

Calculate the detector NEP at the wavelength $\lambda_1 = 0.7$ µm, if the $NEP_{min}(\lambda_2 = 0.9$ µm) is 0.01 pW/Hz$^{1/2}$. The responsivity at λ_1 and λ_2 are R_i ($\lambda_1 = 0.7$ µm) = 0.4 A/W and $R_{imax}(\lambda_2 = 0.9$ µm) = 0.6 A/W, respectively.

Example 3.10

Calculate the minimum detectable power for data from Example 3.9 if the bandwidth Δf is 1 MHz.

REFERENCES

1. M.J. Buckingham, *Noise in Electronic Devices and Systems*, John Wiley, New York, 1983.
2. C.D. Motchenbacher and J.A. Connelly, *Low-Noise Electronic System Design*, John Wiley, New York, 1995.
3. A. Van der Ziel, *Noise in Measurements*, John Wiley, New York, 1976.
4. R.W. Boyd, *Radiometry and the Detection of Optical Radiation*, John Wiley, New York, 1993.
5. C.D. Motchenbacher and F.C. Fitchen, *Low-Noise Electronic Design*, John Wiley, New York, 1973.
6. J.S. Bendat and A.G. Pierson, *Random Data Analysis and Measurement Procedures*, John Wiley, New Jersey, 2000.
7. R.G. Rieke, *Detection of Light: From the Ultraviolet to the Submillimeter*, Cambridge University Press, Cambridge, 1994.
8. C.J. Willers, *Electro-Optical System Analysis and Design. A Radiometry Perspective*, SPIE Press, Bellingham, WA, 2013.
9. B.E.A. Salech and M.C. Teich, *Fundamentals of Photonics*, 3rd edition, John Wiley, 2019.
10. P.W. Kruse, "The photon detector process", in *Optical and Infrared Detectors*, pp. 5–69, edited by R.J. Keyes, Springer, Berlin, 1980.
11. H. Nyquist, "Thermal agitation of electric charge in conductors", *Physical Review* 32(1), 110–113 (1928).
12. A. Van der Ziel, *Fluctuation Phenomena in Semiconductors*. Butterworths, London, 1959.
13. D. Long, "On generation-recombination noise in infrared detector materials", *Infrared. Phys.* 7, 169–170 (1967).
14. N. Sclar, "Properties of doped silicon and germanium infrared detectors", *Prog. Quant. Electron.* 9, 149–257 (1984).
15. F.N. Hooge, "1/f noise sources", *IEEE Trans. Electron Devices* 41(11), 1926–1935 (1994).
16. P. Dutta and P.M. Horn, "Low-frequency fluctuation in solids: 1/f noise", *Rev. Mod. Phys.* 53(3), 497–516 (1981).
17. F.N. Hooge, "1/f noise is no surface effect", *Phys. Lett.* 29A, 123–140 (1969).
18. M. Kinch, "HDVIP™ FPA technology at DRS", *Proc. SPIE* 4369, 566–578 (2001).
19. A. Kolek, Ł. Ciura, K. Czuba, A. Jasik, J. Jureńczyk, I. Sankowska, and J. Kaniewski, "Noise and detectivity of InAs/GaSb T2SL 4.5 µm IR detectors", *Proc. SPIE* 10404, 10404-1–10 (2017).

20. P.W. Kruse, L.D. McGlauchlin, and R.B. McQuistan, *Elements of Infrared Technology*, John Wiley, New York, 1962.
21. A. Smith, F.E. Jones, and R.P. Chasmar, *The Detection and Measurement of Infrared Radiation*, Clarendon, Oxford, 1968.
22. *Managing Noise in the Signal Chain, Part 1: Annoying Semiconductor Noise, Preventable or Inescapable*, www.maximintegrated.com/en/design/technical-documents/tutorials/5/5664.html.
23. R.I. Perez, *Design of Medical Electronic Devices*, Academic Press, San Diego, 2002.
24. Z. Bielecki and M. Brudnowski, "Method of popcorn-noise reduction", *Opto-Electron. Rev.* 11(1), 45–50 (2003).
25. *A Review of Popcorn Noise and Smart Filtering. Application note* (ASN-AN022), 2012. www.advsolned.com/downloads/ASN-AN022.pdf.

4 Fundamentals of Optical Detection

This chapter discusses the fundamental limitations to optical detector performance imposed by the statistical nature of the generation and recombination processes and radiometric considerations. We will try to establish the ultimate theoretical sensitivity limit that can be expected for a detector operating at a given temperature. The models presented here are applicable to any of the detector classes described in next six chapters (Chapters 5 to 10). The main emphasis is put on the methodology, rather than on the detail description. This chapter clarifies and summarises principles of detector technology and combines numerous engineering disciplines necessary for the development of an optical system. This chapter also describes detection mechanisms in most widely used thermal and photon detectors and analysis of the fundamental performance limits to different types of detectors.

4.1 INTRODUCTION

We are not always aware of the fact that the detection of optical signals is inseparable from human life. The visible range of optical radiation is defined by the human eye. At a certain stage of evolutionary development, humans consciously began to expand the range of their ability to communicate over longer distances by using optical signals. The reception of these signals has been in place since the time when light was used to transmit information. Ancient Greeks used mirrors to reflect the sun's rays. The Romans and American Indians used smoke to send signals. The basic detecting element of these primitive means of transmission remained the human eye, while the appropriate signal processing took place in the human brain in a more or less conscious manner. This mode of transmission was slow, the range was limited and there was a high probability of error.

The telegraph and telephone are both wire-based electrical systems. The first working telegraph was built by the English inventor Francis Ronalds in 1816. The telegraph was a very successful communication system for about thirty years before the discovery of the telephone. However, the telegraph was basically limited to receiving and sending one message at a time. The telephone is one invention that changed the world and opened a wide world of communication. It was invented by A.G. Bell in 1876 – he was the first person to register the invention at the patent office. His competitor Elisha Gray registered a similar patent just a few hours after he did. Today, Bell's name is synonymous with the telephone, while Gray is largely forgotten. The very first permanent outdoor telephone wire was completed in 1877. It stretched a distance of just three miles. This was closely followed in the United States by the world's first commercial telephone service.

In 1880 A.G. Bell constructed a light telecommunication system called a photophone. He used sunlight reflected from a thin mirror, vibrating under the influence of his voice, to carry conversations over distance. Modulated sunlight fell into the receiver on a selenium photosensitive cell, which converted the optical signal into electricity. However, this system was not widely used.

DOI: 10.1201/9781003263098-4

The invention of artificial light sources made it possible to build simple optical telecommunication systems, such as flashing signal lamps for ship-to-ship communication, ship-to-shore communication, car directional indicators and so forth. These communication systems had low efficiency of information transmission. Only the invention of the laser in 1960 made it possible to radically increase the link speed. Soon after the invention of the laser, many optical communication systems were developed. Initially, these were systems operating in free space. Their most important feature was the large bandwidth enabling the transfer of large amounts of information. Optical transmission of information requires an optical signal source, a suitable modulation method, a signal transmission method, and a detector to recover the information from the signal. The short wavelength allows light propagation with a very small beam divergence. However, the use of free space in the Earth's atmosphere is limited by such phenomena as scattering and absorption [1]. For the above-mentioned reasons, optical communication in the Earth's atmosphere can only be realised over short distances and in cases where communication interruptions are acceptable. In order to increase the link availability, hybrid systems are used, consisting of a free space optical (FSO) and radio frequency (RF): FSO/RF link [2,3].

Limitations related to interruption of optical communications do not exist in space. The problem, however, is to bring the radiation beam out of the Earth's atmosphere and lead it to relatively small objects in distant space, such as artificial satellites, probes or space stations. Lasers are usually the source of light waves. The first efficient (with low attenuation) optical fibre was developed in 1970 and only since then we have observed dynamic development of fibre telecommunications which, in the last decade of the twentieth century, contributed (among other things) to the worldwide Internet network [4]. In these systems, optical waves are converted into electric current by means of a photodetector. The electrical signal thus obtained is then fed into the signal processing system. In the case of analogue transmission, a signal processor is used to provide amplification and filtering of the signal. In digital systems, the signal processor contains not only amplifiers and filters, but also decision-making systems. The photodetector together with the signal preamplifier is the photoreceiver input stage. Its sensitivity (signal to noise ratio) determines the range of optoelectronic links and the power of transmitters used.

However, optical radiation detection also covers other ranges of electromagnetic radiation, especially infrared and ultraviolet radiation. Successes in the military application of infrared radiation detectors during the Second World War (the Germans first used PbS photoconductive detectors in V-2 rockets) contributed to intensive research and rapid development of detectors. Development of infrared technology, the emergence of new fields such as thermography, laser technology, fibre optics or, more generally, optoelectronics, have made the use of detectors extremely varied and can now be found both in common fire and burglary warning devices, as well as in advanced control systems for industrial equipment.

Military applications, including the adaptation of technology for use in space, are an important field of application that is the main driving force of technological progress. Continuous observation from space makes it possible to detect the launch of any larger rocket as well as to deploy ballistic missiles equipped with nuclear warheads. Thermal imaging devices are installed on Earth's satellites, enabling a synoptic view of the planet, its mineral resources, crops, geography, topography and demographic processes, and it is a view much more insightful than is possible from the surface of the Earth. The highest requirements for infrared detectors are set by thermovision, in which to achieve good image resolution it is necessary to use multielement detectors – large line mosaics and two-dimensional arrays. Precise images of a temperature distribution in the observed objects obtained thanks to these devices are powerful tools for obtaining information and knowledge about these objects. Therefore, these methods are used in almost all fields of industry, research and human activity in general, from military and space technology mentioned above to medicine, construction, heating, energy, electronics and many others.

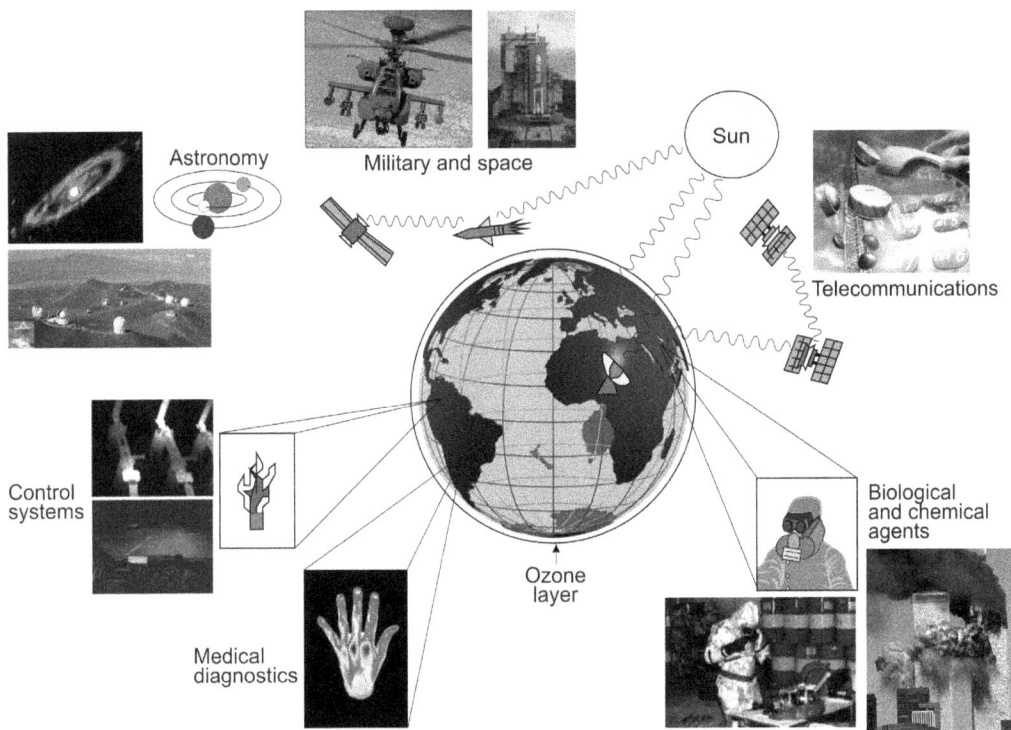

FIGURE 4.1   Examples of applications of electromagnetic radiation detectors.

Ultraviolet detectors are widely used in civil and military applications, including ultraviolet astronomy, high-temperature radiation detectors (e.g., aircraft jet engines), military early warning systems, detection of chemicals and systems installed in space. The ultraviolet spectral range covers the "strategic window" absorption (230–280 nm) of the ozone layer. Detectors that detect ultraviolet radiation against a strong background of visible and infrared radiation are particularly important. For this reason, the technology of detectors with a long-term sensitivity limit close to the edge of the visible spectrum range is being intensively developed; for example, sensor technology with AlGaN ternary alloys.

X-ray and radiation detectors are widely used in medicine, manufacturing industry, astronomy, nuclear industry and research. Examples of industrial applications include measuring the liquids level on filling lines, measuring automobile paint thickness and non-invasive determination of defects in a material structure. Medical applications include commonly used X-rays, computer tomography (CT) images of the heart and dosimetric bone examination.

Figure 4.1 illustrates different areas of an electromagnetic radiation detectors applications.

4.2   CLASSIFICATION OF DETECTORS

Detectors of electromagnetic radiation can be divided into two basic groups: photon detectors and thermal detectors.

In the thermal detector shown schematically in Figure 4.2, the incident radiation is absorbed to change the material temperature, and the resultant change in some physical properties is used to generate an electrical output. The detector is suspended on lags, which are connected to the heat sink. Since radiation can be absorbed in a black surface coating, the spectral response can be very

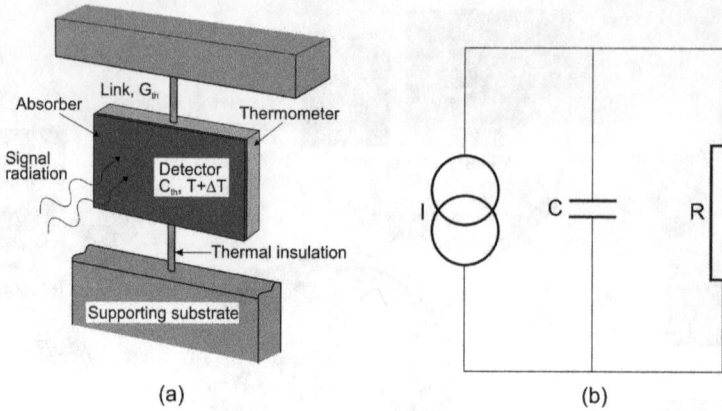

FIGURE 4.2 Thermal detector: (a) scheme of operation and (b) electrical analogue.

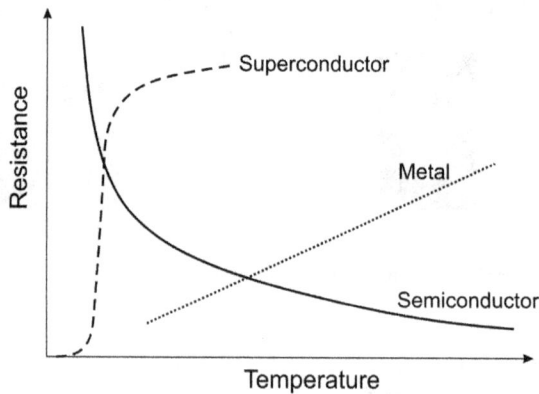

FIGURE 4.3 Temperature dependence of resistance of three bolometer material types.

broad. Attention is directed toward three approaches that have found the greatest utility in infrared technology, namely, bolometers, pyroelectric and thermoelectric effects.

The thermopile is one of the oldest IR detectors, and is a collection of thermocouples connected in series to achieve better temperature sensitivity. In pyroelectric detectors, a change in the internal electrical polarisation is measured whereas, in the case of thermistor bolometers, a change in the electrical resistance is measured. For a long time, thermopiles were slow, insensitive, bulky and costly devices. But with developments in semiconductor technology, thermopiles can be optimised for specific applications. Recently, thanks to conventional complementary metal-oxide semiconductor (CMOS) processes, the thermopile's on-chip circuitry technology has opened the door to mass production.

Usually bolometer is a thin, blackened flake or slab, whose impedance is highly temperature-dependent. Bolometers may be divided into several types. The most commonly used are the metal, the thermistor, and the semiconductor bolometers. A fourth type is the superconducting bolometer. This bolometer operates on a conductivity transition in which the resistance changes dramatically over the transition temperature range. Figure 4.3 shows schematically the temperature dependence of resistance of different types of bolometers.

Many types of thermal detectors are operated in wide spectral range of electromagnetic radiation. The operation principles of thermal detectors are briefly described in Table 4.1.

TABLE 4.1
Thermal Detectors

Detector	Method of operation
Bolometer	Change in electrical conductivity
• Metal	
• Semiconductor	
• Superconductor	
• Ferroelectric	
• Hot electron	
Thermocouple/thermopile	Voltage generation caused by a change in temperature of the junction of two dissimilar materials
Pyroelectric	Changes in spontaneous electrical polarisation
Golay cell	Thermal expansion of a gas
Absorption edge	Optical transmission of a semiconductor
Pyromagnetic	Changes of magnetic properties
Liquid crystal	Changes of optical properties

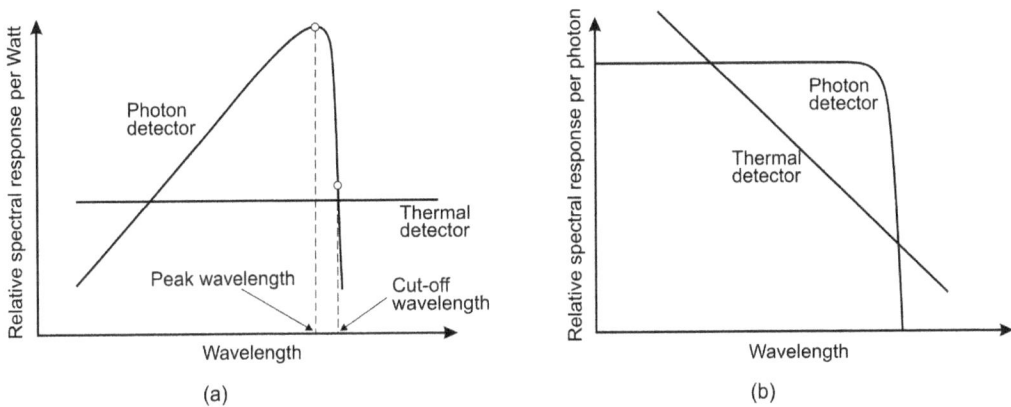

FIGURE 4.4 Relative spectral response for a photon and thermal detector for (a) constant incident radiant power and (b) photon flux, respectively.

The relative response of infrared detectors is plotted as a function of wavelength with either a vertical scale of W^{-1} or $photon^{-1}$ (see Figure 4.4). The signal does not depend upon the photonic nature of the incident radiation. Thus, thermal effects are generally wavelength independent [see Figure 4.4(a)]; the signal depends upon the radiant power (or its rate of change) but not upon its spectral content. In principle, this is not exactly true: it turns out that the layers covering the detector in order to increase the absorption of radiation cause partially selective spectral characteristics of the detector response.

In most cases, thermal detectors work at room temperature. They are characterised by a relatively low sensitivity. Their response rate is also usually low and is of 10^{-3}–10^{-1} s – heating and cooling processes are characterised by high inertia.

Thermal detectors are widely used in low-cost infrared systems that do not require high sensitivity and response rates. As elements with non-selective spectral characteristics, they are often used in spectrometers. Until about 1990, thermal detectors were much less intensively tested compared to photon detectors. The main reason for this was a poorer performance of these detectors: significantly slower response speed and lower sensitivity. However, in the last few decades it has been shown that

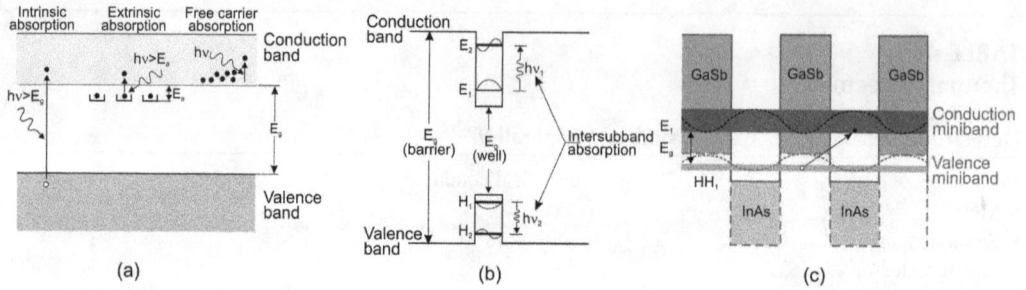

FIGURE 4.5 Fundamental processes of carrier excitation in semiconductor structures: (a) bulk semiconductors, (b) QWs and (c) type-II InAs/GaSb SLs.

a very good thermal image quality can be achieved if large thermal sensor arrays are used, and their speed is sufficient for electronic scanning at a TV frame rate. This fact led to a revolution in a development of cheaper thermal imaging cameras with sensitivity similar to cryogenically cooled (usually to 77 K) cameras containing photon detector arrays. Due to their widespread use, their current global production volume is much larger than that of photon detectors.

However, the development of optical radiation detectors is mainly related to photon detectors made of semiconductor materials. In photon detectors the radiation is absorbed within the material by interaction with electrons either bound to lattice atoms or to impurity atoms or with free electrons. The observed electrical output signal results from the changed electronic energy distribution. The fundamental optical excitation processes in semiconductors are illustrated in Figure 4.5(a) [5]. In quantum wells [Figure 4.5(b)] the intersubband absorption takes place between the energy levels of a quantum well associated with the conduction band (n-doped) or valence band (p-doped). In the case of type-II InAs/GaSb superlattice [Figure 4.5(c)], the superlattice bandgap is determined by the energy difference between the electron miniband E_1 and the first heavy-hole state HH_1 at the Brillouin zone centre. A consequence of the type-II band alignment is spatial separation of electrons and holes.

The photon detectors show a selective wavelength dependence of response per unit incident radiation power. Their response is proportional to the rate of arrival photons as the energy per photon is inversely proportional to wavelength. In consequence, the spectral response increases linearly with increasing wavelength [see Figure 4.4(a)], until the cut-off wavelength is reached, which is determined by the detector material. The cut-off wavelength is usually specified as the long wavelength point at which the detector responsivity falls to 50 per cent of the peak responsivity. Thermal detectors tend to be spectrally flat in the first case (their response is proportional to the energy absorbed), thus they exhibit a flat spectral response [see Figure 4.4(a)], while photon detectors are generally flat in the second case [see Figure 4.4(b)].

Photon detectors exhibit both good signal-to-noise performance and a very fast response. But to achieve this, the photon IR detectors may require cryogenic cooling. This is necessary to prevent the thermal generation of charge carriers. The thermal transitions compete with the optical ones, making non-cooled devices very noisy.

Depending on the nature of the interaction, the class of photon detectors is further sub-divided into different types. Their comparison is given in Table 4.2. The most important are intrinsic detectors, extrinsic detectors, photoemissive detectors (Schottky barriers) and quantum well and superlattice detectors [5]. Examples of spectral characteristics of thermal and photon detectors in a wide spectral range are shown in Figures 4.6 and 4.7.

In general, photon detectors, compared to thermal detectors, are characterised by higher sensitivity and faster response rates. Typically, infrared detectors with a long-term sensitivity limit above 3 μm are normally cooled to below 300 K in order to reduce the speed of thermal processes of

TABLE 4.2
Photon Detectors

Type		Transition	Electrical output	Examples
Intrinsic		Interband	Photoconductive	Si, GaN, InSb, HgCdTe
			Photovoltaic	Si, InGaAs, InSb, HgCdTe
			Capacitance	Si, InSb, HgCdTe
			PEM	InSb, HgCdTe
Extrinsic		Impurity to band	Photoconductive	Si:As, Si:In, Si:Ga, Ge:Cu, Ge:Hg
Free carriers		Intraband	Photoemissive	GaAs/CsO, PtSi, Pt_2Si, IrSi
Quantum wells	Type I	Intersubband	Photoconductive	GaAs/AlGaAs, InGaAs/AlGaAs
	Type II	Miniband to miniband transition	Photoconductive Photovoltaic	InAs/GaSb, InAs/InAsSb
	Type III	Miniband to miniband transition	Photovoltaic	HgTe/CdTe
Quantum dots		Transition in "artificial atoms"	Photoconductive	InAs/GaAs, InGaAs/InGaP, Ge/Si

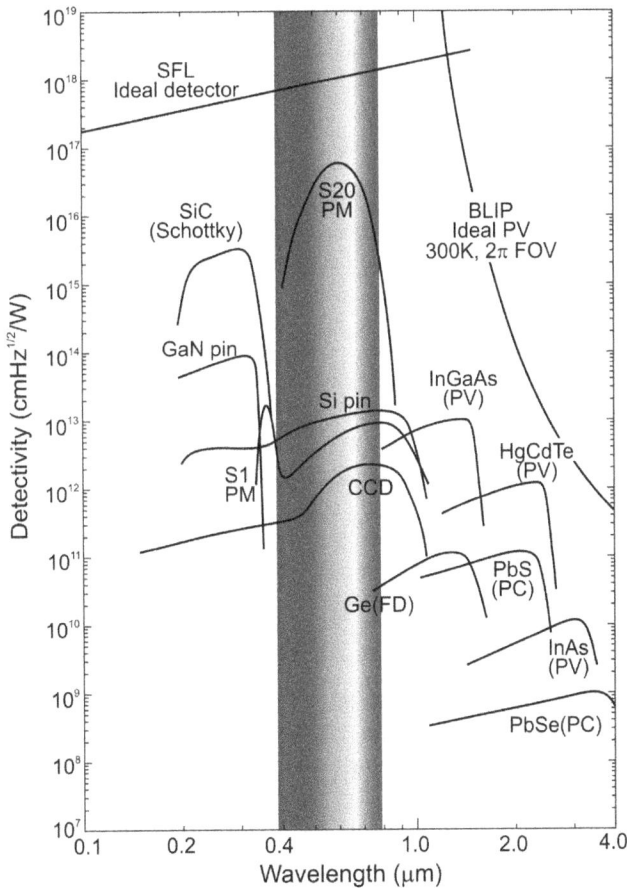

FIGURE 4.6 Detectivity versus wavelength values of 0.1–4 μm photodetectors. PC indicates the photoconductive detector; PV – the photovoltaic detector, and PM indicates the photomultiplier. SFL is the signal fluctuation limit.

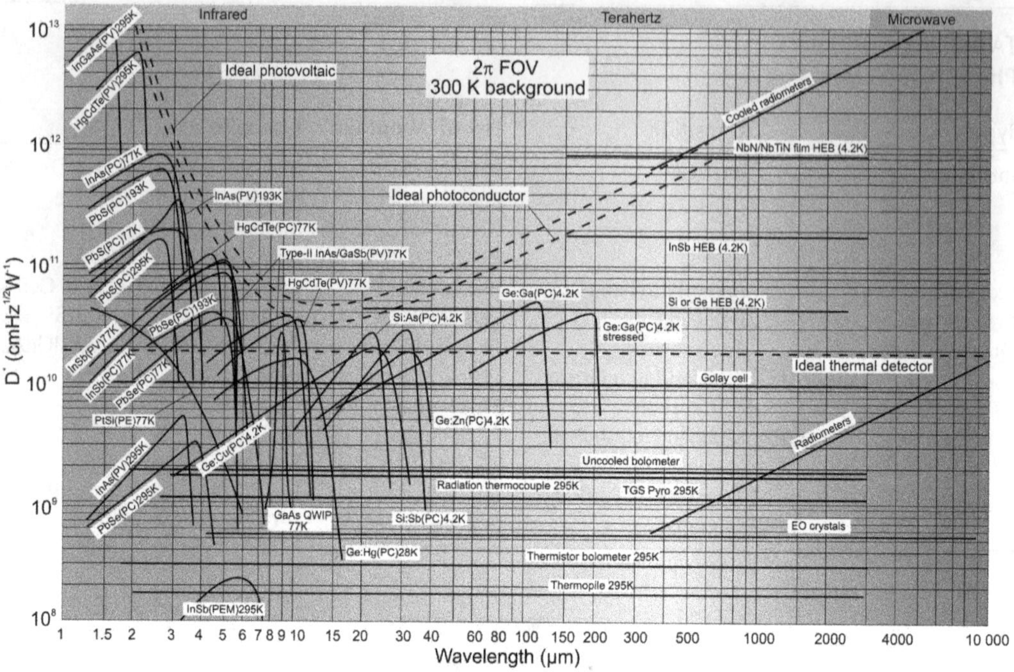

FIGURE 4.7 Comparison of the D^* of various available detectors when operated at the indicated temperature. Chopping frequency is 1000 Hz for all detectors except the thermopile (10 Hz), thermocouple (10 Hz), thermistor bolometer (10 Hz), Golay cell (10 Hz), and pyroelectric detector (10 Hz). Each detector is assumed to view a hemispherical surrounding at a temperature of 300 K. Theoretical curves for the background-limited D^* (dashed lines) for ideal photovoltaic and photoconductive detectors and thermal detectors are also shown. PC: photoconductive detector, PV: photovoltaic detector, PEM: photoelectromagnetic detector, and HEB: hot electron bolometer (after Reference 6).

carrier's excitation. The general trend is illustrated in Figure 4.8 for seven high-performance detector materials suitable for low-background applications: Si, InGaAs, InSb, T2SL, HgCdTe photodiodes, Si:As BIB detectors and extrinsic Ge:Ga unstressed and stressed detectors. The consequence of the need for cooling is the greater mass of the detector set (including the cooling system), higher price, inconvenience in use, and so forth.

In the literature there are many monographs devoted to the theory and technology of optical radiation detectors, working in different ranges of electromagnetic spectrum; for example, References [7–13].

4.3 PHYSICAL BASICS OF THERMAL DETECTORS OPERATION

Analysing the operation of a thermal detector, we will first determine the detector temperature increase due to the incident radiation absorption. Then, we will find a relationship between the temperature increase and the change in a certain property of the detector active substance determining the signal. The first stage of calculations is common for different types of thermal detectors, while the second stage is differentiated depending on the detector type and is presented in further points while discussing different types of detectors.

The idea of the thermal detector is simple. The incident radiation raises the detector temperature while the signal is the result of a change in a certain property dependent on temperature, such as thermoelectric force, resistance or electrical capacity. Figure 4.2 shows the idea of the thermal sensor operation.

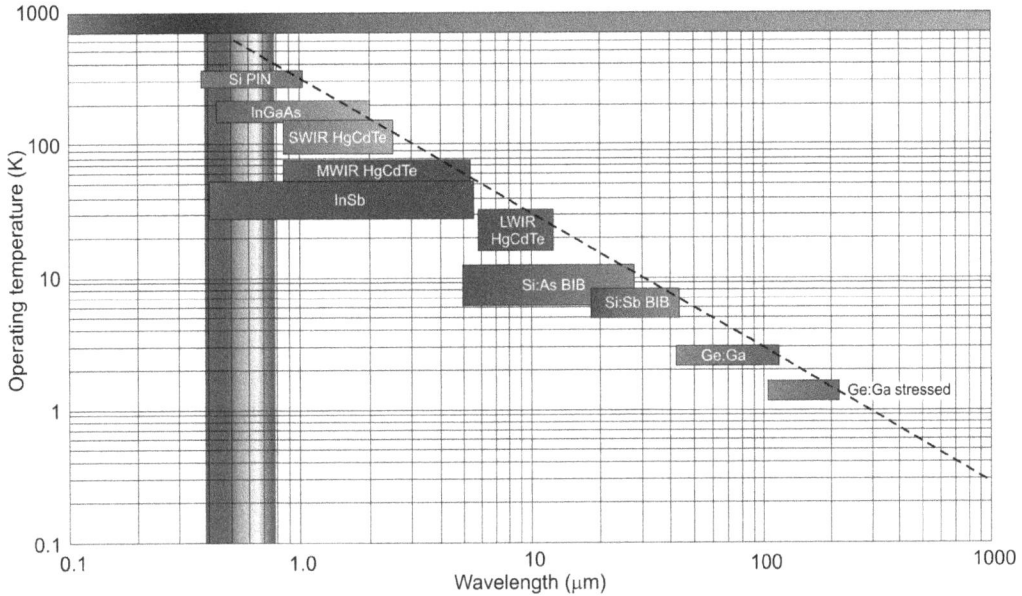

FIGURE 4.8 Operating temperatures of photon detectors. The dashed line indicates the trend toward a lower operating temperature for a longer wavelength detection.

TABLE 4.3
Thermal-electric Analogies

Thermal		Thermal	
Value	**Unit**	**Value**	**Unit**
Heat energy	J	Charge	C
Heat flow	W	Current	A
Temperature	K	Voltage	V
Thermal impedance	K/W	Impedance	Ω
Heat capacitance	J/K	Capacitance	F

The detector is characterised by the thermal capacity C_{th} coupled with the thermal conductivity G_{th}, depending on a method of connecting the detector with the environment. When radiation does not fall on the detector, the average temperature of the detector is T, although this temperature fluctuates around this value. When the radiation is absorbed by the detector, the temperature increase is determined by solving the heat balance equation [7, 13]:

$$C_{th}\frac{d\Delta T}{dt} + G_{th}\Delta T = \varepsilon\Phi, \qquad (4.1)$$

where ΔT is the temperature difference between the detector and the environment caused by the signal Φ, and ε is the emissivity of the detector.

The thermal detector has its own electrical circuit, as shown in Figure 4.2(b). Analogies between thermal and electrical quantities are specified in Table 4.3.

Assuming the radiant power to be a periodic function:

$$\Phi = \Phi_o e^{i\omega t}, \tag{4.2}$$

where Φ_o is the amplitude of sinusoidal radiation, the solution of a differential heat radiation is the following:

$$\Delta T = \Delta T_o e^{-(G_{th}/C_{th})\omega t} + \frac{\varepsilon\Phi_o e^{i\omega t}}{G_{th} + i\omega C_{th}}. \tag{4.3}$$

The first term is the transient part and, as time increases, this term exponentially decreases to zero, so it can be dropped with no loss of generality for the change in temperature. Therefore, the change in temperature of any thermal detector due to incident radiative flux is as follows:

$$\Delta T = \frac{\varepsilon\Phi_o}{\left(G_{th}^2 + \omega^2 C_{th}^2\right)^{1/2}}. \tag{4.4}$$

Eq. (4.4) illustrates several important features of the thermal detector. In order to achieve the highest possible ΔT value, the thermal capacity of the detector C_{th} and its thermal coupling with the environment G_{th} want to be as small as possible. The detector should be constructed in such a way as to isolate it from the environment as much as possible (eliminate any additional thermal connection between the detector and the environment) and reduce the detector weight (dimensions).

Eq. (4.4) shows that as ω is increased, the term $\omega^2 C_{th}^2$ will eventually exceed G_{th}^2 and then ΔT will fall inversely as ω. A characteristic thermal response time for the detector can, therefore, be defined as

$$\tau_{th} = \frac{C_{th}}{G_{th}} = C_{th} R_{th}, \tag{4.5}$$

where $R_{th} = 1/G_{th}$ is the thermal resistance. Then, Eq. (4.4) can be written as:

$$\Delta T = \frac{\varepsilon\Phi_o R_{th}}{\left(1 + \omega^2 \tau_{th}^2\right)^{1/2}}. \tag{4.6}$$

The typical value of a thermal time constant is several milliseconds. This is much longer than a typical photon time constant of a photon detector. Note that for a thermal detector there is a compromise between the sensitivity, ΔT, and the time constant (frequency response). If one wants a high sensitivity, then a low-frequency response is forced upon the detector.

For further discussion, we introduce the coefficient K, which reflects how well the temperature changes translate into the detector electrical output voltage [14]:

$$K = \frac{\Delta V}{\Delta T}. \tag{4.7}$$

Then, the corresponding RMS voltage signal due to the temperature changes ΔT is as follows:

$$\Delta V = K\Delta T = \frac{K\varepsilon\Phi_o R_{th}}{\left(1+\omega^2\tau_{th}^2\right)^{1/2}}. \tag{4.8}$$

The detector voltage responsivity R_v is the ratio of the output signal voltage ΔV to the input radiation power and is given by

$$R_v = \frac{K\varepsilon R_{th}}{\left(1+\omega^2\tau_{th}^2\right)^{1/2}}. \tag{4.9}$$

As the last expression shows, the low-frequency voltage responsivity ($\omega<<1/\tau_{th}$) is proportional to the thermal resistance and does not depend on the heat capacitance. The opposite is true for high frequencies ($\omega>>1/\tau_{th}$). In this case, R_v is not dependent on R_{th} and is inversely proportional to the heat capacitance.

As stated previously, the thermal conductance (thermal resistance) from the detector to the outside world should be small (high). The smallest possible thermal conductance would occur when the detector is completely isolated from the environment under vacuum with only a radiative heat exchange between it and its heat-sink enclosure. Such an ideal model can give us the ultimate performance limit of a thermal detector. This limiting value can be estimated from the Stefan-Boltzmann total radiation law.

If the detector temperature is increased by a small amount dT, the flux radiated is increased by $4A\varepsilon\sigma T^3 dT$. Hence, the radiative component of the thermal conductance is as follows:

$$G_R = \frac{1}{\left(R_{th}\right)_R} = \frac{d}{dT}\left(A\varepsilon\sigma T^4\right) = 4A\varepsilon\sigma T^3. \tag{4.10}$$

In this case,

$$R_v = \frac{K}{4\sigma T^3 A\left(1+\omega^2\tau_{th}^2\right)^{1/2}}. \tag{4.11}$$

When the detector is in thermal equilibrium with the heat sink, the fluctuation in the power flowing through the thermal conductance into the detector is the following:

$$\Delta P_{th} = \left(4kT^2G\right)^{1/2}, \tag{4.12}$$

which will be the smallest when G assumes its minimum value (i.e., G_R). Then, ΔP_{th} will be a minimum and its value gives the minimum detectable power for an ideal thermal detector (detector is perfectly isolated from the environment). Then, we say that ΔP_{th} is equal to the noise equivalent power, *NEP*:

$$\Delta P_{th} = \varepsilon NEP = \left(16A\varepsilon\sigma kT^5\right)^{1/2}, \tag{4.13}$$

or

$$NEP = \left(\frac{16A\sigma kT^5}{\varepsilon} \right)^{1/2}. \tag{4.14}$$

If all the incident radiation is absorbed by the detector, $\varepsilon = 1$, and then,

$$NEP = \left(16A\sigma kT^5 \right)^{1/2} = 5.0 \times 10^{-11} \text{ W}, \tag{4.15}$$

for $A = 1$ cm^2, $T = 290$ K, and $\Delta f = 1$ Hz.

4.3.1   DETECTIVITY AND FUNDAMENTAL LIMITS

The most important parameters of thermal detectors include noise-equivalent power, sensitivity, detectivity and response speed. These parameters are defined in Chapter 2. To determine the detector detectivity, the noise level must be known. In thermal detectors, there are Johnson noise, noise due to fluctuations in detector temperature and background temperature, and $1/f$ noise. The mean square of a total noise voltage is the following:

$$V_n^2 = V_J^2 + V_{th}^2 + V_{1/f}^2. \tag{4.16}$$

According to Eqs. (3.28), (3.40), (4.9) and (4.16), the detectivity of thermal detectors is given by

$$D^* = \frac{K\varepsilon R_{th} A^{1/2}}{\left(1 + \omega^2 \tau_{th}^2 \right)^{1/2} \left(\frac{4kT_d^2 K^2 R_{th}}{1 + \omega^2 \tau_{th}^2} + 4kTR + V_{1/f}^2 \right)^{1/2}}. \tag{4.17}$$

The first factor in the denominator of Eq. (4.17) determines the thermal detector frequency characteristics, while the second factor is the resultant noise which is the sum of temperature noise, thermal noise and $1/f$ noise.

The fundamental limit to sensitivity of any thermal detector is set by a temperature fluctuation noise. Under this condition at low frequencies ($\omega \ll 1/\tau_{th}$), from Eq. (4.17) we obtain

$$D_{th}^* = \left(\frac{\varepsilon^2 A}{4kT_d^2 G_{th}} \right)^{1/2}. \tag{4.18}$$

It is assumed here that ε is independent of a wavelength, so that the spectral detectivity and blackbody detectivity values are identical.

Figure 4.9(a) shows detectivity dependence on temperature, while Figure 4.9(b) shows the detectivity dependence on thermal conductance for three values of the photosensitive areas [15]. It is clearly shown that the improved performance of thermal detectors can be achieved by decreasing the temperature of the detector and increasing thermal isolation between the detector and its surroundings.

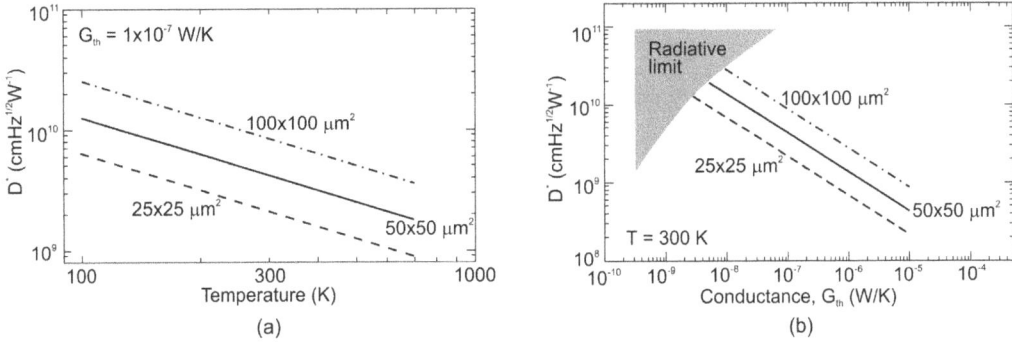

FIGURE 4.9 Temperature fluctuation noise limited detectivity for thermal infrared detectors of different areas plotted (a) as a function of the detector temperature and (b) as a function of the total thermal conductance between the detector and its surroundings (after Reference 15).

If a radiant power exchange is a dominant heat exchange mechanism between the detector temperature T_d and the background temperature T_B, then, the basic type of noise is the noise caused by fluctuations in the radiation exchange. The square value of this noise is the following [7,9]:

$$V_b^2 = \frac{8k\varepsilon\sigma A\left(T_d^2 + T_B^2\right)}{1 + \omega^2 \tau_{th}^2} K^2 R_{th}^2. \tag{4.19}$$

This equation is valid for the detector FOV = 2π.

Using the definition of detectivity (2.11) and Eq. (4.19), we obtain:

$$D_b^* = \left[\frac{\varepsilon}{8k\sigma\left(T_d^5 + T_B^5\right)}\right]^{1/2}. \tag{4.20}$$

As you can see from this equation, D_b^* does not depend on the detector area.

Very frequently the background temperature, T_B, is equal to room temperature. The detectivity determined by Eq. (4.20) should be called detectivity limited by the radiation noise because thermal detectors are sensitive to the power of radiation and not to photons. However, in the literature it is accepted to define it as the photon noise-limited detectivity.

Figure 4.10 shows the photon noise-limited detectivity for an ideal thermal detector operating at different temperatures, as a function of the background temperature. We see that the highest possible D^* for a thermal detector operating at room temperature and viewing a background at room temperature is of 1.98×10^{10} cmHz$^{1/2}$/W [7]. The next figure (Figure 4.11) shows the background-limited detectivity as a function of the sensor temperature, for ideal thermal detector operation.

Photon detectors have higher detectivity compared to thermal detectors because their spectral characteristics are significantly narrowed (Figure 4.7) compared to the spectral characteristics of thermal detectors (and, thus, the photon noise is lower). Spectral characteristics of the detector are limited by means of cooled filters.

In practice, the detectivity achieved by a given detector differs significantly from the values theoretically predicted and presented in Figures 4.10 and 4.11. Even in the absence of other sources of noise, the performance of a radiation noise-limited detector will be worse than that of an ideal

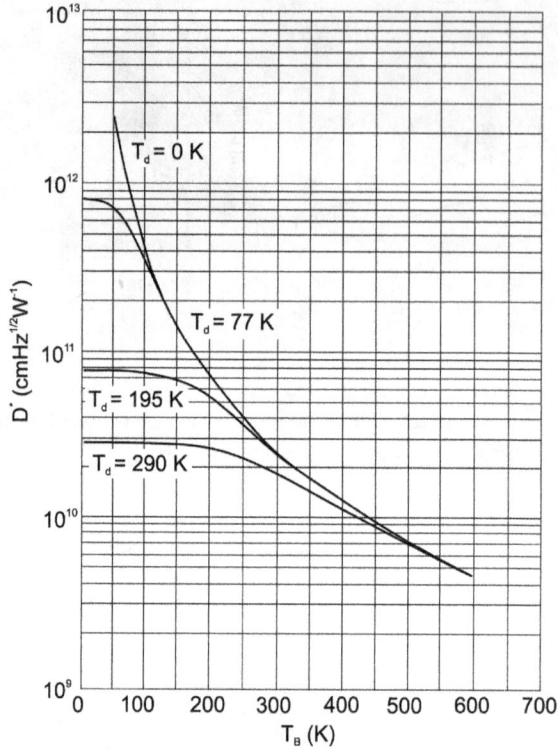

FIGURE 4.10 Temperature fluctuation noise-limited detectivity of thermal detectors as a function of detector temperatures T_d and background temperature T_B for 2π FOV and $\varepsilon = 1$.

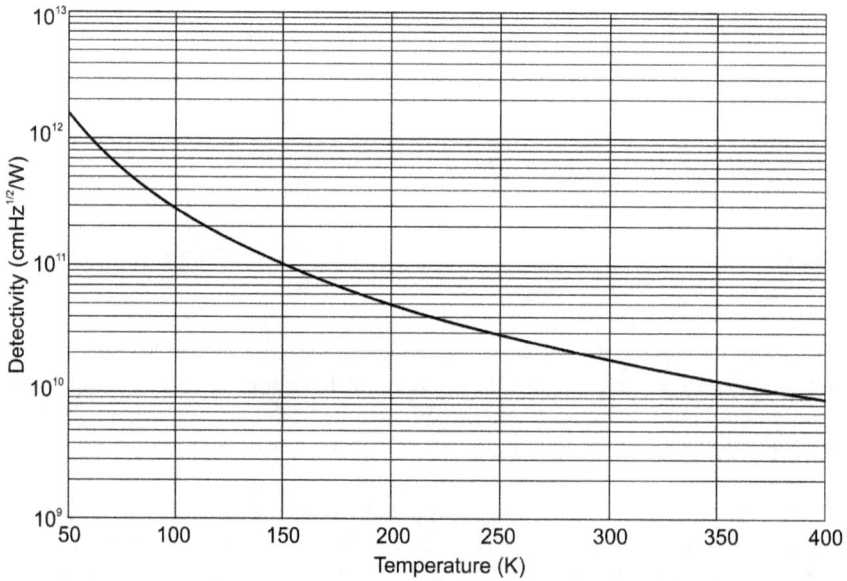

FIGURE 4.11 BLIP detectivity of a thermal detector as a function of the sensor temperature for 2π (2pi) FOV and $\varepsilon = 1$.

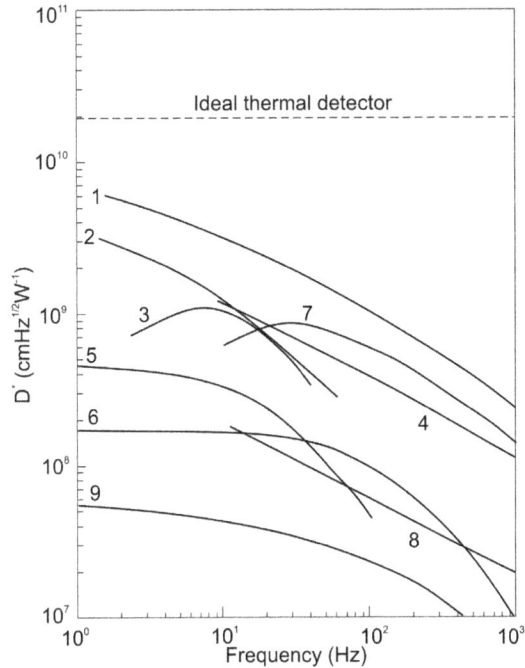

FIGURE 4.12 Performance of uncooled thermal detectors: (1) alaine-doped triglycine sulfate (TGS) pyroelectric detector (A = 1.5 × 1.5 mm²); (2) spectroscopic thermopile (A = 0.4 mm², τ_{th} = 40 ms); (3) Golay cell; (4) TGS pyroelectric detector in a ruggedised encapsulation (0.5 × 0.5 mm²); (5) Sb–Bi evaporated film thermopile (A = 0.12 × 0.12 mm², τ_{th} = 13 ms); (6) immersed thermistor (A = 0.1 × 0.1 mm², τ_{th} = 2 ms); (7) LiTaO$_3$ pyroelectric detector; (8) Plessey lead zirconate titanate (PZT) ceramic pyroelectric detector; and (9) thin film bolometer (after Reference 16).

detector by the factor $\varepsilon^{1/2}$ [see Eq. (4.20)]. Further performance degradation will arise from the following:

- encapsulation of detector (reflection and absorption losses at the window);
- effects of excess thermal conductance (influence of electrical contacts, conduction through the supports;
- influence of any gas – conduction and convection; and
- additional noise sources.

Figure 4.12 shows the performance of a number of thermal detectors operating at room temperature. Typical values of detectivities of thermal detectors at 10 Hz change in the range from 10^8 to 10^9 cmHz$^{1/2}$/W.

The most important thermal detectors are thermopiles, bolometers and pyroelectric detectors. We briefly discuss them below, and will describe them in more detail in Chapter 5.

4.3.2 THERMOPILES

The thermocouple was discovered in 1826 by German physicist J. Seebeck. He noticed a current flow in a closed electrical circuit consisting of two different metals if their contact points are at different temperatures (Figure 4.13). In 1833, Melloni constructed the first thermopiles (a system of serially connected thermocouples) in order to achieve better temperature sensitivity. Nowadays, usually the number of thermocouples ranges from 20 to 120.

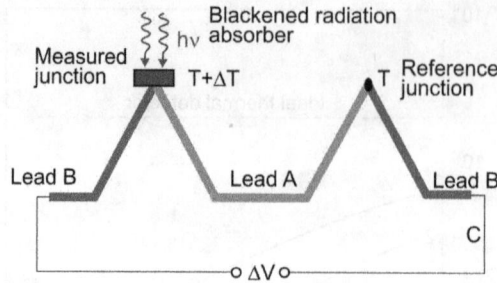

FIGURE 4.13   Thermocouple.

Two other phenomena are connected with a thermoelectric phenomenon. In 1834, C.A. Peltier found that when an electric current flows through a contact of two different metals, depending on the current flow direction, the junction heats up or cools down (not taking into account the Joule heat generated in each conductor). The physical cause of the Peltier phenomenon is a different concentration of free electrons on both sides of the metal contact. In 1854, W. Thomson also noticed that in a single homogeneous conductor along the length of which there is a certain temperature gradient, heat is emitted or absorbed depending on the type of material and the current flow direction. The reason for this phenomenon is a different concentration of free electrons in the conductor, which is determined by the temperature gradient.

Let us consider the operation of the thermocouple shown in Figure 4.13. It is made of two different materials, A and B, connected by the conductor C. The measuring junction is connected to the photosensitive (active) surface on which the radiation falls. This surface is usually a thin absorbent layer fixed directly to the junction.

Under the absorbed radiation influence, the temperature of the active surface increases from T to $T + \Delta T$, causing the joint to heat up. The temperature difference of the connectors results in an electromotive force, the value of which is directly proportional to the temperature difference of these junctions:

$$\Delta V = \alpha_s \Delta T, \tag{4.21}$$

where α_s is the effective Seebeck coefficient expressed in $\mu V/K$. Its value is equal to the difference in Seebeck's coefficients of materials A and B. Thus,

$$\Delta V = \alpha_s \Delta T = \left(\alpha_A - \alpha_B \right) \Delta T. \tag{4.22}$$

Taking into account Eqs. (4.7) and (4.22) we notice that $K = \alpha_s$. Consequently, Eq. (4.9) takes the form of

$$R_v = \frac{\alpha_s \varepsilon R_{th}}{\left(1 + \omega^2 \tau_{th}^2 \right)^{1/2}}. \tag{4.23}$$

At very low frequencies, $\omega^2 \tau^2 tau_{th} \ll 1$, and, then,

$$R_v = \frac{\alpha_s \varepsilon}{G_{th}}. \tag{4.24}$$

It should be noted that the Peltier effect can cause considerable asymmetry in the thermoelectric effect. This phenomenon is reversible, since the absorption and release of heat depend on the current flow direction. There is a close relationship between the Peltier coefficient (which defines the ratio of absorbed heat to electric current) and the Seebeck coefficient:

$$\Pi = \alpha_s T. \tag{4.25}$$

A common value for the Peltier coefficient is 100–300 mV.

Thermocouples are made as single elements, with double or quadruple structures, as 16 or 32 element lines and as mosaics with a small number of elements (e.g., 8×8). These instruments work at room temperature, have a constant sensitivity value as a function of wavelength, no modulation of incident radiation is required; they are durable, cheap and reliable in operation.

4.3.3 BOLOMETERS

Another type of thermal detector is the bolometer. This is a resistor with a very small thermal capacity and a large temperature coefficient so that the absorbed radiation produces larger changes in resistance. However, unlike the photoresistor, there is no direct interaction of photons with electrons – the incident radiation interacts with the crystal lattice of the resistor. In the bolometer's so-called "hot carriers", the radiation is absorbed directly by electrons.

The bolometer model is shown in Figure 4.14. It consists of two integrated parts: a radiation absorber and a temperature-sensitive element (resistor). The absorber is connected to the "surroundings" by means of a thermal conductivity of the lowest possible value. As a result of the absorbed radiation, it is heated, as a result of which the resistance R_d changes, causing a modulation of intensity of the current flowing in the supply circuit.

In contrast to a thermocouple, the bolometer is biased from a DC voltage source. In practice, systems with voltage divider [Figure 4.15(a)] and bridge systems [Figure 4.15(b)] are used. They provide an accurately controlled bias current through the detector and monitoring the output voltage.

The bridge circuit includes two detectors positioned in such a way that one of them is shielded, while the other is illuminated by a useful signal and background radiation. If the radiation does not fall on the detector, the bridge is in balance, and there is no current flowing through the resistor R_2. Illumination of the detector causes a reduction of its resistance and, therefore, an imbalance of the bridge. The change of the bolometer resistance caused by the increase of its temperature is determined by the following equation:

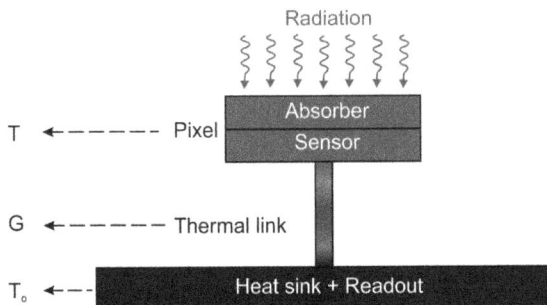

FIGURE 4.14 Bolometer model.

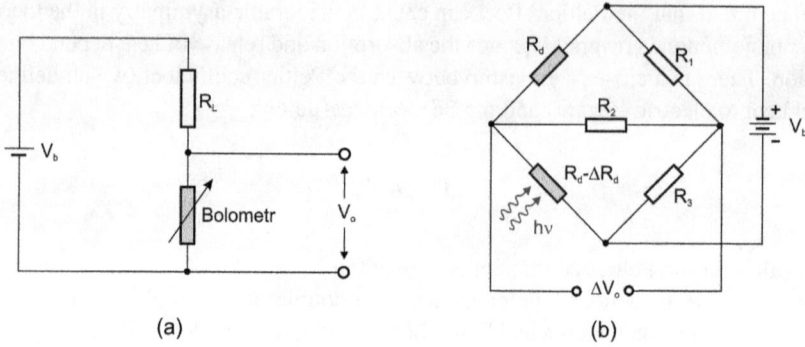

FIGURE 4.15 Bolometer circuits: (a) voltage divider and (b) basic Wheatstone bolometer bridge.

$$\Delta R_d = \frac{dR_d}{dT_d} \Delta T_d, \tag{4.26}$$

where R_d is the bolometer resistance, and ΔT_d is the bolometer temperature increase.

Current flows through the R_2 resistor causing a voltage drop, ΔU_o:

$$\Delta U_0 = \frac{I_1 \Delta R_d R_2}{2R_2 + R_1 + R_3}, \tag{4.27}$$

where I_1 is the current flowing through the bolometer in a bridge circuit in a steady state. The use of the second detector enables compensation of resistance changes due to ambient temperature fluctuations.

The relative temperature coefficient of resistance (TCR) is defined as

$$a = \frac{1}{R_d} \frac{dR_d}{dT_d}, \tag{4.28}$$

and a voltage change of the constant current-biased (I) bolometer is the following:

$$\Delta V = I \Delta R_d = IR_d a \Delta T. \tag{4.29}$$

Thus, in this case, $K = IR_d a$ [see Eq. (4.9)] and the voltage responsivity is as follows:

$$R_v = \frac{IR_d a R_{th} \varepsilon}{\left(1 + \omega^2 \tau_{th}^2\right)^{1/2}}. \tag{4.30}$$

Expressions for voltage responsivity of the bolometer and the thermocouple are similar with α_s replaced by $IR_d a$. The responsivity is proportional to the thermal resistance. The maximum bias current is limited by the maximum allowed element temperature T_{max}. Therefore,

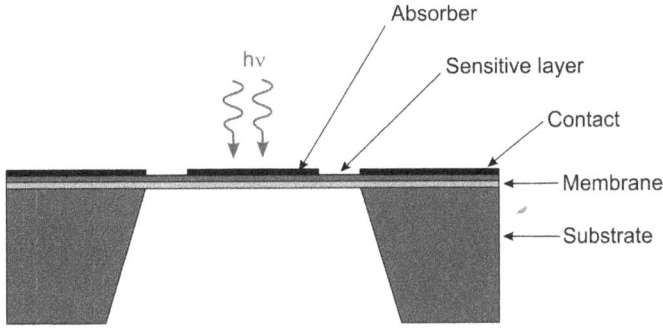

FIGURE 4.16   Schematic cross section of a thin-film bolometer.

$$I^2 R_d = G_{th}\left(T_{max} - T\right),$$ (4.31)

and

$$R_v = \alpha\varepsilon\left[\frac{R_d R_{th}\left(T_{max} - T\right)}{1 + \omega^2 \tau_{th}^2}\right]^{1/2}.$$ (4.32)

The value of R_v is controlled in part by $R_{th} = 1/G_{th}$; bolometers with high thermal conductance are fast [see Eq. (4.5)], but their responsivity is low. The key to developing highly sensitive bolometers is having a high temperature coefficient α, a very low thermal mass C_{th}, and excellent thermal isolation (low thermal conductance G_{th}).

The above considerations are widely used for the simplest model, which omits the Joulean heating of the bias current and assumes a constant electrical bias.

The first bolometer constructed by Langley in 1880 consisted of a blackened thin platinum foil and was used for solar observations. Metallic bolometers, made of thin films or of vapor-deposited layers of nickel, bismuth or antimony, have been used until now. They work at room temperature; however, they are characterised by small temperature coefficients of resistance.

Figure 4.16 shows the cross-section of a thin film-bolometer prepared by a silicon micromachining compatible with the integrated circuit-processing technology that enables the development of very large, low-cost, monolithic two-dimensional arrays. This structure includes an absorber layer, a temperature-sensitive layer, and a membrane. In this case, the detector element is deposited on a thin planar membrane attached to the substrate.

The development of microbolometer detector arrays, initially focused on military applications mainly in night vision systems, has been reinforced in recent years by a much wider range of civil applications (industrial control and control systems, low-cost thermal imaging cameras, systems supporting night vision of car drivers, etc.).

Detailed information about different bolometers is given in chapter 5.

4.3.4   PYROELECTRIC DETECTORS

The pyroelectric phenomenon has been known for several hundred years and is the result of changes in a dielectric polarisation of many crystals under the influence of temperature changes. Although many crystals with a non-centric symmetry of the crystal lattice show a spontaneous electrical polarisation, usually no external electric field is observed. If the material is a conductor, the moving charge carriers undergo an internal statistical decomposition that neutralises the internal dipole moment. However, in many pyroelectric materials, which are also good insulators, the external charge distribution is relatively stable, then, even relatively slow temperature changes in the material cause changes in the crystal lattice and dipole moment. However, if these changes do not cause changes in the surface charge, the changes in the external electric field cannot be measured either. It follows that the value of the temperature coefficient of changes in a dipole moment, called the pyroelectric coefficient, determines the observation of the pyroelectric phenomenon.

It should be noted that pyroelectric detectors differ from other types of thermal detectors in a way that they are sensitive to the temperature change rate, not to the temperature increase – which is the case with most thermal detectors. For this reason, pyroelectric detectors operate under modulated radiation conditions to prevent neutralisation of the induced surface charge.

The pyroelectric detector can be considered as a small capacitor with conductive electrodes mounted perpendicularly to a spontaneous polarisation direction [Figure 4.17(a)]. Figure 4.17(b) shows the equivalent circuit of a detector and a preamplifier. The pyroelectric material contains a large number of separate domains, with their own dipole momentum, differently oriented with a total zero effect. To change the polarisation of the active area, the material is heated, and an electric field is applied. While the detector is in operation, the change in the active area polarisation is revealed by changing the capacitator capacitance and the current generation, the magnitudes of which depend on the temperature change caused by the incident radiation and on the pyroelectric coefficient of the active substance.

The pyroelectric coefficient determines the rate of change of electrical polarisation with temperature. In conventional pyroelectrics, the value of the internal polarisation P is equivalent to the value of the electrical displacement field D, which is stable in the presence of a polarised electric field. The pyroelectric coefficient is defined as follows:

$$p = \frac{dP}{dT} = \left(\frac{dD}{dT} \right)_{E=0}. \tag{4.33}$$

However, a much larger amount of active detector substances used requires an external electric field to amplify the electrical displacement and, therefore, this coefficient can be defined as

$$p(E) = \left(\frac{dD}{dT} \right)_{E}. \tag{4.34}$$

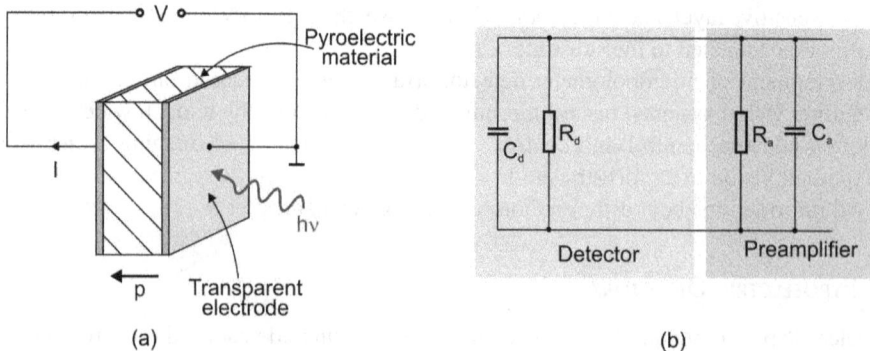

FIGURE 4.17 Pyroelectric detector: (a) geometry of pyroelectric detector and (b) its equivalent electrical circuit.

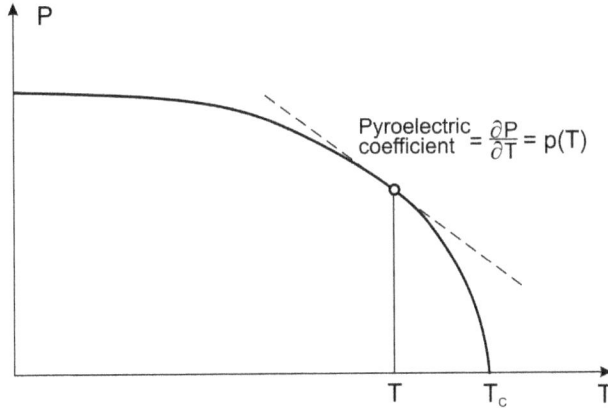

FIGURE 4.18   Dependence of spontaneous polarisation on temperature.

This leads to a stable response of ferroelectric materials operating below Curie T_C temperature. This mode of detector operation is known as a dielectric bolometer, which results in a large pyroelectric coefficient.

Figure 4.18 shows the temperature dependence of a spontaneous polarisation. The derivative of the polarisation curve as a function of temperature characterises the pyroelectric material. Above the Curie temperature, the ferroelectric material is paramagnetic.

The loss of polarisation in ferroelectric materials is the result of aging processes, temperature influences, or mechanical shocks. Such a material can return to a ferroelectric state as a result of an external electric field on a material cooled below the Curie temperature.

The output photocurrent of a pyroelectric detector can be expressed as follows:

$$I_{ph} = Ap\frac{dT}{dt}, \qquad (4.34)$$

where A is the detector area. Taking into account Eq. (4.6), we obtain

$$I_{ph} = \frac{\varepsilon p A \Phi_o \omega}{G_{th}\left(1 + \omega^2 \tau_{th}^2\right)^{1/2}}. \qquad (4.35)$$

An element with the area A and thickness t gives the thermal capacitance $C_{th} = c_{th}At$ (where c_{th} is the volume-specific heat) connected via the thermal resistance R_{th} to a heat sink. This gives the thermal time constant $\tau_{th} = C_{th}R_{th}$.

Taking into account Eq. (4.35), the current responsivity is equal to

$$R_i = \frac{I_{ph}}{\Phi_o} = \frac{\varepsilon p A \omega}{G_{th}\left(1 + \omega^2 \tau_{th}^2\right)^{1/2}}, \qquad (4.36)$$

and for low frequencies ($\omega \ll 1/\tau_{th}$), the response is proportional to ω. At frequencies greater than this value, the response is constant, being

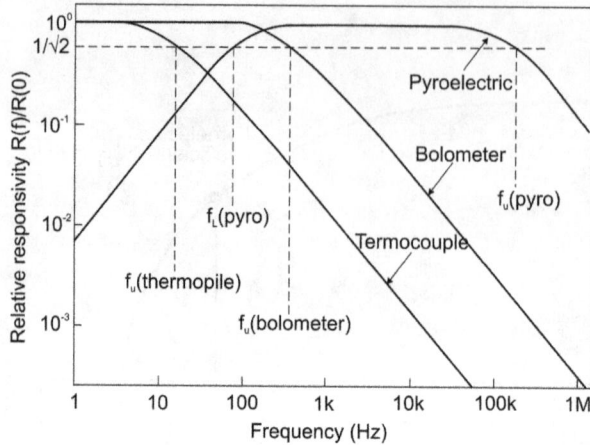

FIGURE 4.19 Typical frequency characteristics of thermocouple, bolometer and pyroelectric detector. For thermocouple and bolometer f_u is the high frequency cut-off due to thermal circuit; for the pyroelectric, the thermal cut-off is moved to the cut-off f_u(pyro) of the preamplifier, but there is a low-pass cut-off at f_L.

$$R_i = \frac{\varepsilon p}{c_{th} t}.$$ (4.37)

If we assume that the thermal time constant of the pyroelectric detector is greater than the electrical time constant, then it determines the lower cut-off frequency f_L as

$$f_L = \frac{1}{2\pi\tau_{th}} = \frac{1}{2\pi R_{th} C_{th}}.$$ (4.38)

Its value is usually less than 1 Hz. On the other hand, the electrical time constant decides about the upper limit frequency, depending on the type of a preamplifier used. For a voltage preamplifier, it depends on the value of resistance and capacitance of the equivalent circuit [Figure 4.17(b)], while using a current preamplifier, its value is determined by a very small load resistance, which is the quotient of the feedback resistance and the voltage gain of the amplifier with an open feedback loop. Usually, it is in the range of 10–1000 Hz.

If we assume that the detector structure has the shape of a cube with the edge length a, then, the thermal capacity is proportional to a^3, the thermal resistance is proportional to $1/a^2$, so the thermal time constant is proportional to a. Reducing the detector dimensions, we obtain a smaller thermal time constant.

Figure 4.19 shows the frequency characteristics of thermal detectors [10]. Thermocouples and bolometers are sensitive to temperature rise and, therefore, their lower cut-off frequency is zero (carries a constant component).

4.4   PHYSICAL PRINCIPLES OF PHOTON DETECTORS

As mentioned, the basis of photon detectors is an interaction of radiation photons with electrons (see Figure 4.5). Effectiveness of this interaction is determined by the radiation absorption, and more precisely, by absorption coefficient and coupling of the incident radiation with the detector.

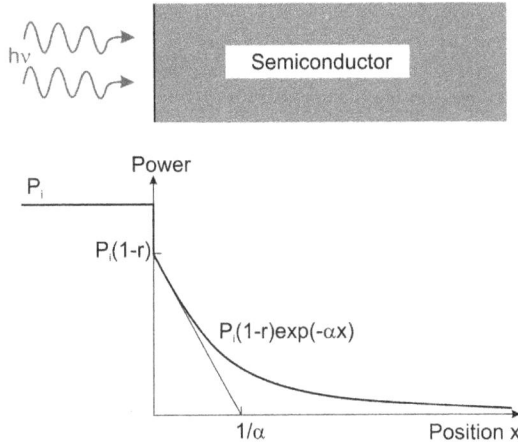

FIGURE 4.20 Radiation absorption in a semiconductor.

4.4.1 RADIATION ABSORPTION

Photon detectors are based on photon absorption in semiconductor materials. Part of the incident radiation is reflected from the front surface. For many semiconductors in the visible and infrared range this reflection is of about 30 per cent. However, when anti-reflective coatings are applied, it is reduced to less than 1 per cent. A signal whose photon energy is sufficient to generate photocarriers will continuously lose energy as the optical field propagates through the semiconductor (see Figure 4.20). Inside the semiconductor, the field decays exponentially as energy is transferred to the photocarriers. The material can be characterised by the absorption length, α, and the penetration depth, $1/\alpha$. Penetration depth is the point at which $1/e$ of the optical signal power remains.

The power absorbed in the semiconductor as a function of position x within the material is then

$$P_a(x) = P_i(1-r)(1-e^{-\alpha x}), \tag{4.39}$$

where P_i is the incident power of radiation and r is the reflectivity.

The number of photons absorbed is the power (in Watts) divided by the photon energy $E = hv$. If each absorbed photon generates a photocarrier, the number of photocarriers generated per number of incident photons for a specific semiconductor is given by

$$\eta(x) = (1-r)(1-e^{-\alpha x}), \tag{4.40}$$

where $0 \leq \eta(x) \leq 1$ is a definition for the quantum efficiency as the number of electron-hole pairs generated per incident photon.

Figure 4.21 shows the quantum efficiency of some of the detector materials used to fabricate ultraviolet (UV), visible and infrared detectors. Photocathodes and AlGaN detectors are being developed in the UV region. Silicon p-i-n diodes are shown with and without antireflection coating. Lead salts (PbS and PbSe) have intermediate quantum efficiencies, while PtSi Schottky barrier types and quantum well infrared photodetectors (QWIPs) have low values. InSb can respond from the near UV out to 5.5 μm at 80 K. A suitable detector material for near-IR (1.0–1.7 μm) spectral range is InGaAs lattice matched to the InP. Various HgCdTe alloys, in both photovoltaic and photoconductive

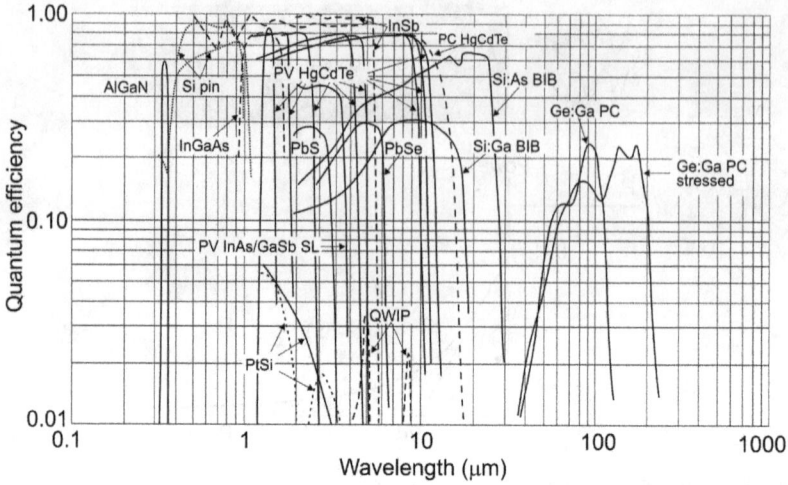

FIGURE 4.21   Quantum efficiency of different detectors (after Reference 5).

TABLE 4.4
Quantum Efficiency of Photon Detectors

Detector type	$\eta(\%)$
Intrinsic photoconductors	≈ 70
Extrinsic photoconductors	≈ 30
Photoconductive QWIP	≈ 20
Intrinsic photodiodes	≈ 70
Superlattice photodiodes	≈ 50
Photoemissive detectors	≈ 20
Photo film	≈ 1

---

configurations, cover from 0.7 μm to over 20 μm. InAs/GaSb strained layer superlattices have emerged as an alternative to the HgCdTe. Impurity-doped (Sb, As, and Ga) silicon BIB detectors operating at 10 K have a spectral response cut-off in the range of 16 to 30 μm. Impurity-doped Ge detectors can extend the response out to 100–200 μm. Table 4.4 compares a typical quantum efficiency of different types of photon detectors.

Figures 4.22 and 4.23 show the spectral relationships of absorption coefficients (with the corresponding penetration depth) for different semiconductors used in the design of photon detectors. In the region of the material maximum usable wavelength, the absorption efficiency drops dramatically. For wavelengths longer than a cut-off wavelength, the values of α are too small to give a considerable absorption. Since α is a strong function of the wavelength, for a given semiconductor the wavelength range in which a considerable photocurrent can be generated is limited.

In the high-energy range (above the energy gap E_g), the absorption coefficient can be approximated by the following relationship [17]:

$$\alpha = \alpha_o \left(h\nu - E_g \right)^{1/2} + \alpha'_o, \tag{4.41}$$

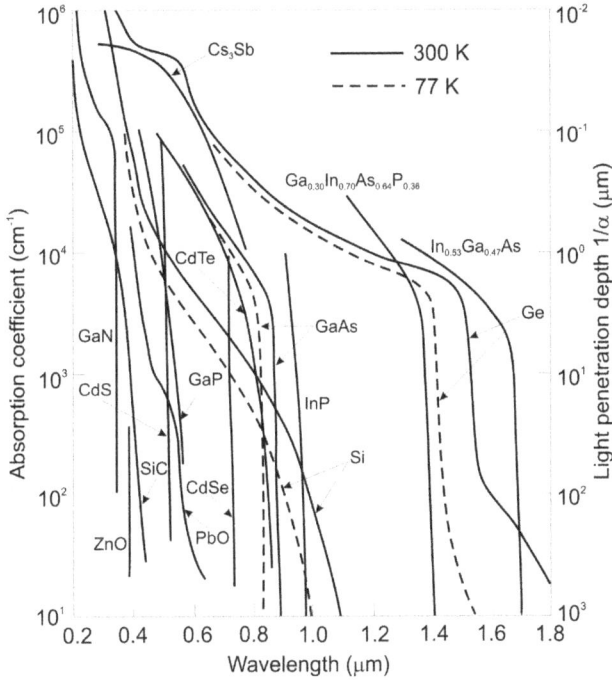

FIGURE 4.22 Absorption coefficient for various photodetector materials in the spectral range of 0.2–1.8 μm.

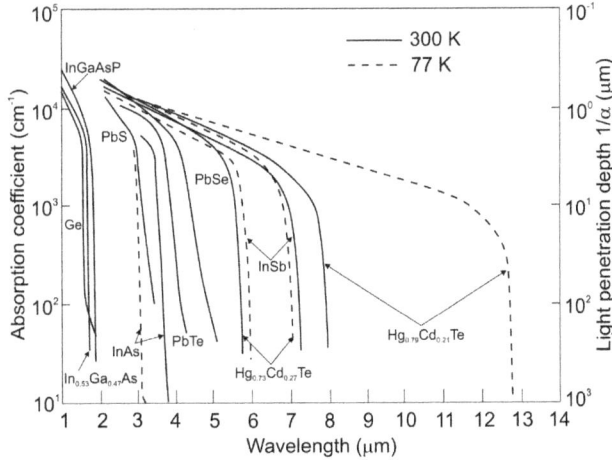

FIGURE 4.23 Absorption coefficient of semiconductors with a narrow bandgap.

and in terms of energy below E_g:

$$\alpha = \alpha'_o \left(\frac{E_g - h\nu}{kT} \right). \tag{4.42}$$

For example, for InSb, the constant values are as follows: $\alpha_o = 1.9 \times 10^4$ cm^{-1} i $\alpha'_o = 800$ cm^{-1}. For the HgCdTe ternary alloy, the values are similar, while for the material with a wide-bandgap type GaN, $\alpha_o = 2{,}3 \times 10^5$ cm^{-1}.

TABLE 4.5
Physical Properties of the Selected Semiconductor Materials

Material	Temperature T (K)	Dielectric constant, ε	Carrier lifetimes τ(s)	Electron mobility μ_e (cm²/Vs)	Hole mobility μ_h (cm²/Vs)	Energy gap E_g (eV)
Si	300	11.8	1×10^{-4}	1.35×10^3	480	1.11
Ge	300	16	1×10^{-2}	3.9×10^3	1900	0.67
GaN	300	9.0	?	9.0×10^2	150	3.39
GaAs	300	13.2	$\geq1\times10^{-6}$	8.5×10^3	400	1.43
$In_{0.53}Ga_{0.47}As$	300	14.6	1×10^{-4}	1.38×10^4	200	0.75
PbS	300	161	2×10^{-5}	5.75×10^2	200	0.37
InSb	77	17.9	1×10^{-7}	1.0×10^6	10000	0.228
$Hg_{0.79}Cd_{0.21}Te$	77	18.0	1×10^{-6}	2.0×10^5	440	0.10
$Hg_{0.72}Cd_{0.28}Te$	77	16.7	1×10^{-6}	8.0×10^4	440	0.25
InAs/GaSb SLs	77	15	1×10^{-7}	2.0×10^4	200	0.10

Other important parameters of semiconductor materials, important from the point of view of a photodetector design, are collected in Table 4.5.

The absorption coefficient, α, for extrinsic semiconductors is given by

$$\alpha = \sigma_p N_i,\tag{4.41}$$

where σ_p is the photoionisation cross-section, and N_i is the neutral impurity concentration.

The upper limit of N_i is set by either a "hopping" or an "impurity band" conduction. Practical values of α for optimised doped photoconductors are in the range of 1–10 cm⁻¹ for Ge and of 10–50 cm⁻¹ for Si. Thus, to maximise quantum efficiency, the detector crystal thickness should not be less than about 0.5 cm for doped Ge and about 0.1 cm for doped Si. Fortunately, for the most extrinsic detectors, the drift length of photocarriers is long enough for quantum efficiencies approaching 50 per cent to be obtained.

The absorption coefficient is considerably modified for low-dimensional solids. Figure 4.24 shows the infrared absorption spectra for different n-doped, 50-period GaAs/Al$_x$Ga$_{1-x}$As quantum well infrared photodetector (QWIP) structures measured at room temperatures [18]. The spectra of the bound-to-bound continuum (B-C) QWIP (samples A, B, and C) are much broader than the bound-to-bound (B-B; sample E) or bound-to-quasibound (B-QB) QWIP (sample F). Correspondingly, the value of the absorption coefficient for the B-C QWIP is significantly lower than that of the B-B QWIP, due to the oscillator strength conservation.

Comparing Figures 4.23 and 4.24 we can notice that the absorption coefficients for a direct band-to-band absorption are higher than those for intersubband transitions. The typical value of α for quantum transitions in GaAs/AlGaAs wells is below 1000 cm⁻¹ and is lower than in bulk semiconductors for interband absorption.

4.4.2 COUPLING OF RADIATION WITH DETECTORS

There are different methods of light coupling in a photodetector to enhance quantum efficiency [19]. A notable example of a method described for thin film solar cells [20] can be applied to photodetectors. In general, these absorption-enhancement methods can be divided into four categories that use optical concentration, antireflection structures, optical path increase, or light localisation, as shown in Figure 4.25.

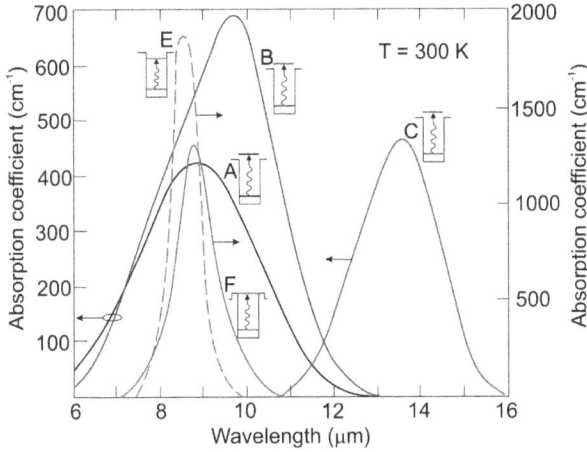

FIGURE 4.24 Absorption coefficient spectra measured at T = 300 K for different GaAs/AlGaAs QWIP samples (after Reference 18).

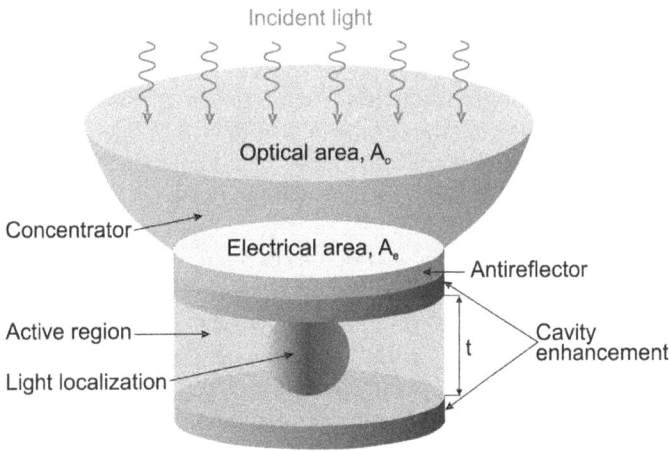

FIGURE 4.25 Different methods of absorption enhancement in a photodetector using an optical concentrator, an antireflection structure, structures for optical path increase (cavity enhancement), and light localisation structures.

Semiconductor materials used for photodetectors have large values of refractive index and thus large values of reflection coefficient at the device surface. This reflection is minimised using antireflection structures. The simplest way to enhance absorption is the use of a backside reflector to double pass of radiation. In thin devices quantum efficiency can be significantly enhanced using interference phenomena to set up a resonant cavity within the photodetector [19,21]. Various optical resonator structures are used. In the simplest method, interference occurs between the waves reflected at the rear, highly reflective surface and at the front surface of semiconductor. The thickness of the semiconductor is selected to set up the standing waves in the structure with peaks at the front and nodes at the back surface. The quantum efficiency oscillates with thickness of the structure, with the peaks at a thickness corresponding to an odd multiple of $\lambda/4n$, where n is the refractive index of the semiconductor. The gain in quantum efficiency increases with n. With the use of interference effects, a strong and highly non-uniform absorption can be achieved even for long wavelength radiation with a low absorption coefficient.

Another possible way to improve the performance of photodetectors is an increase the apparent "optical" size of the detector in comparison with the actual physical size, using a suitable concentrator that compresses impinging radiation. The concentration efficiency can be then defined as the ratio between the optical and the electrical area, minus absorption and scattering losses. This must be achieved without reduction of acceptance angle, or at least with limited reduction to angles required for fast optics systems. Various types of suitable optical concentrators can be used, including optical cones, conical fibres and other types of reflective, diffractive and refractive optical concentrators [22].

An efficient way to achieve an effective concentration of radiation is utilising an immersion lens. There are a number of different structures to serve the same purpose. Roughly, one could divide them into refractive, reflective and diffractive elements, although hybrid solutions are also possible. Microlenses monolithically integrated with detectors are typically used in CCD and CMOS active pixel imagers for visible application, concentrating the incoming light into the photosensitive region when they are accurately deposited over each pixel (see Figure 12.29).

The principle of operation of a hemispherical immersion lens is shown in Figure 4.26. The detector is located at the centre of curvature of the immersion lens. The lens produces an image on the detector. No spherical or coma aberration exists (aplanatic imaging). Due to immersion, the apparent linear size of detector increases by a factor of n. The image is located at the detector plane. The use of a hemispheric immersion lens in combination with an objective lens of an imaging optical system is shown in Figure 4.26(b). The immersion lens plays the role of a field lens, which increases the FOV of the optical system.

Advances in optoelectronics-related materials science, such as metamaterials and nanostructures, have opened doors for new non-classical approaches to device design methodologies, which are expected to offer enhanced performance along with reduced product cost for a wide range of applications. Surface plasmons (SPs) are widely recognised in the field of surface science following the pioneering work of Ritchie in 1950s [23]. The relative ease of manipulating SPs opens an opportunity for their applications to photonics and optoelectronics for scaling down optical and electronic devices to nanometric dimensions. For the first time, it is possible to reliably control light at the nanoscale. Additionally, plasmonics takes advantage of the very large (and negative) dielectric constant of metals, to compress the wavelength and enhance electromagnetic fields in the vicinity of metal conductors. Coupling light into semiconductor materials remains a challenging and active research topic. Micro- and nano-structured surfaces have become a widely used design tool to increase light absorption and enhance the performance of broadband detectors without employing anti-reflection coatings [24, 25]. The smaller volumes of photodetectors provide lower noise, while higher absorption results in a stronger output signal. This leads to miniaturised detector structures with length scales that are much smaller than those being currently achieved.

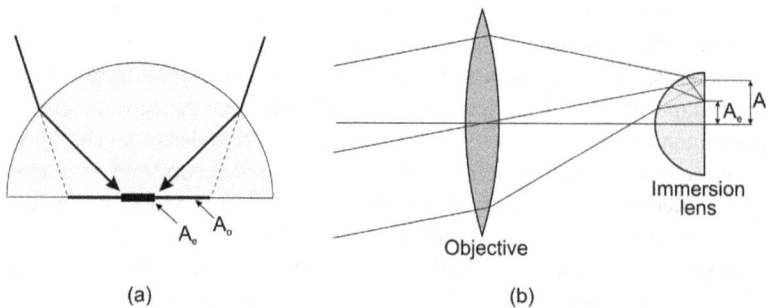

(a)   (b)

FIGURE 4.26 Principle of optical immersion (a), and ray tracing for an optical system with a combination of an objective lens and an immersion lens (b) (after Reference 22).

A plasmon is a quantised electron density wave in a conducting material. Bulk plasmons are longitudinal excitations, whereas surface plasmons (SPs) can have both longitudinal and transverse components [24]. Light of frequency below the frequency of the plasmon for that material (the plasma frequency) is reflected, while light above the plasma frequency is transmitted. SPs on a plane surface are nonradiative electromagnetic modes (EM), that is, they cannot be generated directly by light, nor can they decay spontaneously into photons. However, if the surface is rough or has a grating on it, or is patterned in some way, light around the plasma frequency couples strongly with the surface plasmons, creating what is called a polariton, or a surface plasmon polariton (SPP) – a transverse-magnetic optical surface wave that may propagate along the surface of a metal until energy is lost, either via absorption in the metal or radiation into free-space.

In its simplest form, an SPP is an EM excitation (coupled EM field/charge-density oscillation) that propagates in a wave-like fashion along the planar interface between a metal and a dielectric medium, and whose amplitude decays exponentially with increasing distance into each medium from the interface. Thus, the SPP is a surface EM wave, whose field is confined to the near vicinity of the dielectric-metal interface. This confinement leads to an enhancement of the field at the interface, resulting in an extraordinary sensitivity of the SPP to surface conditions. The intrinsically two-dimensional (2D) nature of SPPs prohibits them from directly coupling to light. Usually, a surface metal grating is required for the excitation of SPPs by normally incident light. Moreover, since the EM field of an SPP decays exponentially with distance from the surface, it cannot be observed in conventional (far-field) experiments unless the SPP is transformed into light by its interaction with a surface grating.

Schematic representation of an electron density wave propagating along a metal-dielectric interface is shown in Figure 4.27. The charge density oscillations and associated electromagnetic fields comprise SPP waves. The local electric field component is enhanced near the surface and decays exponentially with distance in a direction normal to the interface.

The interaction between the surface charge density and the electromagnetic field results in the momentum of the SP mode, $\hbar k_{SP}$, being greater than that of a free-space photon of the same frequency, $\hbar k_o$ ($k_o = \omega/c$ is the free-space wavevector) – see Figure 4.27(c). Solving Maxwell's equations under the appropriate boundary conditions yields the SP dispersion relation, that is the frequency-dependent SP wave-vector [26]

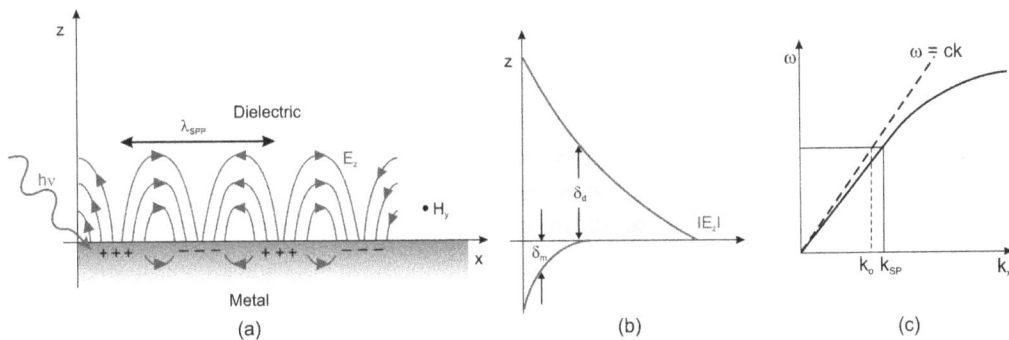

FIGURE 4.27 (a) Schematic illustration of electromagnetic wave and surface charges at the interface between the metal and the dielectric material; the magnetic field (H_y) is perpendicular to the drawing plane and generation of the surface charge requires an electric field perpendicular to the boundary surface, with δ_d and δ_m damping coefficients in dielectric and metal respectively; (b) the local electric field component is enhanced near the surface and decays exponentially with distance in a direction normal to the interface; (c) the surface plasmon dispersion curves indicating the momentum mismatch between the SP (surface plasmon) mode and the dashed line for light ($\omega = ck$) that must be overcome in order to couple the incident photons with the SP mode; for the same frequency ω the momentum SP ($\hbar k_{SP}$) is greater than the photon of light ($\hbar k_o$) in free space.

$$k_{SP} = k_o \left(\frac{\varepsilon_d \varepsilon_m}{\varepsilon_d + \varepsilon_m} \right)^{1/2}. \tag{4.42}$$

The frequency-dependent permittivity of the metal, ε_d, and the dielectric material, ε_m, must have opposite signs if SPs are to be possible at such an interface. This condition is satisfied for metals because ε_m is both negative and complex (the latter corresponding to absorption in the metal). The increase in $\hbar k_{SP}$ momentum is associated with the binding of the SP to the surface (the resulting momentum mismatch between light and SPs of the same frequency must be bridged if light is to be used to generate SPs).

In contrast to the propagating nature of SPs along the surface, the field perpendicular to the surface decays exponentially with distance from the surface. This in nature evanescent field of SPs is a consequence of the bound, non-radiative SPs, which prevents power from propagating away from the surface.

SPs were first studied in the visible region. The vast majority of plasmonics research has focused on the shorter wavelength side of the optical frequency range. In the visible spectrum, silver is the metal with lowest losses, where propagation distances are typically in the range 10–100 μm. In addition, for a longer incident wavelength, such as the near-infrared telecommunication wavelength 1.55 μm, the propagation length of silver increases towards 1 mm. For a relatively absorbing metal such as aluminium, the propagation length is 2 μm at a wavelength of 500 nm [25].

It appears that common metals, such as gold or silver, have plasmon resonances in blue or deep ultra-violate wavelength ranges. Recently, an increased research effort has been directed to the infrared. However, when moving from the visible to the infrared rage, metal films with arrays of holes that ordinarily show optical transmission are quite opaque. There are no metals available whose plasmon resonances are in the IR range under 10 microns in wavelength. Moreover, the integration of plasmonic structure with an active detector region is intrinsically incompatible due to the low-quality metal deposition techniques in comparison with high-quality epitaxial growth of semiconductors or dielectrics. As a result, many intrinsic plasmonic properties can be masked by the poor metal quality or poor semiconductor-metal interfaces. In addition, wavelength tuneability is difficult to realise since the plasmonic resonance frequency is fixed for a given metal.

Different architectures are used to support SPPs on metalo-dielectric structures involving planar metal waveguides, metal gratings, nanoparticles such as islands, spheres, rods and antennas, or optical transmission through one or many sub-wavelength holes in a metal film. However, great challenges still remain to fully realise many promised potentials.

Figure 4.28 presents three popular geometries to enhance the detector's photoresponse: (a) grating couplers to convert incident light to SPPs, which are focused inside a small-scale detector; (b) particle antenna on a small-scale detector; and (c) metallic photonic crystal structures to enhance the photoresponse. The inclusion of an antenna or resonator enhance the photoresponse or make the detector wavelength and polarisation-specific.

In the first architecture, a nanoscale semiconductor photodetector is discussed. Small area photodetectors benefit from low noise levels, a low junction capacitance, and possible high-speed operation. However due to the decrease of the active area of the semiconductor detector under the same optical power density, a lower output is obtained. A nanoantena in close proximity to the active material of a photodetector allows us to take advantage of the concentrated plasmonic fields [27]. Its role is to convert free-space plane waves into surface plasmons bound to a patterned metal surface without reflection. The antenna-like structure to couple incident radiation to surface plasmons is a technique very popular for THz detectors [28].

In Figure 4.28(b) we show an integrating detector nanoscale structure whose photoresponse is enhanced by a local plasmon resonance. Resonant antennas can confine strong optical fields inside a subwavelength volume. By designing the structure in such a way that the region with highly

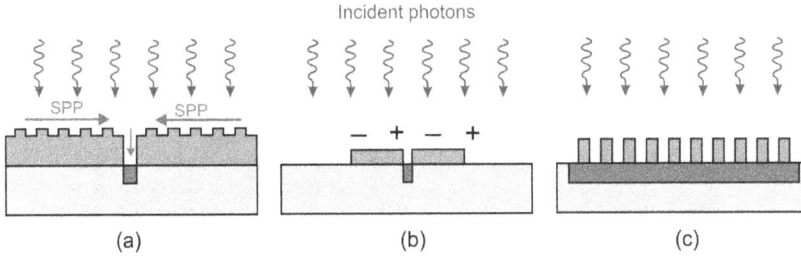

FIGURE 4.28 Different architectures for plasmon-enhanced detectors: (a) grating couplers to focus the generated SPPs inside a small-scale detector, (b) particle antenna on a small-scale detector, and (c) metallic photonic crystal structures.

confined optical fields overlaps with the active region of the photodetector, a strong enhancement of the photocurrent can be achieved using both SPP or localised SPR (LSPP) resonances.

LSSP are charge oscillations that are bound to a small metal particle or nanostructure. These oscillations can be represented by the displacement of charge in the sphere. For example, for a metal sphere in a dielectric, the field inside the metal is given by electrostatic approximation as [29]

$$E_{in} = \frac{3\varepsilon_d E_o}{\varepsilon_m + 2\varepsilon_d},$$
(4.43)

where E_o is the electric field away from the sphere. Ignoring the imaginary contributions to the relative permittivities in Eq. (4.43), it is clear that the field inside the sphere diverges when $\varepsilon_m = -2\varepsilon_d$, which leads to a strong enhancement of the field on the outer surface of the sphere (which is limited in practice by imaginary part of ε_m). The quality of the resonance is limited by the dispersion of the metal and dielectric, as is clear from the field enhancement denominator in Eq. (4.43).

The third way presented of enhancing the photoresponse of a photodetector is shown in Figure 4.28(c). The photoresponse enhancing is achieved by the inclusion of a metallic photonic crystal (PC) on the detector area or arranging the detector structures in a periodic way, forming a PC structure. Integrating of a resonant structure with detector increases the interaction length between the incoming light and the active semiconductor region. This design is interesting for thin film semiconductor detectors with a large absorption length.

Since the absorption coefficient is a strong function of the wavelength, the wavelength range in which an appreciable photocurrent can be generated is limited for a given detector material. So, broadband absorption is usually inadequate due to quantum efficiency roll-off. Research on photonic crystal (PC) structures with a periodic refractive index modulation has opened up several ways for the control of light. Most existing devices are realised as two-dimensional (2D) PC structures, as they are compatible with standard semiconductor processing [28–30].

An important class of 2D PC structures are photonic crystal slabs (PCSs) consisting of a dielectric structure with a periodic modulation in only two dimensions and refractive index guiding in the third. Figure 4.29(a) shows a QWIP fabricated as a PCS structure [30]. The PC structure is underetched by selective removal of the sacrificial AlGaAs layer to create the free-standing PCS. A schematic illustration of the final device is shown in Figure 4.29(b). The photoresponse of the PCS-QWIP shows a wider response peak but additionally displays several pronounced resonance peaks.

4.4.3 Generation and Recombination Mechanisms

The photodetector current sensitivity is determined by the quantum efficiency η and by the photoelectric gain g. The quantum efficiency is determined by the quality of the detector coupling to the incident

(a)

(b)

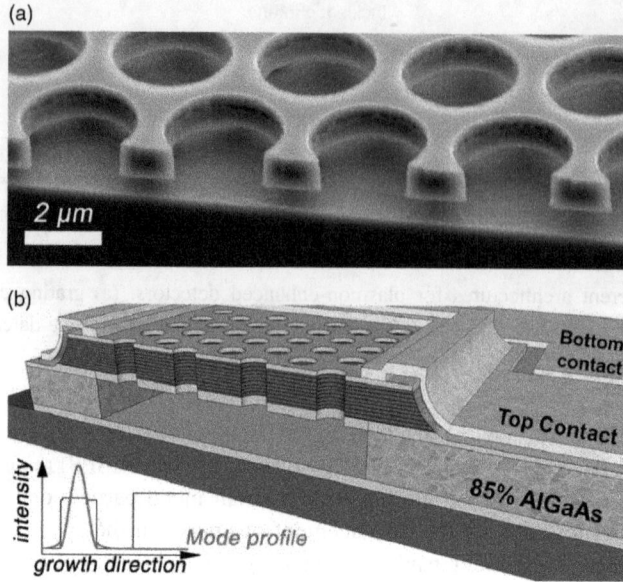

FIGURE 4.29 PCS-QWIP design: (a) SEM image of a cleaved PCS, (b) cross section through the PCS-QWIP structure (after Reference 30).

radiation stream. The photoelectric amplification concept was introduced by Rose in his excellent monograph [31] in order to present a simplified theory of photoelectric conductivity. This term is now commonly used and is understood as the number of carriers leaving the detector electrical contact per one carrier pair generated in the detector. This parameter indicates how the generated electron-hole pairs contribute to the generation of a photocurrent (photocurrent value) of the photodetector. Next, we will assume that both quantum efficiency and photoelectric gain are constant in the detector volume.

The spectral current responsivity is equal to

$$R_i = \frac{\lambda \eta}{hc} qg. \tag{4.44}$$

Assuming that the current gain for the photocurrent and the noise current are the same, the noise current caused by statistical processes of generation and recombination of carriers is determined by the equations [22, 32]:

$$I_n^2 = 2(G + R) A_e t \Delta f q^2 g^2, \tag{4.45}$$

where G and R are the generation and recombination rates, Δf is the frequency band, and t is the detector thickness.

The difference in the generation and recombination terms can be written as [33]:

$$G - R = \sum_k g_k \left(n_o p_o - np \right), \tag{4.46}$$

where $p = p_o + \Delta p$ and $n = n_o + \Delta n$ are the excess carrier concentration, n_o and p_o are the average thermal equilibrium carrier density, and g_k is the factor depending on the type of generation and recombination process.

Under low excitation conditions, when $\Delta n \ll n_o$ ($\Delta p \ll p_o$), the above notation can be reduced to the form of

$$G - R = \sum_k -\frac{\Delta n}{\tau_k},\tag{4.47}$$

where τ_k denotes the lifetime of the k-th process which is independent of the influence of other processes. Under such conditions, the overall lifetime can be defined as follows:

$$\frac{1}{\tau} = \sum_k \frac{1}{\tau_k} = \frac{R - G}{\Delta n}.\tag{4.48}$$

The lifetime of photogenerated electrons and holes is one of the most important parameters of semiconductors used in the construction of photodetectors, because it determines both responsivity of the detector and its response time. Electron-hole pairs recombine in two ways. First, by recombination of the electron from the conduction band with a hole in the valence band and the excess energy is emitted in the form of a photon. This process is called a direct recombination process of the band-to-band type. The second way occurs when the electron initially passes to an energy level lying deep in the forbidden gap, and then intercepts a hole in the valence band. This recombination process is called an "intermediate process" and is often referred to in the scientific literature as the Shockley-Read-Hall (SRH) process. In the recombination process, the released energy is relaxed in the crystal lattice by an interaction with phonons or emitted as a photon.

There is also the third recombination method, in which energy is transferred to the third mobile carrier. This process is called Auger recombination. Note that both Auger recombination and phonon-mediated recombination are non-radiated processes. All three processes are schematically shown in Figure 4.30.

It needs to be highlighted that the SRH process is not an intrinsic, fundamental process because it is related to levels in the forbidden energy gap. Its impact can be limited by reducing a concentration of lattice defects along with a concentration of foreign impurities.

It should be expected that, with a technological progress in obtaining higher quality materials, the SRH process impact on the carrier's lifetime will decrease. On the other hand, the interband radiative and Auger recombination are fundamental processes as they are determined by the band structure of a given semiconductor. There are also non-fundamental processes of radiative and collision recombination with a participation of trap levels in the forbidden gap.

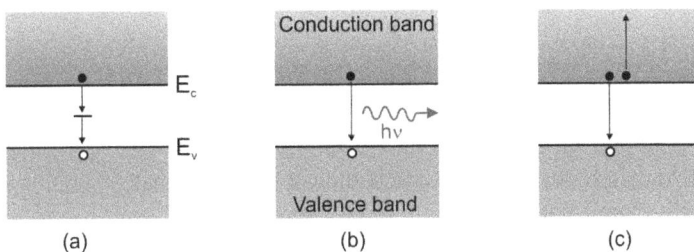

FIGURE 4.30 Mechanisms of carrier recombination in a semiconductors: (a) SRH (trap-assisted) recombination, (b) band-to-band radiative recombination, and (c) Auger recombination.

Detectivity, D^*, is the most important parameter of the detector; it determines the signal-to-noise ratio of the detector normalised to the unit detector area and the unit noise bandwidth and is described by Eq. (2.11). Therefore, according to the Eqs. (4.44) and (4.45) we obtain the following:

$$D^* = \frac{\lambda}{2^{1/2}hc}\left(\frac{A_o}{A_e}\right)^{1/2}\frac{\eta}{t^{1/2}}\frac{1}{(G+R)^{1/2}}. \tag{4.49}$$

It follows that for a given wavelength and operating temperature, the best detector performance will be obtained when the term $\eta/[t(G+R)]^{1/2}$ reaches its maximum value, which corresponds to the condition of obtaining the highest quantum efficiency in the thinnest detector possible, and in addition, the total number of generation and recombination acts per time unit [equal to $(G+R)(A_e t)$] should be as small as possible.

In the following considerations, we will assume that $A_o/A_e = 1$. As for the negligible front and backside radiation reflection, we obtain

$$\eta = 1 - \exp(-\alpha t), \tag{4.50}$$

and

$$D^* = \frac{\lambda}{hc}(1 - e^{-\alpha t})\left[2(G+R)t\right]^{-1/2}. \tag{4.51}$$

The highest detection value for a single radiation transition is obtained when $t = 1.26/\alpha$, for which $(1 - e^{-\alpha t})t^{-1/2}$ reaches the maximum value of $0.62\alpha^{1/2}$. This choice of detector thickness is the best compromise between requirements of high quantum efficiency and low thermal generation in the detector active area. Under optimal conditions $\eta = 0.716$, and then detectivity [32] equals:

$$D^* = 0.45\frac{\lambda}{hc}\left(\frac{\alpha}{G+R}\right)^{1/2}. \tag{4.52}$$

The detectivity can also be increased by a factor of $2^{1/2}$ for a double pass of radiation through the absorber. This can be achieved by the use of a backside reflector. A simple calculation shows that the optimum thickness in this case is half of the single pass case, while the quantum efficiency remains equal to 0.716.

At equilibrium, the generation and recombination rates are equal ($G = R$). In this case we obtain

$$D^* = 0.31\frac{\lambda}{hc}\left(\frac{\alpha}{G}\right)^{1/2}. \tag{4.53}$$

As we can see, the ratio of the absorption coefficient to the thermal generation rates, α/G, is the main figure of merit of any materials for infrared detectors.

Figure 4.31 shows the temperature dependence α/G for four types of the absorber material. It can be seen that, potentially, the best performance is achieved by detectors made of HgCdTe and InAs/GaSb SLs, while lower detectability is obtained for QWIP and extrinsic silicon.

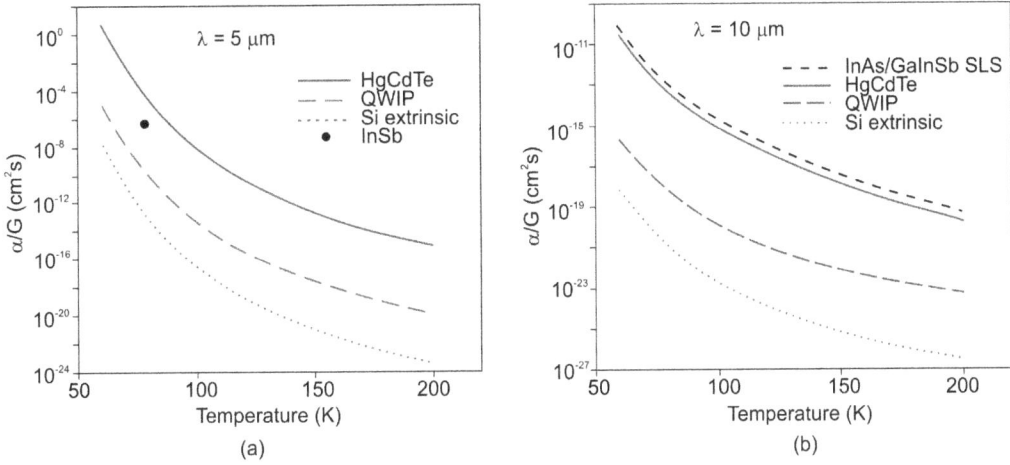

FIGURE 4.31 α/G ratio versus temperature for (a) MWIR ($\lambda = 5\,\mu$m), and (b) LWIR ($\lambda = 10\,\mu$m) photodetectors based on HgCdTe, QWIP, Si extrinsic and type-II superlattice (for LWIR only) material technology.

The α/G ratio versus temperature for various material systems capable of band gap tuning is shown in Figure 4.31 for a hypothetical energy gap equal to 0.25 eV ($\lambda = 5\,\mu$m) and 0.124 eV ($\lambda = 10\,\mu$m). Procedures used in calculations of α/G for different material systems are given in Reference 34. Analysis shows that narrow-gap semiconductors are more suitable for high-temperature photodetectors in comparison to competing technologies such as extrinsic devices, QWIP (quantum well IR photodetector) and QDIP (quantum dot IR photodetector) devices. The main reason for the high performance of intrinsic photodetectors is the high density of states in the valence and conduction bands, which results in strong absorption of infrared radiation.

An optimised photodetector of any type may be a three dimensional (3D) monolithic heterostructure that consists of the following regions [35]: concentrator of IR radiation, absorber of radiation, contacts to the absorber that sense optically generated charge carriers, passivation of the absorber to insulate it from the ambient, and retroreflector to enhance absorption and quantum efficiency The above conditions can be fulfilled using heterojunctions like N$^+$-p-p$^+$ and P$^+$-n-n$^+$ with heavily doped contact regions (symbol "+" denotes strong doping, capital letter denotes a wider gap). Homojunction devices (like n-p, n$^+$-p, p$^+$-n) suffer from surface problems; excess thermal generation results in an increased dark current and recombination which reduces the photocurrent.

The generation rate is the sum of optical and thermal generation:

$$G = G_{th} + G_{op}. \tag{4.54}$$

In order to achieve high detectivity, the thermal generation must be reduced to the lowest possible level. From the Boltzmann's distribution it results that the energy levels occupation is determined by the $\exp(-E_g/kT)$ type, which means that when E_g becomes smaller, the number of thermally induced electrons will increase while maintaining a constant temperature.

It also shows that lowering the detector temperature causes a reduction of the thermal carrier generation. Photodetectors with high sensitivity in the longer wavelength range must be cooled to a lower temperature than detectors with more short-wave sensitivity limit (see Figure 4.8). In practice, it is aimed to achieve such a state of detector operation that the thermal generation is lower than the optical generation caused by the signal and background of the incident radiation. If detectivity is limited by the background of the incident radiation (or more precisely by the fluctuations of the background radiation, that is, the photon noise of the background radiation), which takes place in the case of good quality infrared detectors, then such an ideal state of the detector operation is called BLIP (background limited infrared photodetectors) – see Section 2.3. In Figure 4.7 the theoretical curves of detectivity limited by background radiation fluctuations, for an ideal photoconductive detector, ideal photovoltaic and ideal thermal detector are marked with dotted lines.

Below, we will consider the physical phenomena underlying the operation of photoconductors, photodiodes and photoemission detectors.

4.5 PHOTOCONDUCTIVE DETECTORS

A photoconductive detector, also called a photoconductor or photoresistor, is basically a resistor sensitive to optical radiation; incident radiation changes the material's electrical conductivity. The change in conductivity is measured by means of electrodes attached to the sample. Usually, a transverse geometry of photoresistors is used when the incident radiation is perpendicular to the direction of the biasing current. For a low-resistance material, where a sample resistance is typically 100 Ω, the photoconductor is usually operated in a constant current circuit as shown in Figure 4.32. The series load resistance is large compared to the sample resistance, and the signal is detected as a change in voltage developed across the sample. For high-resistance photoconductors, a constant voltage circuit is preferred, and the signal is detected as a change in current in the bias circuit.

Three fundamental processes of optical excitation of carriers are shown in Figure 4.5(a). The spontaneous process of band-to-band excitation occurs when the photon energy is greater than the energy gap E_g of the semiconductor. In this process both the electron and the hole contribute to the photocurrent. The cut-off wavelength corresponding to the bandgap energy of the intrinsic photoconductors is given by

$$\lambda_c = \frac{hc}{E_g} \text{ which leads to } \lambda_c [\mu m] = \frac{1.238}{E_g [eV]}. \tag{4.55}$$

In the extrinsic conductivity mechanism, the incident radiation energy is too low to excite a free electron-hole pair, but is sufficient to excite the carrier from the impurity level: the electron from the donor level to the conductance band and the hole after capturing the electron from the valence band to the acceptor level. This is shown in Figure 4.5(a). Then, the extrinsic photoconductivity cut-off wavelength is as follows:

$$\lambda_c = \frac{hc}{E_i}, \tag{4.56}$$

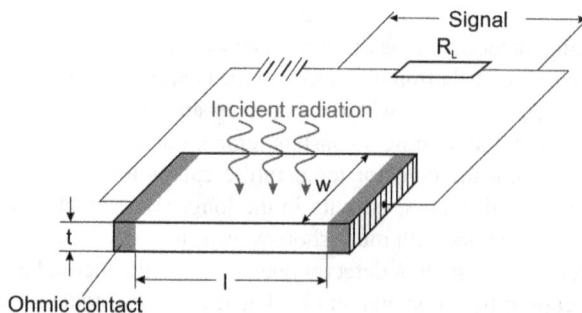

FIGURE 4.32 Geometry and bias of a photoconductor.

where E_i is the impurity ionisation energy. The band-to-impurity absorption is the basis for the operation of very long wavelength infrared detectors with λ_c above 20 μm (see Figure 4.8).

Free carriers' absorption is a secondary phenomenon and is used for detection of very long-wave infrared radiation. In this class of detectors, the radiation falling on a semiconductor with a high carrier mobility (e.g., electrons in InSb) induces intersubband transitions which increase the electrons energy in a conduction band. And since carrier mobility is a function of electron temperature, a change of conductivity is observed. Detectors of this type work at very low temperatures (about 4 K) in order to reduce the speed of energy transfer to the crystal lattice.

In order to determine photoconductor sensitivity, we will assume that the signal photon flux density $\Phi_s(\lambda)$ is incident on the detector area $A = wl$ and that the detector is operated under the constant current condition, that is, $R_L \gg R$. We suppose further that the illumination and the bias field are weak and the excess carrier lifetime τ is the same for majority and minority carriers. To derive an expression for voltage responsivity, we take a one-dimensional approach for simplicity. This is justified for the detector thickness t, which is small with regard to a minority carrier diffusion length. We also neglect the recombination effect at the front and rear surfaces.

The basic expression describing either intrinsic or extrinsic photoconductivity in semiconductors under equilibrium excitation (i.e., steady state) is as follows:

$$I_{ph} = q\eta A\Phi_s g, \tag{4.57}$$

where I_{ph} is the photocurrent at zero frequency (DC) that is the increase in current above the dark current accompanying irradiation.

In general, photoconductivity is a two-carrier phenomenon and, then, the total photocurrent is the sum of electron and hole current:

$$I_{ph} = \frac{wtq\left(\Delta n\mu_e + \Delta p\mu_h\right)V_b}{l}, \tag{4.58}$$

where μ_e is the electron mobility, μ_h is the hole mobility, V_b is the bias voltage, Δn and Δp are excess carrier concentrations, n_o and p_o are the average thermal equilibrium carrier densities, where $n = n_o + \Delta n$ i $p = p_o + \Delta p$.

Taking the conductivity to be dominated by electrons (this is found to be the case in all known high sensitivity photoconductors) and, assuming a uniform and complete absorption of the light in the detector, the rate equation for the excess electron concentration in the sample is the following [36]:

$$\frac{d\Delta n}{dt} = \frac{\Phi_s \eta}{t} - \frac{\Delta n}{\tau}, \tag{4.59}$$

where τ is the excess carrier lifetime. In the steady condition, the excess carrier lifetime is given by the equation

$$\tau = \frac{\Delta nt}{\eta\Phi_s}. \tag{4.60}$$

Comparing Eq. (4.57) to Eq. (4.58) we obtain:

$$g = \frac{tV_b\mu_e\Delta n}{l^2\eta\Phi_s},$$ (4.61)

and invoking Eq. (4.60), we get the following for the photoconductive gain:

$$g = \frac{\tau\mu_eV_b}{l^2} = \frac{\tau}{l^2/\mu_eV_b}.$$ (4.62)

Thus, the photoconductive gain can be defined as

$$g = \frac{\tau}{t_t},$$ (4.63)

where t_t is the transit time of electrons between ohmic contacts. To obtain the last equation, it should be noted that the electron drift speed is determined by the equation

$$v_e = \mu_eE,$$ (4.64)

and the electric field is $E = V_b/l$.

Eq. (4.63) shows that the photoconductive gain is given by the ratio of free carrier lifetime τ to transit time, t_t, between the detector electrodes. The carrier lifetime strongly depends on the semiconductor properties. The photoconductive gain can be less than or greater than a unity depending upon whether the drift length, $L_d = v_d\tau$, is less than or greater than an interelectrode spacing, l.

In many semiconductors, electron mobility is greater than that of holes (see Table 4.5). For large E-fields exceeding approximately 10^5 V/cm, the saturation velocities v_s range from 6×10^6–10^7 cm/s. The application of a higher electric field does not increase the speed.

In most cases, the saturation velocities for electrons and holes are similar, with a tendency towards lower saturation velocities for holes due to their higher effective mass. For this reason, the separate values v_s for electrons and holes are given. In some semiconductors, for example, GaAs, InP and GaN, the electron drift rate reaches a clear maximum for an electric field close to 10^4 V/cm. The electron velocities obtained in these semiconductors are 2×10^7 cm/s. Since the speed of faster carriers determines the transit time of electrons in a photoresistor, sometimes high gain photoresistors operate at a relatively low supply voltage.

The value of $L_d > l$ implies that a free charge carrier swept out at one electrode is immediately replaced by injection of an equivalent free charge carrier at the opposite electrode. Thus, a free charge carrier will continue to circulate until the recombination takes place. Figure 4.33 shows the successive phases of this phenomenon, so called photorecycling effect. After the generation of electron and hole pair, the electron drifts much faster than the hole and therefore leaves the sample quickly. The sample, however, must be neutral, which means another electron must enter the sample from the negative electrode as in (b) (the electrode is ohmic). This new electron also drifts across quickly as in (b) and (c) to leave the sample while the hole is still drifting slowly in the sample. Thus, another electron must enter the sample to maintain neutrality as in (d) and (e), and so on, until either the hole reaches the negative electrode or recombines with one of these electrons entering the sample. The external photocurrent therefore corresponds to the flow of many electrons per absorbed photon, which represents a photoconductive gain. In intrinsic photoconductors, the measured photoconductivity gain reaches the value of 10^6.

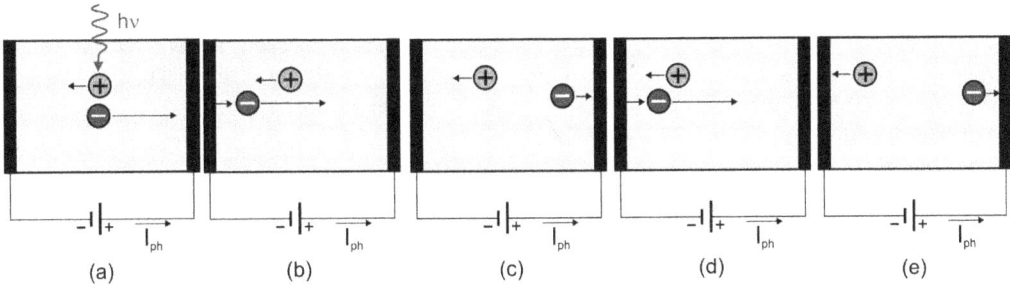

FIGURE 4.33 The idea of photoconductivity enhancement in a photoconductor.

When $R_L \gg R$, a signal voltage across the load resistor is essentially an open circuit voltage:

$$V_s = I_{ph}R_d = I_{ph}\frac{l}{qwtn\mu_e},$$ (4.65)

where R_d is the detector resistance. Assuming that the change in conductivity upon irradiation is small compared to the dark conductivity, the voltage responsivity is expressed as

$$R_v = \frac{V_s}{P_\lambda} = \frac{\eta}{lwt}\frac{\lambda\tau}{hc}\frac{V_b}{n_o},$$ (4.66)

where the absorbed monochromatic power is $P_\lambda = \Phi_s Ah\nu$.

The frequency-dependent responsivity can be determined by the following equation:

$$R_v = \frac{\eta}{lwt}\frac{\lambda\tau_{ef}}{hc}\frac{V_b}{n_0}\frac{1}{\left(1+\omega^2\tau_{ef}^2\right)^{1/2}},$$ (4.67)

where τ_{ef} is the effective carrier lifetime, $\tau_{ef} = \gamma\tau$. The γ coefficient depends on diffusion length, electrons and holes drift length, as well as on the detector length. Because $\gamma \leq 1$, therefore $\tau_{ef} \leq \tau$.

The given simple model takes no account of additional limitations related to the practical conditions of photoconductor operations, such as sweep-out effects or surface recombination. These are specified in Reference 13.

Another parameter of the photoconductor is a current responsivity, defined as the ratio of photo-current to absorbed power. Taking into account Eq. (4.57) we obtain

$$R_i = \frac{I_{ph}}{P_\lambda} = \frac{\eta q}{h\nu}g = \frac{\lambda\eta}{hc}qg.$$ (4.68)

It follows that both voltage and current responsivities increase linearly with the incident radiation wavelength.

Equation (4.66) shows the basic requirements for a high photoconductive responsivity at a given wavelength, λ, are necessary: the high quantum efficiency η, the long excess-carrier lifetime τ, the smallest possible piece of structure lwt, the low thermal equilibrium carrier concentration n_o and the highest possible bias voltage V_b.

A number of internal noise sources are usually operative in photoconductive detectors. The fundamental types are photon noise from the signal and background and detector self-noises such as Johnson–
Nyquist (sometime called thermal) noise and generation-recombination (g-r) noise. The third form of
noise, not amenable to exact analysis, is called 1/f noise because it exhibits a 1/f power law spectrum to a
close approximation. The mean square of a total noise voltage is described in a way similar to Eq. (4.16).

Depending on a dominant influence of individual noise sources, we can distinguish a limitation
of photoconductors detectivity by the generational-recombination noise D_{gr}^*, the background radiation D_B^*, and the surface recombination rate D_s^*.

When the generation-recombination (g-r) noise dominates, the detectivity is determined by the
following equation:

$$D_{gr}^* = \frac{\lambda}{2hc} \frac{\eta}{t^{1/2}} \left(\frac{n+p}{np} \right)^{1/2} \tau^{1/2}.$$ (4.69)

Under conditions of a dominant influence of the background radiation,

$$D_B^* = \frac{\lambda}{2hc} \left[\frac{n(n+p)}{\Phi_B n} \right]^{1/2},$$ (4.70)

and with a strong influence of the surface recombination rate s:

$$D_s^* = \frac{\eta\lambda}{2hc} \left(\frac{n_0 + p_0}{2n_i^2 s} \right)^{1/2}.$$ (4.71)

Detailed analyses of the limitations of photoconductors detectivity can be found in Reference 13.

4.6 PHOTOVOLTAIC DETECTORS

The photovoltaic effect is created in structures containing built-in potential barriers. These phenomena arise when excess carriers are injected into the vicinity of these barriers. Potential barriers
cause oppositely charged carriers to move in opposite directions depending on the external polarisation circuit. The most important photovoltaic phenomena include those observed in the p-n junction,
in Schottky's barriers [metal-semiconductor (MS)], and in metal-insulator-semiconductor (MIS)
structures. Each of the devices, the operation of which is based on these phenomena, has certain
advantages and disadvantages; we will discuss them in the further sections.

4.6.1 P-N JUNCTION PHOTODIODES

The most common device, which is based on the photovoltaic phenomenon, is a p-n junction produced
in a semiconductor. This device is called a photodiode and its principle of operation is presented
in Figure 4.34. Photons with energy greater than the energy gap, incident on the front surface of
the device, create electron-hole pairs in the material on both sides of the junction. By diffusion, the
electrons and holes generated within a diffusion length from the junction reach the space-charge
region. Then electron-hole pairs are separated by the strong electric field; minority carriers are
readily accelerated to become majority carriers on the other side. In this way, a photocurrent is

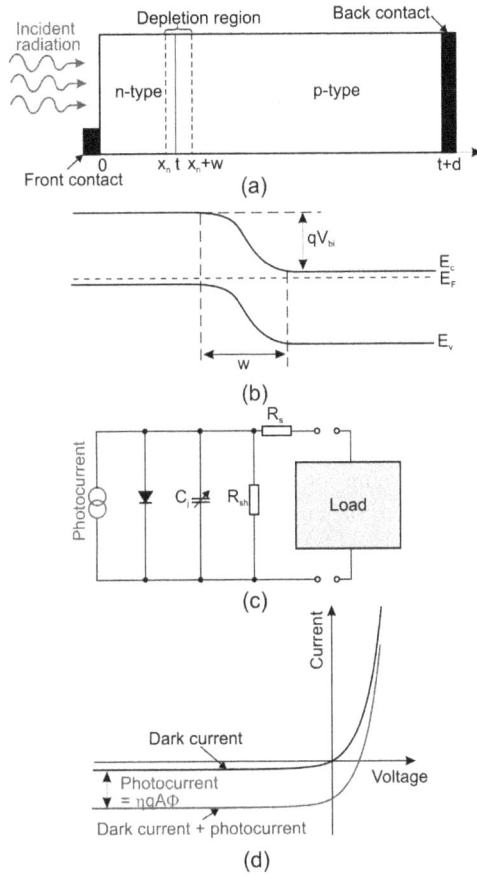

FIGURE 4.34 p-n junction photodiode: (a) geometrical structure of an abrupt junction, (b) energy band diagram, (c) equivalent circuit of a photodiode, and (d) current-voltage characteristics of an illuminated and nonilluminated photodiode.

generated causing a vertical shift of the current-voltage characteristic of the photodiode towards the negative current, as shown in Figure 4.34(d).

It can be shown that in the case of a step junction in the charge region, the built-in electric potential [see Figure 4.34(b)] is determined by the following equation [37]:

$$V_{bi} = \frac{kT}{q} \ln\left(\frac{N_a N_d}{n_i^2} \right),\tag{4.72}$$

where N_a and N_d are the concentrations of acceptors and donors in the p-type and n-type area and n_i is the intrinsic concentration.

The equivalent circuit of a photodiode is shown in Figure 4.34(c), where R_{sh} is the shunt resistance of a photodiode, C_j is the junction capacitance, R_s is the series resistance and R_L is the load resistance. For practical purposes, R_s is much smaller than the load resistance R_L and, for this, can be neglected.

The total current density in the p-n junction can be presented as follows:

$$J(V,\Phi) = J_d(V) - J_{ph}(\Phi),$$ (4.73)

where the dark current density $-J_d$ depends only on V_b and the photocurrent depends only on the photon flux density Φ.

In general, a current gain in a typical photovoltaic detector is equal to 1 (it can be much higher, i.e., in the avalanche photodiode) and then, according to Eq. (4.57), the magnitude of photocurrent equal

$$I_{ph} = \eta q A \Phi.$$ (4.74)

Dark current and photocurrent are linearly independent, even when these currents are significant. If a p-n diode is open-circuited, accumulation of electrons and holes on two sides of the junction produce an open-circuit voltage (Figure 4.34(d)). A current will be conducted in the circuit, if a load is connected to the diode. The maximum current is achieved when an electrical short is placed across diode terminals, which is called the short-circuit current.

Open-circuit voltage can be obtained by multiplying a short-circuit current by the incremental diode resistance $(\partial I / \partial V)^{-1}$ at $V = V_b$ in the following equation

$$V_{ph} = \eta q A \Phi R,$$ (4.75)

where V_b is the bias voltage and $I = f(V)$ is the current-voltage characteristic of a photodiode.

In many direct applications the photodiode is operated at zero-bias voltage as follows:

$$R_0 = \left(\frac{\partial I}{\partial V} \right)^{-1}_{\Big|_{V_b=0}}.$$ (4.76)

A frequently encountered figure of merit for a photodiode is the $R_0 A$ product:

$$R_0 A = \left(\frac{\partial J}{\partial V} \right)^{-1}_{\Big|_{V_b=0}},$$ (4.77)

where $J = I/A$ is the current density.

In radiation detection, the photodiode is operated at any point of a I-V characteristic. Reverse bias operation is usually used for very high-frequency applications to reduce the RC time constant of the devices (C strongly depends on the bias voltage).

Diffusion current is a fundamental current mechanism in a p-n junction photodiode. Figure 4.34(a) presents a one-dimensional photodiode model with an abrupt junction, where the width of spatial charge, w, surrounds the metallographic junction boundary $x = t$, and then, two quasi-neutral regions $(0, x_n)$ and $(x_n+w, t+d)$ are homogeneously doped. The dark current density consists of the electrons injected from the n-side over a potential barrier into the p-side and the analogous current due to holes injected from the p-side into the n-side. Current-voltage characteristic for an ideal diffusion-limited diode is given by the following equation:

$$I_D = AJ_s \left[\exp\left(\frac{qV}{kT}\right) - 1 \right], \tag{4.78}$$

where the saturation current density, J_s, is a complex function of many parameters such as concentration of minority carriers on both sides of the junction, surface recombination velocities at the illuminated surface (for holes in the n-type material), back photodiode surface (for electrons in the p-type material), as well as minority carriers' diffusion lengths and minority carriers' diffusion coefficients, on both sides of the junction. Detailed equations determining the saturation current density are derived in Reference 13.

For a junction with thick quasineutral regions [$x_n \gg L_h$, $(t+d-x_n-w) \gg L_e$], the saturation current density equals

$$J_s = \frac{qD_h p_{no}}{L_h} + \frac{qD_e n_{po}}{L_e}, \tag{4.79}$$

and when the Boltzmann statistic is valid, [$n_o p_o = n_i^2$, $D = (kT/q)\mu$ and $L = (D\tau)^{1/2}$], we obtain

$$J_s = \left(kT\right)^{1/2} n_i^2 q^{1/2} \left[\frac{1}{p_{po}}\left(\frac{\mu_e}{\tau_e}\right)^{1/2} + \frac{1}{n_{no}}\left(\frac{\mu_h}{\tau_h}\right)^{1/2} \right]^{-1}, \tag{4.80}$$

where p_{po} and n_{no} are the hole and electron majority carrier concentrations, τ_e and τ_h are the electron and hole lifetimes in p- and n-type regions, respectively. Diffusion current varies with temperature as n_i^2.

Resistance at zero bias can be obtained from Eq. (4.78) by a differentiation of I-V characteristics:

$$R_0 = \frac{kT}{qI_s}, \tag{4.81}$$

and, thus, the R_0A product determined by a diffusion current is as follows:

$$\left(R_0 A\right)_D = \left(\frac{dJ_D}{dV}\right)^{-1}_{V_b=0} = \frac{kT}{qJ_s}. \tag{4.82}$$

Assuming Eq. (4.80), the R_0A product is presented by the following equation:

$$\left(R_0 A\right)_D = \frac{\left(kT\right)^{1/2}}{q^{3/2} n_i^2} \left[\frac{1}{n_{n0}}\left(\frac{\mu_h}{\tau_h}\right)^{1/2} + \frac{1}{p_{p0}}\left(\frac{\mu_e}{\tau_e}\right)^{1/2} \right]^{1/2}, \tag{4.83}$$

for a diode with thick regions on both sides of the junction.

Three regions contribute to the photodiode quantum efficiency: two neutral regions of different conductivity types and the spatial charge region, η_{DR}:

$$\eta = \eta_n + \eta_{DR} + \eta_p. \tag{4.84}$$

The individual components of quantum efficiency are defined in Reference 38.

Usually, the photodiode is constructed in such a way that most of incident radiation can be absorbed on one side of the junction, for example, on the p-type side of Figure 4.34(a). This can be achieved in two ways: if the photodiode illuminated area is sufficiently thin or by using a heterojunction in which the illuminated area of the n type has a greater energy gap and most of the radiation reaches the junction area.

If the back contact is several lengths of the diffusion path L_e, the quantum yield is as follows:

$$\eta(\lambda) = (1-r)\frac{\alpha(\lambda)L_e}{1+\alpha(\lambda)L_e}. \tag{4.85}$$

If, on the other hand, the rear contact is at a distance shorter than the diffusion length, then:

$$\eta(\lambda) = (1-r)\left[1 - e^{-\alpha(\lambda)d}\right], \tag{4.86}$$

where d is the thickness of the p-type region. In these considerations it is assumed that the back contact has zero surface recombination and the radiation is not reflected from the back contact.

4.6.2 REAL PHOTODIODES

In the above paragraph, we considered an ideal photodiode with a diffusion nature of current carrier transport. However, this behaviour cannot always be observed in practice, especially for wide-gap p-n junctions. Dark current-voltage characteristics of the photodiode can be determined by several additional excess mechanisms as a superposition of current contributions from three diode regions which are bulk, depletion region, and surface. We can distinguish among them:

1. Thermally generated current in the bulk and the depletion region:
   - diffusion current in bulk p and n regions;
   - generation-recombination current in depletion region;
   - band-to-band tunnelling;
   - inter-trap and trap-to-band tunnelling;
   - anomalous avalanche current; and
   - ohmic leakage across depletion region.
2. Surface leakage current:
   - surface generation current from surface states;
   - generation current in a field-induced surface depletion region;
   - tunnelling induced near the surface;
   - ohmic or nonohmic shunt leakage; and
   - avalanche multiplication in a field-induced surface region.
3. Space charge-limited (SCL) current.

Figure 4.35 presents a scheme of these mechanisms [13]. Each component has its own individual relationship with voltage and temperature. In the subsequent sections, we will consider the current contribution of high-quality photodiodes with high $R_o A$ products limited by

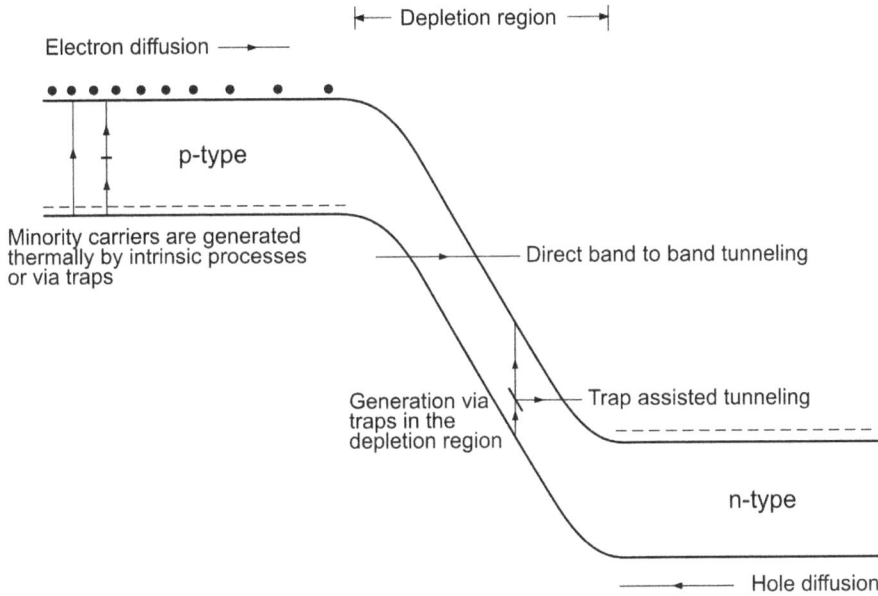

FIGURE 4.35   Schematic illustration of the main mechanisms contributing to the dark current in a reverse biased p-n junction.

- generation-recombination within depletion region;
- tunnelling through depletion region; and
- surface effects.

4.6.2.1   Generation-recombination Current

The generation-recombination current (g-r) in a depletion region can be much greater than the diffusion current, especially at low temperature. Width of the space charge region is, however, much smaller than the minority carrier diffusion length. In reverse bias, the current can be obtained by

$$I = qG_{dep} V_{dep},$$

(4.87)

where G_{dep} is the generation rate and V_{dep} is the volume of the depletion region. The generation rate from traps in the depletion region is particularly given by Shockley–Read–Hall (SRH) equation:

$$G_{dep} = \frac{n_i^2}{n_1 \tau_{eo} + p_1 \tau_{ho}},$$

(4.88)

where n_1 and p_1 are the electron and hole concentrations which could be obtained if the Fermi energy is at the trap energy, also, τ_{eo} and τ_{ho} are the lifetimes in strong n-type and p-type materials. If one of the terms in the denominator of Eq. (4.88) dominates, and for the case of a trap at the intrinsic level $p_1 = n_i$, we can obtain

$$G_{dep} = \frac{n_i}{2\tau_o},$$ (4.89)

and the depletion region g-r current equals

$$J_{GR} = \frac{qwn_i}{2\tau_o}.$$ (4.90)

The comparison of Eqs. (4.80) and (4.90) indicates that the generation rate in the bulk material is proportional to n_i^2, whereas the generation rate in the depletion region is proportional to n_i for a mid-gap state. It follows that the temperature dependence of the g-r current is much weaker than that of the diffusion component, given that $n_i \sim exp(E_g / 2kT)$.

The depletion region width and its volume increase with a reverse voltage. For an abrupt junction, we obtain as follows:

$$w = \sqrt{\frac{2\varepsilon_o \varepsilon_r \left(V_{bi} \pm V_b\right)}{qN_a N_d \left(N_a + N_d\right)}},$$ (4.91)

where N_a and N_d are the acceptor and donor concentrations, respectively. $V_{bi} = (kT/q)\ln(N_a N_d / n_i^2)$ is the built-in voltage and V_b is the applied voltage. Often, one side of the junction is degenerate. For the linearly graded junction, the depletion region width depends on $V_b^{1/3}$.

The theoretical basis of the g-r current generation mechanism was developed by Sah, Noyce and Shockley in 1957 [39], and this theory has been successfully applied to the present day. According to their theory, the doping levels were assumed to be the same on the two sides of the junction, and a single recombination centre located in the gap vicinity was assumed, as well. The g-r current density under reverse-bias voltage, and forward-bias voltage values being less than V_b by several kT/q, was derived as follows:

$$J_{GR} = \frac{qn_i w}{(\tau_{eo}\tau_{ho})^{1/2}} \frac{2sh\left(qV_b / 2kT\right)}{q\left(V_{bi} - V_b\right)/kT} f(b),$$ (4.92)

where τ_{eo}, τ_{ho} are the carrier lifetimes with the depletion region. The function $f(b)$ is a complex expression dependent on the energy of the recombination centre and the bias voltage, and has a maximum value of $\pi/2$, and is often assumed to be 1.

The $R_0 A$ product determined by g-r current has the form of

$$(R_0 A)_{GR} = \left(\frac{dJ_{GR}}{dV}\right)_{V=0}^{-1} = \frac{V_b (\tau_{eo}\tau_{ho})^{1/2}}{qn_i wf(b)}.$$ (4.93)

Further we assume $\tau_{ho} = \tau_{eo} = \tau_o$, $E_t = E_i$ and $f(b) = 1$. Then, Eq. (4.93) becomes as follows:

$$(R_o A)_{GR} = \frac{V_b \tau_o}{q n_i w}.$$ (4.94)

In Eq. (4.94) the greatest uncertain value is τ_o.

4.6.2.2 Tunnelling Current

The third type of dark current component existing is a tunnelling current caused by electrons directly tunnelling across the junction, from the valence band to the conduction band (direct tunnelling) or by electrons indirectly tunnelling across the junction via intermediate trap sites in the junction region – direct tunnelling or trap-assisted tunnelling (TAT); (see Figure 4.35). Usual direct tunnelling calculations assume a particle of a constant effective mass incident on a triangular or parabolic potential barrier. For a triangular potential barrier, we obtain [37]:

$$J_T = \frac{q^2 E V_b}{4\pi^2 \hbar^2} \left(\frac{2m^*}{E_g} \right)^{1/2} \exp\left[-\frac{4(2m^*)^{1/2} E_g^{3/2}}{3q\hbar E} \right].$$ (4.95)

For an abrupt p-n junction, the electric field can be approximated by the following equation:

$$E = \left[\frac{2q}{\varepsilon_o \varepsilon_s} \left(\frac{E_g}{q} \pm V_b \right) \frac{np}{n+p} \right]^{1/2}.$$ (4.96)

The tunnel current is considered to have an extremely strong dependence on energy gap, applied voltage, and an effective doping concentration $N_{ef} = np/(n + p)$. However, it is relatively insensitive to a temperature variation and the shape of the junction barrier. For the parabolic barrier, we obtain [37]

$$J_T \propto \exp\left[-\frac{(\pi m^*)^{1/2} E_g^{3/2}}{2^{3/2} q\hbar E} \right].$$ (4.97)

The indirect tunnelling mechanism is more complex. That is a two-step process in which one step is a thermal transition between one of the bands and the trap, and the second step is a tunnelling between the trap and the other band. The tunnelling process occurs at lower fields than a direct band-to-band (BBT) because electrons have a shorter distance to the tunnel (see Figure 4.35). More information on this subject can be found in Reference 13.

4.6.2.3 Surface Leakage Current

In a real p-n junction, in wide-gap semiconductors and at low temperatures in particular there occurs an additional dark current related to the surface. Surface phenomena play an important part in determining the photovoltaic detector performance. The surface provides a discontinuity resulting in a large density of interface states. These states generate minority carriers by the SRH mechanism and can increase both diffusion and depletion region-generated currents. Surface can also have a net charge affecting the depletion region position at the surface.

In order to eliminate, at least partially, the influence of leakage currents, the p-n junction surface is passivated. The aim is to ensure that coating of the passivating layer (usually native oxides) does not introduce changes in the junction band structure, and that bands on the boundary surface of the semiconductor-passive layer are flat. For silicon, SiO_2 is the ideal oxide.

G-R kinetics through fast surface states is identical to the one through bulk SRH centres. The current in a surface channel is given by the equation:

$$I_{GRS} = \frac{qn_i w_c A_c}{\tau_o},$$

(4.98)

where w_c is the channel width and A_c is the channel area.

Summarising the above discussion, for a well-passivated p-n junction, we can assume that the dark current

$$I_{dark} = I_{diff} + I_{gr} + I_{btb} + I_{tat} + I_{Rsh},$$

(4.99)

can be found as a superposition of diffusion (I_{diff}), generation-recombination (I_{gr}), band-to-band tunnelling (I_{btb}), and trap-assisted tunnelling (I_{tat}) currents. The remaining mechanism is current due to the shunt resistance I_{Rsh}, which originates from surface and bulk leakage current and shows the presence in the reverse-bias region. Possible currents that operate in the photodiode are shown in Figure 4.36. The avalanche current, which occurs in diodes with large depletion widths, and a high reverse bias voltage is omitted in our considerations.

In many practical analyses of I-V characteristics, the dominant mechanism determining their character is decisive. However, this approach is not always right. A better solution is a numerical analysis of individual current components summing them up for comparison with experimental data over a wide range of bias voltage and operating temperature. The latter method of the current component analysis is shown in Figure 4.37(a) for the p-and-n photodiode from the InAs/GaSb superlattice at 160 K, with a long-wave sensitivity limit of about 5 μm. Figure 4.37(b) shows the dependence of the R_0A product as a function of the bias voltage coupled with Figure 4.37(a) by the differentiation operation [see Eq. (4.77)].

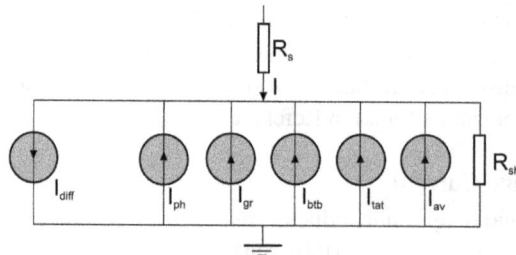

FIGURE 4.36 Possible currents operating in the photodiode. I_{diff} is ideal diffusion current, I_{ph} is the photocurrent, I_{gr} is due to generation-recombination mechanism, I_{btb} is due to band-to-band tunnelling, I_{tat} is due to trap-to-band tunnelling, I_{av} is the avalanche current, and R_{shunt} is due to surface and bulk leakage shunt resistance. Limiting currents act in opposition to diffusion current.

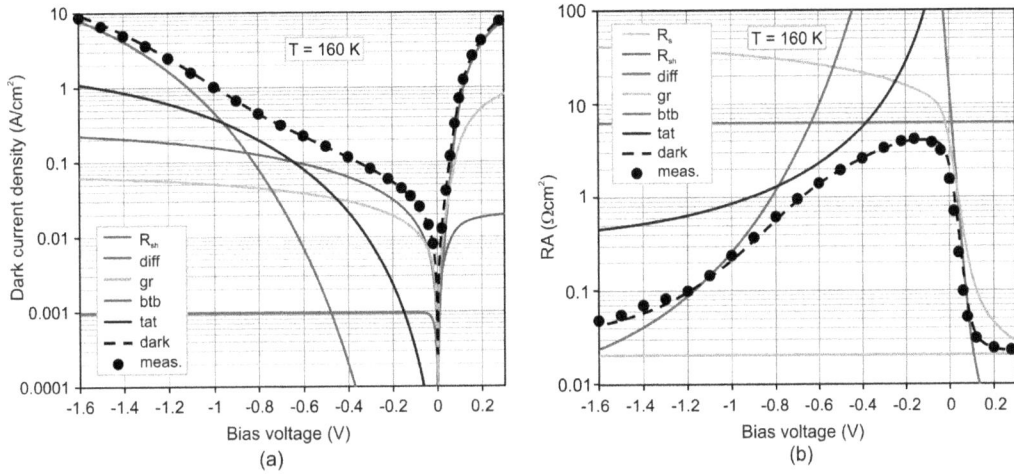

FIGURE 4.37 Measured and modelled characteristics of MWIR p-i-n InAs/GaSb type-II superlattice photodiode ($\lambda_c \approx 5$ μm) at a temperature 160 K: the dark current density (a) and the resistance area product (b) versus bias voltage (after Reference 40).

4.6.3 RESPONSE TIME

The upper-frequency response of a photodiode can be determined by three effects:

- time of carrier diffusion to the junction depletion region, τ_d;
- transit time of carrier drift across the depletion region, τ_s; and
- RC time constant associated with circuit parameters, including the junction capacitance C and the parallel combination of diode resistance and external load (the series resistance is neglected).

The response time of a photodiode can be determined from the following relationship:

$$\tau_{tot} = \left(\tau_d^2 + \tau_s^2 + \tau_{RC}^2 \right)^{1/2}. \tag{4.100}$$

The diode parameters responsible for these three factors are as follows: absorption coefficient α, width of the area of depletion region w_{dep}, junction capacitance C_d, preamplifier input capacitance C_a, load resistance R_L, preamplifier input resistance R_a, and series resistance R_s (see Figure 4.38).

Photodiodes designed for a fast response are generally constructed in a way so that the radiation absorption occurs in the p-type region. This fact ensures that most of photocurrent is carried by electrons being more mobile than holes (by diffusion or drift).

Assuming that the diffusion length is greater than both diode thickness and absorption depth, the cut-off frequency where the response drops by 2, is given by the following equation [13]:

$$f_{diff} = \frac{2.43D}{2\pi t^2}, \tag{4.101}$$

where D is the diffusion constant, and t is the diode thickness.

The depletion region transit time equals

$$\tau_t = \frac{w_{dep}}{v_s},$$

(4.102)

where w_{dep} is the depletion region width and v_s is the carrier saturation drift velocity in the junction field, which has a value of about 10^7 cm/s. For example, assuming typical parameters: $\mu_e = 10^4$ cm²/Vs, $v_s = 10^7$ cm/s, $\alpha = 5 \times 10^3$ cm^{-1} and $w_{dep} = 1$ μm, transit time, as well as diffusion time are of about 10^{-11} s.

Diffusion processes are generally slow in comparison with a drift of carriers in the high-field region. Therefore, in order to have a high-speed photodiode, the photocarriers should be generated in the depletion region or close to it, so that diffusion times are less than (or equal) to the carrier drift times.

If a photodiode capacitance is larger, response time becomes limited by an RC time constant of the load resistor R_L and the photodiode capacitance:

$$\tau_{RC} = \frac{AR_T}{2} \left(\frac{q\varepsilon_o \varepsilon_s N}{V} \right)^{1/2}.$$

(4.103)

$R_T = R_{sh}(R_s + R_L)/(R_s + R_{sh} + R_L)$, where R_s, R_d and R_L are the series, diode, and load resistances. The detector behaves approximately like a simple RC low-pass filter with a 3-dB bandwidth given by the following equation:

$$\Delta f = \frac{1}{2\pi R_T C_T}.$$

(4.104)

Generally, R_T is the combination of a load and amplifier resistance, and C_T is the sum of a photodiode and amplifier capacitance (see Figure 4.38).

The p-n photodiode has two major drawbacks. Its depletion layer capacitance is not small enough to allow for photodetection at high modulation frequencies. Capacitance influences RC time constant. Secondly, its depletion layer is at most a few microns, meaning that the majority of long wavelength photons are absorbed outside the depletion layer with no field to separate and drift the electron-hole pairs. Thus, this fact has an impact on low quantum efficiency at these wavelengths. Those problems are reduced in a p-i-n photodiode.

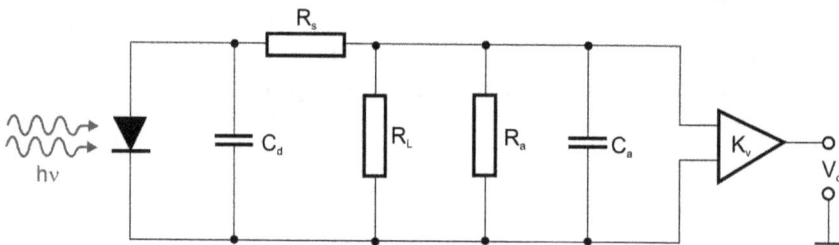

FIGURE 4.38 Equivalent circuit of an illuminated photodiode (the series resistance includes the contact resistance as well as the bulk p- and n-type regions).

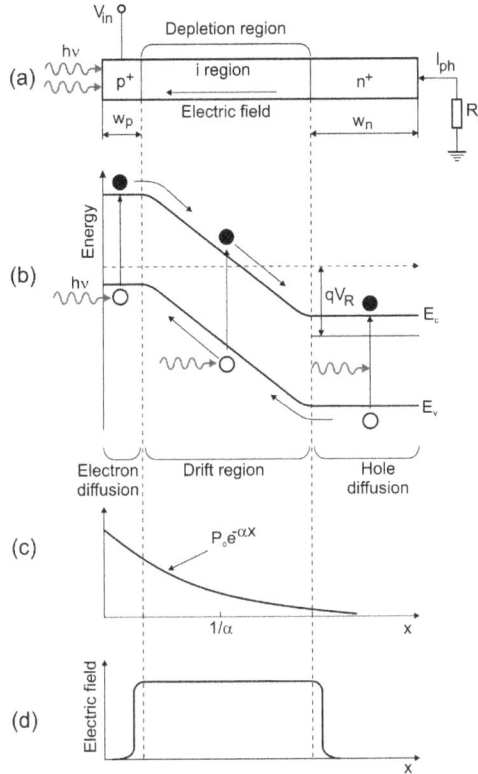

FIGURE 4.39 P-i-n photodiode: (a) geometry, (b) energy band diagram at reverse bias, (c) distribution of the excited carrier concentration, and (d) electric field profile.

4.7 P-I-N PHOTODIODES

P-i-n photodiodes, also called PIN, are currently the most popular light detectors in optical fibre systems. Figure 4.39 shows the schematic representation of a p-i-n diode, energy band diagram under reverse-bias conditions together with optical absorption characteristics. In these photodetectors, between n^+ and p^+ two strongly doped regions, there is a relatively wide (i.e., undoped) layer of conductivity similar to that of the intrinsic "i" one. The type "i" layer is an area with a high resistance compared to type p^+ and n^+ areas. Under normal operating conditions, the p-i-n photodiode is reverse biased. Almost all the voltage applied to the diode is deposited on the intrinsic layer, creating a strong electric field inside an almost constant value. Generally, for a doping concentration of $\sim 10^{14}$–10^{15} cm^{-3} in the intrinsic region, a bias voltage of 5–10 V is sufficient to deplete several micrometres, and the electron velocity reaches the saturation value as well.

Depending on the photon penetration depth, electron-hole pairs can be generated simultaneously in all three layers: p, i, n. Electrons and holes are generated in the intrinsic layer and are quickly separated in a strong electric field and carried towards adjacent layers: electrons towards the n-type layer, holes towards the p-layer. Electrons produced in the p-type layer diffuse towards the p-i junction barrier. After crossing the barrier, they are lifted in the electric field of the barrier layer towards the n-type area. Holes produced in the n-type layer diffuse towards the i-n junction and then in the barrier layer are lifted by the electric field towards the p-type region.

The p-i-n photodiode has a "controlled" depletion layer width, which can be tailored to meet the requirements of photoresponse and bandwidth. A trade-off is necessary between response speed and quantum efficiency. For high response speed, the depletion layer width should be small, but for high quantum efficiency (or responsivity) the width should be large. An external resonant microcavity approach has been proposed to enhance quantum efficiency in such a situation [21]. In this approach the absorption region is placed inside a cavity so that a large portion of the photons can be absorbed even with small detection volume.

Two generic p-i-n photodiodes, front-illuminated and back-illuminated are commonly used (see Figure 4.40). For practical applications, photoexcitation is provided through either an etched opening in the top contact, or an etched hole in the substrate. The latter reduces the active area of the diode to the size of the incident light beam. Sidewalls of mesas are covered using passivation materials such as polyimide. A compromise between quantum efficiency and response can be reached if the light is incident from the side, parallel to the junction as shown in Figure 4.40(d). The light can also be allowed to strike at an angle that creates multiple reflection inside the device, substantially increasing the effective absorption and quantum efficiency. This solution is often used to couple a detector with one-mode fibre.

The heterojunction structures [Figures 4.40(a,b)] are commonly used to improve photodiode performance. Development of modern epitaxial technologies (MBE and MOCVD) allows the use of the so-called gap engineering structures, which in turn enable the construction of optoelectronic devices with more optimal performance parameters: lower dark current and higher quantum efficiency.

For the 1.0–1.55-µm wavelength range suitable for optical communications, Ge and a few III-V compound semiconductor alloys are materials for p-i-n photodiodes, primarily because of their large absorption coefficients (see Figure 4.22). Typical p-i-n photodiode responsivities as a function of wavelength in a NIR spectral region are shown in Figure 4.41 [41]. Representative values are 0.65 A/W for silicon at 900 nm and 0.45 A/W for germanium at 1.3 µm. For InGaAs, typical values are 0.9 A/W at 1.3 µm and 1.0 A/W at 1.55 µm. At present, III-V semiconductors have largely replaced germanium as materials for fibre optical compatible detectors. Due to small bandgap, the dark current of Ge photodiodes degrades the signal-to-noise ratio. Also, passivation technique for Ge photodiodes is not satisfactory. Table 4.6 compares the performance values for p-i-n photodiodes derived from various vendor data sheets.

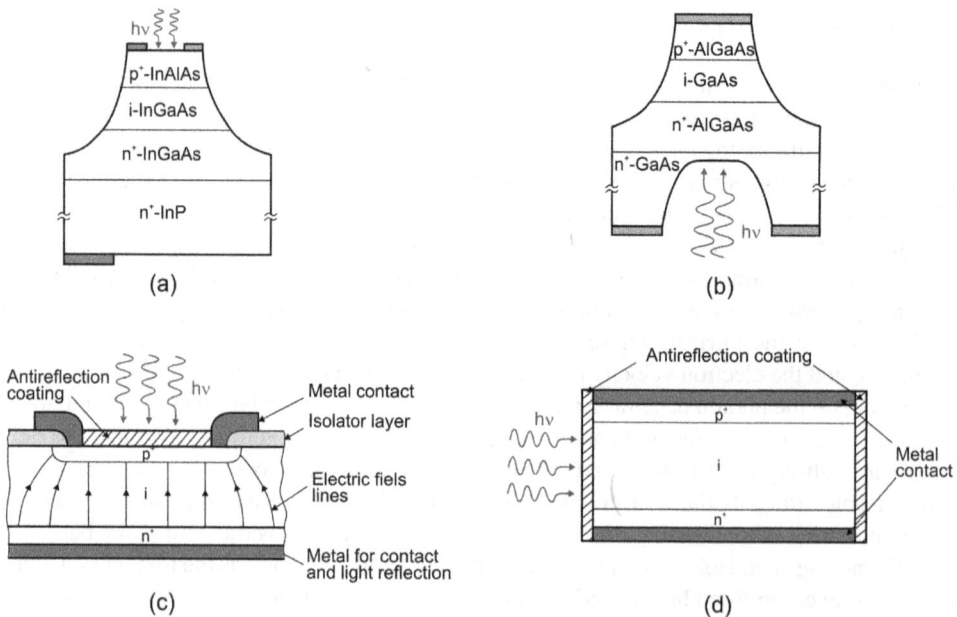

FIGURE 4.40 Device configurations of p-i-n photodiodes: (a) front-illuminated mesa, (b) back-illuminated mesa, (c) front-illuminated planar, and (d) parallel-illuminated planar.

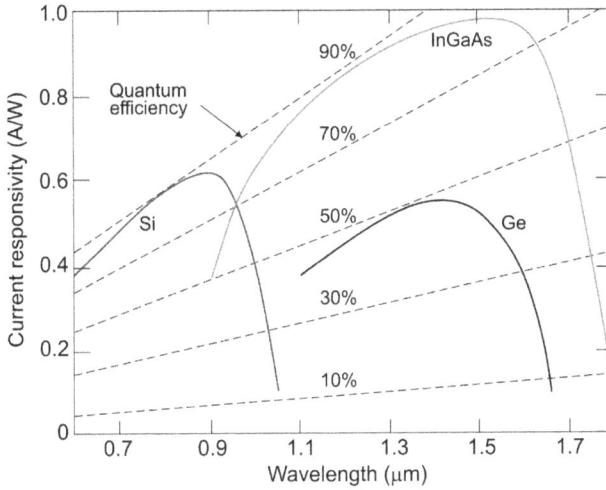

FIGURE 4.41 Comparison of the current responsivity and quantum efficiency as a function of wavelength for p-i-n NIR photodiodes.

TABLE 4.6
Summary of Si, Ge, and InGaAs p-i-n Photodiode Characteristics

Parameter	Si	Ge	InGaAs
Wavelength range (nm)	400–1100	800–1650	1100–1700
Peak wavelength (nm)	900	1550	1550
Current responsivity (A/W)	0.4–0.6	0.4–0.5	0.75–0.95
Quantum efficiency (%)	65–90	50–55	60–70
Dark current (nA)	1–10	50–500	0.5–2.0
Rise time (ns)	0.5–1	0.1–0.5	0.05–0.5
Bandwidth (GHz)	0.3–0.7	0.5–3	1–2
Bias voltage (–V)	5	5–10	5
Capacity (pF)	1.2–3	2–5	0.5–2

The principal source of noise in a p-i-n photodiode is g-r noise; it is larger than the Johnson noise, since the dark current in a reverse-biased junction is very low.

The response speed of a p-i-n photodiode is ultimately limited either by transit time or by circuit parameters. The transit time of carriers across the i-layer depends on its width and the carrier velocity. Usually, even for moderate reverse biases that carriers drift across the i-layer with saturation velocity. The transit time can be reduced by reducing the i-layer thickness. Fabricating the junction close to the illuminated surface can minimise the effect of diffusion of carrier created outside the i-layer. The additional passivation and antireflection layers reduce the surface recombination, which is particularly important in the case of a short-wave radiation detection.

The transit time of the p-i-n photodiode is shorter than that obtained in a p-n photodiode even though the depletion region is longer than in the p-n photodiode case due to carriers traveling at near their saturation velocity virtually the entire time they are in the depletion region (in p-n junction the electric field peaked at the p-n interface and then rapidly diminished). For p and n regions less than one diffusion length in thickness, the response time to diffusion alone is typically 1 ns/μm in p-type silicon and about 100 ps/μm in p-type III-V materials. The corresponding values for n-type III-V materials is several nanoseconds per micrometre due to the lower mobility of holes.

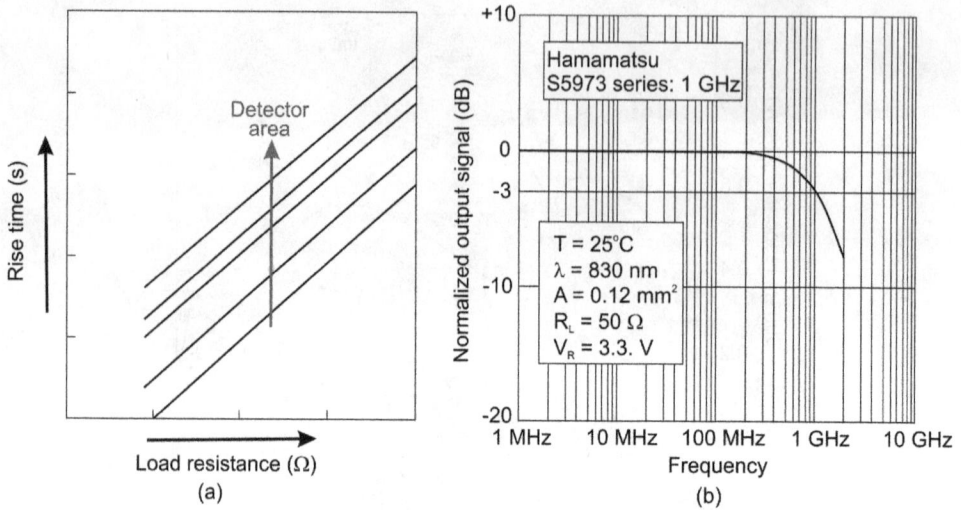

FIGURE 4.42 p-i-n photodiode characteristics: (a) the response time as a function of load resistance for different detector surfaces and (b) frequency characteristic (after Reference 43).

In most cases, the p-i-n photodiode response speed is limited by its capacity (which consists mainly of the diode junction capacity and the holder capacity) and the equivalent resistance [see Eq. (4.103)]. The photodiode response to a rectangular pulse depends on the relation between τ_{RC} constant, diffusion time of carriers τ_d, and transit time of carriers across the i-layer. For long diffusion times there is a clear distortion of both front and back of the pulse. The rise time depends also on photodiode area and load resistance [see Figure 4.42(a)]. As you can see from this figure, both area and load resistance increasing cause a significant increase of the photodiode rise time. Wherever high response rates are required, small load resistances and small area photodiodes should be used. For example, Figure 4.42(b) shows a normalised output signal of an S5973 type silicon photodiode as a function of frequency [42].

High-frequency photodiodes must have capacities of no more than a few picofarads (see Table 4.6). Reducing the photosensitive surface and increasing the reverse bias voltage reduce the voltage responsivity and detectivity. R_L photodiode load resistance also affects the value of voltage responsivity and detectivity. A low value of R_L reduces the value of voltage responsivity and detectivity. These parameters reach the highest values in operation without external load. Thus, a compromise between the photodiode response speed and its responsivity and detectivity is required.

4.8 AVALANCHE PHOTODIODES

For many years, a direct detection of low intensity light signals was possible thanks to the photomultiplier tube (PMT). Despite high sensitivity, a large active area, and amplification of even several million, they have a number of disadvantages: they are characterised by a limited dynamic range of operation and a low quantum efficiency, they work flawlessly in the presence of magnetic fields and have large dimensions and a delicate (not resistant to mechanical influences) construction.

The technology of avalanche photodiode (APD) production was mastered in the late 1960s. It was believed that they would replace photomultipliers. However, the avalanche photodiodes produced at that time were characterised by a very small photosensitive area, which practically limited their use only to detection elements mounted at the end of the optical fibre. Moreover, they were characterised by a low avalanche gain, rarely exceeding 100. In the following years APD structures were modified and improved. In the 1980s, avalanche photodiodes with a photosensitive area comparable to the area of photomultipliers and very good performance parameters were developed.

Avalanche photodiodes can detect an electromagnetic radiation of extremely low intensity. This is possible thanks to the phenomenon of impact ionisation, which allows for obtaining a high internal gain of the generated photocurrent. They are produced from silicon, germanium, III-V semiconductor compounds, the most popular of which is the ternary solid solution of InGaAs, and recently also II-VI compounds, of which the HgCdTe solid solution is the most important. Due to the ability to count single photons and detection in short time intervals, APD photodiodes are widely used in rangefinders, optical radar, and ultra-sensitive spectroscopy. Moreover, APD photodiodes compete with p-i-n photodiodes in optical telecommunications. They work mainly in ultraviolet, all visible range and near infrared spectra. Using scintillation crystals, it is possible to detect X-rays, gamma-rays (γ) or charged particles using APD.

The most common design of the avalanche photodiode is the p^+-π-p-n^+ structure presented in Figure 4.43. Radiation falling on the p^+ region is completely absorbed in the i-region, which leads to the generation of electrons and holes. Under the influence of the internal electric field, the carriers are separated. The holes move through the intrinsic layer and into the extreme p^+-type layer of the

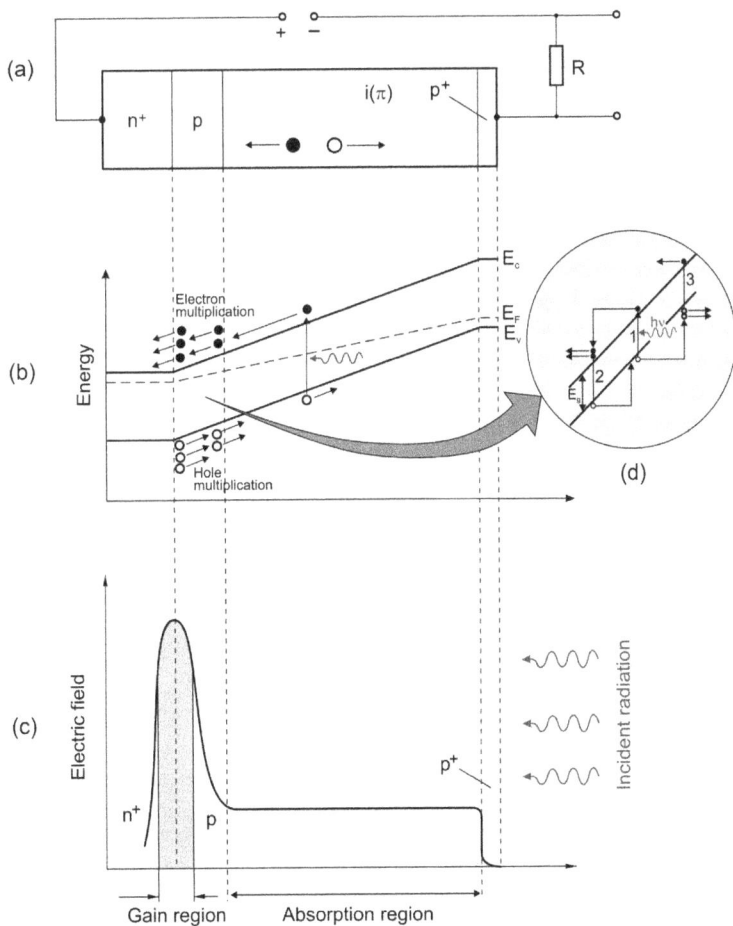

FIGURE 4.43 Avalanche p^+-π-p-n^+ photodiode: (a) structure, (b) energy band diagram, (c) electric field profile, and (d) schematic representation of the multiplication process.

photodiodes, while the electrons move towards the p-n junction. There is a very strong electric field in this junction as a result of applying a relatively high bias voltage to the p-n junction in the reverse direction. Electrons arriving from the absorber i-layer as a result of the existing electric field are rapidly accelerated. Avalanche ionisation occurs as a result of collisions with the semiconductor crystal lattice (in the p-n$^+$ junction area). This process provides new carriers and causes a rapid increase in current flowing in the reverse direction. This current can increase from several hundred to several thousand times. This is a phenomenon of internal signal amplification.

Quantity that characterises the photodiode is the ratio of total current to primary current called the avalanche multiplication factor M. It depends on the photodiode material, its construction, and operating conditions. In the avalanche photodiode, the current efficiency is M-times higher than in the case of a p-i-n photodiode.

The avalanche multiplication process is shown in Figure 4.43(d). A photon absorbed in point 1 creates an electron-hole pair. Under the effect of the strong electric field the electron accelerates. The acceleration process is constantly interrupted by random collisions with the lattice in which the electron loses some of its acquired energy. Those competing processes cause the electron to reach an average saturation velocity. The electron can gain enough kinetic energy which, upon collision with an atom, can break lattice bonds, creating the second electron hole pair. This is called impact ionisation (at point 2). Newly created electron and hole both acquire kinetic energy from the field and create additional electron hole pairs (e.g., at point 3). These, in turn, continue the process by creating other electron hole pairs. This process depends on a semiconductor structure and a lattice scattering (mainly optical phonons). It is thoroughly analysed in Reference [44].

Abilities of electrons and holes to create the phenomenon of collision ionisation are characterised by the ionisation coefficients α_e and α_h. These quantities represent ionisation probabilities per unit length. The ionisation coefficients increase with a depletion layer electric field and decrease with an increasing of the device temperature. The increase with the field is due to additional carrier velocity, while the decrease with temperature is due to an increase in nonionising collisions with thermally excited atoms. For a given temperature, the ionisation coefficients are exponentially dependent on the electric field and have a functional form of

$$\alpha = a\exp\left[-\left(\frac{b}{E}\right)^c\right],\qquad(4.105)$$

where a, b, c are experimentally determined constants, and E is the magnitude of an electric field.

Figure 4.44 presents the curves of α_e and α_h as a function of the electric field for several semiconductors important in APDs. As is presented, starting from a few 10^5 V/cm, the ionisation coefficients steeply increase with a small increase of the electric field, while for the field $< 10^5$ V/cm, ionisation is negligible in all the semiconductor compounds. In some semiconductors, electrons ionise more efficiently than holes (Si, GaAsSb, InGaAs, for which $\alpha_e > \alpha_h$), while in others the reverse is real (Ge, GaAs, where $\alpha_h > \alpha_e$).

An important parameter for characterising the APD performance is the ionisation ratio $k = \alpha_h/\alpha_e$. When holes do not ionise in the appreciable way (i.e., $\alpha_h \ll \alpha_e$; $k \ll 1$), most of the ionisation is achieved by electrons. An avalanching process proceeds then, principally from right to left (i.e., from the p side to n side) as presented in Figure 4.43(d). It terminates sometime later when all electrons arrive at the n side of the depletion layer. If electrons and holes both ionise appreciably ($k \approx 1$), on the other hand, these holes moving to the right create electrons moving to the left, which, in turn, generate further holes moving to the right, in a possibly continuous circuit.

Although this process increases the device gain (i.e., the total generated charge in the circuit per photocarrier pair), it is, however, undesirable for several reasons: it is time-consuming and, therefore, it reduces the device bandwidth. It is random and, therefore, it increases the device noise.

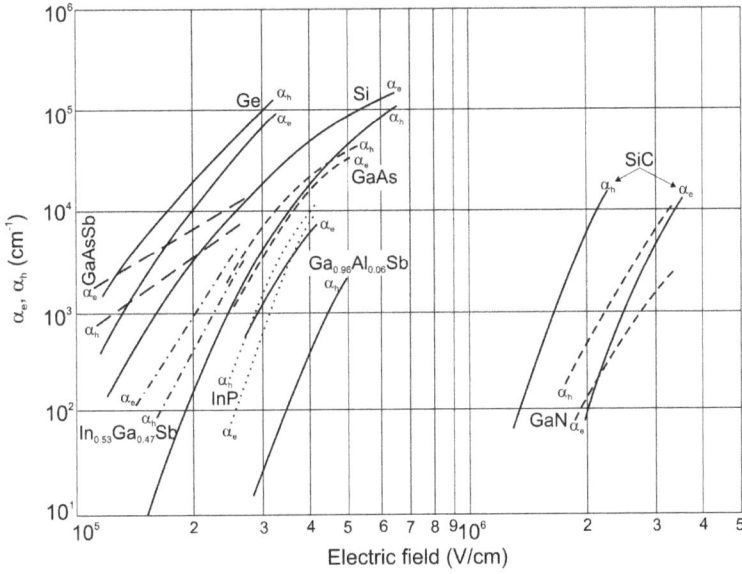

FIGURE 4.44 Ionisation coefficients of electrons (α_e) and holes (α_h) as a function of the electric field for some semiconductors used in avalanche photodiodes.

Also, it can be unstable, thereby causing an avalanche breakdown. Thus, it is desirable to manufacture APDs from materials that permit only one type of carrier (either electrons or holes) for the impact ionisation. If electrons have the higher ionisation coefficient, that is, an optimal behaviour is achieved by injecting the electron of a photocarrier pair at the p-edge of the depletion layer and by using the material which value of k is as low as possible. If holes are injected, the hole of a photocarrier pair should be injected at the n-edge of the depletion layer, and k should be as large as possible. The ideal case of a single carrier multiplication is achieved when $k = 0$ or ∞.

According to the local field model of the avalanche photodiode [45, 46], the mean square value of the noise current per unit bandwidth, assuming the mean value of M avalanche gain and I_{ph} photocurrent, has the form of

$$I_n^2 = 2qI_{ph}M^2F(M),\qquad(4.106)$$

where $F(M)$ is the excess noise factor associated with M that arises from a stochastic nature of the ionisation process.

Under the conditions of a homogeneous electric field and perfect electron ionisation, the excess noise factor can be described as

$$F_e\left(M_e\right) = kM_e + \left(1-k\right)\left(2 - \frac{1}{M_e}\right).\qquad(4.107)$$

This is similar for the case when holes initiate multiplication

$$F_h\left(M_h\right) = \frac{1}{k}M_h + \left(1 - \frac{1}{k}\right)\left(2 - \frac{1}{M_h}\right).\qquad(4.108)$$

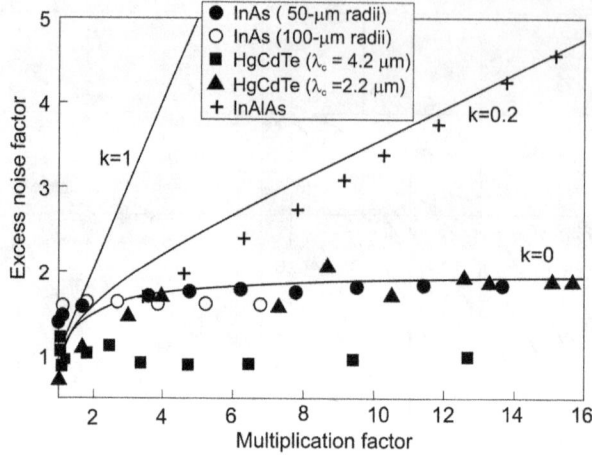

FIGURE 4.45   A comparison between the F_e reported on APDs of different materials including, InAs diodes with a 3.5-μm intrinsic width and radii of 50 μm and 100 μm, HgCdTe photodiodes with cut-off wavelengths of 4.2 μm and 2.2 μm and an InAlAs diode (after Reference 47).

As mentioned above, to achieve a low F, not only must α_e and α_h be as different as possible, but also the avalanche process must be initiated by carriers with the higher ionisation coefficient. According to McIntyre's rule, the noise performance of ADP can be improved by more than a factor of 10 when the ionisation ratio is increased to 5. Most of III-V semiconductors have $0.4 \leq k \leq 2$.

Figure 4.45 presents the excess noise factor versus the multiplication factor in InAs APDs and compares with data for different materials [47]. We notice that experimental data for some avalanche photodiodes (InAs and HgCdTe) fall slightly below the local model prediction for $k = 0$. It turns out that this model does not take into account "dead space" of the diode, where there is no impact ionisation [48]. If the avalanche multiplication area is much thicker than the "dead space" range, then the local field model is a good approximation of the multiplication phenomenon.

Summarising the discussion so far, it should be stated that the conditions for obtaining a small avalanche noise current is a large difference between the values of electrons and holes ionisation coefficients and the possibility of starting the avalanche process by carriers with a higher ionisation coefficient. In order to meet the second condition, in the avalanche photodiode, the photon absorption area is separated from the avalanche multiplication area of carriers, so that only carriers with a higher ionisation coefficient reach the multiplication area.

Taking into account the conditions of the photodiode making a technological process, it is easier to manufacture a detector with the structure opposite to that shown in Figure 4.43, namely n⁺-p-π-p⁺, when the radiation falls on the n^+ type contact layer. Figure 4.46 shows the cross-section of a silicon avalanche photodiode with an epiplanar n⁺-p-π-p⁺ type structure. In this construction the high resistivity absorption area (π type) is separated from the avalanche region – appropriately doped p-type region. Optically generated electron-hole pairs in the absorption area are separated by the region's high electric field. Holes are moved to a p⁺-type region and do not take part in the avalanche process. Electrons are directed into the avalanche region, where they undergo the multiplication process before they reach the n⁺-region. Next, they are registered in an external circuit as a multiplied photoelectric circuit. Generation of electron-pairs in the avalanche region also increases participation of holes in the avalanche process. However, the avalanche regions are 10 to 50 times smaller than the thickness of π region. Moreover, as holes are moved in the direction of the p⁺-region, only very small part of them will be multiplied. The avalanche region is surrounded by the n-type protective ring and the p⁺-type limiting ring that stops space charge at the SiO₂/Si interface. The photodiode active area is coated with an antireflection SiO₂. Inactive regions are coated with a silicon nitrate layer and

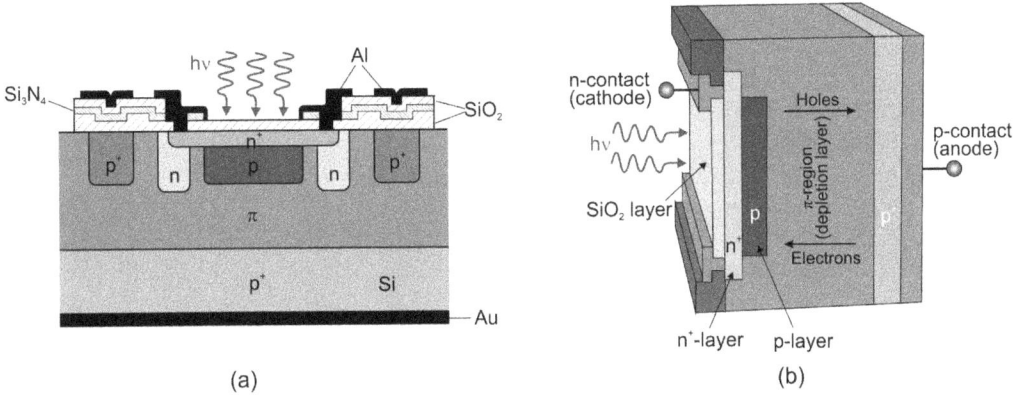

FIGURE 4.46   Silicon avalanche photodiode: (a) cross-section and (b)) spatial views.

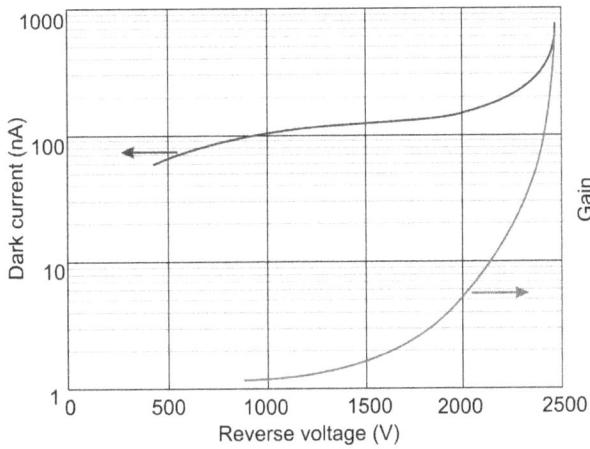

FIGURE 4.47   Typical dark current and gain (*M*) *vs.* reverse bias voltage for a silicon APD.

covered with aluminum. However, avalanche photodiodes of this type have worse noise properties in comparison with the construction p^+-π-p-n^+ presented in Figure 4.43.

In a well-designed and well-fabricated silicon avalanche photodiode, the dominant component of the dark current is the generation and recombination current, the part of which coming from the avalanche area is multiplied similarly to the photoelectric current. The avalanche photodiode output current after taking into account the gain *M* is equal $I_t = MI_{ph} + I_{dr}$, where dark current $I_{dr} = I_{ds} + I_{db}$, is the sum of two currents: surface leakage current I_{ds} and bulk leakage current I_{db}. The second component, I_{db}, is amplified in the same way as the signal current. However, for lower values of bias voltages, the proportion of the I_{ds} current in the total noise is much greater than the I_{db} bulk current. As the reverse bias voltage of the photodiode increases, the avalanche multiplication factor increases, and, thus, the proportion of the I_{db} current becomes dominant in the total current noise.

Figure 4.47 shows the example of a typical dark current and gain dependence on the reverse bias voltage for a silicon APD photodiode. Silicon avalanche photodiodes are characterised by a gain up to 1000 (for $I_n = 1$ pA/Hz$^{1/2}$), gain-bandwidth products above 100 GHz, applied bias above 400 V. *NEP* value achieved in the best photodiodes is over 10^{-14} W/Hz$^{1/2}$.

Two of the most important objectives in APD design are reduction of dark current and enhancement of device speed. In order to obtain the best performance, the device material in which avalanching occurs must be defect free. An essential problem in the device fabrication is the excessive leakage current at the junction edges. In Si APDs the common technique used to alleviate this problem is to incorporate a guard ring, which is an n-p junction created by selective-area diffusion around the periphery of the diode (see Figure 4.46). Very careful regulation of the detector bias is required for stable operation of APDs.

At present the following materials have proved to be appropriate for the fabrication of high-performance avalanche photodiodes (APDs):

- Silicon (for wavelengths of 0.4 to 1.1 μm). The electron ionisation rate is much higher than the hole ionisation rate ($\alpha_e \gg \alpha_h$);
- Germanium (for the wavelengths of up to 1.65 μm). Since the bandgap in Ge is lower than in Si, and the ionisation rates for electrons and holes are approximately equal ($\alpha_e \approx \alpha_h$), the noise is considerably higher, and this limits the applications of Ge-based APDs;
- GaAs based devices. Most compound materials have $\alpha_e \approx \alpha_h$, so designers usually use heterostructures like GaAs/Al$_{0.45}$Ga$_{0.55}$As, for which α_e(GaAs) $\gg \alpha_e$(AlGaAs). The large increase in gain occurs due to the avalanche effect that occurs in GaAs layers. GaAs/Al$_{0.45}$Ga$_{0.55}$As heterostructures are in spectral range below 0.9 μm. Applying InGaAs layers allows the sensitivity to extend to $\approx$ 1.4 μm;
- InP-based devices are used in the wavelength range of 1.2–1.6 μm. In double lattice-matched heterostructure n$^+$-InP/n-GaInAsP/p-GaInAsP/p$^+$-InP either of carriers are injected into the high field region – this structure is essential for low-noise operation. The second structure, p$^+$-InP/n-InP/n-InGaAsP/n$^+$-InP, is similar to the Si reach through devices. The absorption occurs in the relatively wide InGaAsP layers and avalanche multiplication of the minority carriers proceeds in the n-InP layer.
- Hg$_{1-x}$Cd$_x$Te APDs. These devices are electron-initiated, and their operation has been demonstrated for a broad range of compositions from $x = 0.7$ to 0.21 corresponding to cut-off wavelengths from 1.3 μm to 11 μm. Thus, HgCdTe APD at gain = 100 provides 10 to 20 times less noise than InGaAs or InAlAs APDs and 4 time less noise than Si APDs.

Table 4.7 lists the typical parameters of the most widely used avalanche photodiodes for Si, Ge and InGaAs.

TABLE 4.7
Summary of Si, Ge, and InGaAs Avalanche Photodiode Characteristics

Parameter	Si	Ge	InGaAs
Wavelength range (nm)	400–1100	800–1650	1100–1700
Peak wavelength (nm)	830	1300	1550
Current responsivity (A/W)	50–120	2.5–25	–
Quantum efficiency (%)	77	55–75	60–70
Avalanche gain	20–400	50–200	10–40
Dark current (nA)	0.1–1	50–500	10–50 ($M = 10$)
Rise time (ns)	0.1–2	0.5–0.8	0.1–0.5
Gain×Bandwidth (GHz)	100–400	2–10	20–250
Bias voltage (V)	150–400	20–40	20–30
Capacity (pF)	1.3–2	2–5	0.1–0.5

4.9   SCHOTTKY BARRIER PHOTODIODES

Schottky barrier photodiodes are used as light detectors in a wide spectral range from ultraviolet to far infrared. They are characterised by fabrication simplicity, absence of high-temperature diffusion processes, and high-speed response. Schottky barrier photodiodes use a thin translucent metal electrode (Figure 4.48) to form a potential barrier between the metal and the semiconductor (MS). The creation of a barrier at the MS joint is due to the difference in work function of both materials.

Metal electrodes are made of molybdenum, platinum, chromium, tungsten and silicides (e.g., palladium, titanium or platinum silicide), while the semiconductor layer is usually made of n-type silicon. In this case, the metal layer, 1–2-nm thick, replaces a p-type semiconductor in a typical p-n photodiode. If a metalwork function is greater than that of an n-type semiconductor, then more electrons tunnel from the semiconductor to the metal than from the metal to the semiconductor. As a result of this phenomenon, in the n-type area near the junction, there is depletion in electrons, while an excess of electrons appears in the metal. The barrier electric field plays the role of the spatial charge area of a p-n junction and causes a separation of generated carriers. In contrast to the p-n junction, where majority and minority current carriers participate in the current flow, in the Schottky barrier junction the participation of minority carriers in the current flow can be neglected.

Figure 4.49 shows four basic processes of a carrier transport in the n-type Schottky junction under forward bias:

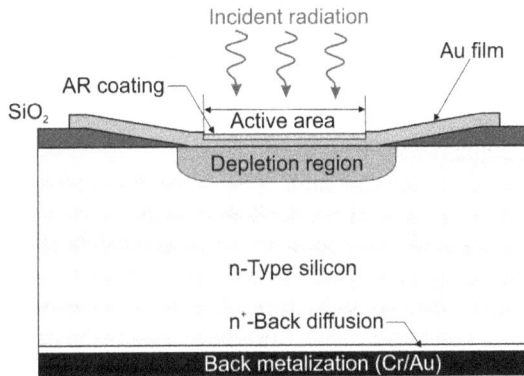

FIGURE 4.48   Example of a photodiode structure with a Schottky junction.

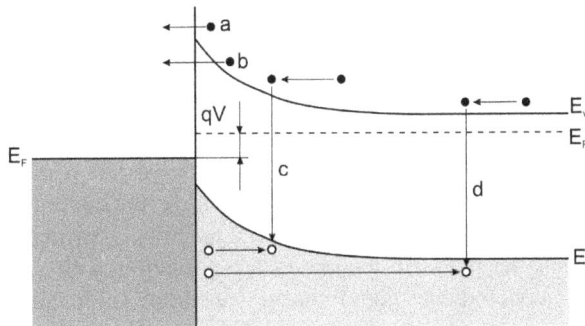

FIGURE 4.49   Four basic transport processes in the forward-biased Schottky barrier on an n-type semiconductor.

(a)   emission of electrons over a semiconductor to metal barrier;
(b)   quantum mechanical tunnelling of carriers through the barrier;
(c)   recombination in the space charge region; and
(d)   recombination in the neutral region (which is equivalent to injecting metal holes into a semiconductor).

Current flow through the metal-semiconductor contact is described by a thermo-emission mechanism above the Schottky junction if the concentration of donors (or acceptors) in the semiconductor does not exceed the level of about 10^{18} cm^{-3}. For higher doping concentrations, the tunnel current through the narrow barrier dominates.

The *I-V* characteristic of the Schottky junction, defined by the thermo-emission mechanism, is described by the following equation:

$$J_{MSt} = J_{st}\left[\exp\left(\frac{qV_b}{\beta kT}\right) - 1\right],$$ (4.109)

where the saturation current density equals

$$J_{st} = A^*T^2 \exp\left(-\frac{\phi_b}{kT}\right),$$ (4.110)

and $A^* = 4\pi q k^2 m^*/h^3$ equals $120(m^*/m)$ Acm^{-2}K^{-2} is the Richardson constant, m^* is the effective mass, ϕ_b is the potential barrier at the interface and β is an empirical constant close to unity. Equation (4.109) is similar to the transport equation for p-n junctions. However, the expressions for the saturation current densities are quite different.

The carrier transport theory in the Schottky barrier junction, initially based on Bethe thermo-emission theories and Schottky diffusion approaches, was generalised by Crowell and Sze in the thermodiffusion model. These and other theories are described in the excellent monograph by Sze [37].

Figure 4.50 shows the band structure of Schottky junctions as a photovoltaic detector. A photon with energy greater than the barrier height $q\phi_b$ is absorbed, causing the generation of an electron-hole pair which is then separated by the barrier electric field. The carriers then pass to a metal electrode or to a semiconductor, creating a photocurrent. A voltage develops across the Schottky junction device with the metal end positive and semiconductor end negative.

Now let us consider the advantages and disadvantages of photoconductive detectors, p-n junction, and Schottky junction photodiodes. An important advantage of photoresistors is their construction simplicity and a possible high photoelectric gain that directly affects the relaxation of preamplifier low noise requirements. Their disadvantage is the participation of recombination processes in noise. The advantages of p-n junctions are the following: low or zero bias voltage, high impedance, and high frequency capability. Also, compared to Schottky junctions, p-n junctions show advantages. The thermo-emission process in Schottky barriers is much more efficient than the diffusion process and, therefore, for a given built-in voltage, the saturation current in a Schottky diode is several orders of magnitude higher than in a p-n junction. Additionally, the built-in voltage of a Schottky diode is smaller than that the one of a p-n junction with the same semiconductor. However, the p-n junction photodiodes high frequency operation is limited by the minority-carrier storage problem.

Schottky-barrier structures are majority-carrier devices and, thus, they have inherently fast responses and large operating bandwidths. In other words, the minimum time required to dissipate

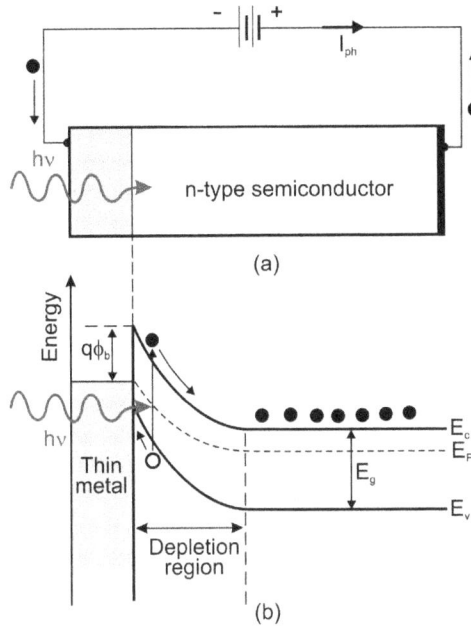

FIGURE 4.50   Metal-semiconductor photodiode: (a) photodiode geometry and (b) band structure.

carriers injected by the forward bias is dictated by the recombination lifetime. In a Schottky barrier electrons are injected from the semiconductor into the metal under forward bias if the semiconductor is n-type. Afterwards, they thermalise very rapidly ($\approx 10^{-14}$ s) by carrier–carrier collisions and that time is not relevant compared to the minority carrier-recombination lifetime. MS photodiodes are characterised by a very fast response rate. There are examples of photodiodes with bandwidths in excess of 100 GHz. Diode is usually operated under a reverse bias.

MS photodiodes are particularly useful in a detection of ultraviolet and visible radiation. In these spectral regions, the absorption coefficients of semiconductors (with wide bandgaps) are very large, of the order of 10^5 cm^{-1} or more (see Figure 4.22), which corresponds to an effective absorption length of $1/\alpha \approx 0.1$ µm or less. By selecting the appropriate metal and the appropriate anti-reflective coating, a large part of the incident radiation is absorbed near the semiconductor surface.

4.10   METAL-SEMICONDUCTOR-METAL PHOTODIODES

Metal-semiconductor-metal (MSM) photodiodes are made by forming two Schottky contacts on an undoped semiconductor layer [Figure 4.51(a)] [49]. This type of construction is characterised by a lower dark current compared to a single Schottky diode and a faster response speed compared to a p-i-n photodiode. Their bandwidth is in the order of hundreds of GHz. The high response speed of MSM photodiodes is due to a short distance between the contacts and, therefore, a short response time of the carriers. For Hamamatsu photodiodes, type G4176, the rise and fall times of the signal are 30 ps and the dark current is 100 pA, with a photosensitive surface of 0.2×0.2 mm^2 [50]. The disadvantage of this type of device is their low sensitivity (approx. 0.3 A/W). MSM photodiode is powered so that one contact is biased in the reverse direction, while the other contact is forward biased [Figure 4.51(b)].

Diagrams of the biased and unbiased energy band states are shown in Figures 4.52(a) and 4.52(b), respectively. At low biases, the electron injection at the reverse-biased contact dominates the conduction mechanism. At higher biases, the conduction is supplemented by the holes injection at

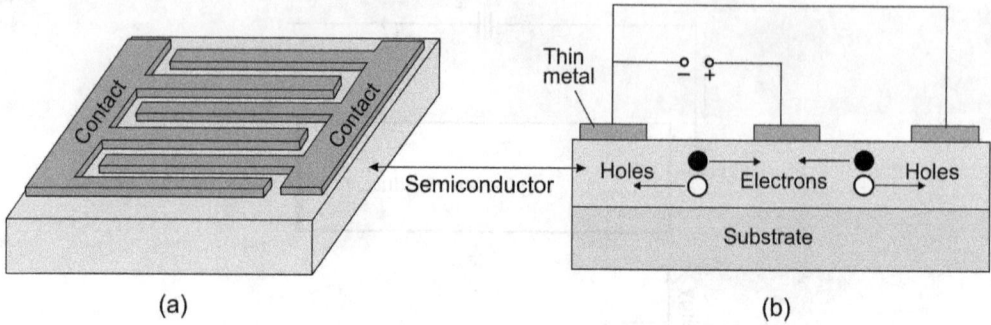

FIGURE 4.51   Metal-semiconductor-metal photodiode: (a) top view, (b) cross section structure.

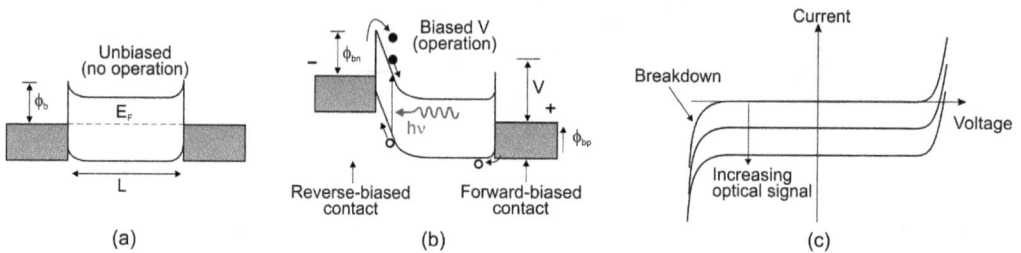

FIGURE 4.52   Metal-semiconductor-metal photodiode: (a) unbiased band diagrams, (b) biased band diagrams, and (c) current-voltage characteristics.

the forward-biased contact. The depletion region at the reverse-biased contact is much larger than the depleted region near the forward-biased contact, but upon meeting, the device is considered to achieve the "reach through" condition. Figure 4.52(c) presents the *I-V* characteristics for an MSM photodiode for three levels of illumination.

4.11   BARRIER PHOTODETECTORS

The first barrier detector was proposed by White in 1983 [51] as a high impedance photoconductor in which a HgCdTe heterostructure with a high-band gap barrier coupled, on both its sides, with two thin wide bandgap layers, that is, contact layer and absorber layer. However, this type of detector has not found a wider application because of the large barrier, so-called band offset resulting from the discontinuity of the heterostructure, for the flow of holes in the valence band.

The barrier detector concept assumes an almost zero one-band offset approximation throughout the heterostructure, allowing for the flow of only minority carriers in a photoconductor. Little or no valence band offset (VBO) was difficult to realise using standard IR detector materials such as InSb and HgCdTe. The situation has changed dramatically in the middle of the first decade of the twenty-first century after the introduction of 6.1 Å III-V material detector family, and when the first high-performance detectors (in InAs and InAsSb) [52,53], as well as FPAs were demonstrated. Unipolar barriers introduction in various designs based on type-II superlattices (T2SLs) drastically changed the IR detectors' architecture [54]. Generally, the unipolar barriers are used to implement the barrier detector architecture to increase the collection efficiency of photogenerated carriers and reduce a dark current generation without inhibiting photocurrent flow. The ability to tune the positions of conduction and valence band edges independently in a broken-gap T2SL is especially helpful in the unipolar barrier's design.

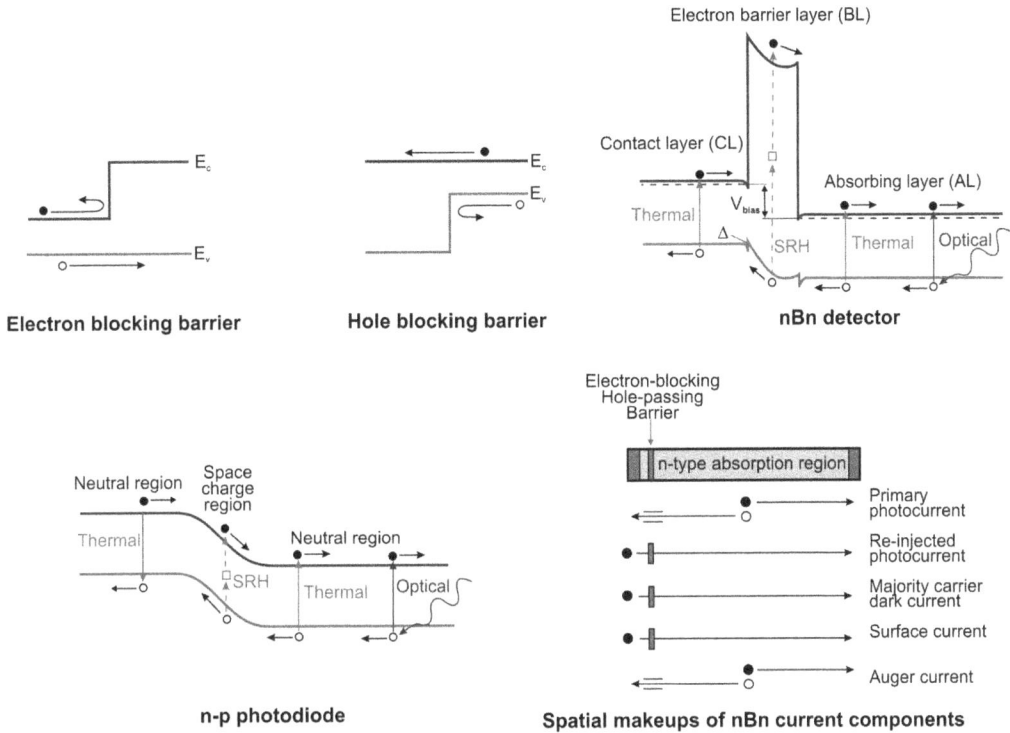

FIGURE 4.53 Illustrations of electron- and hole-blocking unipolar barriers, bandgap diagram of the nBn barrier detector (the valence-band offset, Δ, is shown explicitly), and p-n photodiode. The bottom right side of the nBn barrier detector shows spatial makeups of the various current components and barrier blocking.

The term "unipolar barrier" was coined to describe a barrier that can block one carrier type (electron or hole), but allows for the unimpeded flow of the other. Among different types of barrier detectors, the most popular is the nBn detector, shown in Figure 4.53. The n-type semiconductor on one side of the barrier constitutes a contact layer for device biasing, while the n-type narrow-bandgap semiconductor on the other side of the barrier is a photon-absorbing layer, the thickness of which should be comparable to the light-absorption length in the device, typically several microns.

Figure 4.53. Illustrations of electron- and hole-blocking unipolar barriers, the bandgap diagram of the nBn barrier detector (the valence-band offset, Δ, is shown explicitly), and p-n photodiode. The bottom right side of the nBn barrier detector shows spatial makeups of the various current components and barrier blocking.

The same doping type in the barrier and active layers is very important to maintain a low, diffusion-limited dark current. The barrier needs to be carefully engineered. It has to be nearly lattice matched to the surrounding material and to have zero offset in the one band and a large offset in the other. It should be placed near the minority carrier collector and away from the optical absorption region. Such barrier arrangement allows for photogenerated holes to flow to the contact (cathode) while majority carrier dark current, reinjected photocurrent, as well as surface current are blocked. Adequately, the nBn detector is designed to reduce the dark current (associated with SRH processes) and noise without impeding the photocurrent (signal). Especially, the barrier serves to reduce the surface leakage current because the benefit of the nBn architecture is self-passivation. The spatial makeups of the various current components and barrier blocking in the nBn detector are shown in the bottom right side of Figure 4.53 [55].

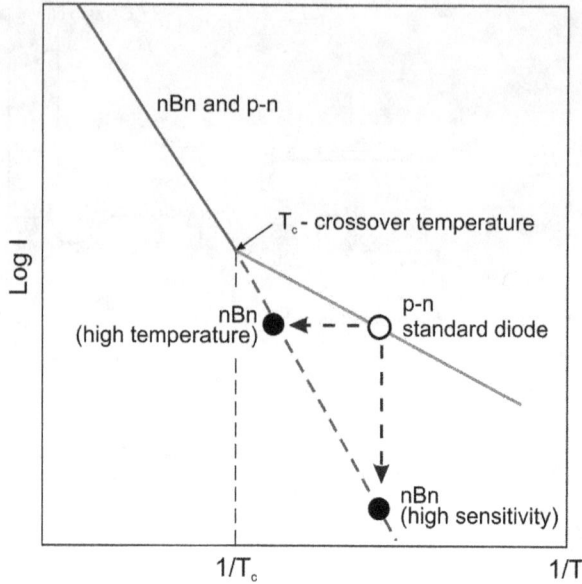

FIGURE 4.54 Schematic Arrhenius plot of the dark current in a standard diode and in an nBn device.

Kleipstein [56] defined criteria for a combination of bias voltage and barrier concentration allowing operation with no depletion region in a narrow-gap absorption layer. The valence band barrier is present for an n-type barrier (see Figure 4.53) that can considerably impede a hole current transport between the absorption layer and the contact layer, which can require large bias voltages to overcome. On the contrary a p-type barrier has no barrier, but rather a potential well for holes in the valence band, which does not impede hole transport between the absorption layer and the contact layer.

The nBn detector is essentially a "minority carrier photoconductor" with unity gain, due to the majority carrier flow absence, and in this regard is similar to a photodiode – the junction (space charge region) is replaced by the electron blocking unipolar barrier (B), and the p-contact is replaced by the n-contact. It can be stated that the nBn design is a hybrid between a photoconductor and a photodiode.

Figure 4.54 presents a typical Arrhenius plot of a dark current in a conventional diode and in an nBn detector. Diffusion current typically varies as $T^3\exp(-E_{g0}/kT)$, where E_{g0} is the band gap extrapolated to zero temperature, T is the temperature, and k is the Boltzmann constant. Generation–recombination current varies as $T^{-3/2}\exp(-E_{g0}/2kT)$ and is dominated by a generation of electrons and holes by SRH traps in the depletion region. Since in the nBn detector there is no depletion region, the generation–recombination contribution to the dark current from the photon-absorbing layer is totally suppressed. The lower portion of the Arrhenius plot for the standard photodiode has a slope that is roughly half of the upper portion. The solid line (nBn) is an extension of the high-temperature diffusion-limited region to temperatures below T_c, which is defined as a crossover temperature at which the diffusion and generation–recombination currents are equal. In a low-temperature region, the nBn detector offers two important advantages. First, it exhibits a higher signal-to-noise ratio than a conventional diode operating at the same temperature. Second, it operates at a higher temperature than a conventional diode with the same dark current. The latter is depicted by the horizontal dashed line in Figure 4.54.

Absence of a depletion region offers a way for materials with relatively poor SRH lifetimes, such as all III-V compounds, to overcome a disadvantage of large depletion dark currents. While the idea

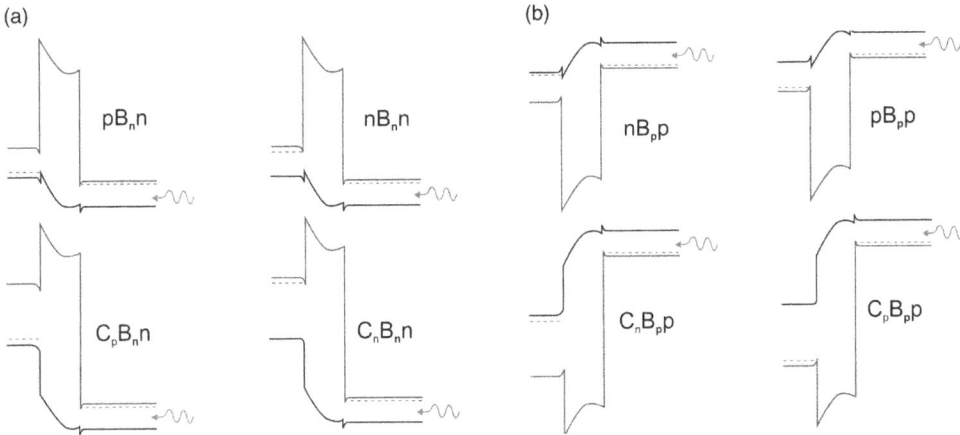

FIGURE 4.55 Schematic band profile configurations under operating bias for $XB_n n$ (a) and $XB_p p$ (b) barrier detector families. In each case, the contact layer (X) is on the left side, and the radiation is incident onto the active layer on the right side. When X is composed of the same material as the active layer, both layers have the same symbol (denoting the doping type), otherwise it is denoted as C (with the doping type as a subscript) (after Reference 57).

of nBn design has originated with bulk InAs materials [53], its demonstration using T2SL-based materials facilitates the experimental realisation of the barrier detector concept with a better control of band edge alignments.

Klipstein *et al.* [57] have studied a wide family of barrier detectors, which they divide into two groups: $XB_n n$ and $XB_p p$ detectors (see Figure 4.55). As far as the former group is concerned, all designs have the same n-type $B_n n$ structural unit but use different contact layers (X), in which either the doping, material, or both are varied. If we consider, for example, $C_p B_n n$ and $nB_n n$ devices, C_p is the p-type contact made from a different material than the active layer, whereas n is the n-type contact made from the same material as the active layer. In the case of a $pB_n n$ structure, the p-n junction can be located at the interface between the heavily doped p-type material and the lower doped barrier, or within the lower doped barrier itself. A pBp architecture should be employed when the materials surface conduction is the p-type and has to be used with the p-type absorbing layer.

The unipolar barriers can also be inserted into a conventional p-n photodiode architecture. There are two possible placements into which the unipolar barrier can be implemented: (i) outside the depletion layer in the p-type layer or (ii) near the junction, but at the edge of the n-type absorbing layer (see Figure 4.56).

Depending on barrier placement, different dark current components are filtered. For instance, placing the barrier in the p-type layer blocks surface current, but currents due to diffusion, generation–recombination, TAT and BBT cannot be blocked. If the barrier is placed in the n-type region, junction-generated currents and surface currents are effectively filtered out. The photocurrent shares the same spatial makeup as the diffusion current, which is shown in Figure 4.57.

Unipolar barriers can seriously improve the performance of IR photodiodes. Figure 4.58 compares the temperature-dependent $R_0 A$ product data for an n-side unipolar barrier photodiode with that of a conventional p-n photodiode. Unipolar barrier photodiode shows performance near "Rule 07" with an activation energy near the bandgap of InAs indicating a diffusion-limited performance and six orders of magnitude higher $R_0 A$ value in a low-temperature range than that of the conventional p-n junction. "Rule 07" criterion manifests the performance of p-on-n HgCdTe photodiode architecture, which is limited by the Auger 1 diffusion current from 10^{15} cm^{-3} n-type material [59], and is the popular reference mark to compare the performance of any type of detector with the HgCdTe

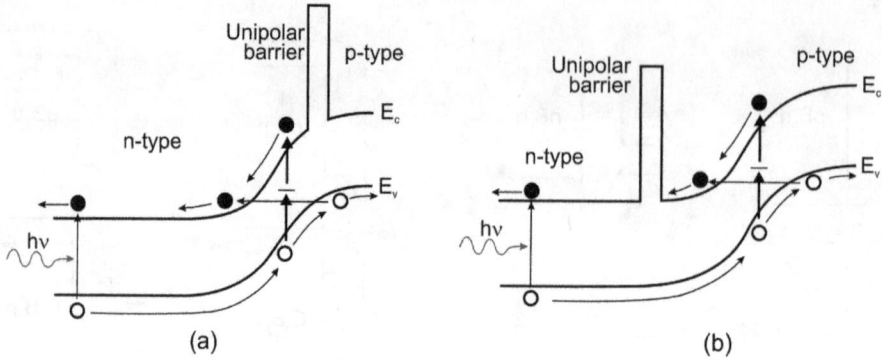

FIGURE 4.56 Band diagrams of a *p*-side (a) and an *n*-side (b) unipolar photodiode under bias (after Reference 58).

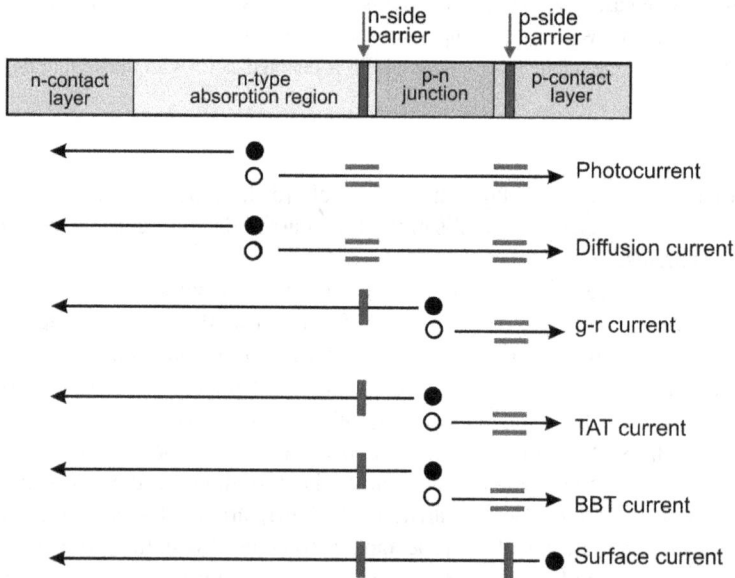

FIGURE 4.57 Placing the barrier in a unipolar barrier photodiode results in the filtering of surface and junction-related currents. Diffusion current is not filtered because it shares the same spatial makeup as the photocurrent (after Reference 58).

state of the art. Any detector architecture that is limited by Auger 7 p-type diffusion, or by depletion currents will not behave according to "Rule 07." In fact, the appropriate criterion to be used for comparative studies is the detector dark current relative to the system flux current.

4.12 PHOTOEMISSIVE DETECTORS

Both the photoconductive and photovoltaic phenomena can be classified as phenomena with an internal photoelectric effect. At this point, we will look at detectors with an external photoelectric effect.

Photoelectric effect is the emission of electrons when the optical radiation hits a photocathode. The high-energy electron has sufficient kinetic energy, greater than the vacuum level barrier, to exit

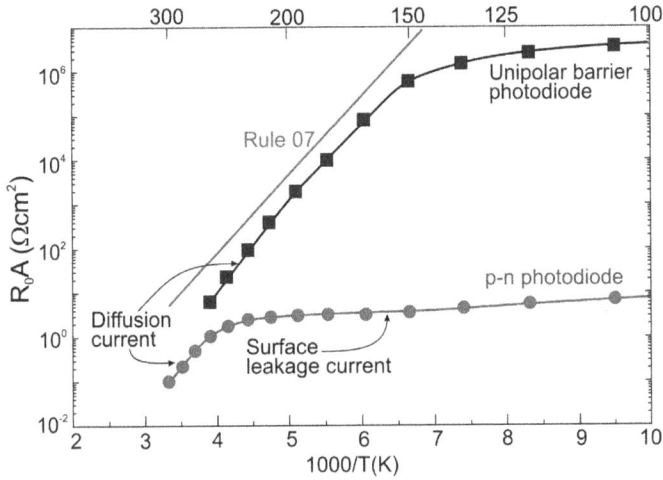

FIGURE 4.58 Comparison of R_0A product of a conventional InAs photodiode with an implemented n-side barrier photodiode (after Reference 58).

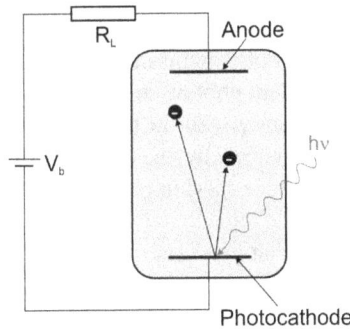

FIGURE 4.59 Classic photoemission vacuum diode.

the photocathode and be emitted as a free electron (e.g., from the photocathode to the anode – see Figure 4.59. Electrons emitted in such a way are called photoelectrons. If we add a large electric field between the cathode and the anode, the emitted electrons are accelerated in the space between the cathode surface and the anode, and they are collected by the anode producing a photocurrent proportional to incoming photons intensity. Current through the device is typically of the order of a few microamperes.

Vacuum photodiode shown in Figure 4.59 is basically a vacuum or a gas-filled tube (a phototube or a photo-emissive cell). Phototubes were previously more widely used but are now replaced by solid-state photodetectors.

Photocathodes can be classified by the electron emission process into the reflection mode and transmission mode photocathodes. The reflection mode photocathode is usually formed on a metal plate, and photoelectrons are emitted from the photocathode in the opposite direction to the incident light. Transmission mode photocathode is usually deposited as a thin film on an optically transparent flat plate, and photoelectrons are emitted in the same direction as the incident light. The photocathode should be characterised by a high absorption coefficient, a large diffusion length (allowing the excited electron to reach the surface), and a low work function. Only if these conditions are met by the photocathode material can we obtain a good quality photoemission detector.

The light wavelength range over which the device is sensitive depends on a material used for the photoemissive cathode. Metals are characterised by a large work function in the 4–5 eV range. Only high-energy ultraviolet radiation can release electrons from metal photocathodes. Most photocathodes are made of a compound semiconductor consisting mainly of alkali metals with a low work function. By changing the photocathode materials, it is possible to achieve sensitivity in various wavelengths from soft X-rays to near IR-radiation. In order to increase the long-term limit of sensitivity, the cathode surface is covered with cesium, which has a lower work function (1.92 eV); therefore, the photocathode is more sensitive in the visible range. Gas-filled devices are more sensitive, but frequency response to a modulated illumination falls off at lower frequencies compared to the vacuum devices.

A further increase in sensitivity can be achieved by modifying the photoemission by generating more electrons in the process of secondary emission from cathode to anode. Thus, a modified vacuum photodiode is a photomultiplier, and modern constructions of such devices are called microchannel plate (MCP), as is described in chapter 6.

4.12.1 Internal Photoemission Process

The original electron photoemission model from metals into vacuum was described by Fowler in the 1930s [60]. In the 1960s Fowler's photo yield model was modified based on studies of internal photoemission of hot electrons from metal films into a semiconductor [61,62]. Cohen et al. modified the Fowler emission theory to account for emission into semiconductors [63].

As illustrated in Figure 4.60, internal photoemission resembles electron emission from metal to vacuum by photon irradiation. The incident photons are absorbed in the metal and generate electron-hole pairs. The excited electrons randomly walk in the metal films until they reach the interface between the metal and the semiconductor. Finally, the electrons surmount the barrier and are emitted into the semiconductor. The internal photoemission process involves three steps:

- photoabsorption in the electrode that gives rise to a hot carrier gas;
- hot carrier transport in the electrode and in the semiconductor prior to barrier emission; and
- emission over the Schottky barrier.

Unlike intrinsic detectors, the QE of the Schottky-barrier detector depends on the photon energy because of the strong dependence of the emission probability on the energy of the excited electron.

Assuming that the probability of electron excitation is independent of the energy of the initial and final states and that there is an abrupt transition from filled to empty states at the Fermi level (see Figure 4.61), the total number of possible excited states is given by

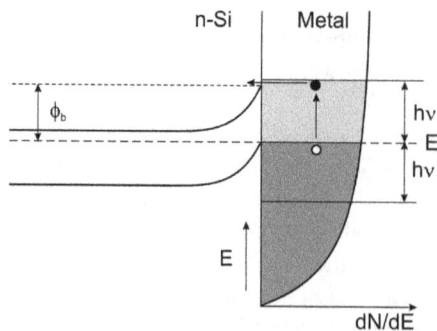

FIGURE 4.60   Internal photoemission in Schottky-barrier detector.

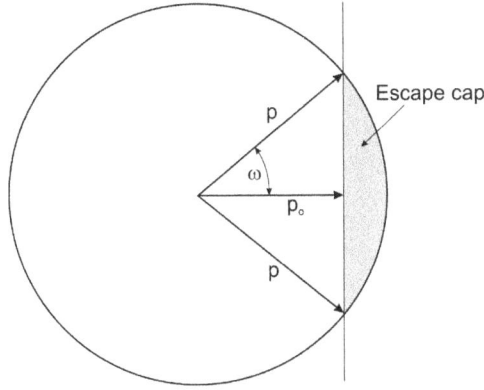

FIGURE 4.61 Momentum criterion for internal photoemission. p_o is the momentum corresponding to the barrier height. The excited electrons with momentum included within the escape cap are emitted into the semiconductor.

$$N_T = \int_{E_F}^{E_F+h\nu} \frac{dN}{dE} dE,$$ (4.111)

where dN/dE is the density of states of the metal, E_F is the Fermi energy, $h\nu$ is the incident photon energy, and E is the electron energy with respect to the metal conduction band edge. The photoemission occurs when an electron is excited to a state for which the component of the momentum normal to the interface corresponds to a kinetic energy equal to or greater than the barrier. Therefore, the number of states that meet the momentum criterion is

$$N_E = \int_{E_F+\phi_b}^{E_F+h\nu} \frac{dN}{dE} P(E) dE,$$ (4.112)

where $P(E)$ is the photoemission probability for the electron with an energy E, and ϕ_b is the height of the barrier. If the momentum distribution of the electrons is isotropic, $P(E)$ can be calculated as shown in Figure 4.61. In this figure, p is the momentum of the excited electron and p_o is the momentum corresponding to the barrier height:

$$p = \sqrt{2m^* E},$$ (4.113)

$$p_o = \sqrt{2m^* \left(E_F + \phi_b \right)},$$ (4.114)

where m^* is the effective mass of the electron. $P(E)$ is the ratio of the surface area of the sphere included within the escape cap to the total surface area of the sphere and is equal to

$$P(E) = \frac{1}{2}(1 - \cos\omega) = \frac{1}{2}\left(1 - \sqrt{\frac{E_F + \phi_b}{E}} \right).$$ (4.115)

For further discussion we assume that dN/dE can be considered to be independent of the energy over the energy range of interest because the Fermi energy is much greater than the photon energy. Then Eqs. (4.111) and (4.112) become

$$N_T = \frac{dN}{dE} h\nu, \tag{4.116}$$

$$N_E = \frac{dN}{dE} \frac{\left(h\nu - \phi_b\right)^2}{8E_F}. \tag{4.117}$$

Here we assume that there are no collisions of electrons or energy losses before the excited electron reaches the interface. Thus, the internal quantum efficiency, which is the ratio of N_E to N_T, is given by

$$\eta_i = \frac{1}{8E_F} \frac{\left(h\nu - \phi_b\right)^2}{h\nu}. \tag{4.118}$$

This simple theory described by Cohen et al. [63] was later extended by Dalal [64], Vickers [65] and Mooney and Silverman [66]. Following theses authors, the general form for the quantum efficiency for internal photoemission is given by

$$\eta = C_f \frac{\left(h\nu - \phi_b\right)^2}{h\nu}, \tag{4.119}$$

where C_f is the Fowler emission coefficient. The Fowler coefficient provides an energy independent measure of the efficiency of the internal photoemission. Its value may be approximated by

$$C_f = \frac{H}{8E_F}, \tag{4.120}$$

where H is a device and a voltage dependent factor.

Equation (4.119) converted to wavelength variables is given by

$$\eta = 1.24 C_f \frac{\left(1 - \lambda/\lambda_c\right)^2}{\lambda}. \tag{4.121}$$

C_f depends upon the physical and geometric parameters of the Schottky electrode. Values of λ_c and C_f as high as 6 μm and 0.5 (eV)$^{-1}$, respectively, have been obtained in PtSi-Si [67]. Schottky photoemission is independent of such factors as semiconductor doping, minority carrier lifetime, and alloy composition and, as a result of this, has spatial uniformity characteristics that are far superior to those of other detector technologies. Uniformity is limited only by the geometric definition of the detectors.

4.12.2   SILICIDE PHOTOEMISSIVE DETECTORS

There are five silicides used for Schottky-barrier IR detectors: palladium silicide (Pd_2Si), platinum silicide (PtSi), iridium silicide (IrSi), cobalt silicide (Co_2Si) and nickel silicide (NiSi).

Figure 4.62 compares the spectral quantum efficiency of the typical photon detectors. From this figure, it seems reasonable to choose high-η intrinsic photodetectors. The effective η of Schottky-barrier detectors in the 3–5 μm atmospheric window is very low, of the order of 1 per cent, but useful sensitivity is obtained by means of near full frame integration in area arrays. An extension of this technology to the long wavelength band is possible using IrSi (see Figure 4.61), but this will require cooling below 77 K [68].

The current responsivity [see Eq. (4.44) with $g = 1$] can be expressed as

$$R_i = qC_f\left(1 - \frac{\lambda}{\lambda_c}\right)^2.$$

(4.122)

Two specific properties of photoemissive detectors follow from the last two equations. The photoresponse decreases with wavelength and the quantum efficiency is low, compared to that of bulk detectors. Both of these properties are a direct result of conservation of momentum during carrier emission over the potential barrier. The majority of excited carriers, which do not have enough momentum normal to the barrier, are reflected and not emitted. Figure 4.63 shows typical spectral responses of Pd_2Si, PtSi, and IrSi Schottky-barrier detectors [69].

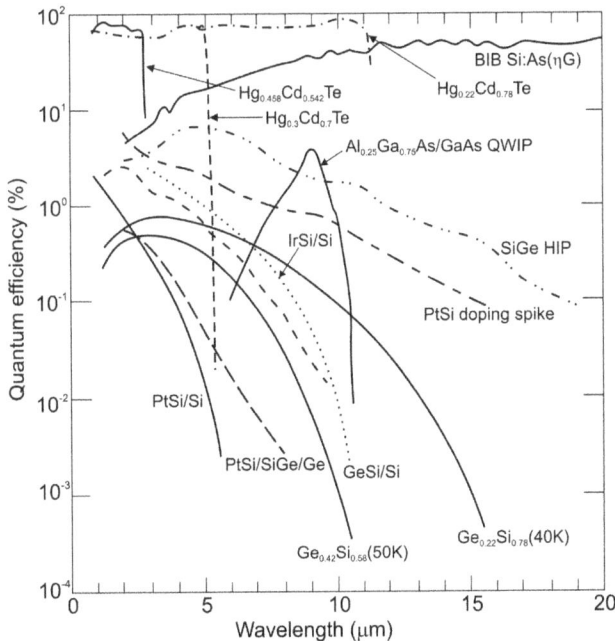

FIGURE 4.62 Quantum efficiency versus wavelength for several detector materials. The detectors include HgCdTe intrinsic photodiodes, blocked impurity band (BIB) extrinsic detectors, GaAs-based quantum well infrared photodetectors (QWIPs), and Si-based photoemissive detectors (PtSi, IrSi, PtSi/SiGe, PtSi doping spike, and SiGe heterojunction internal photoemission).

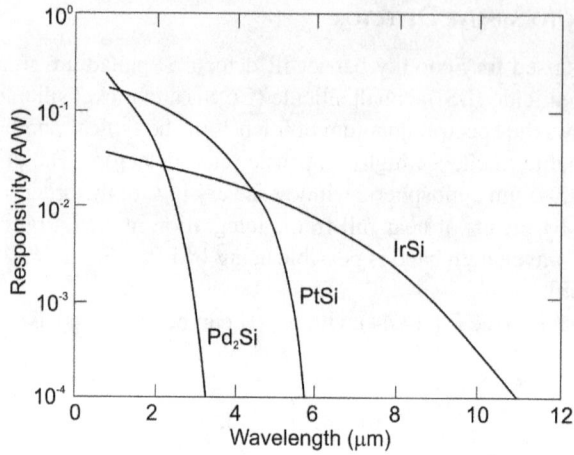

FIGURE 4.63   Spectral response of Pd$_2$Si, PtSi, and IrSi Schottky-barrier detectors (after Reference 69).

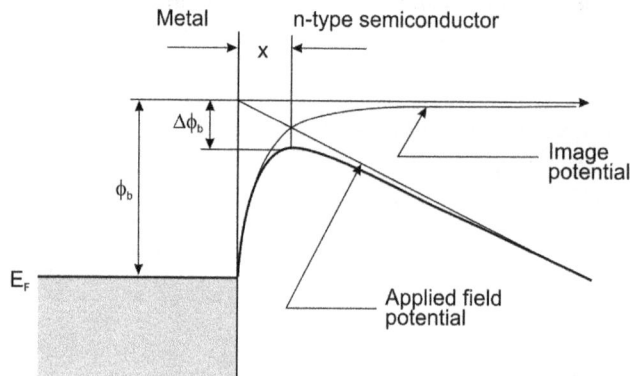

FIGURE 4.64   Barrier lowering by Schottky effect. The attraction force between the emitted electron and the induced positive charge reduces the barrier height by $\Delta\phi_b$.

Figures 4.49 and 4.60, which are often given as the energy band diagram for a Schottky barrier, are misleading because they give the impression that the peak of the Schottky barrier potential occurs at the semiconductor-electrode interface. The electric field near the Schottky barrier has influence on the barrier height. When the carrier is injected into the semiconductor, it feels an attractive force called the image force. As a result, the effective barrier height is reduced. This lowering is called the Schottky effect. As a result of this effect, the peak potential always occurs in the semiconductor, typically at a depth of 5 to 50 nm (see Figure 4.64 [37]).

The magnitude of the barrier lowering $\Delta\phi_b$ is given by [37]

$$\Delta\phi_b = \sqrt{\frac{qE}{4\pi\varepsilon_o\varepsilon_s}}, \tag{4.123}$$

where q is the electron charge, E is the electric field near the barrier, ε_o is the permittivity of free space, and ε_s is the dielectric constant of silicon. The electric field is given by

$$E = \sqrt{\frac{2qN_d}{\varepsilon_o \varepsilon_s}\left(V + V_{bi} - \frac{kT}{q}\right)}, \qquad (4.124)$$

where N_d is the impurity concentration of silicon, V is the applied voltage, and V_{bi} is the built-in potential. The last equation indicates that the barrier height can be controlled by the reverse bias voltage and the impurity concentration of the substrate. The distance between the interface and potential maximum becomes shorter for larger electric fields, and this shift of the potential maximum enhances the quantum efficiency coefficient.

From Eq. (4.119) we find that the quantum efficiency of the Schottky-barrier detector is expressed by two parameters: the barrier height and the Fowler emission coefficient. We can determine those two parameters from the plot of $\sqrt{\eta \times h\nu}$ versus $h\nu$. This type of analysis is known as a Flower Plot. The Flower coefficient is determined from the square of the slope and the barrier potential from the intercept of the plot. Figure 4.65 shows the Fowler plot based on spectral responsivity data from a PtSi/p-Si detector [70]. Image lowering improves the emission efficiency and extends the spectral response to longer wavelengths with increased voltage.

The current flowing through the barrier in silicide Schottky-barrier diodes is dominated by thermionic emission current. The thermionic emission theory gives the current-voltage characteristic expressed by Equation (4.109). The effective Richardson constant for holes in silicon, A^*, is about 30 A/cm²K² in a moderate electric field range [37].

The Schottky-barrier diode is operated under reverse bias in the IR focal plane arrays (FPAs). In the reverse biased condition, barrier lowering due to the Schottky effect has to be taken into consideration. For a reverse bias greater than $3kT/q$, from Eq. (4.110) we get

$$J_{st} = A^* T^2 \exp\left[-\frac{q(\phi_b - \Delta\phi_b)}{kT}\right], \qquad (4.125)$$

where $\Delta\phi_b$ is the magnitude of the barrier lowering calculated by Eq. (4.123). By the last equation we can determine the effective barrier height at a certain reverse bias from the plot of J_{st}/T^2 versus $1/T$. Figure 4.66 is a Richardson analysis for the PtSi diode of Figure 4.65, biased at 1 V [70]. The

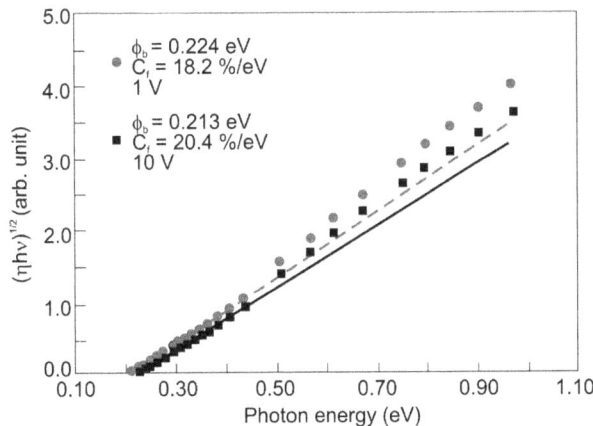

FIGURE 4.65 Flower photoemission analysis for PtSi/p-Si Schottky diode, with $\lambda_c = 5.5$ µm at 1 V bias and $\lambda_c = 5.8$ µm at 10 V (after Reference 70).

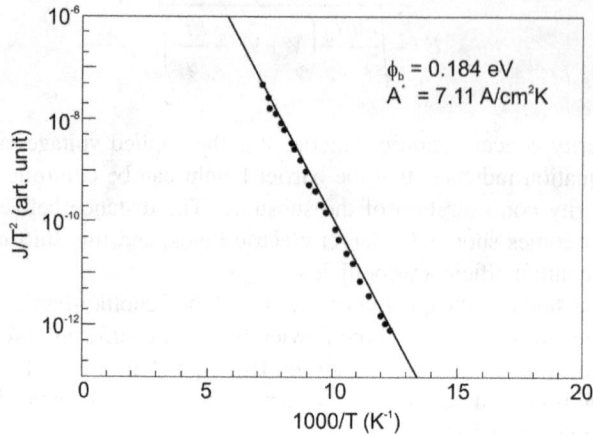

FIGURE 4.66 Richardson thermionic emission analysis PtSi/p-Si diode, at 1 V bias. Note difference in barrier potential compared to Flower analysis in Figure 4.65 (after Reference 70).

Richardson constant is determined with less accuracy from the vertical intercept. The Richardson analysis is often linear over more than five orders of magnitude. The presence of any leakage current or excess series resistance causes this plot to saturate. Thus, the Richardson analysis allows assessment of data quality. It is important to note that the barrier height obtained from the electrical measurement (ϕ_{bt}) is lower than that from the optical measurement (ϕ_{bo}) as discussed previously:

$$\phi_{bt} = \phi_{bo} - nhv, \tag{4.126}$$

where nhv is the average energy loss by electron-phonon scattering. The typical measured value of this energy loss is from 20 to 50 meV. The lower values are observed in the most efficient devices where elastic scattering is dominant.

PROBLEMS

Example 4.1

Consider the silicon p-n photodiode as shown in figure below. The photodiode has a depletion layer width of $w = 40$ μm, $L_e = 3$ μm, $L_h = 10$ μm, and has a p-type undepleted region thickness $t = 4$ μm. Calculate the photodiode internal efficiency at 700 nm, neglecting the losses due to the radiation reflection from the illuminated photodiode surface.

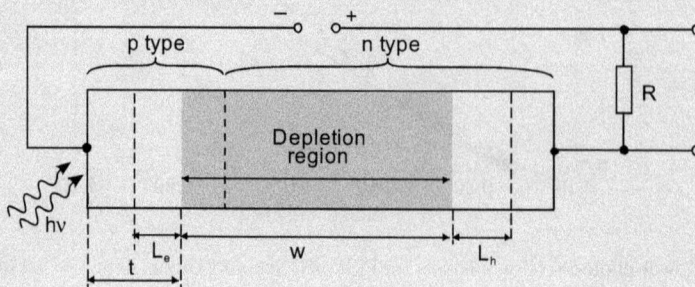

Example 4.2

Calculate the photocurrent and gain when 5×10^{12} photons/s are arriving at the surface of a photoconductor of $\eta = 0.8$. The minority carrier lifetime is $\tau = 0.5$ ns, and the device has mobility $\mu_e = 2500$ cm^2/Vs, the electric field $E = 5000$ V/cm, and the length $l = 10$ μm.

Example 4.3

Consider the photodiode InGaAs shown in Figure 4.41. What is quantum efficiency at peak responsivity? What is quantum efficiency at 900 nm (maximum responsivity for a Si photodiode)?

Example 4.4

Consider a hypothetical HgCdTe photodiode with an active area of 50×50 μm^2, $R_o = 500$ kΩ, quantum efficiency 60 per cent operating at 80 K. Calculate the device detectivity at 8 μm wavelength

Example 4.5

Consider the Si p-i-n photodiode (S15137 type) with an active area of 5 mm in diameter. It generates a photocurrent of 140 μA, when radiation with a wavelength of 1000 nm and an irradiance of 1 mW/cm^2 is incident. What is the responsivity and external quantum efficiency of a photodiode at 1000 nm?

Example 4.6

An avalanche photodiode (G 8931-10 type) has a current responsivity of 0.9 A/W at 1550 nm in the absence of multiplication. It is biased to operate with a multiplication of 30. Calculate the quantum efficiency and the photocurrent if the radiant flux is 10 nW. What is the current responsivity when the multiplication factor is $M = 30$?

Example 4.7

A silicon APD (S14643-02 type) has a quantum efficiency of 78 per cent at 760 nm in the absence of multiplication. The APD is biased ($V_R = 100$ V, at 20°C) to operate with $M = 200$. What is the photocurrent when the radiant flux is 5 nW?

Example 4.8

An InGaAs photodiode has an "i" layer with a width of 10 μm. The p$^+$ layer on the illumination side is very thin. The photodiode is reverse biased $V_R = 50$ V and illuminated with a very short optical pulse of $\lambda = 1550$ nm. What is the response time of the photocurrent if absorption occurs over "i" layer?

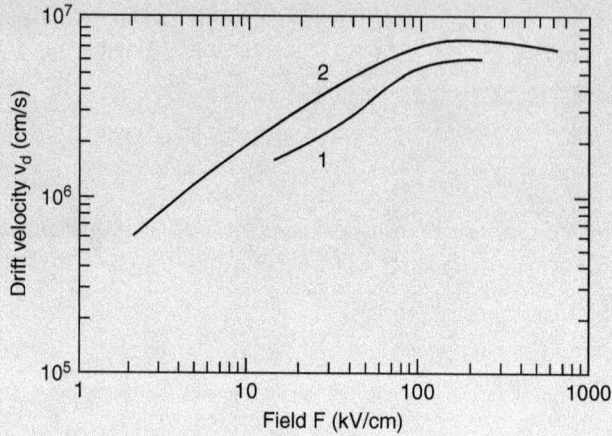

Example 4.9

Consider a Si APD with a width absorption region of $w_d = 50$ μm, width multiplication region $w_m = 0.5$ μm, electron velocity $v_e = 10^7$ cm/s, hole velocity $v_h = 5 \times 10^6$, gain $g = 100$, and electron injection $k = 0.1$.

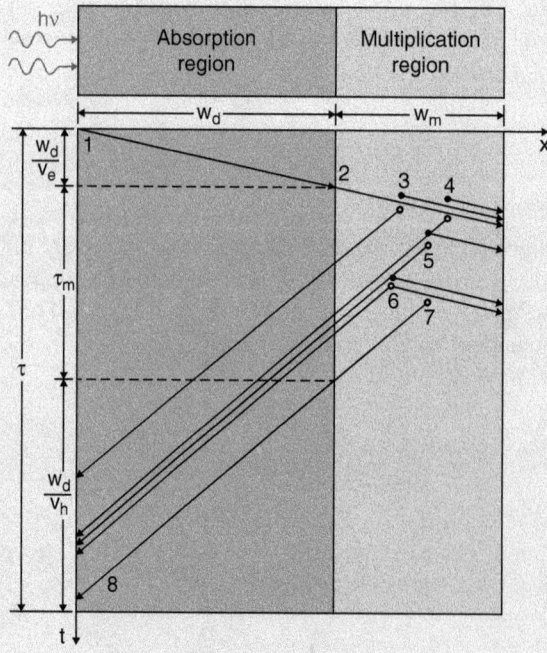

Example 4.10

5×10^{12} photons fall on the PbS photoconductor surface. Calculate the photocurrent and the photoconductive gain. The photoconductor is biased $V_R = 50$ V, the lifetime $\tau = 20$ µs, the quantum efficiency $\eta = 0.8$, the carrier mobility $\mu_e = 5.75 \times 10^2$ cm²/Vs, and the length of photoconductor $l = 1$ mm.

REFERENCES

1. A.G. Alkholidi and K.S. Altowij, "Free space optical communications – Theory and practices", in *Wireless Communications*, pp.159–212, edited by M. Khatib, InTech, 2014, http://dx.doi.org/10.5772/58884.
2. A.K. Majumdar, *Advanced Free Space Optics (FSO)*, Springer, New York, 2016.
3. J. Mikołajczyk, Z. Bielecki, M. Bugajski, J. Piotrowski, J. Wojtas, W. Gawron, D. Szabra, and A. Prokopiuk, "Analysis of free-space optics development", *Metrology and Measurement Systems* 24(4), 653–674 (2017).
4. A. Yariv and P. Yeh, *Photonics: Optical Electronics in Modern Communications*, Oxford University Press, Oxford, 2006.
5. A. Rogalski, M. Kopytko, and P. Martyniuk, *Antimonide-Based Infrared Detectors – A New Perspective*, SPIE Press, Bellingham, WA, 2018.
6. A. Rogalski, "Progress in focal plane array technologies", *Prog. Quant. Electron.* 36, 342–473 (2012).
7. W. Kruse, L.D. McGlauchlin, and R.B. McQuistan, *Elements of Infrared Technology*, John Wiley, New York, 1962.
8. I.R. Keyes, *Optical and Infrared Detectors*, Springer, Berlin, 1980.
9. E.L. Dereniak and G.D. Boreman, *Infrared Detectors and Systems*, John Wiley, New York, 1996.
10. S. Donati, *Photodetectors. Devices, Circuits, and Application*, Hoboken, NJ, Wiley-IEEE Press, 2020.
11. G.H. Rieke, *Detection of Light: From Ultraviolet to the Submillimeter*, Cambridge University Press, Cambridge, 2003.
12. J.D. Vincent, S.E. Hodges, J. Vampola, M. Stegall, and G. Pierce, *Fundamentals of Infrared and Visible Detector Operation and Testing*, John Wiley, Hoboken, NJ., 2016.
13. A. Rogalski, *Infrared and Terahertz Detectors*, 3rd edition, CRC Press, Boca Raton, 2019.
14. J. Piotrowski, "Breakthrough in infrared technology–The micromachined thermal detector arrays", *Opto-Electron. Rev.* 3, 3–8 (1995).
15. P.G. Datskos and V. Lavrik, "Detectors: Figures of merit," in *Encyclopedia of Optical Engineering*, ed. R. Driggers, 349–357, CRC Press, New York, 2003.
16. E.H. Putley, "Thermal detectors," in *Optical and Infrared Detectors*, ed. R. J. Keyes, 71–100, Springer, Berlin, 1977.
17. J.I. Pankove, *Optical Properties of Semiconductors,* Dover, New York, 1971.
18. B.F. Levine, "Quantum-well infrared photodetectors", *J. Appl. Phys.* 74, R1–R81 (1993).
19. Z. Jakšić, *Micro and Nanophotonics for Semiconductor Infrared Detectors*, Springer, Heidelberg, 2014.
20. S.J. Fonash, *Solar Cell Device Physics*, Elsevier, Amsterdam, 2010.
21. M.S. Ünlü and S. Strite, "Resonant cavity enhanced photonic devices," *J. Appl. Phys.* 78, 607–639 (1995).
22. J. Piotrowski and A. Rogalski, *High-Operating-Temperature Infrared Photodetectors*, SPIE Press, Bellingham, WA, 2007.
23. R.H. Ritchie, "Plasma losses by fast electrons in thin films", *Phys. Rev.* 106, 874–881 (1957).
24. S.A. Maier, *Plasmonic: Fundamentals and Applications*, Springer, New York, 2007.
25. J. Zhang, L. Zhang, and W. Xu, "Surface plasmon polaritons: physics and applications", *J. Phys. D: Appl. Phys.* 45, 113001 (2012).
26. J.R. Sambles, G.W. Bradbery, and F.Z. Yang, "Optical-excitation of surface-plasmons – an introduction", *Contemp. Phys.* 32, 173–183 (1991).
27. P. Biagioni, J.-S.Huang, and B. Hecht, "Nanoantennas for visible and infrared radiation," *Rep. Prog. Phys.* 75, 024402 (2012).

28. K. Ishihara, K. Ohashi, T. Ikari, H. Minamide, H. Yokoyama, J.-I. Shikata, and H. Ito, "Therahertz-wave near field imaging with subwavelength resolution using surface-wave-assisted bow-tie aperture," *Appl. Phys. Lett.* 89, 201120 (2006).

29. U. Kreibig and M. Vollmer, *Optical Properties of Metal Clusters*, Springer, Berlin, 1995.

30. S. Kalchmair, H. Detz, G.D. Cole, A.M. Andrews, P. Klang, M. Nobile, R. Gansch, C. Ostermaier, W. Schrenk, and G. Strasser, "Photonic crystal slab quantum well infrared photodetector", *Appl. Phys. Lett.* 98, 011105 (2011).

31. A. Rose, *Concept in Photoconductivity and Allied Problems,* Interscience, New York, 1963.

32. J. Piotrowski and A. Rogalski, Comment on "Temperature limits on infrared detectivities of InAs/$In_xGa_{1-x}Sb$ superlattices and bulk $Hg_{1-x}Cd_xTe$" [*J. Appl. Phys.* 74, 4774 (1993)], *J. Appl. Phys. 80*(4), 2542–2544 (1996).

33. S. Blakemore, *Semiconductor Statistics,* Pergamon Press, Oxford, 1962.

34. A. Rogalski, "Quantum well photoconductors in infrared detectors technology", *J. Appl. Phys.* 93, 4355–4391 (2003).

35. J. Piotrowski and A. Rogalski, "New generation of infrared photodetectors", *Sens. Actuator* A67, 146–152 (1998).

36. R.A. Smith, *Semiconductors,* Cambridge University Press, Cambridge, 1978.

37. S.M. Sze, *Physics of Semiconductor Devices,* John Wiley, New York, 1981.

38. F. Van De Wiele, "Quantum efficiency of photodiode", in *Solid State Imaging*, pp. 41–76, eds. P. G. Jespers, F. Van De Wiele, and M. H. White, Noordhoff, Leyden, 1976.

39. C.T. Sah, R.N. Noyce, and W. Shockley, "Carrier generation and recombination in p-n junctions and p-n junction characteristics", *Proc. IRE* 45, 1228–1243 (1957).

40. J. Wróbel, E. Plis, W. Gawron, M. Motyka, P. Martyniuk, P. Madejczyk, A. Kowalewski, M. Dyksik, J. Misiewicz, S. Krishna, and A. Rogalski, "Analysis of temperature dependence of dark current mechanisms in mid-wavelength infrared pin type-II superlattice photodiodes", *Sens. Mater.* 26(4), 235–244 (2014).

41. G. Kreiser, *Optical Fiber Communications*, McGraw Hill, Boston, 2000.

42. *Photodiodes.* Hamamatsu, 1993.

43. Si photodiodes. Technical note. Hamamatsu. Cat. No. KSPD 9001E01, 2020 www.hamamatsu.com/resources/pdf/ssd/si_pd_kspd9001e.pdf.

44. F. Capasso, "Physics of avalanche diodes", in *Semiconductors and Semimetals*, Vol. 22D, pp. 2–172, edited by W.T. Tang, Academic Press, Orlando, 1985.

45. R.J. McIntryre, "Multiplication noise in uniform avalanche diodes", *IEEE Trans. Electron Devices* 13, 164–168 (1966).

46. R.J. McIntyre, "The distribution of gains in uniformly multiplying avalanche photodiodes: Theory", *IEEE Trans. Electron. Devices* ED-19, 703–713 (1972).

47. A.R.J. Marshall, "The InAs electron avalanche photodiode, in advances in photodiodes", ed. by G.F.D. Betta, InTech, 2011. www.intechopen.com/books/advances-in-photodiodes/the-inas-electron-avalanche-photodiode.

48. J.P.R. David and C.H. Tan, "Material considerations for avalanche photodiodes", *IEEE J. Sel. Top. Quant. Electron.* 14, 998–1009, 2008.

49. S.B. Alexander, *Optical Communication Receiver Design*, SPIE Optical Engineering Press, Bellingham, WA. 1997.

50. http://hamamatsu.com.cn/UserFiles/DownFile/Product/G4176E.pdf.

51. A.M. White, "Infrared detectors", *U.S. Patent* 4,679,063, 22 September, 1983.

52. P.C. Klipstein, "Depletionless photodiode with suppressed dark current and method for producing the same", *U.S. Patent* 7,795,640 (2 July 2003).

53. S. Maimon and G. Wicks, "nBn detector, an infrared detector with reduced dark current and higher operating temperature", *Appl. Phys. Lett.* 89, 151109-1–3 (2006).

54. D.Z.-Y. Ting, A. Soibel, L. Höglund, J. Nguyen, C.J. Hill, A. Khoshakhlagh, and S. D. Gunapala, "Type II superlattice infrared detectors, in Semiconductors and Semimetals", Vol. 84, pp. 1–57, edited by S.D. Gunapala, D.R. Rhiger, and C. Jagadish, Elsevier, Amsterdam, 2011.

55. G.R. Savich, J.R. Pedrazzani, D.E. Sidor, and G.W. Wicks, "Benefits and limitations of unipolar barriers in infrared photodetectors", *Infrared Physics & Technol.* 59, 152–155 (2013).

56. P. Klipstein, "XBn barrier photodetectors for high sensitivity operating temperature infrared sensors", *Proc. SPIE.* 6940, 69402U-1–11 (2008).

57. P. Klipstein, D. Aronov, E. Berkowicz, R. Fraenkel, A. Glozman, S. Grossman, O. Klin, I. Lukomsky, I. Shtrichman, N. Snapi, M. Yassem, and E. Weiss, "Reducing the cooling requirements of mid-wave IR detector arrays", *SPIE Newsroom* 10.1117/2.1201111.003919, 2011.

58. G.R. Savich, J. R. Pedrazzani, D. E. Sidor, S. Maimon, and G. W. Wicks, "Dark current filtering in unipolar barrier infrared detectors", *Appl. Phys. Lett.* 99, 121112 (2011).

59. W.E. Tennant, D. Lee, M. Zandian, E. Piquette, and M. Carmody, "MBE HgCdTe technology: A very general solution to IR detection, described by 'Rule 07', a very convenient heuristic", *J. Electron. Materials* 37, 1406–1410 (2008).

60. R.H. Fowler, "The analysis of photoelectric sensitivity curves for clean metals at various temperatures", *Phys. Rev.* 38, 45–57 (1931).

61. C.R. Crowell, W.G. Spitzer, L.E. Howarth, and E.E. Labate, "Attenuation length measurements of hot electrons in metal films", *Phys. Rev.* 127, 2006 (1962).

62. R. Stuart, F. Wooten, and W.E. Spicer, "Monte-Carlo calculations pertaining to the transport of hot electrons in metals", *Phys. Rev.* 135(2A), 495–504 (1964).

63. J. Cohen, J. Vilms, and R. J. Archer, "Investigation of semiconductor Schottky barriers for optical detection and cathodic emission", Air *Force Cambridge Research Labs. Report* No. 68-0651 (1968) and No. 69-0287 (1969).

64. V.L. Dalal, "Simple model for internal photoemission", *J. Appl. Phys.* 42, 2274–2279 (1971).

65. V.E. Vickers, "Model of Schottky-barrier hot electron mode photodetection", *Appl. Opt.* 10, 2190–2192 (1971).

66. J.M. Mooney and J. Silverman, "The theory of hot-electron photoemission in Schottky barrier detectors", *IEEE Trans. Electron Devices* ED-32, 33–39 (1985).

67. F.D. Shepherd, "Schottky diode based infrared sensors", *Proc. SPIE* 443, 42–49 (1984).

68. F.D. Shepherd, "Silicide infrared staring sensors", *Proc. SPIE* 930, 2–10 (1988).

69. M. Kimata and N. Tsubouchi, "Schottky barrier photoemissive detectors," in *Infrared Photon Detectors*, ed. A. Rogalski, 299–349, SPIE Optical Engineering Press, Bellingham, WA, 1995.

70. F.D. Shepherd, "Infrared internal emission detectors", *Proc. SPIE* 1735, 250–261 (1992).

5 Thermal Detectors

The history of thermal detectors is fascinating if we now realise the well-known fact that two snake families (from the rattlesnake families) feel temperature differences between animals and the environment, which allows them to locate their food prey. Nature has equipped them with miniature thermal imaging cameras (using the pyroelectric effect), which form the infrared images in the range of 8–14 μm, thus giving the snakes a greater advantage over their prey. Around 2300 BC the Greeks already knew tourmaline, the magical mineral that, when heated, would charge and cause unexpected shocks. This effect was also the result of a pyroelectric phenomenon.

5.1 INTRODUCTION

Infrared radiation was discovered by Herschel in 1800 [1], using a typical liquid-containing thermometer with a specially blackened radiation-absorbing bubble. By examining the excellent split radiation through the prism, he observed that the thermometer moving outside the visible split light range still indicated a temperature rise. The thermometer became the first of three, an infrared detector commonly used until the First World War. The other types of detectors were the thermocouple and the bolometer. In 1821, Seebeck discovered the thermoelectric phenomenon [2]. The first thermostat was constructed by Nobili in 1829 by connecting many thermocouples in series [3]. In 1833 Macedonio Melloni modified the technology by combining thermocouples in a series of several thermocouples. The third detector was a bolometer discovered by Langley in 1881. Langley constructed a bolometer much more sensitive than thermocouples in those years. Already after the Second World War it was proposed to use a gas thermometer, the so-called Golay cell, until now quite commonly used in spectrometers.

Photoconductivity (the photon phenomenon) was first observed by Smith in 1873, during experiments with selenium used as an insulator in underwater cables [4]. This discovery significantly increased interest in photoelectric phenomena for many decades to come, but the quality of this research was largely questionable.

In the 1930s and 1940s the physical foundations of the solid-state theory were developed, which initiated a development of semiconductor devices in the 1950s. We have been observing their further dynamic development until now. However, it should be clearly noted that, in the field of optical radiation detectors, this development is mainly related to photon detectors. Nevertheless, after 1990, there was a significant progress in the technology and performance of thermal detectors, especially infrared microbolometers, due to the adaptation of the silicon micromechanics technique to the technological process of obtaining these detectors.

The principles of thermal detectors theory, and characterisations are given in Chapter 4. Typical properties of thermal detectors operating at room temperature are summarised in Table 5.1. In this

DOI: 10.1201/9781003263098-5

TABLE 5.1
Typical Properties of Thermal Detectors Operating at Room Temperature

Type	A [mm²]	R_v [V/W]	D^* [cmHz$^{1/2}$/W]	R [Ω]	τ [ms]	Remarks
Bulk thermopile	0.20×0.20	2	3×10^8	10	20–30	Perkin Elmer
Thin film thermopile	1.0×1.0	50	2×10^8	2000	30–50	Dexter
Thin film thermopile	0.12×0.12	280	3.6×10^9	5000	13	SBRC
Si thermopile	1.2×1.2	50	1.3×10^8	125×10^3	20	Hamamatsu
Thin film thermopile (72 elements)	Ø 0.5 mm	70	3.44×10^8	20×10^3	35	Electro Opt. Comp., Inc.
Metallic bolometer Ni	1×1	3	3×10^8	6–8	20–30	$I = 20$ mA
Thermistor	1×1	75	5×10^7	10^6	4	$I = 50$ µA
Pyroelectric detector TGS	1×1	10^5	5×10^8			$f = 10$ Hz
	1×1	10^3	5×10^7			$f = 1000$ Hz
Pyroelectric detector LiTaO$_3$	1×1	10^5	3×10^8			$f = 10$ Hz
	1×1	10^3	3×10^7			$f = 1000$ Hz
Golay cell		10^6	2×10^{-10} (*NEP*)			

chapter the main efforts are directed towards describing their specific properties: thermocouples, bolometers and pyroelectric detectors.

5.2 THERMOPILES

The general theory of a thermocouple is presented in Section 4.3.1. We will complete it at this point.

The main source of a thermocouple noise in the frequency range from 0.1 to 1000 Hz is the Johnson-Nyquist noise. Then, according to the detectivity definition [Eq. (4.17)] and $K = \alpha_s$, we have

$$D^* = \frac{\alpha_s \varepsilon A_d^{1/2}}{G_{th}\left(4kTR\right)^{1/2}}.$$ (5.1)

In order to achieve a high detectivity, the junction thermal capacity, G_{th}, must be low and the radiation absorption should be effective. With a careful design of the thermocouple, a radiation absorption of 99 per cent can be achieved over a wide spectral range (from visible to far infrared; of about 40 µm).

The spectral responsivity of the thermocouple depends also on the type of a housing window material. The most commonly used are wide-spectrum silicon filters (6–14 µm), with CaF$_2$ (1–10 µm), sapphire (2–5 µm) and narrow-spectrum filters used in gas detection systems.

A single thermocouple is not used as a detector in practice. If N thermocouples are placed in series, the responsivity is increased by N:

$$R_v = \frac{N\alpha_s \varepsilon}{G_{th}(1+\omega^2\tau_{th}^2)^{1/2}}.$$ (5.2)

Such a device is called a thermopile (Figure 5.1). In order for the thermopile to be characterised by low thermal inertia, thin wires or very thin foil strips are used. The hot junction side (photosensitive area) is designed to be a thermally isolated structure on which an absorption film is attached. To

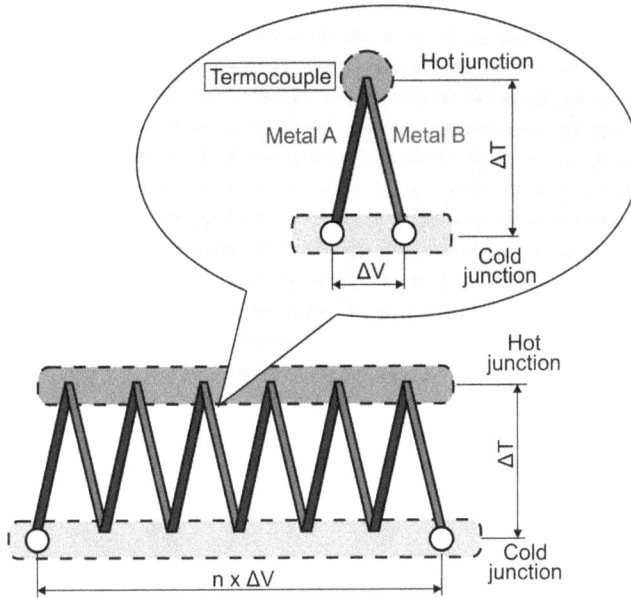

FIGURE 5.1   Diagram of the thermopile.

make the thermally isolated structure, microelectromechanical system (MEMS) technology is used to process the membrane (thin film) to make it float in a hollow space.

5.2.1   THERMOELECTRIC MATERIALS

Materials used for thermocouples should be characterised by

- large Seebeck coefficient α_S;
- large thermal resistance R_{th} (to minimise the heat transfer between hot and cold junctions);
- low volume resistivity (to reduce the noise and heat developed by the current's flow);
- high melting point;
- high permissible temperature of continuous operation;
- continuous and linear dependence of thermoelectric force on temperature.

Keep in mind that by scaling down a device by a certain percentage the surface area only decreases with the square root [see Eq. (5.1)], the miniaturisation of the thermopile is an appropriate way to increase the overall detectivity. Unfortunately, these requirements are incompatible in view of the Wiedemann-Franz law relating the thermal conductivity G_{th} and the electrical resistivity ρ:

$$\frac{G_{th}\rho}{T} = L. \tag{5.3}$$

The L is known as the Lorentz number and has very nearly a constant value for most materials, especially metals, except at very low temperatures. This leads naturally to the well-known criterion of figure-of-merit for thermoelectric materials in which a maximum value of

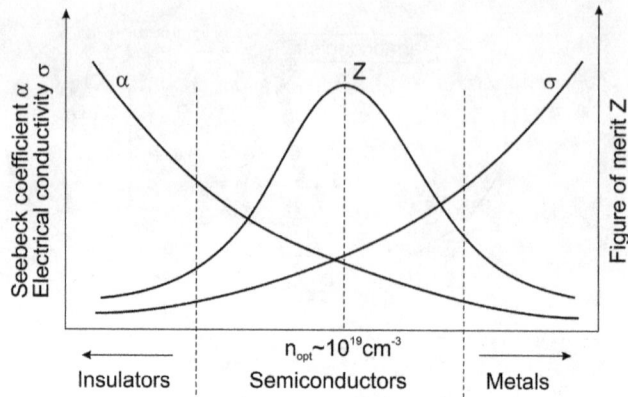

FIGURE 5.2 Thermoelectric properties of metals, semiconductors, and insulators.

$$Z = \frac{\alpha_S^2}{\rho G_{th}} \qquad (5.4)$$

is sought [5]. It is important to note that this thermoelectric figure-of-merit is defined in terms of output power delivered into an optimum load resistance, rather than the open-circuit voltage that enters directly into the definition of the responsivity [see Eq. (5.2)].

Equation (5.1) indicates that the thermocouple materials should be chosen from low-resistivity materials. However, a lower ρ value also gives a lower Seebeck coefficient. Therefore, an optimum point needs to be determined considering all these parameters based on the figure-of-merit. Figure 5.2 shows a graph for the visual interpretation of the thermoelectric properties of metals, semiconductors and insulators [6]. An optimum value for the figure-of-merit for semiconductors is achieved at a doping value about 10^{19} cm^{-3} for single crystal silicon and polysilicon materials. A similar conclusion was predicted by Ioffe more than sixty years ago [7].

It should be noted that when the number of thermocouples is increased to obtain a high output voltage, it also increases the thermal conduction between the hot and cold junctions and the series electrical resistance and thermal noise. This means that care should be taken to optimise the number of thermocouples for a thermopile. Increasing the number of thermocouples does not necessarily increase the performance.

Table 5.2 lists the parameters for selected thermoelectric materials [8,9]. The bismuth/antimony (Bi/Sb) thermocouple is the most classical material pair in conventional thermocouples, and not only from a historical point of view [10]. The Bi/Sb also has the highest Seebeck coefficient and the lowest thermal conductivity of all metal thermocouples. After doping these materials with Se or Te, an improvement of the α_s coefficient up to 230 μV/K is achieved. We can see that good current conductors, such as gold or silver, have a very low thermoelectric coefficient.

In order to compare the properties of individual metals used in the thermocouples production, the thermoelectric force of individual metals and alloys against platinum, taken as a reference at a temperature difference of 100°C, is also given. Adoption of the platinum standard is conditioned by its high resistance to weather conditions, stability of physical properties and high melting point. Dependence of the thermoelectric force of individual metals and alloys in relation to platinum in the entire temperature range of their operation is shown in Figure 5.3.

Despite the long tradition of metal thermocouples, new advantages can be found by using semiconducting materials, such as silicon (crystalline, polycrystalline) for thermoelectric materials due

TABLE 5.2
Parameters of Selected Thermoelectric Materials at Near Room Temperature (after References 8 and 9)

Sample	α_a (µV/K)	Reference electrode	ρ (µΩm)	G_{th} (W/mK)
p-Si	100–1000		10–500	≈150
p-poly-Si	100–500		10–1000	≈20–30
p-Ge	420	Pt		
Sb	48.9	Pt	18.5	0.39
Cr	21.8			
Fe	15		0.086	72.4
Ca	10.3			
Mo	5.6			
Au	1.94		0.023	314
Cu	1.83		0.0172	398
In	1.68			
Ag	1.51		0.016	418
W	0.9			
Pb	−1.0			
Al	−1.66		0.028	238
Pt	−5.28		0.0981	71
Pd	−10.7			
K	−13.7			
Co	−13.3	Pt	0.0557	69
Ni	−19.5		0.0614	60.5
Constantan	−37.25	Pt		
Bi	−73.4	Pt	1.1	8.1
n-Si	−450	Pt	10–500	≈150
n-poly-Si	−100 to −500		10–1000	≈20–30
n-Ge	−548	Pt		

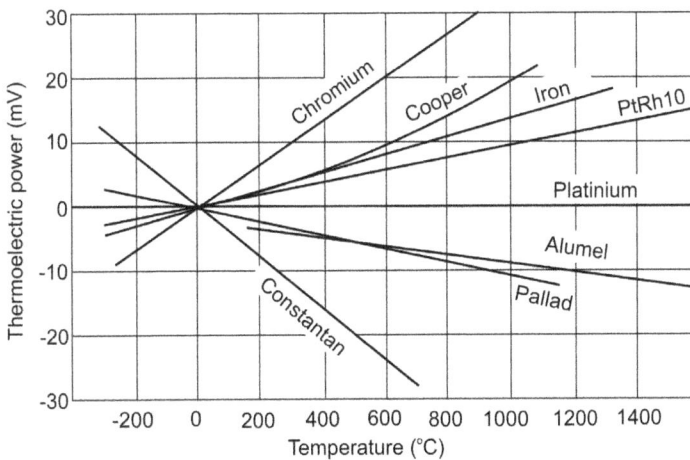

FIGURE 5.3 Dependence of the thermoelectric power of metals and alloys as a function of temperature related to platinum.

to the possibility of using standard integrated circuit processes. The Seebeck coefficient of semiconductor materials depends on the variation of the Fermi level of the semiconductor with respect to temperature; therefore, for semiconductor thermopiles, the magnitude and sign of the Seebeck coefficient and resistivity can be adjusted in the doping type and doping level.

For practical silicon sensor design-purposes it is very convenient to approximate the Seebeck coefficient as a function of electrical resistivity [11]:

$$\alpha_s = \frac{mk}{q} ln\left(\frac{\rho}{\rho_o}\right),$$ (5.5)

with $\rho_o \cong 5\times10^{-6}$ Ωm and $m \cong 2.6$ as constants. Typical values of the Seebeck coefficient of silicon are 500–700 μV/K for the optimum compromise between low resistance and high Seebeck coefficient. Eq. (5.3) suggests that the Seebeck coefficient of a semiconductor increases in magnitude with increased resistivity, and therefore, with decreasing doping level. However, a thermopile material with very low electrical resistivity is not necessarily the best choice for a particular infrared detector, as the Seebeck coefficient is only one of the parameters influencing its overall performance.

For a wide variety of surface micromachined devices, polysilicon has rapidly become the most important material [12,13]. Polysilicon's popularity in this area is a direct result of its mechanical properties and its relatively well-developed deposition and processing technologies. These characteristics along with the capability of utilising established IC processing techniques make it a natural selection.

The measured Seebeck coefficient for polysilicon is shown in Figure 5.4 [14]. The Seebeck coefficient for p-type polysilicon and n-type polysilicon are almost the same, but the signs are opposite. The value of this coefficient greatly depends on impurity concentration. The used impurity concentrations are between 10^{19} and 10^{20} cm^{-3}.

The use of silicon enables the use of a standard technology with a large scale of integration in the construction of two-dimensional arrays of detectors. Significant advances in the sensor technology are due to the development of silicon micromechanics. Technique is based on a fabrication of small, permanent structures with a submicron precision using a combination of photolithography techniques and selective etching. This technique can be used for many materials, but silicon is privileged because many micromechanical techniques are similar in nature to those used in the

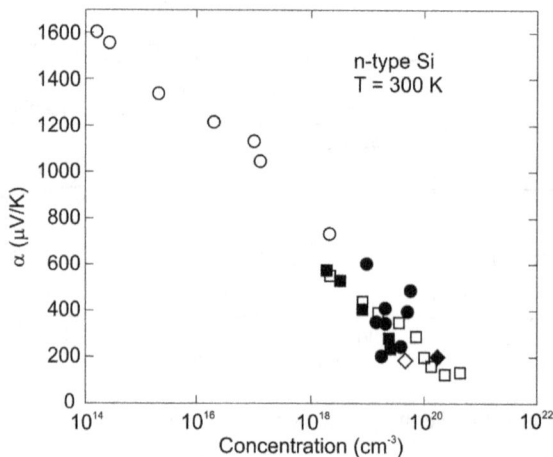

FIGURE 5.4   Seebeck coefficient for polysilicon (after Reference 14).

production of large-scale integration circuits. Silicon also enables a monolithic connection of detectors with processors reading the signal in two-dimensional arrays of detectors. Basic techniques of silicon micromechanics are discussed in the monograph by Ristica [13].

5.2.2 TECHNOLOGY AND PROPERTIES OF THERMOCOUPLES

As already mentioned, the first thermocouples were constructed from thin metal wires. The most popular combinations were copper-constantan, bismuth-silver and bismuth-bismuth/tin alloy. Advances in the semiconductor technology with a higher Seebeck coefficient have made it possible to design more sensitive thermocouples. However, the production of thin wires from semiconductor materials was difficult. Schwartz proposed a new thermocouple design. The positive electrode was made of an alloy (33% Te, 32% Ag, 27% Cu, 7% Se, 1% S) and the negative electrode of an alloy (50% Ag_2Se, 50% Ag_2S). The structural bond between these electrodes was constituted by a gold foil. Sensitivity of thermocouples made in this way increased by almost an order of magnitude (3×10^9 cmHz$^{1/2}$/W). The detectors were mounted in vacuum-tight housings filled with gas of a low thermal conductivity (e.g., xenon). Response time of these detectors was usually 30 ms. Their response rate increased as the element's thickness was reduced. However, as the thickness was reduced, the resistance increased and hence the effect of Johnson noise.

Although the sensitivity of metal thermocouples is much lower than that of semiconductor elements, these detectors are still often used due to their advantages (durability, stability and operational reliability). They are still used in many ground-based metrology instruments and industrial pyrometers.

High-speed thermocouples are made by a vacuum deposition of metal junctions using advanced photolithography techniques to produce small parts. Bismuth and antimony are the most commonly used vapor-deposited materials on an insulating substrate with a good thermal conductivity (e.g., sapphire or beryllium oxide). The resulting thermocouples sometimes have responses of less than 30 ms. Unfortunately, they have a relatively low sensitivity of 5×10^{-6} V/W and a detectivity of 10^6 cmHz$^{1/2}$/W. Thermocouples obtained by evaporation of vacuum bismuth and antimony on thin corundum or plastic substrates show a better performance.

In recent years, there has been a huge progress in the development of integrated thermocouples made of semiconductor materials using planar and micromechanical technologies. Connection between "hot" and "cold" areas is formed on a very thin (several-micron) silicon membrane [see Figure 5.5(a)] or on a cantilever beam with the embedded thermocouple. Heat generated in the "hot" area, flowing through the membrane (or beam) to a cold area with ambient temperature, causes a temperature difference to appear across the thermal resistance of the membrane (or beam). Figure 5.5(b) shows the cross-section of a MEMS thermocouple, which may contain a single, double or quadruple structure.

The most widely used approach is n-polySi/Al thermopiles. Although Al has a very low Seebeck coefficient, this approach is used widely, as it is easy to implement with post-CMOS (Complementary

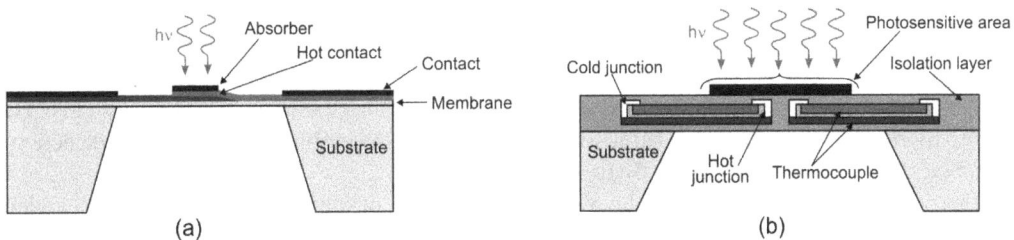

FIGURE 5.5 Cross-section of the thermocouple: (a) thin layer, (b) with a single/dual structure (after Reference 15).

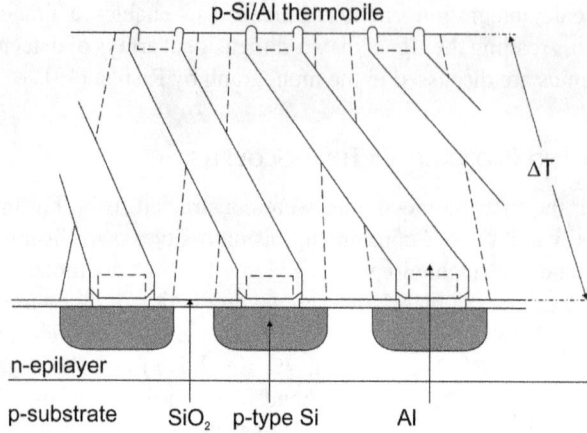

FIGURE 5.6 Integrated Al/p-Si thermopile.

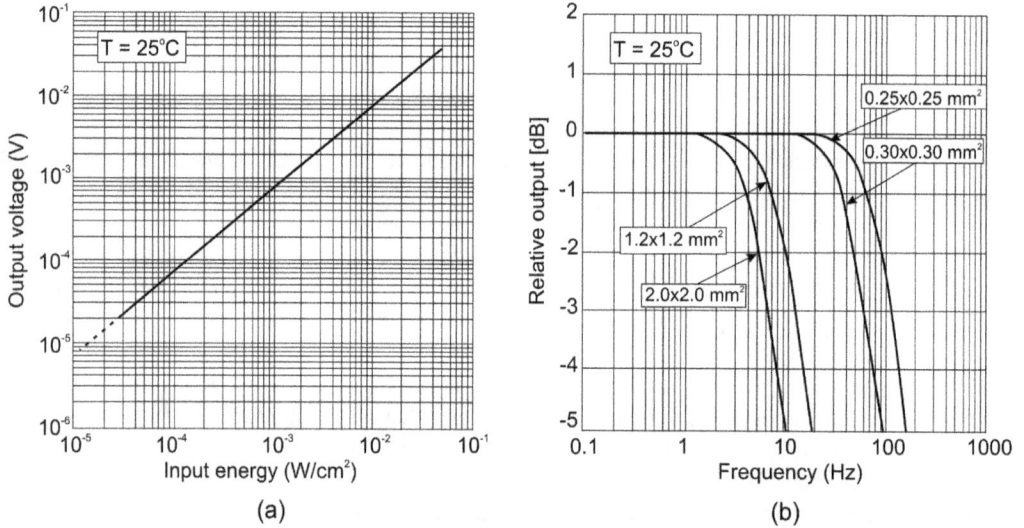

FIGURE 5.7 Characteristics of Hamamatsu T11262 thermocouples: a) dependence of the thermocouple output voltage on the incident radiation power density, b) relative frequency response (after Reference 15).

Metal-Oxide-Semiconductor) processes. Very attractive is the p-polySi/n-polySi approach, as it provides relatively high Seebeck coefficient. Polysilicon's popularity in this area is a direct result of its mechanical properties and its relatively well-developed deposition and processing technologies. These characteristics along with the capability of utilising established IC processing techniques make it a useful selection. The scheme of a silicon thermocouple is shown in Figure 5.6. The structure is made of p-type strips in the n-type epitaxial layer, connected to aluminum strips [11]. The sensitivity of a thermocouple consisting of 44 thermocouples was about 6 V/W, and the detectivity for a blackbody at 500 K was about 5×10^7 cmHz$^{1/2}$W^{-1}.

Thermocouples are characterised by a linear dependence of the output voltage on the incident radiation power density [Figure 5.7(a)], and their upper limit frequency decreases with the increase of the active surface [Figure 5.7(b)] [15]. Table 5.3 presents some representative parameters of different micromachined CMOS thermopiles [8].

TABLE 5.3
Characteristics Data of Different Micromachined Thermopiles (after Reference 8)

Sort	Area (mm²)	D^* (10⁷ Jones)	R (µV/W)	Material system	τ (ms)	α_t (µV/K)	Couples	Atm.	Data
CB	0.013	0.68	10	Al/poly		58	20		Sim
CB	0.77	1.5	25	Al/poly		58	200		Sim
CB	15.2	5		p-Si/Al	300	700	44	Air	Meas
MB	15.2	10	>10	p-Si/Al		700	44	Vac	Meas
MB	0.12	1.7	12	Al/poly	10	−63	4×10		Meas
MB	0.3	2	44	n,p poly	18	200	4×12		Meas
MB	0.15	2.4	72	n,p poly	10	200	4×12		Meas
MB	0.15	2.4	150	n,p poly	22	200	4×12	Kr	Meas
MB	0.12	1.74	12	Al/poly AMS	10	65	10	Air	Meas
MB	0.12	1.78	28	Al/poly AMS	20	65	2×24	Air	Meas
MB	0.42	4.4	11	InGaAs/InP				Air	Meas
M	0.42	71	184	InGaAs/InP				Vac	Meas
M	4	6	6	Bi/Sb	15	100	60		Meas
M	4	3.5	7	n-poly/Au	15		60		Sim
M	4	4.8	9.6	p-poly/Au	15		60		Sim
M	0.25	9.3	48	p-poly/Al	20		40		
M	3.28	13	12	p-poly/Al	50		68		
M	0.2	55	180	Bi/Sb	19	100	72	Air	Meas
M	0.2	88	290	Bi/Sb	35	100	72	Kr	Meas
M	0.2	52	340	$Bi_{0.50}Sb_{0.15}Te_{0.35}/$ $Bi_{0.87}Sb_{0.13}$	25	330	72	Air	Meas
C	0.2	77	500	$Bi_{0.50}Sb_{0.15}Te_{0.35}/$ $Bi_{0.87}Sb_{0.13}$	44	330	72	Kr	Meas
C	9	26	14.8	Bi/Sb	100		72	Ar	Meas
C	0.785	29	23.5	Bi/Sb	32		15	Ar	Meas
C	0.06	25	194	Si	12		20	Ar	Meas
C	0.37	5.6	36	CMOS	<6				Meas
C	1.44	8.7	27	CMOS	<6				Meas
C	0.37	5.6	36	CMOS	<6				Meas
C	1.44	4.6	12	CMOS	30				
C	0.2	45	200		20		72	N₂	Meas
C	1.44	35	100		30		200	N₂	Meas
C	0.49	21	110	BiSb/NiCr	40		100		Meas
C	0.49	6	35	CMOS	25				Meas
C	1.44	8	20	CMOS	35				Meas
C	0.6	24	80	CMOS	<40			Vac	Meas

CB: cantilever beam thermopile, MB: micro bridge thermopile, M: membrane thermopile, C: commercial thermopile, Sim: simulated data, Meas: measured data.

Thermopiles are widely used, mostly as single-point detectors, in many low-power applications such as in the automotive industry (e.g., in reliability tests of electronic modules, windscreen defrosting systems or tire temperature measurement), medicine (e.g., for measuring temperature inside the ear, in blood flow measurement systems), agriculture (e.g., for determining disease state of plants and arable fields), household appliances (e.g., in control systems in refrigerators, air conditioners, electric irons) and gas sensors [16].

With recent improvements in the resolution and sensitivity of thermopile IR FPA, the thermopile detector has been regarded as among the best cost–performance ratio solutions for thermal imager development. Compared with the microbolometer, the thermopile has a large advantage in price and is easy to obtain from the market. Thermopiles have very useful characteristics; they are highly linear, require no optical chopper – however, they have D^* values lower than bolometers and pyroelectric detectors. They operate over a broad temperature range with little or no temperature stabilisation. They have no electrical bias, leading to negligible $1/f$ noise and no voltage pedestal in their output signal. However, array implementations of thermopiles are limited, and much less effort has been made in their development. This is mainly owing to the large pixel size required for implementing each thermopile pixel. Because of poor sensitivity, the pixel pitch is limited to ~ 100 μm, which especially limits their use for large format detector arrays. Their responsivity (of the order of 5–15 V/W) and noise are orders of magnitude less and thus their applications in thermal imaging systems require very low-noise electronics to realise their potential performance.

Figure 5.8 shows an example of a thermopile pixel structure and an SEM photo of a thermopile pixel. The cavity formed in the substrate reduces the thermal conductance and enhances the responsivity. To thermally isolate the pixels, front-access process is needed.

At present various infrared array sensors based on thermopile technology are adopted by some low-end markets, such as home appliances. Table 5.4 gathers their typical performance. Lapis Semiconductor and Heimann Sensor are selling relatively large format arrays.

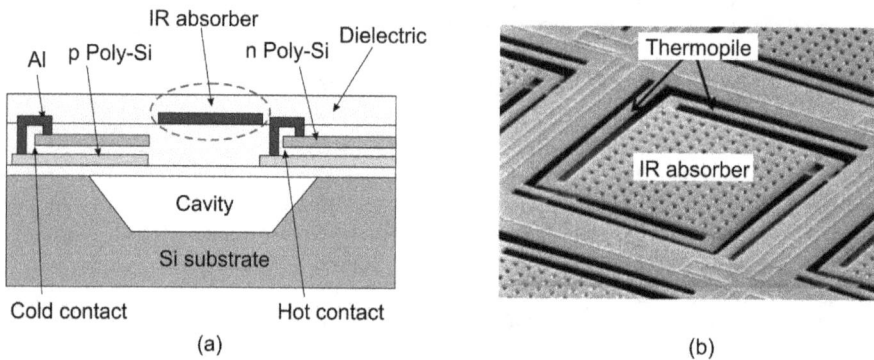

FIGURE 5.8 Typical pixel structure for thermopile infrared array: (a) cross-sectional pixel structure and (b) SEM photo of thermopile pixel (adapted after Reference 17).

TABLE 5.4
Thermopile Focal Plane Arrays

Company	Lapis	Heimann	Excelitas	Melexis
Array format	48×47	80×64	32×32	32×24
Pixel pitch (μm)	100	90	220	100
NEDT (K)	0.5	0.1	0.8	0.1
Field of view (deg)	N.A.	41×33	60	110
Frame rate/Time constant	6 Hz	30 Hz	115 ms	64 Hz
Packaging	Vacuum	Vacuum	Atmospheric pressure (N_2)	Atmospheric pressure

5.3 BOLOMETERS

The second widely used thermal detector is a bolometer. The bolometer is a resistance element made of a material with a very low heat capacity and a high temperature coefficient of resistance, so that as a result of the absorbed radiation, the structure heats up and the detector resistance changes. The general theory of the bolometer is described in Section 4.3.3.

Taking into account the type of material from which the bolometers are made, we divide them into

- metal;
- thermistor bolometers (thermistors);
- semiconductor;
- composite; and
- superconductive.

The most numerous groups are metal, thermistor and semiconductor bolometers. Composite bolometers are used in low-noise and low-temperature detection systems. In order to achieve high detectivity and detection of very small radiation fluxes, cryogenically cooled bolometers (e.g., superconducting bolometers) are used to a temperature below liquid helium.

Kruse carried out the analysis of bolometer operation including the Joulean heating and constant electrical bias [18]. It appears that the behaviour of the detector seriously depends on temperature dependence of bolometer resistance upon temperature.

The resistance of a piece of semiconductor can be shown to be the form

$$R = R_o T^{-3/2} \exp\left(\frac{b}{T}\right),$$
(5.6)

where R_o and b are constants. For a semiconductor at room temperature

$$\alpha = -\frac{b}{T^2}.$$
(5.7)

For a metal that has a linear dependence of resistance on temperature; that is

$$R = R_o\left[1 + \gamma\left(T - T_o\right)\right],$$
(5.8)

and thus

$$\alpha = \frac{\gamma}{1 + \gamma\left(T - T_o\right)}.$$
(5.9)

Here γ is the temperature coefficient of the detector material.

In the case of bolometer operation under constant electrical bias and Joulean heating, the solution of a heat balance equation is similar to that described by Eq. (4.3) [4] and has the form

$$\Delta T = \Delta T_o e^{-(G_e/C_{th})t} + \frac{\varepsilon\Phi_o e^{i\omega t}}{G_e + i\omega C_{th}}.$$
(5.10)

The first term of Eq. (5.10) represents a transient, whereas the second term is a periodic function. Here G_e is the "effective" thermal conductance defined as

$$G_e = G - G_o \left(T_1 - T_o\right) \alpha \left(\frac{R_L - R_B}{R_L + R_B}\right), \tag{5.11}$$

where G_o is the average thermal conductance through a detector medium in temperature range between T_1 and T_o, and G is the thermal conductance when the bolometer is at temperature T. Here R_B and R_L are the bolometer and load resistances, respectively. Eq. (5.11) indicates that G_e is the difference in two terms. The G_e is positive if

$$G > G_o \left(T_1 - T_o\right) \alpha \left(\frac{R_L - R_B}{R_L + R_B}\right), \tag{5.12}$$

and then the transient term goes to zero with time, and only the periodic function remains. However, in the case when

$$G < G_o \left(T_1 - T_o\right) \alpha \left(\frac{R_L - R_B}{R_L + R_B}\right), \tag{5.13}$$

where G_e is negative, that means the bolometer temperature will increase exponentially with time [see Eq. (5.10)] reaching burnout. This can happen with semiconductors but not with metals [19].

Assuming that $R_L >> R_B$, it can be shown that the responsivity is given by

$$R_v = \frac{\alpha I_b R_B \varepsilon}{G_e \left(1 + \omega^2 \tau_e^2\right)^{1/2}}, \tag{5.14}$$

where τ_e is defined as

$$\tau_e = \frac{C_{th}}{G_e}. \tag{5.15}$$

Here, τ_e is known as the "effective thermal response time." The dependence of thermal capacity and τ on temperature due to bias current heating is termed the "electrothermal effect."

Usually, when large focal plane arrays are implied, the electrical bias is pulsed rather than continuous, heating is due to the electrical bias (Joulean), and the incident absorbed radiant flux. In this situation the heat transfer equation is nonlinear and numerical solutions must be obtained [20].

In addition to radiation noise and temperature noise associated with the thermal impedance of the element, Johnson noise associated with resistance R is one of the most important noise sources. With room temperature bolometers, amplifier noise should not be important but with cryogenic devices it is usually the dominant noise source. With some types of bolometers, low frequency current noise is important and is the principal factor limiting current.

5.3.1 METAL BOLOMETERS

Metal bolometers are mainly made of nickel, platinum, bismuth, antimony, niobium, or titanium. They are characterised by a high, long-term stability and a positive temperature coefficient of resistance. A typical value of this coefficient is about 0.3%/°C. Being made from metal, these bolometers need to be small so that the heat capacity is low enough to allow a reasonable sensitivity. Most metal bolometers are formed as film strips, about 100–500 Å thick, and with a resistance in the order of 1–5 MΩ. They are often coated with a black absorber such as evaporated gold or platinum black.

The unquestionable advantage of these detectors is their resistance to high power densities of incident radiation, parameter stability and low noise. They are used to detect mid-infrared and far-infrared radiation as well as terahertz radiation. The metal bolometers operating at room temperature reach an NEP of a few $pW/Hz^{1/2}$ and detectivities of about 1×10^8 $cmHz^{1/2}/W$. The time constant of these detectors is in the order of 10 ms. For uncooled bolometers, these parameters depend mainly on the type of metal used and geometric dimensions of the detection structure. Such devices are manufactured as discrete elements and as small two-dimensional arrays due to power consumption and amplifier design constraints associated with matching the low detector impedance.

Between metals, titanium films are more frequently used in the bolometers due to the following reasons: titanium can be used in a standard silicon process line, low thermal conductivity (0.22 W/Kcm in bulk material – far lower than that of most other metals), and low $1/f$ noise [21, 22]. However, metal in thin-film form has a temperature coefficient resistance of 0.004 %/K, considerably lower than for competitor materials, which causes it to be of little use in uncooled bolometer arrays.

Figure 5.9 shows the pixel structure of a microbolometer matrix of 256×256 [22]. It consists of three layers: active layer (absorber), layer supporting the absorber and layer containing the signal-reading systems. The active layer of the detector was made of titanium in the form of a meander and protected with SiO_2. The absorber supporting layer consists of two bridges containing electrically conductive paths connecting the active part of a pixel with the readout circuit obtained in a CMOS technology. This detector has a sensitivity of about 9000 V/W (at 70 µA bias current) and a detectivity of 2.4×10^9 $cmHz^{1/2}/W$.

5.3.2 THERMISTORS

Thermistors have found a wide range of applications, ranging from burglary and fire warning systems to industrial temperature-measuring systems, space-sensor systems and radiometric ones. They have become convenient sensors for radiometric measurements where a uniform spectral response is desired. Thermistors are constructed from a sintered-made mixture of various semiconducting oxides (manganese, cobalt and nickel oxides) mounted on sapphire type insulating substrates. In turn, the substrate is mounted on a metallic heat sink mainly to control the time constant of the instrument.

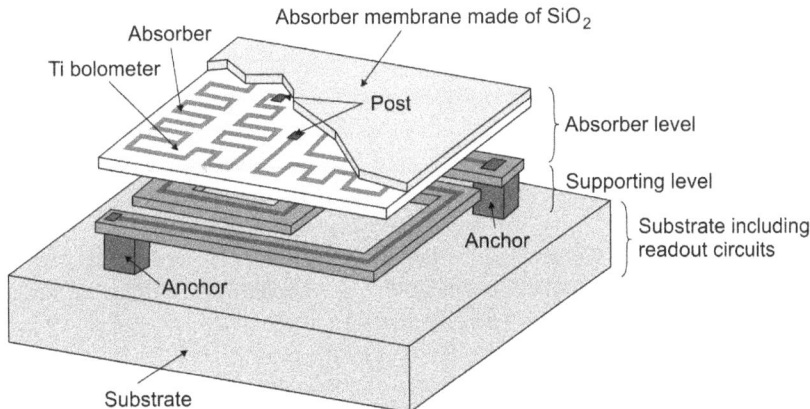

FIGURE 5.9 Pixel structure of a microbolometer matrix with the Ti active layer.

The detector active part is blackened to increase the absorption of radiation. Typically, thermistors are made in the form of rectangular plates with photo-sensitive surface dimensions ranging from 0.05×0.05 mm^2 to 5×5 mm^2, a thickness of about 10 μm and a resistivity ranging from 250 Ωcm to 2500 Ωcm. The negative temperature coefficient of resistance is high, from 2 to 4 %/°C, and the time constant from 1 to 10 ms. The negative temperature coefficient depends on a band gap, impurity states and dominant conduction mechanism. This coefficient is not constant, but varies as T^{-2} which is a result of the semiconductor resistivity exponential dependence.

For a single unit, the usual construction uses a matched pair of devices (Figure 4.15(b). One of the thermistors pairs needs to be shielded from radiation and fitted into a bridge in such a way that it operates as the load resistor. Such arrangement allows for optimising the signal by compensating ambient temperature changes. It can result in a dynamic range of a million to one. Device sensitivity and response time cannot be optimised at the same time as improved heat sinking in order to reduce the time constant preventing the detector from reaching its maximum temperature, which reduces the responsivity. Considerations conducted by Astheimer [23] indicate that the Johnson noise-limited detectivity of this bolometer type at room temperature can be described by the following equation:

$$D^* = 3 \times 10^9 \, \tau^{1/2}, \quad [\text{cmHz}^{1/2} \, / \, \text{W}], \tag{5.16}$$

where τ is the detector response time. Their sensitivity closely approaches that of the thermopile for frequencies higher than 25 Hz. At lower frequencies, there may be excess or $1/f$ noise.

Achieving greater detectivity is possible by using radiation concentrators (high refractive index immersion lenses n_r). This causes the apparent increase of the detector surface, n_r times (or n_r^2 in the case of hyper-hemispherical lenses), which is shown in Figure 4.26. Also, immersion reduces the bias power dissipation by the factors n_r^2 (or n_r^4), thus reducing the cooler's heat load and enabling the higher bias power dissipation densities in order to be achieved. The lens material requirements are such that it should have as large refraction index as possible, as well as it should be electrically insulating in order not to short the thermistor film. Germanium, silicon, and arsenic triselenide are among the most useful materials. Thermistor detectors are especially adaptable to the immersion because a low thermal impedance inherent in immersion allows for a higher bias voltage to be applied.

Thermistor detectors are mainly fabricated by bonding thermistor material thin flakes with a substrate. These detectors are manufactured using modern silicon microelectronics and micromechanics. This makes it possible to obtain dyes with a very large number of elements and ensures high reliability and low production costs. One- and two-dimensional arrays of thermistor bolometers are also produced using MEMS technology [24]. The MEMS technology produces higher performance devices – reduced crosstalk between pixels, higher fill factor and better thermal management. An example of such a matrix array is shown in Figure 5.10.

5.3.3 Semiconductor Bolometers

Increasing bolometers' detectivity can be achieved by lowering their operating temperature. At lower temperatures, relative changes in resistance caused by the incident radiation flux are much greater than at room temperature. When the temperature is lowered, the material specific heat is reduced, so that the detection element can be thicker without increasing the heat capacity. This, in turn, increases the absorption of radiation. Sensitivity of a cooled detector may be several orders of magnitude greater than that of a room-temperature detector.

The semiconductor bolometers are considered to be the most highly developed form of thermal detectors for low-light levels, as well as detectors of choice for many applications, in the infrared and submillimetre spectral range in particular. They must be constructed carefully to ensure that they are isolated from the thermal surroundings, and the techniques typically used to construct them do not lend themselves to efficient development of large arrays.

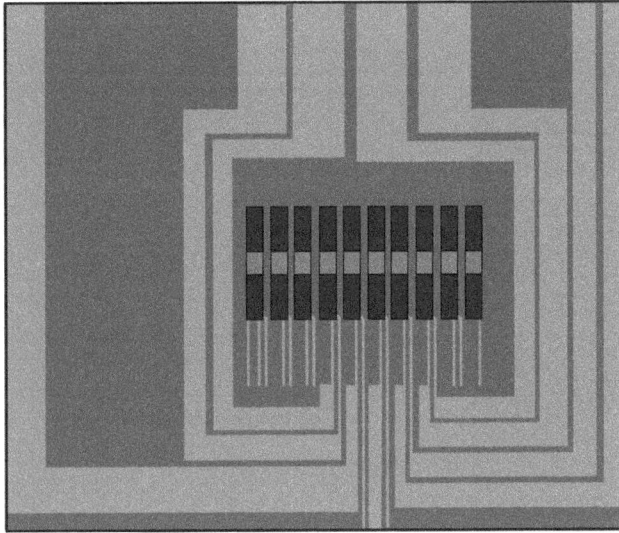

FIGURE 5.10   A typical thermistor bolometer array used in an imaging application.

The temperature dependence of semiconductor resistance is described by Eq. (5.6). However, at very low temperatures (<10 K), the semiconductor material must be doped more heavily than assumed in Eq. (5.6) so that the dominant conductivity mode is hopping. This mechanism freezes out relatively slowly; the resistance is given by an empirical expression of the form

$$R(T) = R_0 \exp\left(\sqrt{\frac{T_0}{T}} \right). \tag{5.17}$$

The constants T_0 and R_0 are of the order of 2–10 K and 0.1–0.5 Ω. The corresponding temperature coefficient of resistance is where typically $a \approx 4$. We then have

$$\alpha(T) = \frac{1}{R}\frac{dR}{dT} = -\frac{1}{2}\sqrt{\frac{T_0}{T^3}}. \tag{5.18}$$

Note that $\alpha < 0$ and has strong temperature dependence. This is in contrast to superconducting bolometers, which have positive α allowing for electrothermal feedback. An excellent agreement between Eq. (5.17) and experimental data was found for Ge bolometers [25, 26].

Initially, in the 1950s, the most popular solid-state bolometer used as a thermometer and operating at low temperatures was carbon. In bolometer development, the most important step with a superior performance was the invention of a low-temperature bolometer that was based on heavily gallium-doped and compensated germanium with sensitivity close to the theoretical limits (Figure 5.11) over the wavelength range from 5 to 100 µm. Currently, silicon bolometers with a spectral sensitivity ranging from 2 µm to 3000 µm are more popular. Compared to germanium, silicon has a lower specific heat (about five times) and is easier to process. Silicon bolometers reach *NEP* below 1×10^{-14} W/Hz$^{1/2}$ at a temperature of about 1 K [27].

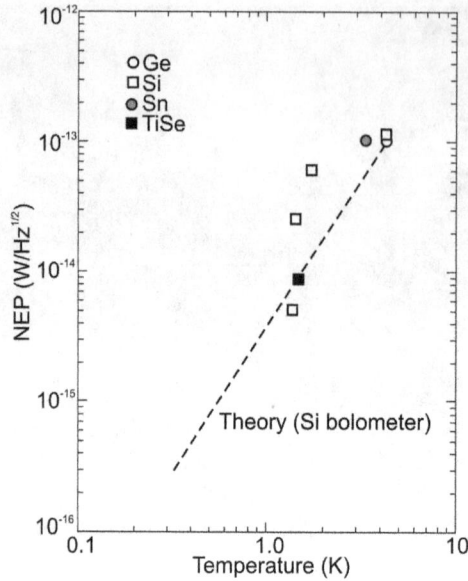

FIGURE 5.11 *NEP* dependence in the low temperature range for germanium, silicon, tin and titanium selenide bolometers. The dashed line represents theoretical *NEP* for silicon bolometers in the absence of background.

In p-type detectors, the absorbed energy is immediately transferred to the crystal lattice, causing an increase in the detector temperature (proportion of free carriers is insignificant). For small aperture detectors operating at 4.2 K, the proportion of Johnson noise and photon noise is comparable. As the aperture area increases, the photon noise will outweigh the detector self-noise. Due to their high stability and a low noise level, the semiconductor bolometers are used in infrared astronomy as well as in laboratory infrared spectroscopy. The performance of far infrared bolometers is comparable to that of the best photon detectors.

Bolometer structures described earlier combine the functions of radiation adsorption and temperature sensors. These two functions are difficult in a practical implementation at the same time, especially for chip bolometers designed for millimetre and submillimetre wavelengths. To obtain good absorption properties, the bolometer should have a thickness of one or several millimetres. This condition fulfilment causes an increase in thermal capacity, and thus a decrease in detector sensitivity.

In order to overcome those limitations, composite bolometers are manufactured to lower heat capacity and to reduce consistently the time constant. They consist of three parts: radiation-absorbing material, substrate determining its active area, as well as temperature sensor as shown in Figure 5.12. An absorber is made of a thin film of which thickness and composition are adjusted in a way that the emissivity is very high – into hundreds of microns' wavelength region. Black bismuth and nichrome absorbers usually have been used. A temperature sensor (e.g., germanium) is bonded mechanically and thermally to the substrate through an epoxy or varnish. Therefore, substrate and film combination operate as an efficient absorbing element of a large effective area, as well as a low heat capacity for a temperature sensor that could be made very small. It is, therefore, possible to make a detector with a larger effective area without worsening its frequency characteristics.

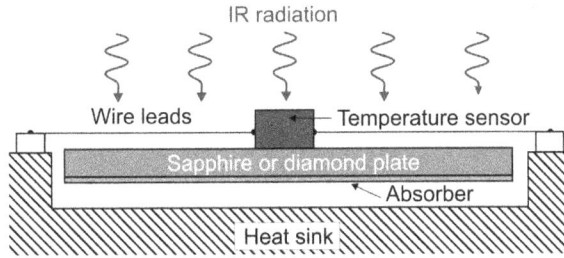

FIGURE 5.12   Composite bolometer.

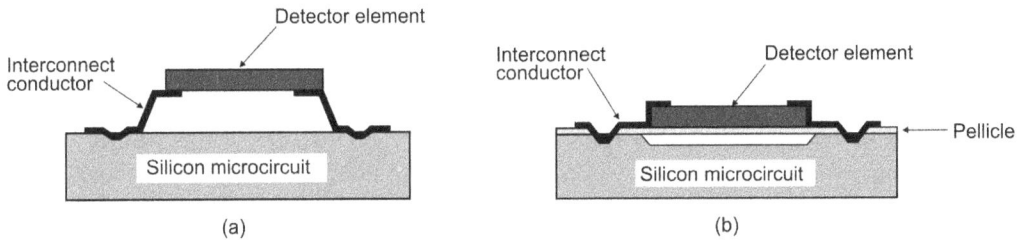

FIGURE 5.13   Thermal detector element design: (a) microbridge detector element, and (b) pellicle supported detector element.

5.3.4 MICROBOLOMETERS

In 1979, Honeywell scientists in Minneapolis, initiated intensive development of silicon micromachining technology for the bolometer construction [28, 29]. This technology can be used for many materials, but silicon is clearly favoured due to the fact, that many micromechanical processes are compatible with the technology used in the design of silicon integrated circuits. The use of silicon also enables a monolithic connection of readout with the microstructures made. Moreover, by using micromechanics, the extremely high thermal resistances in structures can be achieved. This makes it possible to miniaturise bolometers, microbolometers, and their manufacturing with a thermal insulation close to the physical limit of about 1×10^8 °C/W for a square detector of 50×50 μm^2. It has been demonstrated that a microbolometer with an order of lower thermal insulation (1×10^7 °C/W) detects a 10-nW signal, and then, the indicated temperature change of the bolometer is of 0.1°C.

Two options for the bolometers' structure are used: microbridge and pellicle-supported designs (see Figure 5.13) [30]. The former comprises detector elements that are supported on legs above the plane of the microcircuit. The legs are designed to have a high thermal resistance and carry electrical conductors from the detector to the microcircuit. This approach was implied in the Honeywell microbolometer design [28,29]. The second concept consists of detector elements deposited onto a thin dielectric pellicle that is coplanar with the surface of the wafer and is the basis of original Australian monolithic detector technology [30].

A typical microbolometer pixel structure is shown in Figure 5.14 [31]. A detecting area is defined by a thin membrane on which a thin-film detecting material is deposited. The microbolometer consists of a 0.5-μm Si_3N_4 thick bridge which is suspended about 2 μm above an underlying silicon substrate. Two narrow Si_3N_4 legs support the bridge. Thermal isolation between the microbolometer and the heat-sink readout substrate is provided by Si_3N_4 legs. The detector active material is vanadium oxide (usually VO_2) vaporised on a plate. Temperature changes on the plate are indicated by monolithically integrated electrical circuits located below the bridge and electrically connected by

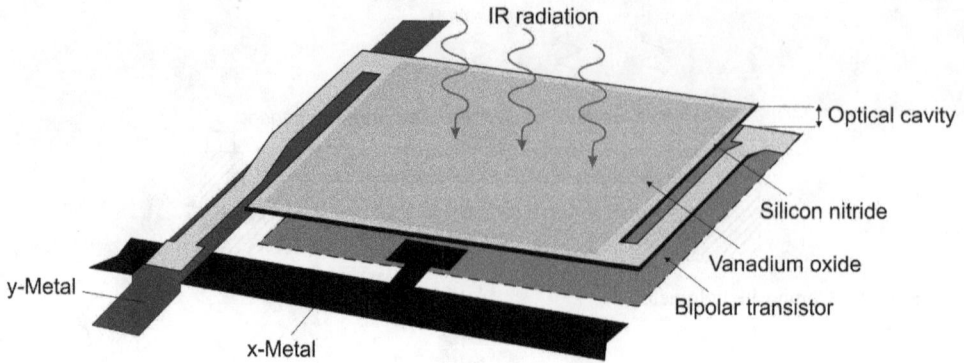

FIGURE 5.14 Bridge structure of the Honeywell microbolometer.

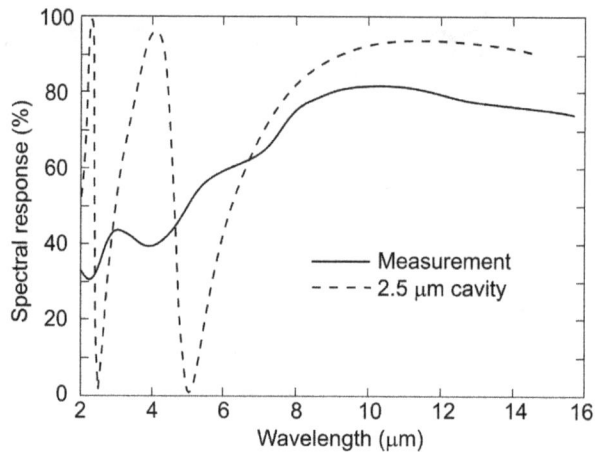

FIGURE 5.15 Quarter-wave cavity spectrum of the ULIS amorphous silicon bolometer.

thin metallic layers (Ni-Cr with a thickness of 500 Å) deposited on "legs". Bipolar input amplifiers obtained with a biCMOS processing technology are usually used to read out the signal.

Approximately 2.5 micron spacing between the membrane and the thin reflective layer on the silicon substrate below provides a quarter-wave resonant optical cavity for a wavelength of about 10 μm. Structures obtained in this way are extremely durable; they are not destroyed at shocks of several thousand g-forces. In order to increase the thermal resistance and, thus, the sensitivity of the microbolometer, a vacuum (typically of 0.01 mbar) is provided in the cavity or else filled with noble gas.

The use of a quarter-wave cavity increases the absorption of radiation in the detector's active material, but also narrows its spectral characteristics. Figure 5.15 shows a comparison of the ULIS microbolometer spectral sensitivity with the theoretically calculated sensitivity [32].

In the early 1990s Honeywell was a monopolist in vanadium oxide bolometer technology. Since these microbolometers were not licensed outside the United States, several research teams around the world developed the microbolometer bridge technology with the amorphous silicon (a-Si) as the active area (similar design to that shown in Figure 5.14).

The most popular thermistor material used in fabrication of the micromachined silicon bolometers is vanadium oxide, VO_x. A thin film of the mixed oxides sputtered on a Si_3N_4 microbridge substrate was originally developed at Honeywell. Vanadium is a metal with a variable valence forming a large

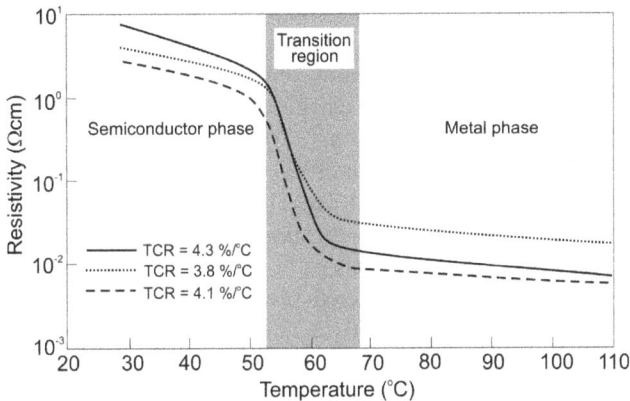

FIGURE 5.16   Resistivity versus temperature characteristics of three VO_2 films (after Reference 33).

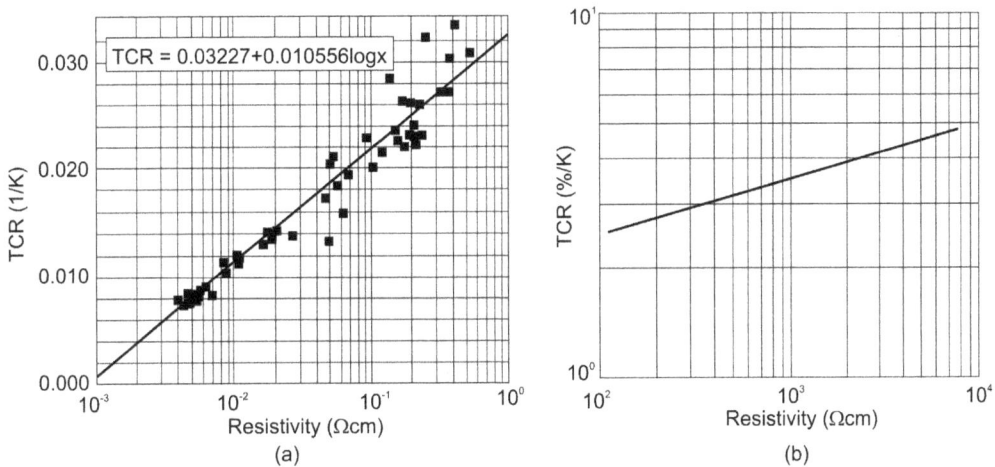

FIGURE 5.17   Temperature coefficient of resistance versus resistivity for thin films of (a) mixed vanadium oxides (after Reference 29) and (b) amorphous silicon (after Reference 34).

number of oxides. Preparation of these materials in both bulk and thin-film forms is very difficult given the narrowness of the stability range of any oxide. Some of the vanadium oxides – among the best-known being VO_2, V_2O_3 and V_2O_5 – show a temperature-induced crystallographic transformation that is accomplished by reversible semiconductor (low-temperature phase) to metal (high-temperature phase) phase transition with a significant change in electrical and optical properties (Figure 5.16). Vanadium dioxide undergoes their transition in the temperature range from about 50 to 70°C.

Figure 5.17 shows the TCR in dependence on resistivity for thin films of mixed vanadium oxides [29] and amorphous silicon (a-Si) [34]. From the point of view of infrared imaging application, the most important property of VO_x is its high negative TCR at ambient temperature, which exceeds 3 per cent per degree. However, there are two reasons for not using VO_x material with higher x-values and substantially higher TCR. In the region of higher x-value, the reproducibility of oxide property suffers due to scatter of experimental data. In addition, Joule heating becomes a problem with high resistivity films. This aggravates the nonlinear temperature versus time problem during the pulse duration [29].

For a-Si, the room temperature TCR values ranging from –0.025 °C^{-1} for doped, low resistivity films to 0.06 °C^{-1} for high resistivity materials have been reported. However, high-resistivity a-Si is characterised by unacceptable levels of $1/f$ noise. Properties of the a-Si films depend upon the method of preparation and the type of dopant. Amorphous hydrogenated silicon (a-Si:H) has a metastable state caused by defects arising from prolonged illumination (Staebler and Wronski effect). This is an undesirable feature that requires a specific annealing cycle during preparation (methodology for reliability enhancement is described in [35]). Because the typical resistivity of a-Si films is several orders of magnitude higher than that of VO_x, a-Si finds application in uncooled arrays in which the bias is continuous rather than pulsed. This choice is dictated by the fact that the bolometer signal depends on $I_b \alpha R$, whereas the power dissipation, which causes the rise in detector temperature, depends on $I_b^2 R$ (here I_b is the bias current).

Currently, microbolometer arrays with different pixel dimensions are manufactured. A reduction in pixel dimensions has been achieved from 50 μm in the 1990s to 8 μm in 2020 with formats up to several megapixels. Detailed information on the detector matrices can be found in chapter 12.

For temperature sensing, the forward biased p-n junction or Schottky-barrier junction can be also used [36]. To explain the operation of a diode sensor, Figure 5.18 shows forward I-V characteristics of a diode for two different temperatures. When the p-n junction is operated in a constant-current mode, the forward voltage measured across the junction reflects the temperature of the device. The forward voltage is determined by J_s, the intersection with the current axis and the gradient q/kT. The forward voltage becomes smaller as the temperature rises.

If the detector is constructed with diodes serially connected by metal straps, the forward current is given by

$$I = AJ_s \exp\left(\frac{qV}{nkT}\right), \tag{5.19}$$

and the temperature coefficient of forward current can be expressed by

$$\left.\frac{dV}{dT}\right|_{I=const} \approx n\frac{(V/n)-E_g}{qT} \tag{5.20}$$

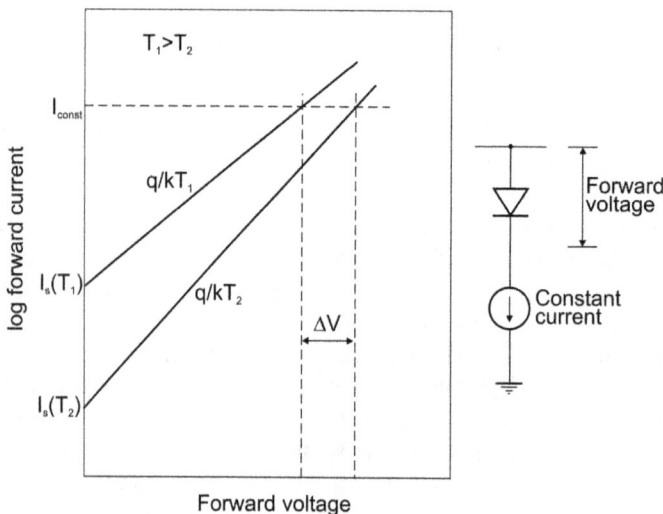

FIGURE 5.18   Operation of forward-biased p-n junction sensor.

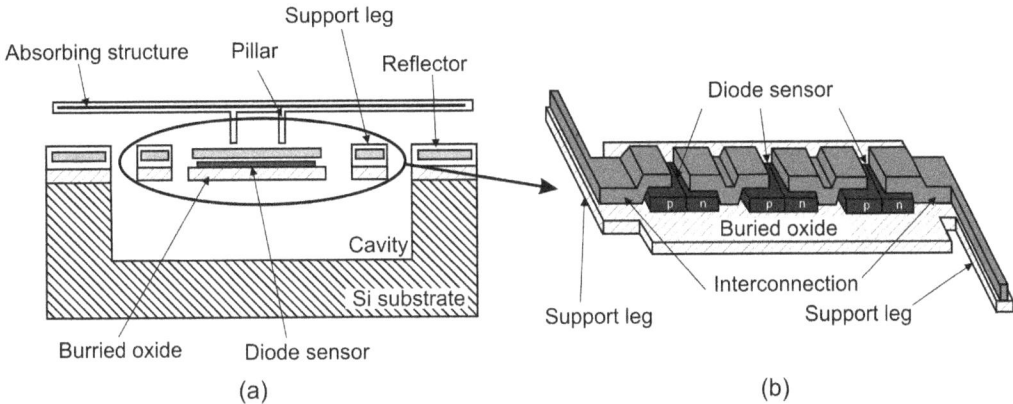

FIGURE 5.19   Pixel structure of SOI diode uncooled infrared FPA, showing cross section (a) and p-n junction temperature sensor (b) (after Reference 38).

where n is the number of series. From the last equation we know that the temperature coefficient of forward voltage is proportional to the number of series.

The main noise in p-n junction is shot noise, which is result of the statistical process of carriers flowing over a potential barrier. It can be given by the following equation:

$$V_n = \sqrt{2qI} \frac{dV}{dI}.$$

(5.21)

In addition to the shot noise, two additional types of noise should be taken into account: the Johnson noise associated with the resistance and $1/f$ noise. The diodes with low $1/f$ power law noise can be manufactured in a standard CMOS technique.

Uncooled FPAs with p-n junction sensors have been successfully developed, and IR camera with some of these devices is commercially available [36, 37]. For example, Figure 5.19 shows a pixel structure with a p-n junction uncooled sensor on an SOI wafer, which was proposed by Ishikawa *et al.* [38]. Using silicon-on-insulator (SOI) technology, it was possible to fabricate a freestanding structure with diode sensor, support legs, horizontal addressing lin, and vertical signal line placed on the same level. The IR absorbing structure consists of a thin absorbing metal and a dielectric film for maintaining the shape of this metal. An interference absorber is formed with this absorbing structure and the reflector deposited on the lower level. A 90 per cent fill factor is feasible with this SOI diode pixel.

5.3.5   SUPERCONDUCTING BOLOMETERS

Superconductivity was discovered in 1911 by H. Kamerlingh-Onnes. For many decades, the practical application of this phenomenon was very difficult due to the need to achieve extremely low temperatures. In the 1940s, work was initiated to design superconducting bolometers [39]. Initially, superconductive bolometers made of niobium compounds were most commonly used. Their usefulness was limited due to the required very low critical temperature and poor radiation absorption. In spite of tremendous progress accomplished in cryogenic technology, superconductivity has been used either when no classical alternative was available or when the required performances were impossible to achieve using a non-superconducting solution. The performance was generally limited by amplifier noise rather than radiation fluctuations. The first bolometer to actually utilise

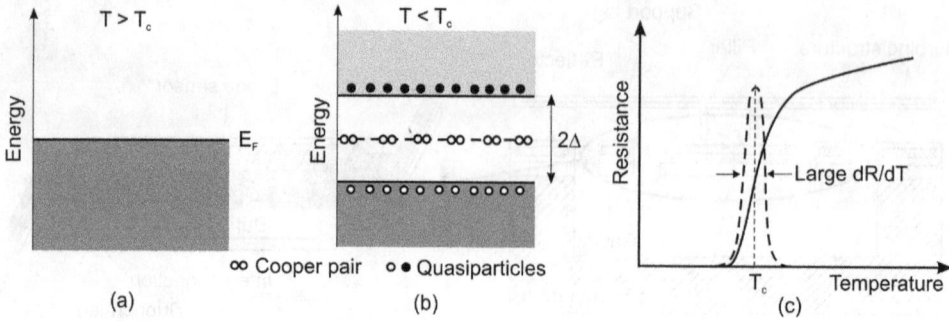

FIGURE 5.20 Operation of superconductor bolometer near transition edge: energy diagram (a) above and (b) below the transition, (c) typical resistance versus temperature plot with the derivative dR/dT superimposed on the transition edge.

the superconducting transition was a composite structure using a blackened aluminium foil absorber in conjunction with tantalum temperature sensor [40].

Figure 5.20 explains fundamentals of superconductor transitions. Below a certain temperature, defined as the critical temperature T_c, the electrons at the Fermi energy condense into a coherent state made up of Cooper pairs, as shown in Figure 5.20(b). The parameter 2Δ is the superconducting energy gap. According to Bardeen-Cooper-Schrieffer theory, the value of 2Δ is given by $3.53kT_c$, which is in reasonably good agreement with the measured value of $(3.2–4.6)kT_c$ for superconducting elements [41]. For a transition temperature of 90 K (typical for YBaCuO), the energy gap predicted from this relationship is 27 meV. Often, given the scatter in the experimental data for different materials, the precise value of the energy gap cannot be determined. As in an ordinary bolometer, there is not a direct photon–lattice interaction, so response is slow, but is independent of wavelength.

The theory, construction principles and performance of superconductor bolometers are considered in several reviews [26, 41–44]. General theory of bolometers described in Section 4.3 is also relevant for superconducting bolometers.

Figure 5.20(c) shows the relationship between the resistance R and the derivative dR/dT near the edge of the phase transition for a superconducting substance. This detector is usually called a transition-edge sensor (TES). Due to the step change of resistance near the critical temperature T_c, a small change in temperature causes a large change in resistance and, therefore, dR/dT is large (in the narrow temperature range of 0.001 K) [45]. It was shown [46] that the value of D^* depends on the time constant of the detector: $D^* = const \times \tau^{1/2}$ [for comparison, see Eq. (5.16)]. The bolometer detectivity values measured experimentally by different authors are presented in Table 5.5 [47, 48].

The most sensitive and slowest bolometers are well insulated from the environment, and their design is precisely developed. This is achieved by using a thin nylon fibre (samples 1–2 in Table 5.5) or a thin membrane supporting the active element [Figure 5.21(a); samples 3–5 in Table 5.5]. A higher response rate is obtained when the bolometer is placed directly on a solid substrate, for example, sapphire [Figure 5.21(b); sample 7 in Table 5.5]. The antenna-coupled design [Figure 5.21(c)] gives an effective way of increasing the sensitivity of thermal radiation detectors while retaining a fast response. In this case, a thin-film antenna deposited onto a substrate receives the radiation, which induces displacement currents in it having a frequency corresponding to the radiation wavelength. The high-frequency currents heat the thin-film bolometer, which fulfils the role of converting thermal power into an electrical signal. The fabrication of microbolometers [see Figure 5.21(d)], using conventional lithography and micromachining techniques, reaches time constants in the μs range and good detectivity. In this case, an antenna with rather large effective area can feed a superconducting microbridge of a much smaller area (a few μm²).

TABLE 5.5
Parameters of Superconductor Thermal Radiation Detectors

Material	Element size (mm²)	Temperature (K)	Sensitivity (V/W)	Time constant (s)	D^* (cmHz$^{1/2}$W^{-1})	NEP (W/Hz$^{1/2}$)	Remarks (Substrate/ Antenna)
1. Sn	3×2	3.05	850	10^{-2}	3.6×10^{11}	7×10^{-13}	
2. Al	4×4	1.27	3.5×10^4	8×10^{-2}	1.2×10^{14}	7×10^{-13}	
3. Ni+Sn	1×1	0.4	2.2×10^6	10^{-3}	2.2×10^{13}	3.4×10^{-15}	
4. Pb+Sn	–	4.8	10^4	6×10^{-3}	–	4.5×10^{-15}	
5. NbN	0.1×0.1	6.5	5×10^5	10^{-4}	–	–	
6. Sn	0.15×0.15	3.7	10^4	6×10^{-3}	10^{10}	1.6×10^{-12}	
6. Pb+Sn	1×1	3.9	24	7×10^{-9}	1.2×10^9	8.4×10^{-11}	
7. Sn	10×10	3.63	1	2×10^{-8}	10^9	10^{-9}	
8. Ag+Sn	2.3×2.3	2.1	2.2	5×10^{-9}	2.6×10^9	9×10^{-10}	
9. Sn	1×1	3.3	4200	2×10^{-6}	5×10^{10}	2×10^{-12}	
10. Pb+Sn	0.02×0.00225	4.7	5700	2×10^{-8}	–	3×10^{-13}	
11. Mo:Ge	–	0.1	10^9	10^{-6}	1×10^{16}	1×10^{-18}	
12. Pb	–	3.7	10^5	10^{-8}	5×10^{11}	2×10^{-14}	Sapphire
13. Au+Pb+Sn	–	3.7	6000	2×10^{-8}	2×10^{11}	5×10^{-14}	Quartz/V antenna
14. YBaCuO	1×1	20	0.1	4×10^{-7}	2.5×10^6	4×10^{-13}	
15. YBaCuO	1×1	86	40	1.3×10^{-2}	6.7×10^7	1.5×10^{-9}	
16. YBaCuO	0.01×0.09	40	4×10^3	10^{-3}	10^8	2.5×10^{-11}	
17. YBaCuO	0.1×0.1	86	15	1.6×10^{-4}	3.3×10^7	3×10^{-10}	
18. YBaCuO	0.1×0.1	80	10^3 (A/W)	6×10^{-2}	3×10^8	10^{-10}	
19. YBaCuO	–	90	2000	10^{-6}	2×10^9	5×10^{-12}	YSZ
20. YBaCuO	–	91	480	2×10^{-5}	2.2×10^9	4.5×10^{-12}	YSZ/Log-periodic
21. YBaCuO	–	90	4000	2×10^{-7}	4×10^9	2.5×10^{-12}	Si_3N_4/ Suspended bridge
22. YBaCuO	–	88	2180	1×10^{-5}	1.1×10^9	9×10^{-12}	Si_3N_4/Log-periodic
23. YBaCuO	–	85	240	3×10^{-7}	8.3×10^8	1.2×10^{-11}	$NdGaO_3$/ Bow-tie

5.3.6 HIGH-TEMPERATURE SUPERCONDUCTING BOLOMETERS

The important discovery by Müller and Bednorz of a new class of superconducting materials [49, 50], so called high-temperature superconducting bolometers (HTSCs), is undoubtedly one of the major breakthroughs in material science at the end of the twentieth century. Figure 5.22 shows the progression of the superconducting transition temperatures from the discovery of the phenomenon in mercury by Onnes in 1911. Between 1911 and 1974, the critical temperatures of metallic superconductors steadily increased from 4.2 K in mercury up to 23.2 K in sputtered Nb_3Ge films. Nb_3Ge held the record for the critical temperature in metallic superconductors until the unexpected discovery of superconductivity at 39 K in the intermetallic MgB_2. The first superconducting oxide $SrTiO_3$ characterised by transition temperature as low as 0.25 K, was discovered in 1964. Discovery of high-temperature superconductivity in the cuprate $(La,Ba)_2CuO_4$ ($T_c \approx 30$ K) opened a new field of research. Within less than a year a critical temperature well above 77 K was achieved in $YBa_2Cu_3O_{7-x}$. So far, at atmospheric pressure the highest transition temperature of 135 K has been found in $HgBa_2Ca_2Cu_3O_{8+x}$.

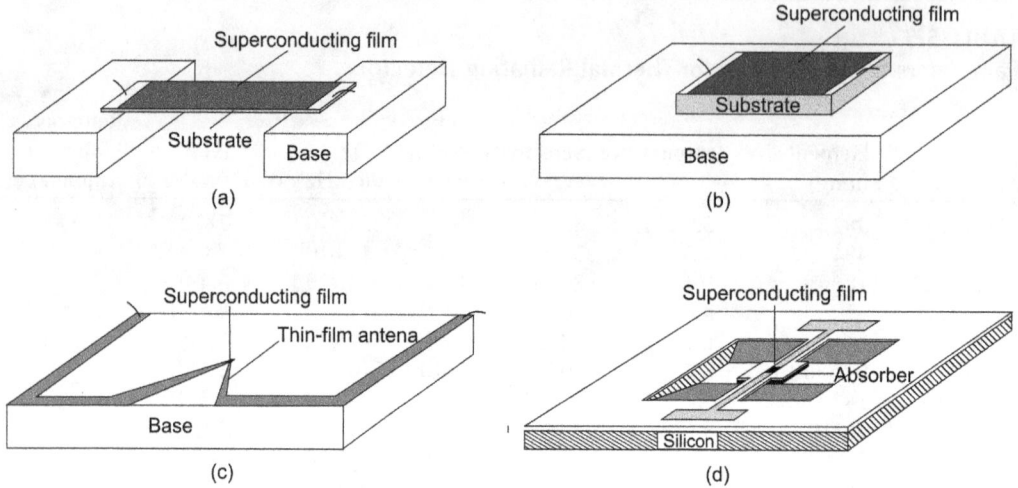

FIGURE 5.21   Superconductor bolometers: (b) non-isothermal bolometer, (b) bolometer on solid substrate, (c) antenna-coupled bolometer, and (d) micromachined bolometer.

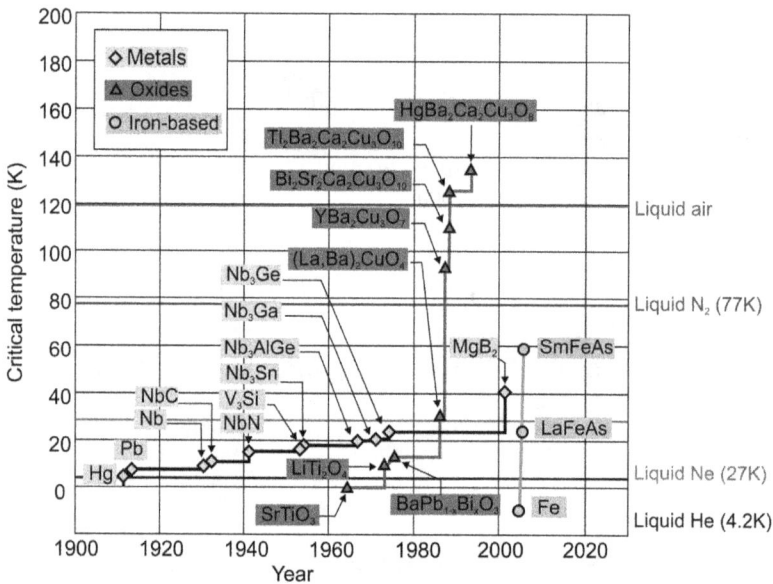

FIGURE 5.22   Evolution of the superconductive transition temperature subsequent to the discovery of the phenomenon.

All compounds showing high-temperature superconductivity belong to the group of so-called unsaturated perovskites with a basic crystal structure similar to $CaTiO_3$. The main research effort is focused on the compound $YbBa_2Cu_3O_{7-x}$ (YBaCuO). The properties of the compound in terms of its use in the infrared radiation detection were carried out by Kruse [51]. Since the phase transition temperature for good layers with YBaCuO is of about 90 K, the temperature of liquid nitrogen (77 K) is convenient for detectors with this compound.

The comparison of HTSC YBaCuO detectors with different types of photon detectors was made in Reference [52], which is shown in Figure 5.23. We can see that D^* falls at short wavelengths

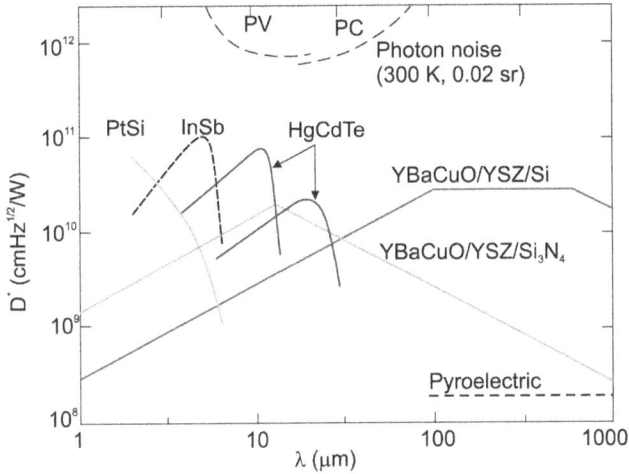

FIGURE 5.23 Detectivity as a function of wavelength for diffraction-limited pixels with FOV = 0.02 sr (*f*/6 optics) and τ = 10 ms. The thick lines show the predicted D^* for HTSC bolometers on silicon and Si_3N_4 membranes using YBaCuO films. These lines were calculated using estimates for the minimum achievable heat capacity and thermal conductance and using measurements of voltage noise in HTSC bolometers. Typical values of D^* for InSb, PtSi, and HgCdTe detectors in FPAs operated at 77 K are shown for comparison. Also are shown the photon noise limits for photovoltaic and photoconductive detectors which view 300 K radiation in a 0.02 sr FOV (after Reference 52).

because the membrane technology is not able to provide a small enough G_{th} for a small detector area, and τ becomes shorter than 10 ms assumed in estimation. It also falls at long wavelengths because the resistance fluctuation noise becomes important in large area detectors. The figure shows that the YBaCuO layers on Si_3O_4 membranes have a potential comparable to that of HgCdTe for a wavelength close to 10 µm. The maximum sensitivity of the YBaCuO layers on silicon membranes is shifted into a longer-term spectral range.

It is generally accepted that good-quality HTSC films require high-quality dielectric substrates, which combine desired dielectric properties with a good lattice match, enabling epitaxial growth of the films. Except for diamond, most suitable substrate materials have similar volume specific heat at 77–90 K. In all cases, it is very much higher than is seen at liquid helium temperatures. Consequently, the thermal time tends to be long. Therefore, one important requirement for substrate material is strength, so that it can be made very thin. Some substrates that are favourable for film growth, such as $SrTiO_3$ and $LaAlO_3$ are too weak to produce thin layers of millimetre dimensions.

In the early 1990s, the adaptation of the silicon micromechanics technique was initiated in order to develop the technology of superconducting detector arrays. Figure 5.24 shows the structure of a superconducting microbolometer from the YBaCuO epitaxial layer deposited on the YSZ epitaxial buffer layer on a silicon substrate [53]. Thus, obtained bolometers with the dimensions of 140×105 µm² were characterised by a detectivity of $(8 \pm 2) \times 10^9$ cmHz$^{1/2}$W^{-1} for the bias current of 2 µA. The detector time constant was 105 ms. Due to the lower than expected performance of superconducting microbolometers compared to the performance of photon detectors operating at a liquid nitrogen temperature, further work on microbolometer arrays operating in the range of 8–14 µm was abandoned.

5.4 PYROELECTRIC DETECTORS

Whenever a pyroelectric crystal undergoes a change of temperature, surface charge is produced in a particular direction as a result of the change in its spontaneous polarisation with temperature. This

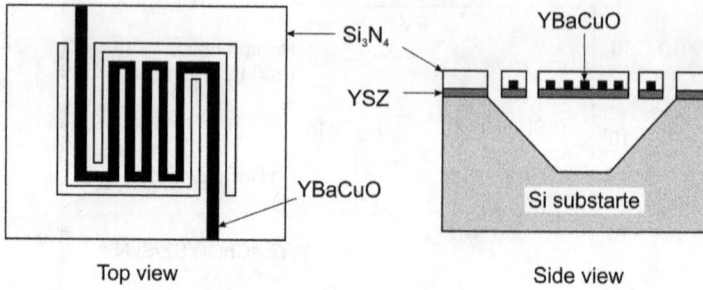

Top view   Side view

FIGURE 5.24 Schematic diagram of YBaCuO microbolometer using epitaxial YBaCuO on an epitaxial YSZ buffer layer on a silicon substrate (after Reference 53).

effect has been known as a physically observable phenomenon for many centuries, being described by Theophrastus in 315 BC [54]. Its name "pyroelectricity" was introduced by Brewster [55]. The concept of using the pyroelectric effect for detecting radiation was proposed very early by Ta [56], but in practice little progress was made due to the lack of suitable materials. The importance of the pyroelectric effect in infrared detection was becoming obvious about sixty years ago. The pyroelectric phenomenon, which is the basis for the operation of pyroelectric detectors, is discussed in section 4.3.4. In this section the performance of pyroelectric detectors will be presented more closely.

5.4.1 RESPONSIVITY

If we assume that the pyroelectric detector is connected to a high-impedance amplifier whose equivalent diagram is shown in Figure 4.17(b), then the observed signal is equal to the voltage caused by the charge, Q. The detector is represented by the capacitance C_d, the resistance R_d and the conductance $G = 1/R_d$. Then, the generated voltage is equal to

$$V = \frac{I_{ph}}{\left(G^2 + \omega^2 C^2\right)^{1/2}},$$
(5.22)

and the voltage responsivity equals

$$R_v = \frac{V}{\Phi_o} = \frac{R_d \varepsilon p A \omega}{G_{th}\left(1 + \omega^2 \tau_{th}^2\right)^{1/2}\left(1 + \omega^2 \tau_e^2\right)^{1/2}},$$
(5.23)

where $\tau_e = C/G$ is the electrical time constant. The last equations are simplified at frequencies that are high compared with τ_{th}^{-1} and τ_e^{-1}; then:

$$R_v = \frac{\varepsilon p}{\varepsilon_o \varepsilon_r c_{th} A \omega},$$
(5.24)

where ε_o is the dielectric permittivity of vacuum, ε_r is the relative permittivity of pyroelectric.

Equation (5.24) indicates that at high frequencies the voltage responsivity of the pyroelectric detector is inversely proportional to the frequency. In the low-frequency range, the responsivity

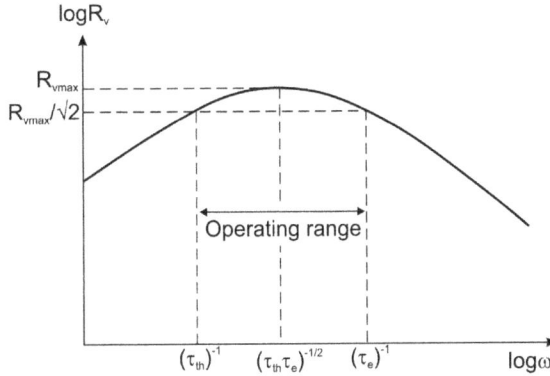

FIGURE 5.25 Frequency dependence of voltage responsivity of a pyroelectric detector.

is modified by the electrical and thermal time constants [see Eq. (5.23)], as shown in Figure 5.25. It appears that the maximum responsivity is for a frequency equal to $(\tau_e \tau_{th})^{-1/2}$ and is as follows:

$$R_{vmax} = \frac{\varepsilon p A R_d}{G_{th}\left(\tau_e + \tau_{th}\right)}.$$ (5.25)

Equation (5.25) shows that the maximum responsivity is achieved with the minimum value of G_{th}. The thermal capacity should also be reduced in order to maintain an appropriate thermal value of the time constant τ_{th}. At the frequencies $\omega = (\tau_e)^{-1}$ and $(\tau_{th})^{-1}$, we obtain

$$R_v = \frac{R_{vmax}}{\sqrt{2}}.$$ (5.26)

It is not possible to distinguish between τ_e and τ_{th} from the measurements of frequency dependence of responsivity. Typical τ_{th} values are from 0.01 to 10 s. In turn, τ_e can vary between 10^{-12}–100s depending on the detector size, capacity and shunt resistance. When the detector operates in the high frequency range (e.g., to characterise laser pulses), one of the time constants (usually τ_e) is reduced to such a value that its inverse is greater than the maximum required frequency. This is usually achieved by reducing the detector electrical capacity and loading the output with a resistance of 50-Ω line. Because the pyroelectric detector speed is limited only by the frequency of the crystal lattice vibrational polarisation (about 10^{12} Hz), this type detectors have the potential to be extremely fast.

The above considerations of the detector response do not take into account the input resistance of the amplifier (R_a) that will appear in parallel with the resistor R_d. For low-frequency detectors, $R_a \gg R_d$ and R_a can be ignored in this case. For fast detectors, $R_a \ll R_d$ and, thus, R_a determines the electrical time constant and the device responsivity.

Figure 5.26 shows, for example, the frequency dependence of the voltage responsivity for different load-resistance values R_L (parallel connection R_d and R_a). For higher values of R_L resistance, an increase of voltage responsivity is observed. However, this causes a decrease in the upper limit frequency of the detector [57].

More rigorous analyses of pyroelectric detectors have been performed by many authors, taking into account the effects of mounting techniques and black coatings [58, 59]. The above treatment, however, is adequate for the majority of applications.

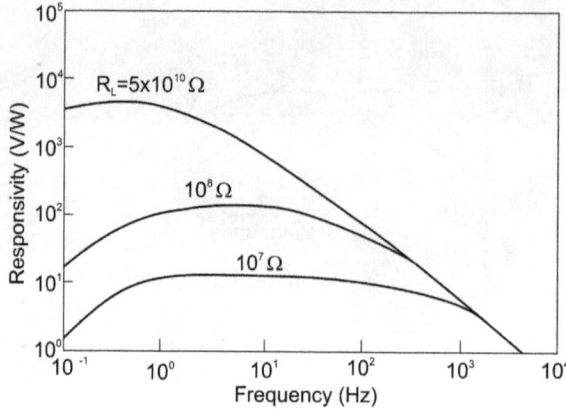

FIGURE 5.26 Frequency dependence voltage responsivity for different load resistance values of the PLT522 detector by GEC-Marconi Infra-Red Limited.

5.4.2 NOISE AND DETECTIVITY

Using a pyroelectric detector we can distinguish in the photoreceiver three basic noise sources:

- thermal fluctuation noise;
- Johnson noise; and
- amplifier noise.

The first two types of noises are described in Chapter 3. The Johnson noise is connected with a detector shunt resistor. However, in most devices at operation moderate frequencies (1 Hz–1 kHz) the noise is dominated by the AC electrical conductance of the detector element. Device AC conductance has two components: frequency-independent component R^{-1} and frequency dependent component G_d:

$$G_d = \omega C \tan \delta, \tag{5.27}$$

where $\tan\delta$ is the loss tangent of the detector material.

For frequencies much less than $\omega = (RC \tan \delta)^{-1}$, the Johnson noise is simply given by

$$V_{Jr}^2 = \frac{4kTR\Delta f}{1 + \omega^2 \tau_e^2}, \tag{5.28}$$

which leads to a ω^{-2} dependence at the frequencies of $\omega \gg \tau_e^{-1}$.

For frequencies much greater than $\omega = (RC \tan \delta)^{-1}$, the noise generated by the detector element AC conductance will dominate, so that

$$V_{Jd}^2 = 4kT\Delta f \frac{\tan\delta}{C} \frac{1}{\omega} \quad \text{for} \quad C \gg C_a. \tag{5.29}$$

This type of noise, also called dielectric noise, dominates at high frequencies.

Figure 5.27 shows the dependence of various noise components on frequency for a typical pyroelectric detector. It has been assumed that both thermal and electrical time constants are longer than 1 s. In nearly all practical detectors the thermal noise is insignificant and is often ignored in

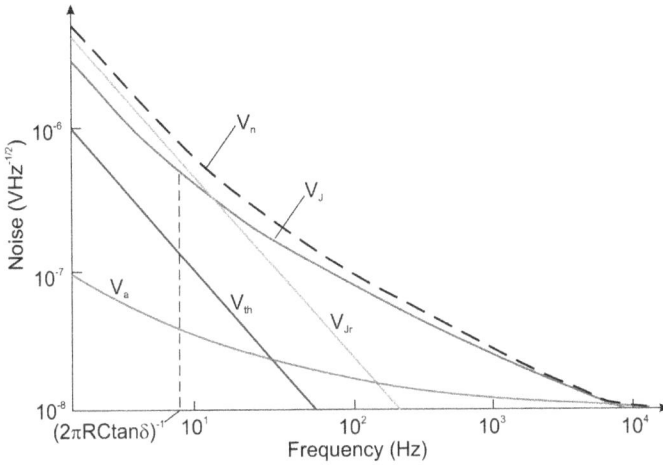

FIGURE 5.27 Relative magnitudes of noise voltages in a typical pyroelectric detector.

calculations. It can be seen that the loss-controlled Johnson noise V_{Jd} dominates above 20 Hz while, below this frequency, the resistor-controlled Johnson noise and the amplifier current noise (V_{Jr}) contribute almost equally significantly to the total noise. At very high frequencies, the amplifier voltage noise (V_a) dominates [60].

At high frequencies (greater than τ_e^{-1} and $(RC tan\delta)^{-1}$), the detectivity [from Eqs. (2.11), (5.24) and (5.29)] is given by the following equation:

$$D^* = \frac{\varepsilon t}{\left(4kT\right)^{1/2}} \frac{p}{c_{th}\left(\varepsilon_o \varepsilon_r tan\delta\right)^{1/2}} \frac{1}{\omega^{1/2}}. \tag{5.30}$$

The fall in detectivity with a frequency of $\omega^{-1/2}$ means that the D^* will be at the maximum of a rather higher frequency than R_v [see Eq. (5.24)] and falls more slowly (as $\omega^{-1/2}$) than R_v (as ω^{-1}) above this maximum. For most detectors, D^* maximises in the 1–100 Hz range [61] and a reasonably flat D^* can be achieved in the range of a few Hz to several hundred Hz (Figure 5.28).

However, the greatest limitations in the use of pyroelectric detectors are related to the phenomenon of microphonics. Microphoning results from the very nature of the pyroelectric material. It is based on the fact that vibrations and acoustic noise generate an undesirable signal at the detector output. If the detector is placed in an environment where there are high vibrations, the microphonics noise may dominate other noise sources. In general, the phenomenon of microphonics can be minimised by an appropriate ("non-rigid") mounting of the detector, by selecting a low microphone feedback material and by using an additional compensation element.

The compensating element [see Figure 5.29(a)] is connected, both in series and in reverse, to the active element and is covered with a radiation-reflective electrode or is mechanically shielded from incident radiation [62]. It is required that the compensating element is placed in an environment similar to that of the active detector, so that the signal conditioned by temperature change or mechanical stress is eliminated [Figure 5.29(b)]. There are also designs in which the detector and the compensating element are connected in parallel. For details, see Section 11.5.2.

There are two other sources of noise found in pyroelectric detectors. If a pyroelectric detector is subjected to ambient temperature changes, fast pulses are sometimes observed and superimposed on the normal pyroelectric response. Those pulses occur in a random fashion, but their number and amplitude are increased with the rate of increasing temperature. Also, it is suggested that those spurious noise signals are due to ferroelectric domain wall movements. They can be minimised by

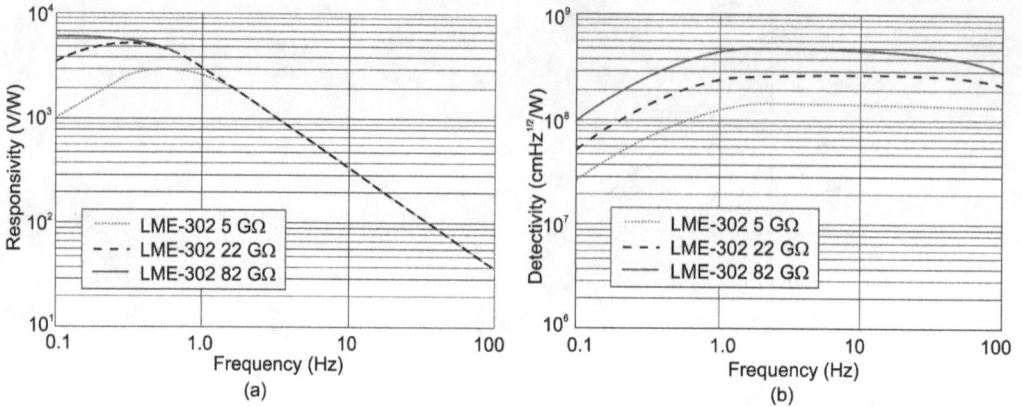

FIGURE 5.28 Examples of frequency characteristics of the IntraTec pyroelectric detector: (a) voltage responsivity and (b) detectivity for three resistance values in the gate circuit (load).

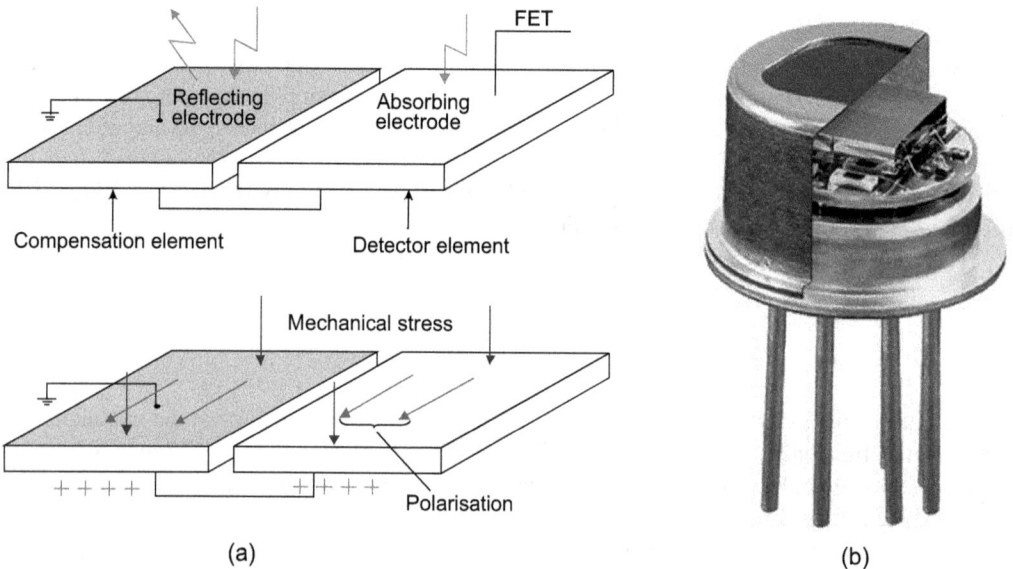

FIGURE 5.29 Pyroelectric detector with compensation element: (a) connection diagram, (b) photo.

a selection of good materials and appear to be lower in ceramics than some of the single crystal materials such as $LiTaO_3$. Finally, the electromagnetic interference is a source of unwanted signals.

5.4.3 PYROELECTRIC MATERIAL SELECTION

Many pyroelectric materials have been investigated to be used in detector applications. However, the choice is difficult because it depends on many factors, including detector size, operating temperature and operation frequency.

It is quite possible to formulate a number of figures of merit (FoM) describing a contribution of the material physical properties in the device performance. For example, the current responsivity [see Eq. (4.37)] is proportional to the following:

$$F_i = \frac{p}{c_{th}}. \qquad (5.31)$$

Instead, the voltage responsivity [see Eq. (5.24)] is proportional to

$$F_v = \frac{p}{\varepsilon_o \varepsilon_r c_{th}}. \qquad (5.32)$$

In the case of a detector dominated by the AC Johnson noise [see Eq. (5.30)], the detectivity is proportional to

$$F_d = \frac{p}{c_{th}(\varepsilon_o \varepsilon_r \tan\delta)^{1/2}}, \qquad (5.33)$$

which forms the FoM for pyroelectric detectors. Here ε_o is the permittivity of free space, and ε_r is the relative permittivity of the pyroelectric material.

A useful FoM including the effect of the circuit input capacitance with which the detector is used is as follows:

$$F = \frac{1}{C_d + C_L} \frac{p}{c_{th}}. \qquad (5.34)$$

This equation reduces to F_i or F_v when C_L is comparatively small or large, respectively.

The relevant figure-of-merit for the materials used in pyroelectric vidicons is F_{vid}:

$$F_{vid} = \frac{F_v}{G_{th}}, \qquad (5.35)$$

where G_{th} is the pyroelectric thermal conductivity. Dependence of F_{vid} on G_{th} can be eliminated by dicing a thermal imaging target into individual islands (by using a reticulation process).

An ideal material should have a large pyroelectric coefficient, low dielectric loss, low dielectric constant and low volume-specific heat. The possibility of fulfilling these requirements in a single material is not promising. It is generally true that a large pyroelectric coefficient and a small dielectric constant are desirable but, it is also true that these two parameters are not independently adjustable. Thus, it is considered that materials having a high pyroelectric coefficient also have a high dielectric constant, and materials having a low dielectric constant also have a low pyroelectric coefficient.

Most ferroelectric detectors operate at temperatures below Curie T_C, where polarisation is not affected by changes in ambient temperature. It is possible for the detectors to operate at temperatures above T_C, in the case of using a polarisation voltage. Then, the detectors work in the dielectric bolometer mode (see Section 5.4.4).

Pyroelectric materials can roughly be classified into three categories: single crystals, ceramics (polycrystalline) and polymers. Their characteristics are presented in Table 5.6. Figure 5.30 shows the frequency dependence of detectivity of selected pyroelectric detectors [63].

Among the single crystals, the most well-known and widespread is TGS [$(NH_2CH_2COOH)_3H_2SO_4$]. It possesses the attractive properties, high pyroelectric coefficient, reasonably low dielectric constant and thermal conductivity (high value of F_v). However, despite these properties, this material is rather

TABLE 5.6
Properties of pyroelectric materials (after Reference 60)

| Material | Temperature [°C] | Structure | p [10^{-4}Cm^{-2}K^{-1}] | Dielectric properties & 1 kHz | | c_{th} [10^{6}Jm^{-3}K^{-1}] | K [10^{-7}m^{2}s^{-1}] | T_c [°C] | F_v [m^{2}C^{-1}] | F_d [10^{-5}Pa$^{-1/2}$] | F_{vid} [10^{-6}sC^{-1}] |
				ε_r	tanδ						
TGS	35	Crystal	5.5	55 (1kHz)	0.025 (1 kHz)	2.6	33	49	0.43	6.1	1.3
DTGS	40	Crystal	5.5	43 (1kHz)	0.020 (1 kHz)	2.4	3.3	61	0.60	8.3	1.8
TGFB	60	Crystal	7.0	50 (1kHz)	0.028 (1 kHz)	2.6	3.3	73	0.61	7.6	1.8
ATGSAs	25	Crystal	7.0	32 (1kHz)	$\leq$0.010 (1 kHz)	–	–	51	0.99	16.6	3.0
PVDF	25	Polymer	0.27	12 (10Hz)	0.015 (10 Hz)	2.43	0.62	80	0.1	0.88	1.6
LiTaO$_3$	25	Crystal	2.3	47	10^{-4} to 5×10^{-3}	3.2	13.0	665	0.17	35.2–4.9	0.13
SBN-50	25	Crystal	5.5	400	3×10^{-3}	2.34	–	121	0.07	7.2	–
PZFNTU	25	Ceramic	3.8	290 (1kHz)	2.7×10^{-3} (1 kHz)	2.5	–	230	0.06	5.8	–
PCWT-4/24	25	Ceramic	3.8	220 (1.5kHz)	0.011 (1.5 kHz)	2.5	–	255	0.08	3.3	–
PGO	25	Crystal	1.1	40	5×10^{-4}(100 Hz)	2.0	3.0	178	0.16	13.1	0.5
PGP:Ba$_3$	25	Crystal	3.2	81	1×10^{-3}(100 Hz)	2.0	3.0	70	0.22	8.4	0.7

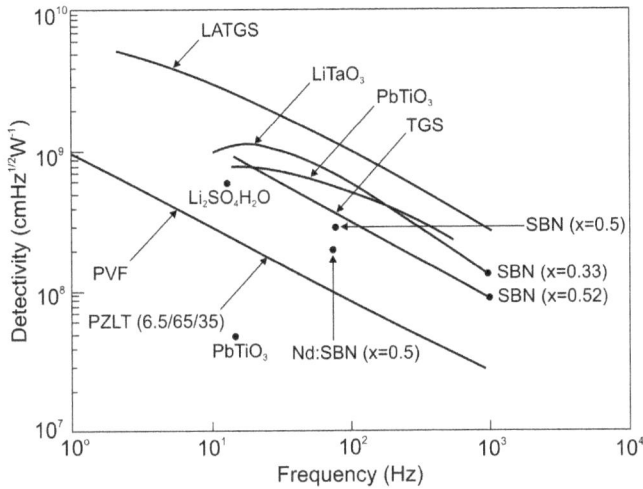

FIGURE 5.30 Frequency dependence of pyroelectric detectors detectivity.

hygroscopic, difficult to handle, and shows poor long-term stability, both chemically and electrically. Its major disadvantage is a low Curie temperature, particularly for detectors that are required to meet military specifications. In spite of the above-mentioned problems, TGS is frequently used for high-performance single element detectors and has become the preferred material for vidicon targets.

LiTaO$_3$, lithium tantalate has worse properties than TGS, due to its lower pyroelectric coefficient and slightly higher relative permittivity (lower value of F_v). Its advantages are the following: high chemical stability, very low loss (so F_d is favourable), very high Curie temperature and is insoluble in water. The material is widely used for single-element detectors, although there are sometimes problems associated with thermally induced transient noise spikes from this material when used in very low-frequency devices. Because of its low permittivity, it is not particularly favourable to use for thermal imaging arrays. Its thermal conductivity is quite high, which makes it not a good material for pyroelectric vidicons.

SBN, strontium barium niobate is the next single crystal pyroelectric material. In fact, there is a family name for a range of solid solutions defined by the equation Sr$_{1-x}$Ba$_x$Nb$_2$O$_6$, in which x can be varied from 0.25 to 0.75. SBN-50 ($x = 0.50$) has a favourable F_d FoM. It shows very good properties if it works in a dielectric bolometer mode. It was used for the production of large infrared imaging arrays. However, due to inferior parameters of these arrays compared to bolometric arrays, their further development was abandoned.

Another group of materials is polycrystalline ferroelectric ceramics, which offer a number of advantages over the materials listed earlier:

- they are relatively cheap to manufacture in large areas using standard mixed-oxide processes;
- they are both mechanically and chemically robust (they can be processed into thin wafers);
- they possess a high Curie temperature;
- they do not suffer from thermally induced noise spikes; and
- they can be modified by the selected dopant elements inclusion into the lattice to control such parameters as: p, εr, $tan\delta$, Curie temperature, electrical impedance, and mechanical properties (controlling grain size of material).

The most important ceramic materials are PZ (lead zirconate, PbZrO$_3$) and PT (lead titanate, PbTiO$_3$) solid solutions. Resistivities of ceramic detectors cover the range of 10^9–10^{11} Ωcm^2 and detectivity is of about 10^8 cmHz$^{1/2}$W^{-1}.

Using bulk pyroelectrics in fabrication of infrared detectors leads to several drawbacks: the material must be cut, lapped and polished to make a thin, well-insulated and sensitive layer. In addition, the array fabrication requires metallisation on both faces and bonding to a silicon readout circuit to yield a complete hybrid array. On account of this, there has been a growth of interest in integration of pyroelectric thin films directly onto silicon substrates as a means for both reducing array fabrication costs and increasing performance through reduced thermal mass and improve thermal isolation [64].

Properties of thin-film materials differ from those of bulk materials in as much as microstructure and substrate influence are of importance [65]. In contrast to bulk ceramics, thin films can be grown textured or even completely oriented in the case of epitaxy. The performance similar to the single-crystal materials is obtained for the optimal texture when the polar axis stays perpendicular to the electrodes everywhere in the film.

The oxide materials (modified lead zirconate titanates or the dielectric bolometer materials) possess the right properties (high ε and high F_d) as ceramics sintered around 1200°C. However, for integrating ferroelectric thin films directly on silicon places, a very important constraint on the temperature at which the ferroelectric can be grown. The interconnect metallisation on the chips should not be taken above 500°C for any length of time, and this places an upper limit on the ferroelectric layer process temperature.

5.4.4 Dielectric Bolometers

Conventional materials discussed above are ferroelectrics operated below T_C, where polarisation is not permanently affected by changes in ambient temperature. However, it is possible to operate ferroelectrics above T_C, with an applied bias field, in the mode of a dielectric bolometer.

In general, the case for ferroelectric materials, the electrical displacement, D, is a sum of contribution from the spontaneous (zero field) polarisation, P_s, and the field-induced polarisation (i.e., $\varepsilon_o \varepsilon_r E$). It is also important to realise that the permittivity around the transition is nonlinear, hence an integral is required:

$$D(E,T) = P_s(T) + \int_0^E \left(\frac{\partial D}{\partial E}\right)_T dE' = P_s(T) + \varepsilon_o \int_0^E \varepsilon_r(E',T) dE', \qquad (5.36)$$

where ε_o is the permittivity of free space and ε_r is the relative permittivity of the pyroelectric material.

The pyroelectric coefficient is the change in displacement with temperature

$$p = \left(\frac{\partial D}{\partial T}\right)_E = p_o + \varepsilon_o \int_0^E \frac{\partial \varepsilon_r}{\partial T} dE', \qquad (5.37)$$

where p_o is the pyroelectric coefficient for $E = 0$.

To obtain high pyroelectric coefficients from dielectric bolometer materials it is desirable to have a large variation in permittivity with temperature and/or high bias fields should be applied. The bias field generally reduces the permittivity variation and even introduces positive slopes; hence, there is a limit to the benefits gained from simply applying high fields.

Below T_C, p_o is large compared with the second term in Eq. (5.37), thus D and p_o are often used interchangeably. However, it is clear from Figure 5.31(b) that the maximum pyroelectric effect (i.e., the maximum slope of P versus T) occurs near T_C, and therefore it seems desirable to operate there.

From Eq. (5.37) results that the induced part of the pyroelectric coefficient depends not only upon the temperature rate of change of the permittivity, but also upon the field dependence of the rate

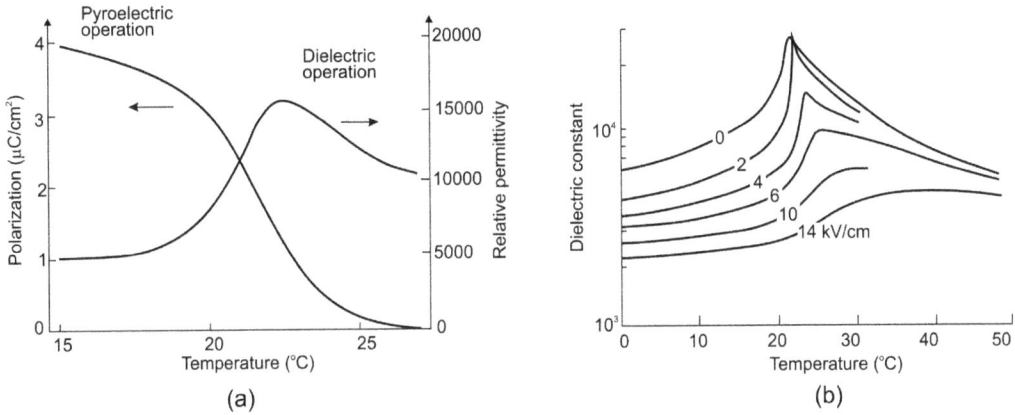

FIGURE 5.31 Barium strontium titanate ceramic: operating mode for (a) ferroelectric ceramic and (b) dielectric constant (after Reference 66).

change. At all temperatures, the dielectric behaviour is nonlinear; that is, the gradient of permittivity varies with the applied field and the dielectric peak and $d\varepsilon/dT$ are both depressed with increasing field [see Figure 5.31(b)]. Note that the pyroelectric coefficient maximum is somewhat lower in temperature than the peak capacitance value. The capacitance data represents a biased sample, and both the dielectric constant and pyroelectric coefficient maxima occur at temperatures above the Curie temperature. As the operating point continues to diverge from the Curie temperature, dielectric contributions to polarisation become dominant. Thus, the electric field application gives several benefits to the detector performance:

- It adds induced polarisation to the spontaneous polarisation;
- It suppresses dielectric permittivity, especially as it peaks near the transition;
- It broadens response peak, easing temperature-control limits;
- It suppresses dielectric loss, by reducing noise; and
- It stabilises polarisation near transitions, providing predictable performance.

Several materials have been examined in dielectric bolometer mode, including potassium thallium niobate, $KTa_xNb_{1-x}O_3$ (KTN), lead zinc niobate, $Pb(Zn_{1/3}Nb_{2/3})O_3$ (PZN), barium strontium titanate, $Ba_{1-x}Sr_xTiO_3$ (BST), lead magnesium niobate, $Pb(Mg_{1/3}Nb_{2/3})O_3$, (PMN), and lead scandium tantalate, $Pb(Sc_{1/2}Ta_{1/2})O_3$ (PST). Dielectric bolometers require stringent bias and temperature stabilisation.

Properties of pyroelectric materials with transitions near ambient and operating with an electric field are shown in Table 5.7. BST ceramics have the best properties. BST crystals are obtained by the Czochralski method, but it is difficult to obtain good-quality single crystals. When the Sr content decreases from 40 per cent to 0 per cent, the T_C changes from 0 to 120 °C. The dielectric constant BST values are greater than 30,000 (see Figure 5.31).

Pyroelectric detector arrays from BST were also successfully used for the construction of thermal imaging cameras operating in the long-term infrared spectrum range of 8–14 μm. However, unlike monolithic bolometric arrays, these arrays are hybrid arrays requiring the mastery of a more complex and costly technology.

Figure 5.32 shows the details of pixels in a two-dimensional pyroelectric detector array (format 245×328) manufactured by Texas Instruments [66, 68]. Pixels of about 50×50 μm² were obtained by laser cutting (Nd-YAG laser) of BST ceramics, its etching (to remove surface damage to the ceramics) and appropriate heat treatment. The illuminated surface is specially made (covered with

TABLE 5.7
Properties of Pyroelectric Materials (Externally Polarised) (after Reference 67)

	T_C [°C]	Pole [V/μm]	ε_r	tanδ [%]	$p \times 10^{-4}$ [C/m²K]	$F_d \times 10^{-5}$ [Pa⁻¹²]
Doped LMN	-20	6	1650	0.1	8.5	8.3
BST	17	4	1500	0.4	18	9.2
PST	25	4	3400	0.4	4.3	14.6
Cathode-sprayed PST (1.5 μm)	6	4	4100	0.48	32	9.1
Cathode-sprayed PbTiO₃ (2.1 μm)	540	0	200	1.0	-5	4.8

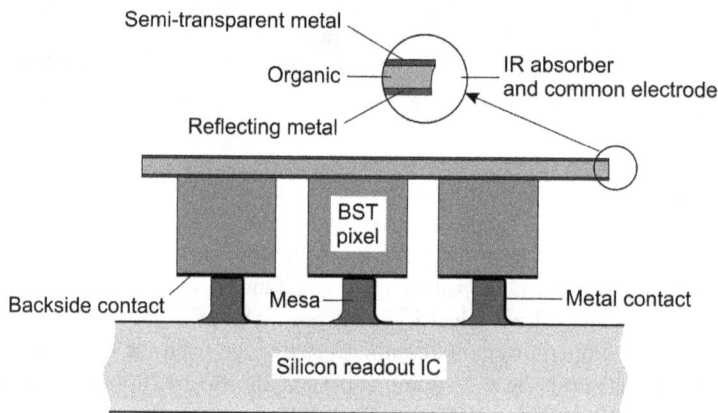

FIGURE 5.32 BST dielectric bolometer pixels (after Reference 68).

a quarter-wave organic layer with two metallic layers) in order to obtain a resonance cavity effect. In this way, more than 90 per cent absorption of infrared radiation in the wavelength range from 7.5 μm to 13 μm was achieved. After thinning and polishing, the final pixel thickness is about 20 μm. Pixel hybridisation with a silicon readout processor was carried out using organic compound posts (in order to obtain high thermal resistance) with edge metallisation. Operating near room temperature, ferroelectric BST pixels hybridised with a silicon readout integrated circuit consistently yield devices with system *NEDT* of 47 mK with *f*/1 optics.

The hybrid arrays have been also demonstrated by BAE Systems in the United Kingdom. In this case the dielectric bolometers are Pb(Sc$_{0.5}$Ta$_{0.5}$)O$_3$ biased at 4–5 V/μm (higher than for BST) with F_d levels between 10 to 15×10⁻⁵ Pa⁻¹/². Conventional unbiased pyroelectrics give values of about 4×10⁻⁵ Pa⁻¹/². The details of fabrication procedures of these arrays are described by Whatmore and Watton [64]. The performance of hybrid arrays is listed in Table 5.8.

A further development of the pyroelectric detectors arrays was related to the progress of work in the monolithic arrays field in which pixels are constructed similarly to silicon microbolometers. In this case, the active pyroelectric material is deposited on a bridge similar to that shown in Figure 5.14. The most effective development has been achieved in fabrication of thin-film ferroelectric (TFFE) detectors. However, there are several key features that distinguish it from bolometer technology. Since the ferroelectric device is a capacitor rather than a resistor (as in a bolometer), the electrodes are located above and below the face of the pixel, are transparent, and do not obscure the active optical area. This enables the use of thin, poorly conducting electrode materials to minimise thermal conductance. A key feature of the design is that the ferroelectric film is self-supporting;

TABLE 5.8
Hybrid Arrays Demonstrated in the UK (DERA/BAE Systems) Programme (after Reference 64)

Array elements	Pitch (μm)	ROIC size (mm²)	Package atmosphere	*NEDT* (mK)	Array *MTF* at Nyquist
100×100	100	15.3×13.4	N_2	87	65%
256×128	56	17.0×12.4	Xe	90	45%
384×288	40	19.7×19.0	Xe	140	35%

TABLE 5.9
Typical Properties of Linear Arrays (after Reference 71)

Number of elements	1×128	1×128	1×128	1×256	1×510
Size of elements [μm²]	90×100	90×500	90×1000	42×100	20×100
Pitch [μm]	100	100	100	50	25
Responsivity R_v [V/W]	230 000	540 000	230 000	620 000	680 000
Noise voltage (mV)	0.7	0.8	1.1	0.7	0.9
NEP (nW)	3.0	1.5	4.9	1.1	1.3
MTF ($R = 3$ lp/mm)	0.6	0.6	0.6	0.6	0.8
Uniformity of R_v (%)	5	5	5	5	10

there is no underlying membrane necessary to provide mechanical support. In such a way, with the use of transparent oxide electrodes, the ferroelectric material can dominate thermal conductance. The *NEDT* of TFFE devices with 48.5 μm pixels is typically about 80–90 mK including all system losses [69]. However, it turned out that the performance of monolithic arrays made in such way was inferior to that of bolometric arrays, because most ferroelectric materials lose physical properties as their thickness is reduced. This is also the case with BST. However, some ferroelectric materials retain their properties, such as $PbTiO_3$ used in fabrication pyroelectric linear arrays.

5.4.5 Pyroelectric Linear Arrays and Multi-colour Detectors

Linear arrays are particularly suitable for applications where there is relative motion between the sensor head and the objects being imaged (e.g., intruder alarms and pushbroom linescan). Arrays from a few tens of elements up to many hundreds are required, but because of the absence of detector scanning along the direction of the array, bandwidths are low. A thin polished wafer of pyroelectric material, about 20 μm thick, is bonded down to a substrate. The manufacture of pyroelectric linear arrays based on $LiTaO_3$ with thicknesses of the self-supporting responsive elements of less than 5 μm has become possible by the development of special thinning techniques (ion-beam etching) [70]. Table 5.9 shows essential properties of different types of $LiTaO_3$ linear arrays.

Figure 5.33 shows the principal design of a pyroelectric linear array that includes a lithium tantalate chip with up to 510 elements [71]. The pixel size is several tens of microns in width, *a*, and up to 1 mm in length, *b*. The chopped radiation signal, Φ_s, strikes the active surface of the pyroelectric material where it is absorbed. The signals generated in the sensitive elements are processed in a CMOS circuit that contains both analogue and digital sections. Sensitivity of the detector array is maximised by reducing the thickness of pyroelectric chips (typical to 5 μm), fabricated ion-beam etching techniques.

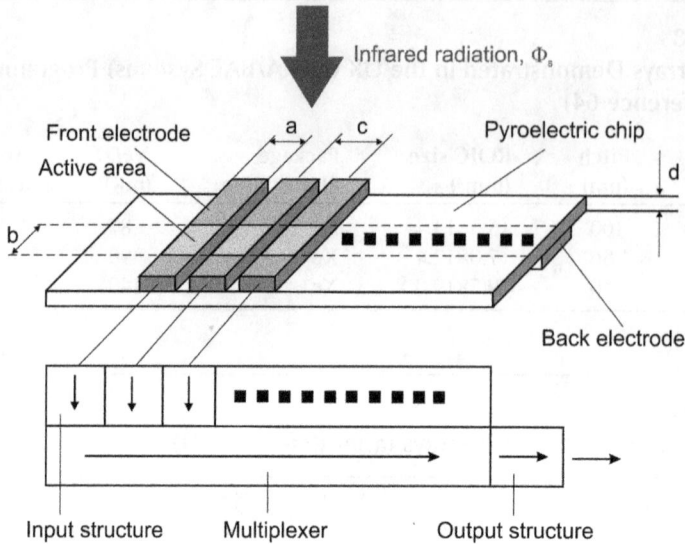

FIGURE 5.33   Principal design of a pyroelectric linear array (adapted after Reference 72).

The pyroelectric $LiTaO_3$ sensors have the optimum signal-to-noise ratio typically between 5 Hz and 10 Hz modulation frequency. However, because of the high thermal crosstalk in sensor chips with a pixel spacing of 5–10 μm, modulation frequencies below 80 Hz are generally not useful.

Readout of charge from pyroelectric detectors is by means of conventional FETs. Each detector is connected to its own source follower FET that acts as an impedance buffer. Outputs of these transistors go to a multiplexer that samples the elements in turn at a rate dependent upon the particular applications.

Recent interest in the use of thin pyroelectric films is justified by their potential for making low thermal mass elements. Arrays that have been demonstrated include the linear arrays fabricated using bulk micromachining techniques with sputtered $PbTiO_3$, La-$PbTiO_3$, PVDF-TrEE, and $Pb(Zr_{0.15}Ti_{0.85})O_3$ on silicon substrates [73].

Using MEMS technology, IntraTec has developed two types of multi-colour pyroelectric detectors:

- multi-colour detector with integrated beam splitter, and
- tunable-colour detector with integrated Fabry-Perot filter.

The principle of the multi-colour detector with integrated beam splitter is shown in Figure 5.34. The infrared (IR) radiation entering through the entrance window is divided by a beam splitter into four independent tracks. Then, after going through IR filters with different spectral characteristics, it hits a pyroelectric detector chip. The beam splitters are made of gold-plated microstructures to achieve a homogeneous distribution of the radiance. The filters are arranged under a certain angle to obtain a normal incidence of the radiation. This type of construction allows obtaining electrical signals from particular spectral ranges at the same time. Detailed information about these detectors can be found in the paper [74, 75].

An interesting construction is a pyroelectric detector integrated with a MEMS tunable Fabry-Perot filter shown in Figure 5.35. The fixed-bottom carrier is equipped with control electrodes, whereas the upper reflector is suspended by springs [Figure 5.35(a)]. There are two-plane parallel mirrors acting as a resonator. Applying the voltage V_c to the electrodes creates an electrostatic force which decreases the resonator gap and, consequently, tunes the filter wavelength. This occurs as a result of the phenomenon of multiple interference of waves, which are the total size of half the

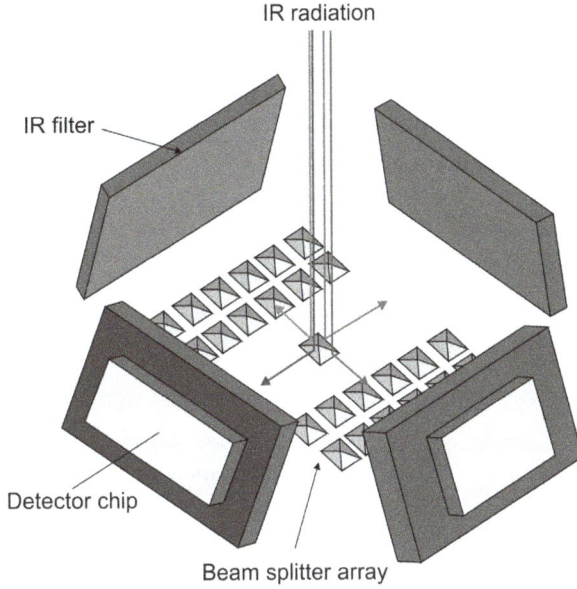

FIGURE 5.34 Example of a four-colour detector with integrated beam splitter: (a) work principle, (b) construction (after Reference 74).

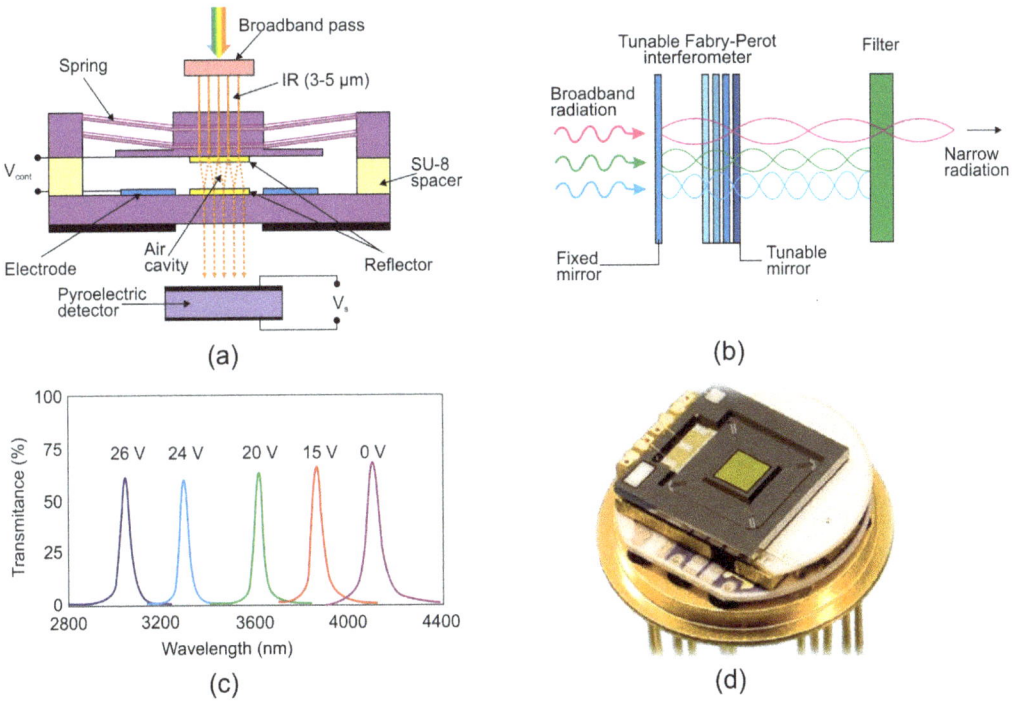

FIGURE 5.35 Pyroelectric detector with a tunable filter: (a) construction of the detector, (b) idea of the filter operation, (c) spectral characteristics, and (d) photo of the detector (after References 75 and 76).

TABLE 5.10
Comparison of Multi and Tunable Colour Pyroelectric Detectors

Specification	Multi-colour detector	Tunable colour detector
Principal	Beam splitter	Tunable Fabry-Perot filter
Filtering	Parallel	Serial
Radiation flux per channel	25 or 50%	100%
Filter	Single and multi-cavity	Single tunable air cavity
Spectral range	(3–25) µm	(4.3–3.0)/(5.0–3.7) µm
Current mode	Yes	Yes
Voltage mode	Yes	Yes
Thermal compensation	No	Yes

wavelength [Figure 5.35(b)]. The electrical signals corresponding to the individual spectral ranges are obtained at different times [Figure 5.35(c)].

Comparison of the parameters of the multi-colour detectors of both technological solutions is given in Table 5.10. These types of detectors are used in gas sensors, scientific research and in special applications.

PROBLEMS

Example 5.1

A thermopile with a sensitivity of $R_v = 20$ V/W and a field of view of 84° was placed in front of a blackbody (BB) with a temperature of 200°C (473 K). Calculate the voltage at the output of the thermopile which is 10 cm from BB.

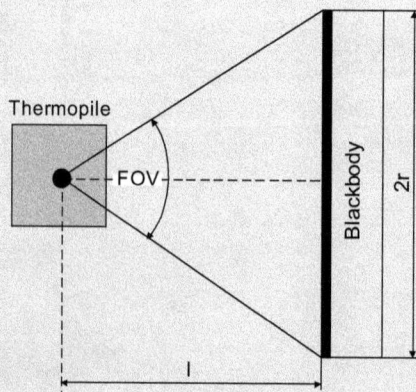

Example 5.2

How many times will the voltage at the detector output decrease if the FOV is reduced twice. Data as in Example 5.1.

Example 5.3

How many times will the voltage at the detector output increase if the detector temperature is reduced to 273 K. Data as in Example 5.1.

Example 5.4

Let us estimate the proportion of background radiation in the output signal in relation to the signal received from the IR source. The source temperature is 473 K, background temperature – 313 K, and detector temperature – 293 K. Other data: $r = 9$ cm, $s = 5$ cm, $l = 10$ cm.

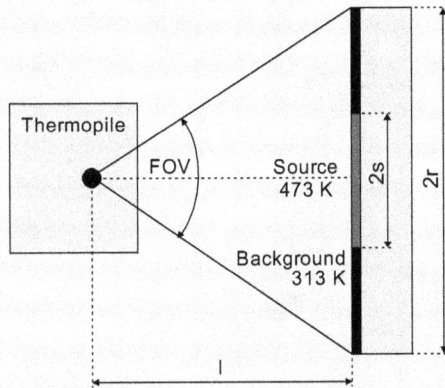

Example 5.5

Consider the poly SiGe microbolometer with a thermal conduction of 3.3×10^{-6} W/K. Calculate the bolometer temperature change when a radiant flux of 1 μW is incident.

Example 5.6

Consider the vanadium oxide (VO_x) bolometer with a temperature coefficient of $\alpha = -0.027$ 1/K, thermal conductance $G_{th} = 2.05 \times 10^{-7}$ W/mK, and resistance $R_d = 50$ kΩ. The detector works in a voltage divider circuit (see Figure 4.15). This circuit is biased by $V_b = 5$ V. Resistor value $R_L = 50$ kΩ. Calculate the voltage sensitivity of this bolometer in a low-frequency range.

Example 5.7

The thermal conductance from the detector to the outside world should be low. The lowest possible thermal conductance would occur when the detector is completely isolated from the environment under vacuum with only a radiative heat exchange between the environment and its heat-sink enclosure. Such an ideal model can give us the ultimate performance limit of a thermal detector. Estimate this limiting value from the Stefan-Boltzmann total radiation law.

Example 5.8 (Adapted after H. Budzer and G. Gerlach, *Thermal Infrared Sensors. Theory Optimization and Practice*, John Wiley & Sons, 2011)

Determine the radiant flux and the voltage responsivity of the microbolometer array. We assume, that the array is at the distance of $l = \# = 50$ mm in front of a blackbody. The temperature of the blackbody $T_s = 30°C$, $f/\# = 1$, pixel size $A = 25 \times 25 \ \mu m^2$, and $\varepsilon = 0.98$.

Example 5.9 (Adapted after H. Budzer and G. Gerlach, *Thermal Infrared Sensors. Theory Optimization and Practice*, John Wiley & Sons, 2011)

Calculate the pyroelectric detector output voltage for the following data: detector area $A = 1 \ mm^2$, temperature $T = 25°C$, blackbody radius $r = 10$ mm, temperature $T_B = 500$ K, FOV = 30°, chopper frequency 10 Hz, and voltage responsivity $R_v = 100$ V/W. The second blackbody temperature is the chopper temperature equal to 300 K. The detector and blackbody distance is $l = 5$ cm.

Example 5.10

Does it make sense to fabricate an infrared detector with a detectivity surpassing the D^*_{BLIP} value? Can a detector operate at a D^* larger than this limit?

REFERENCES

1. W. Herschel, "Experiments on the refrangibility of the invisible rays of the Sun", *Phil. Trans. Roy. Soc. London* 90, 284–292 (1800).
2. J.T. Seebeck, "Magnetische Polarisation der Metalle und Erze durch Temperatur-Differenz", *Abhandlung der deutschen Akademie der Wissenschaften zu Berlin*, 265–373 (1822).
3. A. Rogalski, "History of infrared detectors", *Opto-Electr. Rev.* 14, 279–308 (2012).
4. W. Smith, "Effect of light on selenium during the passage of an electric current", *Nature* 7, 303 (1873).
5. I.B. Cadoff and E. Miller, *Thermoelectric Materials and Devices*, Reinhold, New York, 1960.
6. F. Voelklein, "Review of the thermoelectric efficiency of bulk and thin-film materials", *Sens. Mater.* 8, 389–408 (1996).
7. A.F. Ioffe, *Semiconductor Thermoelements and Thermoelectric Cooling*, Infosearch, London, 1957.
8. A. Graf, M. Arndt, M. Sauer, and G. Gerlach, "Review of micromachined thermopiles for infrared detection", *Meas. Sci. Technol.* 18, R59-R75 (2007).
9. J. Schieferdecker, R. Quad, E. Holzenkampfer, and M. Schulze, "Infrared thermopile sensors with high sensitivity and very low temperature coefficient", *Sens. Actuator A* 46–47, 422–427 (1995).
10. F. Völklein, A. Wiegand, and V. Baier, "High-sensitive radiation thermopiles made of Bi-Sb-Te films", *Sens. Actuator* 29, 87–91, 1991.
11. A.W. van Herwaarden and P.M. Sarro, "Thermal sensors based on the Seebeck effect", *Sens. Actuator* 10, 321–346, 1986.
12. T. Kanno, M. Saga, S. Matsumoto, M. Uchida, N. Tsukamoto, A. Tanaka, S. Itoh, A. Nakazato, T. Endoh, S. Tohyama, Y. Yamamoto, S. Murashima, N. Fujimoto, and N. Teranishi, "Uncooled infrared focal plane array having 128×128 thermopile detector elements", *Proc. SPIE* 2269, 450–459 (1994).
13. *Sensor Technology and Devices*, ed. L. Ristica, Artech House, Boston, 1994.
14. E.M. Barrentine, A.D. Brown, C. Kotecki, V. Mikula, R.A. Reid, S. Yoon, and A.T. Joseph, "Uncooled uoped-Si thermopiles for thermal land imaging applications", *Proc. SPIE* 10980, 109800E-1-10 (2019).
15. *Thermal detectors*. Chapter 07. Hamamatsu Catalogue. www.hamamatsu.com/resources/pdf/ssd/e07_handbook_Thermal_detectors.pdf.

16. www.amphenol-sensors.com.

17. M. Kimata, "Trends in small-format infrared array sensors", *Conference Sensors*, IEEE, 2013, doi: 10.1109/ICSENS.2013.6688495.

18. P.W. Kruse, *Uncooled Thermal Imaging. Arrays, Systems, and Applications*, SPIE Press, Bellingham, 2001.

19. W. Kruse, L.D. McGlauchlin, and R.B. McQuistan, *Elements of Infrared Technology,* Wiley, New York, 1962.

20. C. Jansson, U. Ringh, and K. Liddiard, "Theoretical analysis of pulse bias heating of resistance bolometer infrared detectors and effectiveness of bias compensation", *Proc. SPIE* 2552, 644–652 (1995).

21. A. Tanaka, S. Matsumoto, N. Tsukamoto, S. Itoh, K. Chiba, T. Endoh, A. Nakazato, K. Okuyama, Y. Kumazawa, M. Hijikawa, H. Gotoh, T. Tanaka, and N. Teranishi, "Infrared focal plane array incorporating silicon IC process compatible bolometer", *IEEE Trans. Electron Devices* 43, 1844–1880, 1996.

22. S.B. Ju, Y.J. Yong, and S.G. Kim, "Design and fabrication of a high fill-factor micro-bolometer using double sacrificial layers", *Proc. SPIE* 3698, 180–189 (1999).

23. R.W. Astheimer, "Thermistor infrared detectors", *Proc. SPIE* 443, 95–109 (1984).

24. A. Doctor, "MEMS technology based sensors for payload instruments and attitude control for small satellites", *14th Annual/USU Conference on Small Satellites*, 2000. https://digitalcommons.usu.edu/cgi/viewcontent.cgi?article=2055&context=smallsat.

25. E.E. Haller, "Physics and design of advanced ir bolometers and photoconductors", *Infrared Phys.* 25, 257–66 (1985).

26. P.L. Richards, "Bolometers for infrared and millimeter waves", *J. Appl. Phys.* 76, 1–24 (1994).

27. E.H. Putley, "Thermal detectors", in *Optical and Infrared Detectors*, pp. 71–100, edited by R.J. Keyes, Springer, Berlin. 1977.

28. R.A. Wood, "Uncooled thermal imaging with monolithic silicon focal planes", *Proc. SPIE* 2020, 322–329 (1993).

29. R.A. Wood, "Monolithic silicon microbolometer arrays", in *Semiconductors and Semimetals*, Vol. 47, pp. 45–121, edited by P.W. Kruse and D.D. Skatruda, Academic Press, San Diego, 1997.

30. K.C. Liddiard, "Thin film monolithic arrays for uncooled thermal imaging", *Proc. SPIE* 1969, 206–216 (1993).

31. R.A. Wood, C.J. Han, and P.W. Kruse, "Integrated uncooled IR detector imaging arrays", *Proc. IEEE Solid State Sensor and Actuator Workshop*, 132–135, Hilton Head Island, SC, June 1992.

32. B. Fieque, J.L. Tissot, C. Trouilleanu, A. Crates, and O. Legras, "Uncooled microbolometer detector: recent developments at Ulis", *Infrared Phys. & Technol.* 49, 187–191 (2007).

33. H. Jerominek, T.D. Pope, M. Renaud, N.R. Swart, F. Picard, M. Lehoux, S. Savard, G. Bilodeau, D. Audet, L.N. Phong, and C. N. Qiu, "64×64, 128×128 and 240×320 pixel uncooled IR bolometric detector arrays", *Proc. SPIE* 3061, 236–247 (1997).

34. J.L. Tissot, F. Rothan, C. Vedel, M. Vilain, and J.-J. Yon, "LETI/LIR's amorphous silicon uncooled IR systems", *Proc. SPIE* 3379, 139–44 (1998).

35. J. L. Tissot, J. L. Martin, E. Mottin, M. Vilain, J. J. Yon, and J. P. Chatard, "320×240 microbolometer uncooled IRFPA development", *Proc. SPIE* 4130, 473–479 (2000).

36. M. Kimata, M. Ueno, M. Takeda, and T. Seto, "SOI diode uncooled infrared focal plane arrays", *Proc. SPIE* 6127, 6127-1-11 (2006).

37. M. Kimata, "IR imaging", in *Comprehensive Microsystems*, Vol. 3, 113–162, edited by Y. B. Gianchandani, O. Tabata, and H. Zappe, Elsevier, Amsterdam, 2008.

38. T. Ishikawa, M. Ueno, K. Endo, Y. Nakaki, H. Hata, T. Sone, and M. Kimata, "Low-cost 320×240 uncooled IRFPA using conventional silicon IC process", *Opto-Electr. Rev.* 7, 297–303 (1999).

39. J. Clarke, G.I. Hoffer, P.L. Richards, and N.H. Yeh, "Superconductive bolometers for submillimeter wavelengths", *J. Appl. Phys.* 48, 4865–4879 (1977).

40. D.H. Andrews, R.M. Milton, and W. DeSorbo, "A fast superconducting bolometer", *J. Optical Society of America* 36, 518–524, (1946).

41. C.P. Poole, H.A. Farach, and R.J. Creswick, *Superconductivity*, Academic Press, San Diego, 1995.

42. K. Rose, C.L. Bertin, and R.M. Katz, "Radiation detectors", in *Applied Superconductivity*, Vol. 1, pp. 268–308, edited by V.L. Newhouse, Academic Press, New York, 1975.

43. J. Zmuidzinas and P.L. Richards, "Superconducting detectors and mixers for millimeter and submillimeter astrophysics", *Proc. IEEE* 92, 1597–616 (2004).

44. G. H. Rieke, "Infrared detector arrays for astronomy", *Annu. Rev. Astron. Astrophys.* 45, 77–115 (2007).

45. D.J. Benford and S.H. Moseley, "Superconducting transition edge sensor bolometer arrays for submillimeter astronomy", *Proceedings of the International Symposium on Space and THz Technology*. www.eecs.umich.edu/~jeast/benford_2000_4_1.pdf.

46. K. Rose, "Superconductive FIR detectors", *IEEE Trans. Electron Devices* ED-27, 118–25 (1980).

47. I.A. Khrebtov, "Superconductor infrared and submillimeter radiation receivers", *Sov. J. Opt. Technol.* 58, 261–270 (1991).

48. A.J. Kreisler and A. Gaugue, "Recent progress in HTSC bolometric detectors at terahertz frequencies", *Proc. SPIE* 3481, 457–68 (1998).

49. K.A. Müller and J.G. Bednorz, "The discovery of a class of high-temperature superconductors", *Science* 237, 1133–1139 (1987).

50. J.G. Bednorz and K.A. Müller, "Possible high T_c superconductivity in the Ba-La-Cu-O system", *Zeitschrift fur Physik B-Condensed Matter* 64, 189–93, 1986; "Perovskite-type oxides-the new approach to high-T_c superconductivity", *Rev. Modern Phys.* 60, 585–600 (1988).

51. P.W. Kruse, "Physics and applications of high-T_c superconductors for infrared detectors", *Semicon. Sci. Technol.* 5, S229–S329 (1990).

52. S. Verghese, P.L. Richards, K. Char, D.K. Fork, and T.H. Geballe, "Feasibility of infrared imaging arrays using high-T_c superconducting bolometers", *J. Appl. Phys.* 71, 2491–2498 (1992).

53. M.C. Foote, B.R. Johnson, and B.D. Hunt, "Transition edge $Yba_2Cu_3O_{7-x}$ microbolometers for infrared staring arrays", *Proc. SPIE* 2159, 2–9 (1994).

54. S.B. Lang, "Pyroelectricity: A 2300-year history", *Ferroelectrics* 7, 231–34, 1974.

55. D. Brewster, "Observation of pyroelectricity of minerale", *Edinb. J. Sci* 1, 208–14, 1824.

56. Y. Ta, "Action of radiations on pyroelectric crystals," *Comptes Rendus* 207, 1042–44, 1938.

57. *Infrared detectors*, Application Notes, GEC-Marconi Infra-Red Limited, Southampton 1998.

58. R.L. Peterson, G.W. Day, P.M. Gruzensky, and R.J. Phelan, Jr., "Analysis of response of pyroelectric optical detectors", *J. Appl. Phys.* 45, 3296–303 (1974).

59. S.T. Liu and D. Long, "Pyroelectric detectors and materials", *Proc. IEEE* 66, 14–26 (1978).

60. R.W. Whatmore, "Pyroelectric devices and materials", *Rep. Prog. Phys.* 49, 1335–1386 (1986).

61. *InfraTec Detector and Filter Overview*, www.infratec.eu/sensor-division/pyroelectric-detectors/.

62. www.doitpoms.ac.uk/tlplib/pyroelectricity/infrared.php.

63. L.E. Ravich, "Pyroelectric detectors and imaging", *Laser Focus/Electro-Optics*, 104–115. July 1986.

64. R.W. Whatmore and R. Watton, "Pyroelectric materials and devices", in *Infrared Detectors and Emitters: Materials and Devices*, edited by P. Capper and C.T. Elliott, 99–147, Kluwer Academic Publishers, Boston, 2000.

65. P. Muralt, "Micromachined infrared detectors based on pyroelectric thin films", *Rep. Prog. Phys.* 64, 1339–1388 (2001).

66. H. Betatan, C. Hanson, and E. G. Meissner, "Low cost uncooled ferroelectric detector", *Proc. SPIE* 2274, 147–156 (1994).

67. R. Watton, "PyX3:IR bolometers and thermal imaging: the role of ferroelectric materials", *Ferroelectrics* 133, 5–10 (1992).

68. C.M. Hanson, "Uncooled thermal imaging at Texas Instruments", *Proc. SPIE* 2020, 330–339 (1993).

69. C.M. Hanson, H.R. Beratan, and J.F. Belcher, "Uncooled infrared imaging using thin-film ferroelectrics", *Proc. SPIE* 4288, 298–303 (2001).

70. V. Norkus, T. Sokoll, G. Gerlach, and G. Hofmann, "Pyroelectric infrared arrays and their applications," *Proc. SPIE* 3122, 409–419 (1997).

71. www.dias-infrared.de/pdf/pyrosens_arrays_eng_mail.pdf.

72. V. Norkus, G. Gerlach. DIAS Infrared GmbH, Publication No 8. www.dias-infrared.de/pdf/p008.pdf.

73. A. Rogalski, *Infrared and Terahertz Detectors*, CRC Press, Boca Raton, 2019.

74. N. Neumann, M. Ebermann, K. Schreiber, and M. Heinze, "Multi-colour and tunable-colour pyroelectric detectors", InfraTec GmbH, Dresden, 2008.

75. N. Neumann, M. Ebermann, S. Kurth, and K. Hiller, "Tunable infrared detector with integrated micromachined Fabry-Perot filter", *J. Micro/Nanolith. MEMS MOEMS* 7(2), 021004 (2008).

76. Infra Tec, *Pyroelectric & Multispectral Detectors*. Catalog 2013.

6 Photoemissive Detectors

In 1887, Hertz observed the photoemission effect for the first time when negatively charged particles were emitted from a conductor if it was irradiated with ultraviolet (UV). Two years later, Elster and Geitel [1] revealed a similar effect when they experiment with an alkali metal electrode and visible radiation. Satisfactory explanation of this effect, called photoemission, was given by Einstein in 1905 in terms of electron emission induced by the incident radiation. Further studies indicated that spectral response of many materials is characterised by different threshold wavelengths. For a long time, however, due to very low quantum efficiencies (below 10^{-4} electrons per incident photon), practical application the photoemission effect was limited. The situation suddenly altered in 1929 after the discovery of the AgOCs photocathode by Koller [2] and Campbell [3]. This discovery inaugurated a new era in photoemissive devices since quantum efficiency of AgOCs was two orders of magnitude above anything previously studied.

6.1 INTRODUCTION

Photoemissive detectors are generally the detectors of choice in ultraviolet (UV), visible and near infrared (NIR) where high efficiency is available. In the spectral range below 600 nm, the photo-multiplier has close to ideal sensitivity; that is, selected photomultipliers are capable of detecting single photon arrivals (but at best only with 30 per cent quantum efficiency) and amplifying the photocurrent (pulse) enormously without seriously degrading the signal-to-noise ratio.

The process of photoemission from any material can be considered in three stages (see Figure 6.1):

- the excitation of the photoelectron;
- its diffusion to the emitting surface; and
- the escape of the photoelectron into surrounding vacuum.

The electrons in any material are bounded to the lattice by the ionisation energy, and any electron at the surface that is excited to an energy level greater than the ionisation energy has a high probability of escaping. In the case of a metal the reflectivity is high in the visible region (90–99%) and near infrared region of the spectrum; as a result the energy loss of any excited carrier will be rapid, and the quantum efficiency of any metal photocathode will be low. Using a semiconductor as the photocathode with higher absorption efficiency and longer relaxation time for energy losses, considerably improvement in quantum efficiency is achieved. Also, their lower ionisation potential allows longer wavelength operation.

In a metal electron, scattering is the dominant process, and the mean free path of carriers is short due to its high density. Consequently, only those electrons created within a few atomic layers

DOI: 10.1201/9781003263098-6

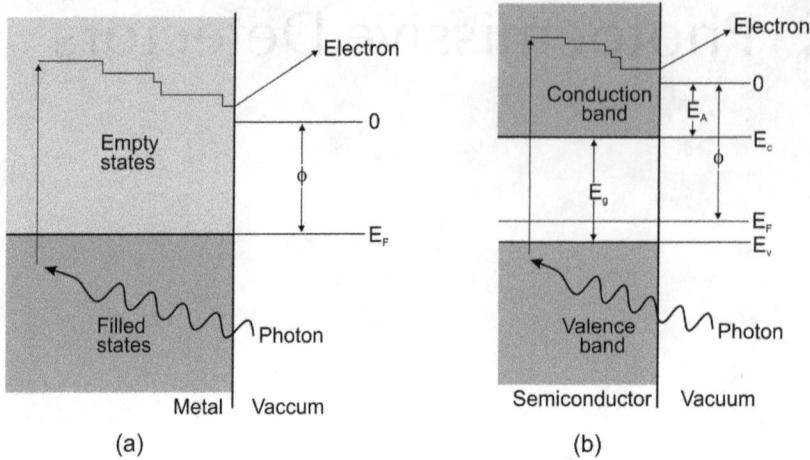

FIGURE 6.1   Energy band diagrams of the photoemissive effect in (a) a metal and (b) a semiconductor.

of the surface can escape. However, for the semiconductor this loss mechanism is negligible, and photoelectrons lose energy by electron-hole pair production (impact ionisation) and by lattice scattering (phonon creation). The loss of energy per scattering is small, typically 0.01 eV, and the mean free path is 30–40 Å. At depths of several hundred Å, sufficient energy for photoemission is possible in the absence of electrons pair production. However, if an electron has an energy above a threshold limit, E_{th}, it can lose energy by creating an electron-hole pair. Usually, the threshold energy is several times larger than the energy gap, E_g.

Finally, the photoelectron must have sufficient energy when it reaches the interface to be able to overcome the surface potential. In the case of metals, it is work function defined as the energy difference between the Fermi level and the minimum free energy of an electron at rest within the vacuum. Metals have relatively high work functions. Most, in fact, range between 4 and 5 eV, which corresponds to a wavelength of 311 to 249 nm. In the case of semiconductors, the level of doping alters the position of the Fermi level, and a better parameter is the electron affinity, E_A, which is defined as the difference in energy between the bottom of the conduction band and the vacuum level.

6.2   CONVENTIONAL PHOTOCATHODES

Figure 6.2 shows three different conditions depending on the relation between E_{th} and E_A:

(a) $E_{th} > E_A$; an electron has a high probability to escape even after producing a secondary electron-hole pair;

(b) $E_A > E_{th}$; any electron with sufficient energy to escape can also create an electron-hole pair, and due to the very short mean free path of pair production only electrons generated near to the surface can escape;

(c) $E_{th} \geq E_A - E_{th}$ slightly larger than E_A; only electrons are able to escape if they have an energy greater than E_A but less than E_{th}, quantum efficiency is moderately low.

The minimum energy required in photoemission process is $E_g + E_A$, unless high density of electrons in the conduction band. In the case when $E_g + E_A < 3$ eV, the emission is in the visible region of the spectrum. However, by appropriate choice of the semiconductor materials, the spectral threshold has been extended into the near infrared. The photon absorption of semiconductors is more efficient, and their relaxation time for energy losses is longer.

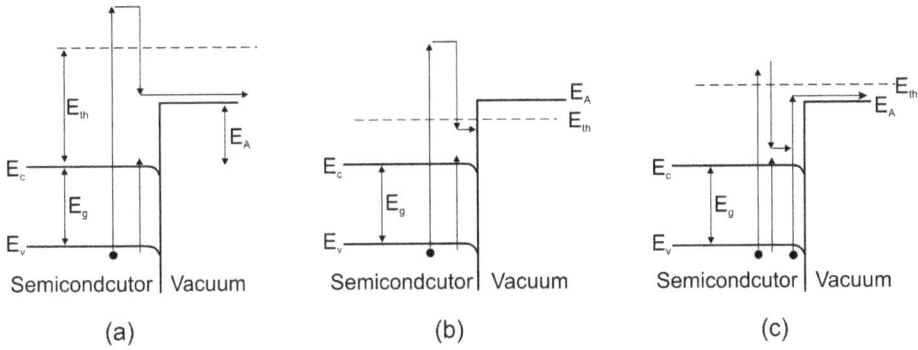

FIGURE 6.2 The photoemission processes for a conventional photocathode in dependence on the relative value of the threshold energy, E_{th}, and the electron affinity, E_A.

TABLE 6.1
Composition and Typical Characteristics of Photocathodes (after Reference 5)

Type of response	Composition	Type of window	Photo-emission threshold (nm)	Wavelength at maximum sensitivity (nm)	Radiant sensitivity at λ_{max} (mA/W)	Quantum efficiency at λ_{max} (%)
S1	AgOCs	1	1100	800	2.3	0.4
S4	SbCs$_3$	1,2,3	680	400	50	16
S11	SbCs$_3$	1	700	440	80	22
S13	SbCs$_3$	2	700	440	80	22
S20	SbNa$_2$KCs	1	850	420	70	20
S20	SbNa$_2$KCs	2	850	420	70	20
S20R (ERMA*)	SbNa$_2$KCs	1	900	550	35	8
Bialkali	SbKCs	1	630	400	90	28
Bialkali	SbKCs	2	630	400	90	28
Bialkali (GEBA**)	SbKCs	1	700	440	100	28
Bialkali	SbNaK	1	700	400	50***	16***
Solar blind	CsTe	2	340	235	20	10

Windows: 1. Borosilicate or lime glass or equivalent. 2. Fused silica. 3. Internal (opaque) cathode.
  *ERMA = Extended-red multialkali, sometimes called S25 **GEBA = Green-extended bialkali
***The SbNaK bialkali cathodes are intended for high-temperature operation and the sensitivity and quantum efficiencies
  are given for 130 °C.

The quantum efficiency of photoemissive materials is controlled by many factors, and some of the results obtained before development of modern vacuum technology are questionable (e.g., variation of the work function in dependence of small quantities of absorbed gasses). More information on this topic can be found in Sommer's monograph [4].

To simplify the identification of photocathodes, each combination has been given an internationally agreed S number, as specified by the Electronic Industries Association (1954). The S designations refer to the total spectral response, including the effect of the input window. They do not identify specific types of cathode or cathode materials, or absolute sensitivities, although they are often so used. A list of the more important photocathodes with their characteristics is collected in Table 6.1, while typical spectral sensitivity curves are shown in Figure 6.3.

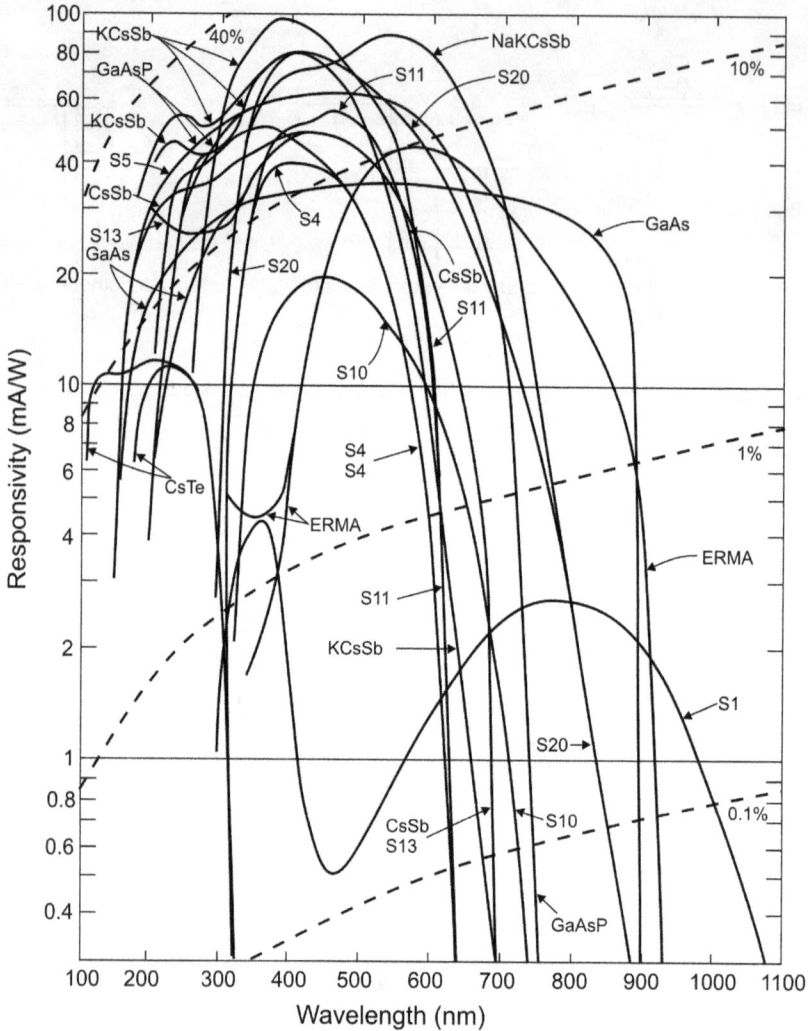

FIGURE 6.3 Typical spectral sensitivity curves of various photoemitters. Dotted lines indicate photocathode quantum efficiency. Chemical formulas are abbreviated to conserve space. S1 = AgOCs with lime or borosilicate crown-glass window; S4 = Cs$_3$Sb with lime or borosilicate crown-glass window (opaque photocathode); S5 = Cs$_3$Sb with ultraviolet-transmitting glass window; S8 = Cs$_3$Bi with lime or borosilicate crown-glass window; S10 = AgBiOCs with lime or borosilicate crown-glass window; S11 = Cs$_3$Sb with fused-silica window (semitransparent photocathode); S13 = Cs$_3$Sb with fused-silica window (semitransparent photocathode); S19 = Cs$_3$Sb with fused-silica window (opaque semicathode); S20 = Na$_2$KCsSb with lime or borosilicate glass window. ERMA = extended red multialkali (after Reference 6).

The material of the input window limits the spectral sensitivity in the short wavelength region. The cut-off wavelengths of borosilicate glass (hard glass) and lime glass (soft glass) are between 250 and 300 nm, and UV-transparent glass and fused silica – below 250 nm [5]. Lithium fluoride operates down to 105 nm. For wavelengths less than 105 nm, there is no transparent material, and windowless photocathodes must be used in evacuated systems, which is possible for some applications, such as space.

The first semiconductor photocathode, developed by Keller in 1929, consists of a layer of cesium on oxidised silver [7]. These cathodes are generally fabricated by depositing a thin layer of silver on a glass carrier, which is then oxidised by a glow discharge, or radio frequency (r.f.) heating. The layer is then sensitised with cesium vapour and heated to about 130°C. The S1 is sensitive in the ultraviolet region down to 300 nm throughout the visible and near infrared region of spectrum. However, the quantum efficiency is slow, typically 1–2 per cent, and the cathodes show long-term decay after storage and rapid deterioration under conditions of high illumination. Due to critical fabrication procedure and low yield, the S1 devices are not widely used if an alternative is available.

The cesium-antimony photocathode is one of the most widely used due to its high quantum efficiency. Its fabrication is relatively simple: an antimony film is evaporated onto a faceplate, which is then activated by evaporating cesium onto the antimony, which is maintained at elevated temperature [4]. After cooling to room temperature, a highly stable film of Cs_3Sb is formed with an energy gap of 1.6 eV and an electron affinity of 0.45 eV. The threshold voltage is approximately 2 eV. It appears that the sensitivity of these tubes can be increased if a small amount of oxygen is introduced and the cathode reheated. Depending on the window material and if the cathode is deposited onto opaque or semitransparent substrate, the $SbCs_3$ tubes have been given a range of S numbers, including S4, 5, 11, 13, 17 and 19.

A large number of multialkali antimonide photocathodes have been produced. $SbNa_2K$ has peak sensitivity in the blue region and, although its quantum efficiency is lower than other multialkali antimonides it can be used at temperatures of up to 150°C. By introducing a small amount of cesium, its response can be extended into the near infrared, and when used with lime glass window this is the S20 photocathode.

Generally, the multialkali cathodes have high quantum efficiencies but are difficult to prepare; consequently, their use has been limited to more specialised photomultipliers and image intensifier tubes. There are approximately ten kinds of photocathods currently used in practical applications. They are operated in transmission (semitransparent) or reflection (opaque) modes. A review of the most popular photocathodes, describing their fabrication methods and sensitivities, has been given by Zwieker [8] and Ghosh [9]. Also, the Hamamatsu's handbook provides reader comprehensive information on photocathods and photomultiplier tubes [10].

6.3 NEGATIVE ELECTRON AFFINITY DEVICES

To improve the photoemission yield and extend the wavelength sensitivity, the electron affinity should be reduced, or ideally become effectively negative. Spicer [11] has predicted that, by using a heavily doped material, an effective negative electron affinity (NEA) cathode could be fabricated. The mechanism and band structures of various NEA photoemitters has been reviewed by Bell, Spicer [12–14] and Zwicker [8].

Usually, NEA devices are fabricated from p-type degenerately doped semiconductors. The band structure for such a device is shown in Figure 6.4. It is shown that although an electron at the surface has an energy lower than E_A, there is a region in the bulk for the p-type material where the energy of an electron at the bottom of the conduction band exceeds the vacuum potential – such situations cannot occur with a conventional photocathode. The region, in which the band bending can be small with respect to the electron escape depth and the optical absorption length, is formed by increasing the doping level. A significant improvement of sensitivity was achieved with a layer of cesium and cesium oxide.

The first NEA devices were fabricated in 1967 on GaAs [15] and GaP [16] substrates with a monolayer of caesium. Further studies showed reduction of the electron affinity and increase of the sensitivity by using thicker layer of Cs and CsO. The threshold energy extends into near infrared to about 1 μm.

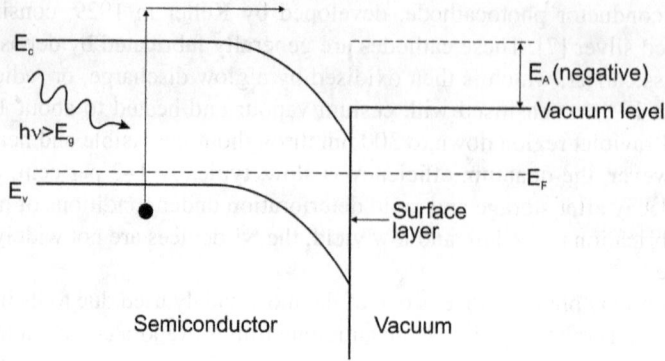

FIGURE 6.4 The photoemission process and energy band structure for a p-type NEA photocathode.

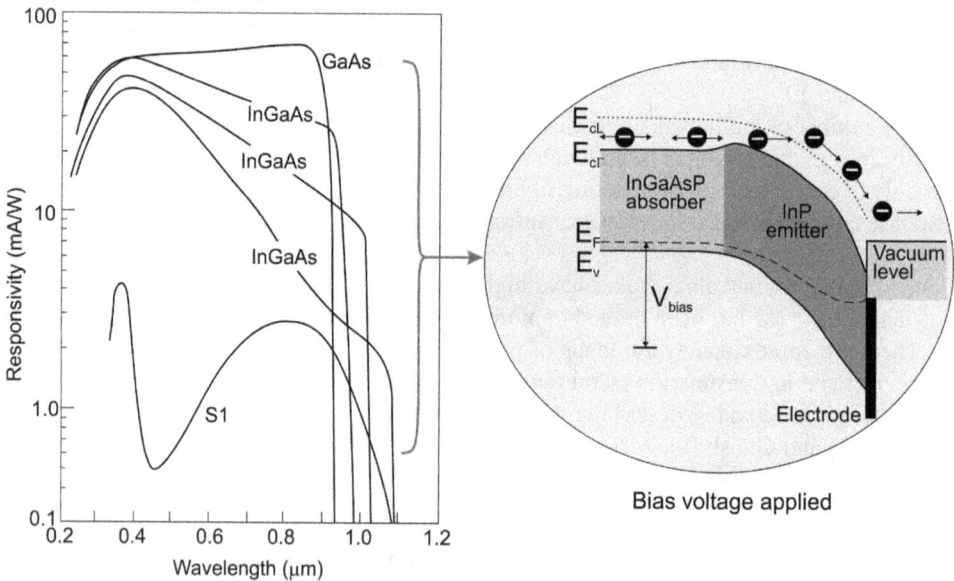

FIGURE 6.5 Responsivity of four members of the InGaAs family of photocathodes. The S1 curve is included for reference. Applying a bias voltage to InP/InGaAs heterostructure (right side), the conduction band barrier lowers what allows for higher sensitivity at long wavelength extending to 1.7 μm.

The best-quality NEA devices have been fabricated using ternary and quaternary III-V alloys, since their band gaps can be varied by adjusting composition, and consequently the wavelength response of photocathodes. Figure 6.5 shows spectral responsivity of four members of the InGaAs family of photocathodes. Quantum efficiencies of 9 per cent and 5.4 per cent for InGaAs and InGaAsP cathodes have been reported. Although by reducing the energy gap, response beyond 1.1 μm can be obtained; the quantum efficiency drops rapidly due to the interface potential barrier of InP/InGaAsP heterostructure. Responsivities are approximately two orders of magnitude greater than obtained from classical photoemitters. However, these photocathods are characterised by large dark current when used at room temperature, and they must be cooled to between −60°C and −80°C.

Typical spectral sensitivity curves of various photocathodes charged with typical transmittance of window materials together with a list of important photocathodes are shown in Figure 6.6. Ternary

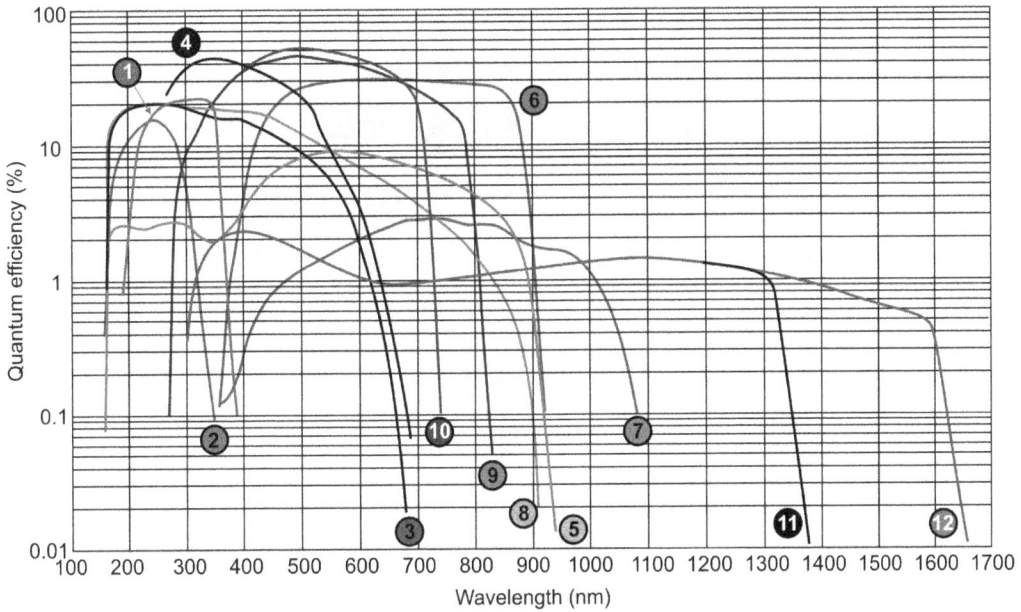

Suffix	Photocathode	Input window
1	GaN	Synthetic silica
2	CsTe	Synthetic silica
3	Bialkali	Synthetic silica
4	Ultra-bialkali	Synthetic silica
5	Enhanced red multialkali	Synthetic silica
6	GaAs	Synthetic silica
7	InGaAs	Borosilicate glass
8	Multialkali (S20)	Borosilicate glass
9	Enhanced red GaAsP	Borosilicate glass
10	GaAsP	Borosilicate glass
11	InGaAs	Borosilicate glass
12	InGaAs	Borosilicate glass

FIGURE 6.6 Spectral sensitivity curves of various photocathodes.

AlGaN alloys are excellent photocathode materials due to their low electron affinity, chemical stability and direct bandgap. A quantum efficiency of 45 per cent around 400 nm is achieved by an ultra-bialkali (UBA) photocathode. Gallium arsenide phosphide (GaAsP) photocathods reach a quantum efficiency of 50 per cent in the visible region. Longer wavelengths sensitive are photocathods based on indium gallium arsenide (InGaAs).

6.4 PHOTOMULTIPLIERS

The photoemissive devices are used for the detection of very low intensity signals, high speed pulses of radiation and for uses requiring high spatial resolution, such as imaging.

Photodetectors based on photoemission usually take the form of vacuum tubes called phototubes. Electrons are emitted from the surface of a cathode and travel to an electrode (anode), which is maintained at a higher electric potential (Figure 4.59). As a result of the electron transport between the cathode and anode, an electric current proportional to the photon flux incident on the photocathode

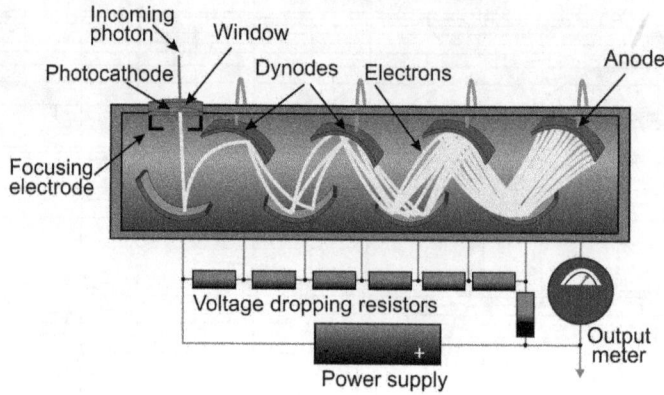

FIGURE 6.7 Schematic presentation of a photomultiplier tube.

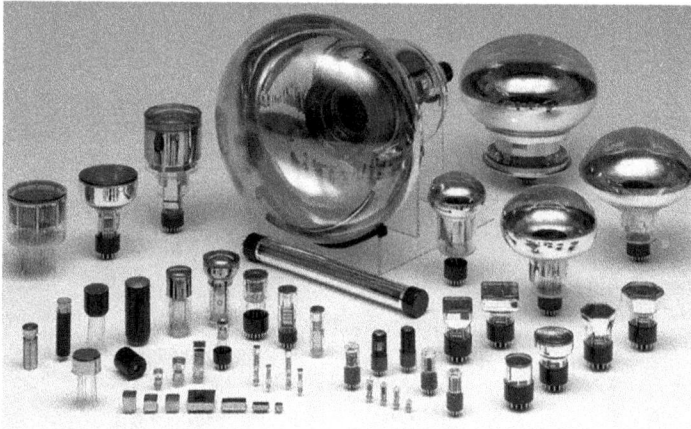

FIGURE 6.8 A representative selection of different PMT types fabricated by Hamamatsu. The custom-designed large 20-in. diameter PMTs (the largest in this figure) are fabricated for use in neutrino SuperKamiokande observatory in near Hida, Japan. The SuperKamiokande facility employs 11,200 PMTs paving the walls of a 40-metre diameter tank of water that probes the neutrinos.

is created in the circuit. The photoemitted electrons may also impact other specially placed metal or semiconductor surfaces in the tube, called dynodes, from which a cascade of electrons is emitted by the process of secondary emission. A photomultiplier tube (PMT) generally contains between ten and fifteen dynodes and approximately 100 V is maintained between successive dynode plates. The result is an amplification of the generated electric current by a factor as high as 10^9. This device illustrated in Figure 6.7, is known as a photomultiplier tube. To meet market demands, different photomultiplier tubes have been developed. Hamamatsu has developed hundreds of different photomultiplier tubes and their representative selection is shown in Figure 6.8 [20].

The photocathode in photomultiplier (PM) devices is usually a semitransparent photoemissive material deposited onto the inside surface of the end face of the tube. This allows direct coupling of the source and detector, thus reducing any light loss. The choice of material for the photocathode is determined by the wavelength of operation. Both a high quantum efficiency as well as a low thermionic emission (to reduce the dark current) in operation spectral region are required. Developments in photocathodes employed in PMTs and summary of their sensitivities is given by Yokozawa [19].

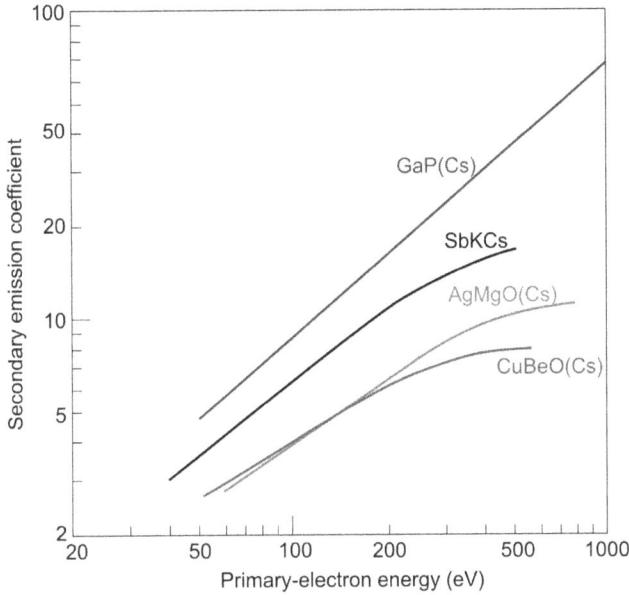

FIGURE 6.9 Secondary emission coefficient of some dynode materials as a function of the primary electron energy (or interdynode voltage).

The gain of a PMT is a function of the applied voltage. Typical emission curves for several materials as a function of incident electron energy are shown in Figure 6.9. The secondary emission process depends on the incident energy of the primary electron, as the number of electrons generated with sufficient energy to escape from the surface increases. If the penetration of accelerated electrons to the dynode is very deep (more than several atoms), the likelihood of secondary electrons escaping a classical dynode becomes low. An optimum bias voltage can, therefore, be found that trades off electron energy with dynode penetration to achieve maximum gain. A NEA dynode is not very likely to trap secondary electrons once these electrons are excited to the conduction band, however. Therefore NEA dynodes show nearly linear increase in gain with applied voltage, what is shown in Figure 6.9 for GaP(Cs).

The most popular materials for PM dynodes are $SbCs_3$, AgMgO and oxidised copper containing about 2 per cent beryllium. $SbCs_3$ offers a high gain at relatively low applied voltages but has poor high temperature stability. AgMgO can be operated at higher currents and temperature but requires increased applied voltages. The third material is similar in performance to the AgMnO system, but is easier to fabricate. As an alternative to coated dynodes, thin plates have been constructed that allow the secondary electrons to be emitted from the back of each plate. Stable operation has been achieved using magnesium oxide.

Typically, secondary emission coefficients, δ, of between 2 and 3 are observed. Higher gain, about five, with an inter dynode voltage of approximately 5 kV has been achieved using potassium chloride [7]. Assuming PMT with n dynodes, transfer efficiency between each dynode of g, and collection efficiency between the photocathode and first dynode as f, the overall amplification of the tube is given by

$$G = f \left(\delta g \right)^n . \tag{6.1}$$

To eliminate heating of the anode and limit an upper current of dynodes, the stable gain is generally limited to 10^7; for pulsed operation to 10^8 [7].

TABLE 6.2
Characteristics of Head-on Photomultiplier Tubes

Dynode type	Rise time (ns)	Pulse linearity at 2% deviation (mA)	Magnetic immunity (mT)	Uniformity	Collection efficiency	Features
Circular-cage	0.9–3.0	1–10	0.1	Poor	Good	Compact, high speed
Box-and-grid	6–20	1–10	0.1	Good	Very good	High collection efficiency
Linear-focused	0.7–3	10–250	0.1	Poor	Good	High speed, high linearity
Venetian blind	6–18	10–40	0.1	Good	Poor	Suitable for large-diameter tubes
Fine mesh	1.5–5.5	300–1000	500–1500*	Good	Poor	High magnetic field, high linearity
Microchannel plate	0.1–0.3	700	1500*	Good	Poor	High speed
Metal channel	0.65–1.5	30	5**	Good	Good	Compact, high speed
Bombardment type	Depends on internal semiconductor	-		Very good	Very good	High photoelectron resolution

*in magnetic field parallel to tube axis
**metal package PMT

The construction of the tube and dynode configuration should ensure that all the electrons emitted by one dynode strike the succeeding one and thus do not miss any stage of amplifications, nor should they collide with any other part of the tube. Their characteristics depend not only on the dynode type but also on the photocathode size and focusing system. The tubes can be devoted as focussed and or unfocussed systems. Table 6.2 summarises typical performance characteristics of photomultipliers [10]. The more popular constructions are shown in Figure 6.10. Focussed tubes are constructed in the conventional linear manner or more simply in a circular fashion, which enables a very compact tube using an opaque photocathode to be assembled. The electrons are finally collected at the anode, which often consists of just a thin wire or grid mounted close to or inside the final dynode, thus enabling any strong capacitance effects to be minimised. The prime features of the circular-cage are compactness and fast time response. The box-and-grid system is often used in tubes of smaller diameter and consists of a train of quarter cylindrical dynodes and is widely used in head-on type PMT because of its relatively simple dynode design and improved uniformity, although time response may to be too slow in some applications. This arrangement has the highest dynode efficiency, but tends to saturate at high anode currents, due to space charge effects. If the plates are curves, a focussing field is obtained, and the electrons are directed towards the centre of each dynode, what is realised in a linear-focused PMT. Generally, the electric field strength at the dynode surface is greater in this type of tube than the more unfocussed one. Consequently, the spread in transit time is less, and output pulses with rise times below 1 ns have been achieved. In a venetian blind system, each dynode consists of small plates mounted at 45° to the axis of the tube, the plates of each succeeding dynode slope in opposite directions. This system offers better uniformity and a large pulse output current and is usually used when time response is not a prime consideration. In box-and-grid and venetian blind tubes there is no focussing of the secondary electrons between stages. The mesh type has a structure of fine mesh electrodes stacked in close proximity. This type provides high immunity to the magnetic field, as well as good uniformity and high pulse linearity. In addition, it has position-sensitive capability when used with cross-wire anodes or multiple anodes. In 1-mm thickness of microchannel plate (MCP) dynodes

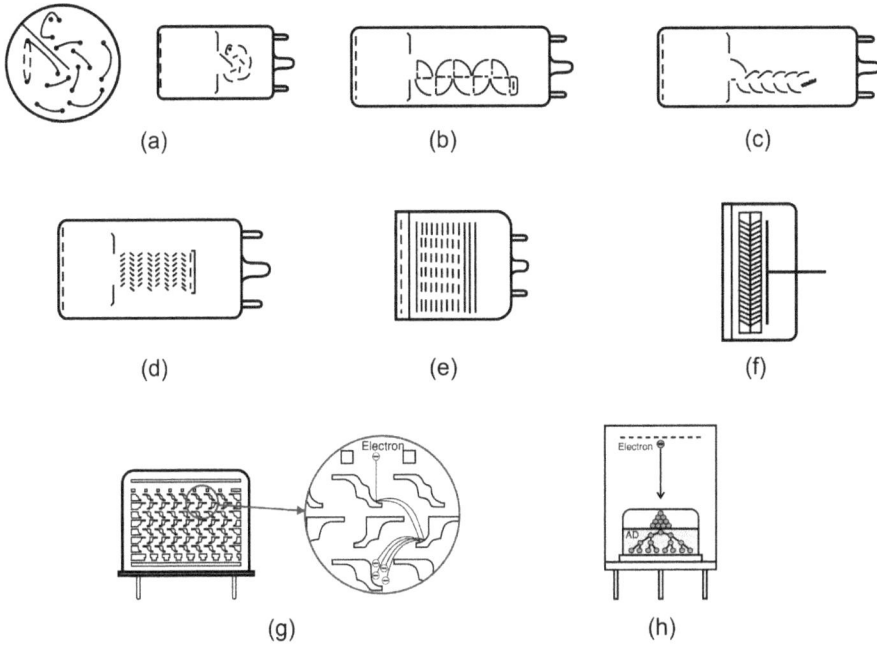

FIGURE 6.10 Photomultiplier tube constructions: (a) circular-cage, (b) box-and-grid, (c) linear-focused, (d) venetian blind, (e) fine mesh, (f) microchannel plate, (g) metal channel, and (h) electron bombardment.

exhibit dramatic improvement in time resolution. Like the mesh type dynode, MCP ensures stable gain in magnetic fields. The metal channel dynode consists of extremely thin and precisely stacked electrodes in close proximity to one other. This structure ensures excellent time characteristics and stable gain. In the electron bombardment structure, photoelectrons are accelerated by a high voltage to strike a semiconductor. Next, the photoelectron energy is transferred to semiconductor to produce gain. In consequence, this dynode structure assures small noise, excellent uniformity, and high linearity.

The linear dynamic range of a PMT is typically 10^8 limited by dark current at the low end of the range and space-charge effects at the high end (see Figure 6.11). Space-charge limiting of current occurs when the electron density between the last dynode and the anode becomes so high that the negative space charge due to the electron cloud significantly repels electrons leaving the dynode. The dark current is due to contributions from leakage current (region a), regenerative effects (including α, β, and γ particles which cause secondary electron emission), and the thermionic emission of electrons (region b). At a high voltage (region c) dominate the field emission and glass or electrode support scintillation. In the PMT pulse operation a problem is with elimination of ion feedback and noise originating from cosmic rays and radioisotopes.

The thermionic emission is often the dominant source of dark current and can be described by

$$J_{st} = A^* T^2 \exp\left(-\frac{q\phi_b}{kT}\right). \tag{6.2}$$

where A^* is the Richardson constant, ϕ_b is the work function, q is the electron charge, k is the Boltzmann constant, and T is the temperature. The last equation indicates that thermionic emission current is a strong function of the photocathode work functions and temperature. For these reasons, photocathodes with low work function (e.g., alkali metals like AgOCs) are sensitive in a longer wavelength range but have high dark current. In contrast, photocathodes with higher work function (e.g., CsTe, CsI)

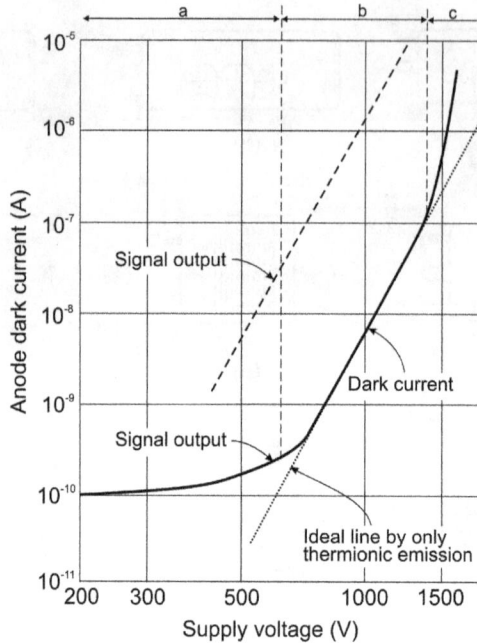

FIGURE 6.11   Typical anode dark current versus supply voltage (after Reference 10).

operate in the ultraviolet region and exhibit low dark current. Summarising, cooling a PMT (typically to $-40°C$) reduces the thermionic contribution below the other sources of dark current.

The response of a photomultiplier is determined by the spread in times of flight of electrons between each stage, and with careful design of the dynode chain, bandwidths of 100 MHz can be obtained. Rise time given in Table 6.2 is the time required for the PMT output to rise from 10 per cent to 90 per cent of peak amplitude when the entire photocathode is illuminated by a light pulse of less than 50 ps.

The PMT is a vacuum tube and, therefore, shot noise is dominant source of noise. However, due to internal amplification, G, the shot noise will now increase G times. The Johnson noise in the anode resistor will be unaltered.

Detectivity as a meaningful figure of merit for detectors, must be used with caution for PMT because, although modern phototubes are generally dark-noise limited devices, they are often limited by signal fluctuation noise. Serious errors in predicting the detection capability of phototubes will arise if noise in the signal is ignored and is presumed to be the important limiting parameter. Very little reliable data are presently available on detectivity of PMT.

With the emergence of photolithographic silicon based PMT and large format high resolution position sensing readouts, considerable progress has been made towards the next generation of microchannel plate detectors. Silicon based PMTs have qualities that make them preferable to glass PMTs (very low intrinsic background, low fixed pattern noise). The fabrication has been scaled to 6-inch wafers so larger MCPs are possible. In the micro-PMT, dynodes are fabricated using MEMS technology by deep etching (about 1mm) on a silicon substrate [see Figure 6.12(a)]. The device structure contains a silicon substrate sandwiched between two glass substrate. Anode bonding of a silicon and glass substrate secures vacuum airtightness. The final wafer-shaped product contains about 100 micro-PMTs. After wafer separation into chips through a dicing process, the size of each chip is about 10 mm and weighs about 0.5 g – see Figure 6.12(b).

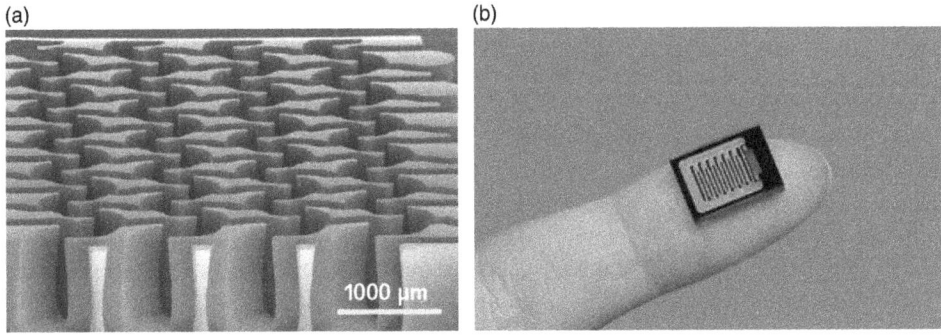

FIGURE 6.12 Micro-PMTs: (a) silicon PMT detector produced on 6" wafer, and (b) separated micro-PMT on a finger tip (after Reference 20).

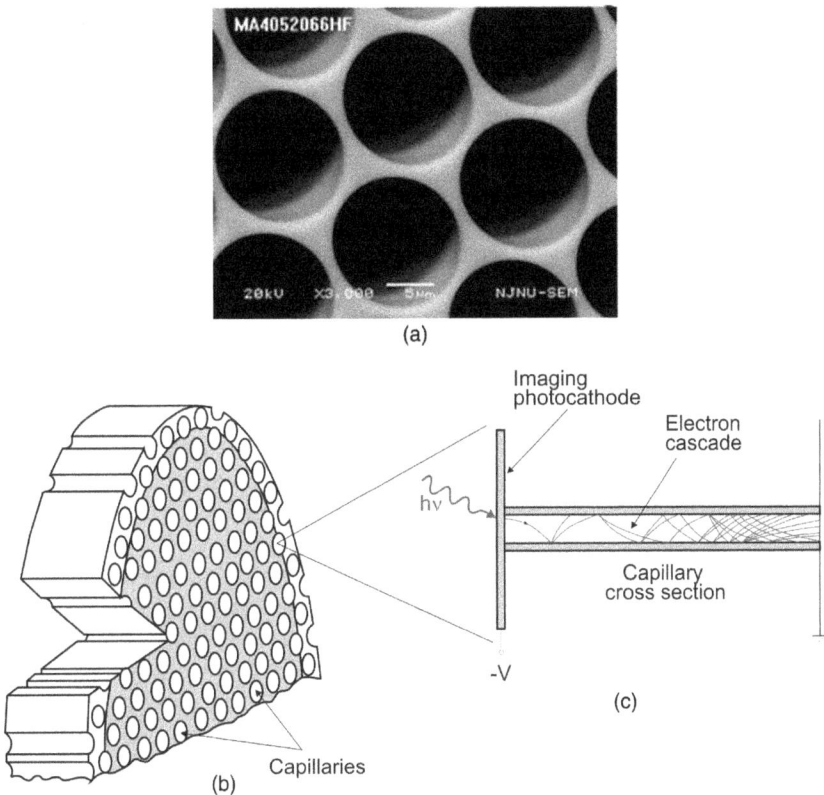

FIGURE 6.13 Schematic presentation of a microchannel plate: (a) SEM view of microtubes set, (b) cutaway view, and (c) a single capillary.

6.5 MICROCHANNEL PLATES

The secondary emission is also used in a modern imaging device called the microchannel plate. It consists of an array of millions of capillaries (of internal diameter ≈ 10 μm) in a glass plate of thickness ≈ 1 mm. Both faces of the plate are coated with thin metal films that act as electrodes and a voltage are applied across them [see Figure 6.13]. The interior walls of each capillary are coated with a secondary-electron-emissive material and behave as a continuous dynode, multiplying the photoelectron current emitted at that position [Figure 6.13(c)]. In such a way, the local photon flux can be converted into a substantial electron flux that can be measured directly. Furthermore, the electron flux can be reconverted into an optical image by using a phosphor coating as the rear electrode to provide electroluminescence; this combination provides an image intensifier.

The microchannel plate (MCP) is a disk consisting of millions of micro glass tubes (channels) fused in parallel with each other. The channels made of combination of oxides of silicon, lead, and alkali compounds in mixture are used to obtain design resistivity in the approximate range of 10^{10}–10^{15} Ωcm^2. Each channel acts as an independent electron multiplier. Its diameter is between 10 μm and 25 μm and length of 0.5 mm and then is possible incorporate 2.5 million of them in a 25 mm plate. They are operated at approximately 1 kV with a typical amplification of 3000. Channel-diameter uniformity of about 2 per cent and hence 4 to 5 per cent gain uniformity is commonly achieved. The MCP offers much faster time response than the other discrete dynodes. It also features good immunity from magnetic fields and two-dimensional detection ability when multiple anodes are used. The electron gain of the channel depends on the applied voltage, the ratio of the channel length to the diameter and the secondary emission characteristics of the channel surface. A gain up to 10^8 for 3 keV applied field is achieved. However, the gain is limited by ionic feedback, which arises due to electron impact ionisation of the residual gas molecules. The positive ions are accelerated back down the tube where they may gain sufficient energy to generate secondary electrons if they collide with the well. To overcome this effect two solutions are used: the tubes are coated with a thin aluminium film (typically 30Å thick), which act as a barrier to the positive ions; or a single-channel multiplier is constructed in a circular configuration. In the last case, any ions now formed are only to be able to move a short distance down the tube before striking the wall and, hence, have not sufficient energy to generate electrons.

It should be noticed that alternative designs of tubes have been considered using magnetically focussed multipliers. In this type of tube the multiplication is obtained from continuous film deposited onto an insulator and biased such that an electron striking one end of the film generates secondaries which are accelerated along the tube and strike the film further along its length [7,21].

A photocathode, electron focusing optics, and a phosphor output screen or a suitable recording medium can be combined in a number of ways to intensify light while retaining imaging information. Phosphor output image intensifiers are reviewed in depth by Csorba [22]. The image (visible, ultraviolet or infrared) is focused onto semitransparent photocathode, and photoelectrons are emitted with a spatial intensity distribution, which matches the focused image. In image intensifiers the electrons are then accelerated towards a phosphor screen where they reproduce the original image with enhanced intensity. Three common forms of image tube are shown in Figure 6.14.

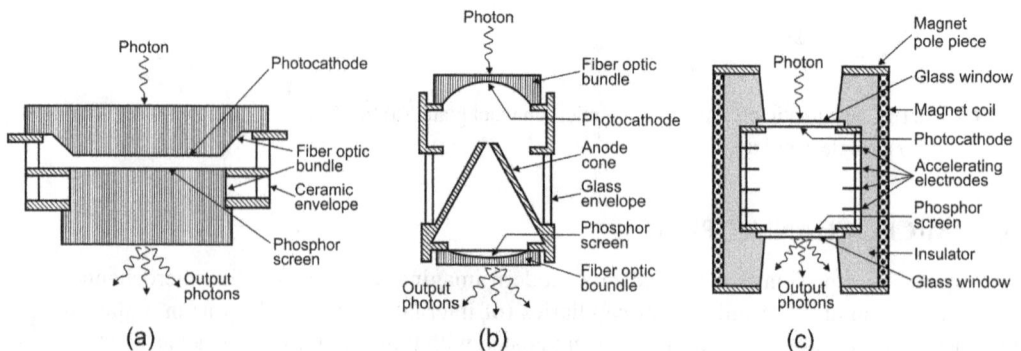

FIGURE 6.14 Cross-sectional diagrams of a variety of image intensifier types: (a) proximity focused, (b) electronically focused and (c) magnetically focused.

In a "proximity-focused" tube, a high electric field (typically 5 kV), and a short distance between the photocathode and the screen limit spreading of electrons to preserve an image. This form of tube is compact, the image is free from distortion and only a simple power supply is required. However, the resolution of such a tube is limited by the field strength at the photocathode, and the resolution is highest when the distance between cathode and screen is small.

An electrostatically focused tube is based upon a system of concentric spheres (cathode and anode, typical bias voltage of 15 kV). In practice, the electrodes depart radically from the simple spherical concept. Additional electrodes can be introduced to provide focusing control and reduce the image distortion, while fibre-optic windows at input and output can be used to improve image quality and provide a better matching to objective and coupling optics. Power suppliers are very simple and lightweight, so this type of tube is widely used in portable applications.

A magnetically focused system gives very high-resolution images with little or no distortion. The focusing coil, however, is usually heavy and power consuming. For the best picture quality, the power suppliers for both tube and coil must be stable. This type of tube is used in applications where resolution and low distortion are vital and weight and power consumption do not create unacceptable problems.

6.6   IMAGE INTENSIFIER SYSTEMS

Night-vision systems can be divided into two categories: those depending upon the reception and processing of radiation reflected by an object and those which operate with radiation internally generated by an object. These devices gather existing ambient light (starlight, moonlight or infra-red light) through the front lens. This light, which is made up of photons, goes into a photocathode tube that changes the photons to electrons.

The human visual perception system is optimised to operate in daytime illumination conditions. The visual spectrum extends from about 420 to 700 nm and the region of greatest sensitivity is near the peak wavelength of sunlight at around 550 nm (see section 1.2). However, at night fewer visible light photons are available and only large, high-contrast objects are visible. It appears that the photon rate in the region from 800 to 900 nm is five to seven times greater than in the visible region around 500 nm. Moreover, the reflectivity of various materials (e.g., green vegetation, because of its chlorophyll content) is higher between 800 and 900 nm than at 500 nm. It means that at night more light is available in the NIR than in the visual region and that against certain backgrounds more contrast is available.

The early concepts of image intensification were not basically different from those today. However, the early devices suffered from two major deficiencies: poor photocathodes and poor coupling. Later development of both cathode and coupling technologies changed the image intensifier into much more useful device. The concept of image intensification by cascading stages was suggested independently by number of workers in the early 1930s, as is noted in Section 6.2.

A considerable improvement in night-vision capability can be achieved with night viewing equipment which consists of an objective lens, image intensifier and eyepiece (see Figure 6.15). Improved visibility is obtained by gathering more light from the scene with an objective lens than the unaided eye; by use of a photocathode that has higher photosensitivity and broader spectral response than the eye; and by amplification of photo-events for visual sensation.

The image intensifiers are classed by generation (Gen) numbers. Gen 0 refers to the technology of the Second World War, employing fragile, vacuum-enveloped photon detectors with poor sensitivity and little gain. Further evolution of image intensifier tubes is presented in Table 6.3. Gen1 represents the technology of the early Vietnam era, the 1960s. In this era, the first passive systems, able to amplify ambient starlight, were introduced. Though sensitive, these devices were large and heavy. Gen1 devices used tri-alkali photocathodes to achieve gain of about 1,000. By the early 1970s, the MCP amplifier was developed comprising more than two million microscopic conducting channels of hollow glass, each of about 10 μm in diameter, fused into a disc-shaped array. Coupling the MCP with multi-alkali photocathodes capable of emitting more electrons per incident photon, produced

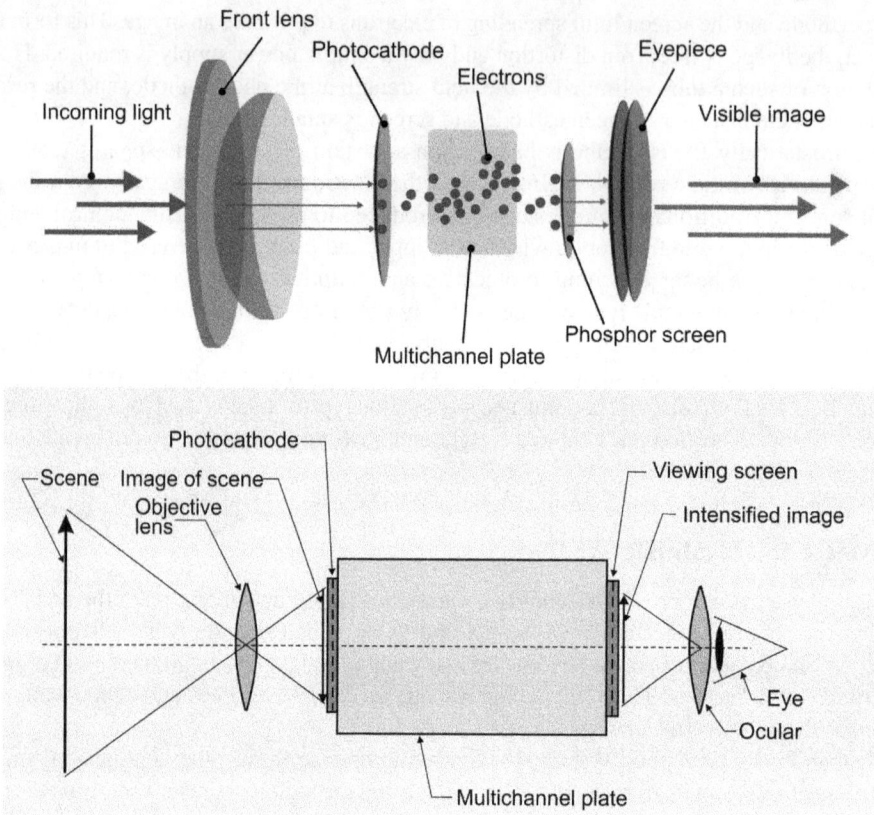

FIGURE 6.15   Diagram of an image intensifier.

TABLE 6.3
Image Intensifier Tubes

Gen 1	Gen 2	Gen 3	Gen 3 filmless

Gen 1	Gen 2	Gen 3	Gen 3 filmless
• Vietnam War • SbCs and SbNa$_2$KCs photocathodes (S10,S20) • electrostatic inversion • photosensivity up to 200 mA/lm	• 1970s • multialkali photocathodes (S25) • microchannel plate (MCP) • photosensivity up to 700 mA/lm • operational time to 4,000 h	• early 1980s • GaAs photocathodes • ion barrier to microchannel plate • photosensivity up to 700 mA/lm • operational time to 10,000 h	• late 1990s • multialkali photocathodes • "filmless" tube • photosensivity up to 1,800 mA/lm • operational time to 10,000 h

TABLE 6.3 (Continued)
Image Intensifier Tubes

Gen. No.	Cathode material	Photocathode sensitivity (µA/lm)	Design type	Luminance gain (lm/lm)	Resolution (lp/mm)	SNR
0	S1	< 60	Inverter tube	< 200	20–60	—
I	S20	< 160	Inverter tube	< 800	20–60	—
I+	S20	< 160	Cascade inverter tube	< 20,000	20–30	5–8
II	S25	< 350	Inverter MCP tube	< 50,000	24–43	12–17
II+	Improved S25	< 700	Proximity focus MCP tube	< 70,000	43–81	16–24
III	GaAs/GaAsP	< 1600	Proximity focus MCP tube with protecting film	< 70,000	36–64	18–25
III+ Thin film	GaAs/GaAsP	< 1800	Proximity focus MCP thin film tubes	< 70,000	57–71	24–28
III Filmless	GaAs/GaAsP	< 2200	Proximity focus MCP filmless tubes	< 80,000	57–71	24–31

Source: K. Chrzanowski, *Opto-Electron. Rev.* **21**, 153–182 (2013) [23].

Gen II. Gen II devices boasted amplifications of 20,000 and operational lives to 4,000 h. Interim improvements in bias voltage and construction methods produced the Gen II+ version. Substantial improvements in gain and bandwidth in the 1980s heralded the advent of Gen III. Gallium arsenide photocathodes and internal changes in the MCP design resulted in gains ranging from 30,000 to 50,000 and operating lives of 10,000 h.

Figure 6.16 shows the response of a typical Gen III image intensifier superimposed on the night sky radiation spectrum [24]. This figure also shows the CIE photopic curve illustrating the spectral response of the human visual perception system, and the Gen II response.

Image intensifiers were primarily developed for night-time viewing and surveillance under moonlight or starlight. At present, image intensifier applications have spread from night-time viewing to various fields, including industrial product inspection and scientific research, especially when used with CCD cameras – the so-called intensified CCD or ICCD [see Figure 6.17(a)]. Gate operation models are also useful for observation and motion analysis of high-speed phenomena (high-speed moving objects, fluorescence lifetime, bioluminescence and chemiluminescence images). Figure 6.17(b) shows an example of a Gen III night-vision goggle.

Image intensifiers are widespread in many military applications. The advent of night vision devices and helmet-mounted displays places additional constraints on the helmet, which is now an important element of the cockpit display system, providing weapon aiming and other information – such as aircraft attitude and status – to the pilot. For example, Figure 6.18 illustrates the TopOwl imaging system developed for airborne applications by Tales [25]. The helmet-mounted sight and display system incorporates a night vision system with a 100 per cent overlapped projection of a binocular image on the visor. TopOwl projects the night scene and associated symbology onto two circular reflective surfaces with a fully overlapped, 40°, binocular field of view (FOV). Standard symbology is used to display flight and weapon management data, helping to reduce crew workload.

6.7 SCHOTTKY BARRIER PHOTOEMISSIVE DETECTORS

In 1973, Shepherd and Yang of Rome Air Development Center proposed the concept of silicide Schottky-barrier detector focal plane arrays (FPAs) as much more reproducible alternative to

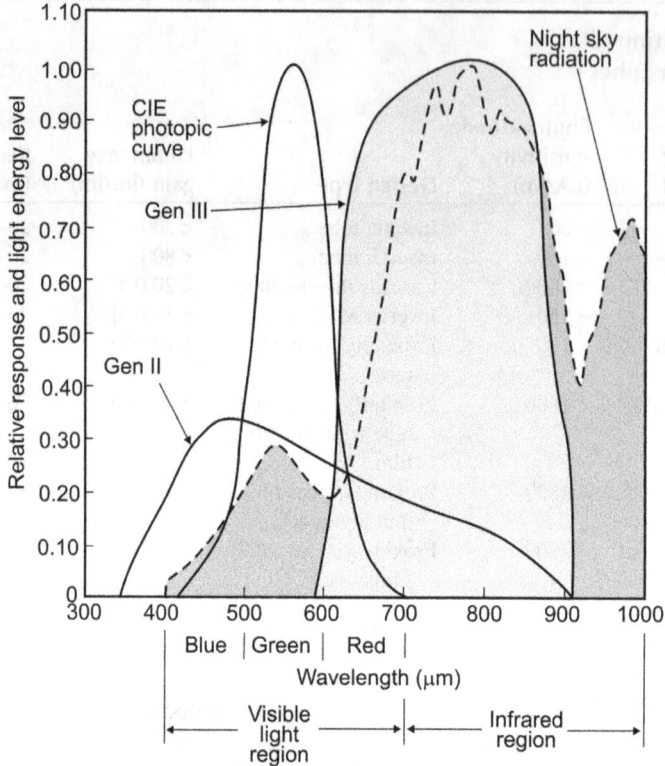

FIGURE 6.16 Image intensifier tube spectral response curves (after Reference 24).

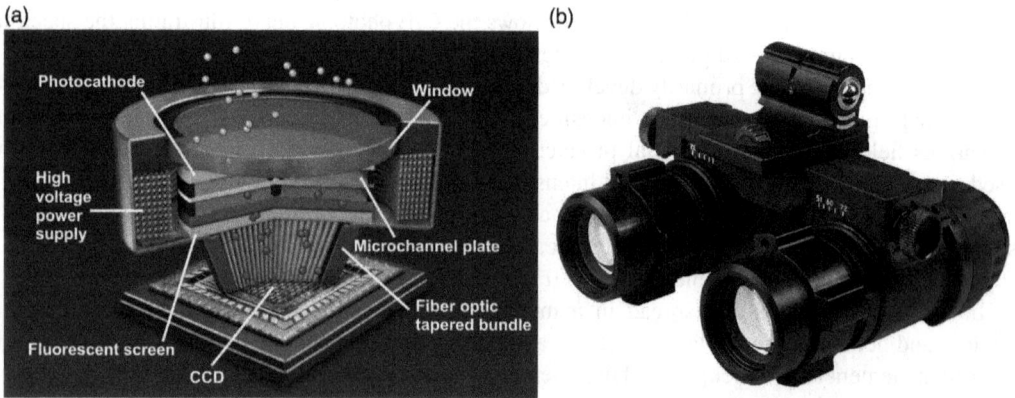

FIGURE 6.17 Night vision device: (a) proximity-focused image intensifier and (b) Gen III night vision goggles AN/AVS-9 (ITT Night Vision).

HgCdTe focal plane arrays (FPAs) for infrared thermal imaging [26]. For the first time it became possible to have much more sophisticated readout schemes – both detection and readout could be implemented in one common silicon chip. Since then, the development of the Schottky-barrier technology progressed continuously and currently offers large IR image sensor format. Such attributes as monolithic construction with standard large scale integration processing and uniformity in responsivity and signal to noise and absence of discernible $1/f$ noise make Schottky-barrier devices a formidable contender to the main-stream infrared systems and applications [27, 28].

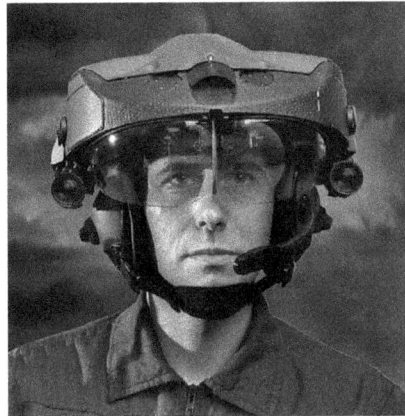

FIGURE 6.18 Tales TopOwl helmet incorporates an optical combiner assembly for each eye, allowing the pilot to view the cockpit and the outside world directly with the night imagery superimposed on it. TopOwl has a 40° FOV and a total head-borne weight of 2.2 kg in full configuration (after Reference 25).

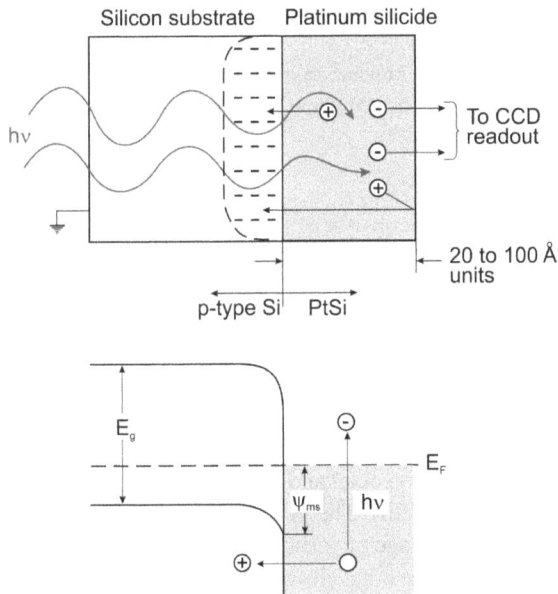

FIGURE 6.19 Operation of a PtSi/p-Si Schottky-barrier detector (after Reference 29).

The most popular Schottky-barrier detector is the PtSi detector, which can be used for the detection in the 3–5 μm spectral range (see Figure 4.63) [27]. Figure 6.19 shows the basic construction and operation of the PtSi detector integrated with a silicon CCD. It is typically operated in backside illumination mode. Radiation is transmitted through the p-type silicon and is absorbed in the metal PtSi (not in the semiconductor), producing hot holes which are then emitted over the potential barrier into the silicon, leaving the silicide charged negatively. The negative charge of silicide is transferred to a CCD by the direct-charge injection method.

The effective quantum efficiency in the 3–5 μm atmospheric window is very low, of the order of 1 per cent, but useful sensitivity is obtained by means of near full frame integration in area arrays. The quantum efficiency has been improved by thinning PtSi film. The thinning is effective down to the PtSi thickness of 2 nm. Another means of improving responsivity is implementation of an "optical

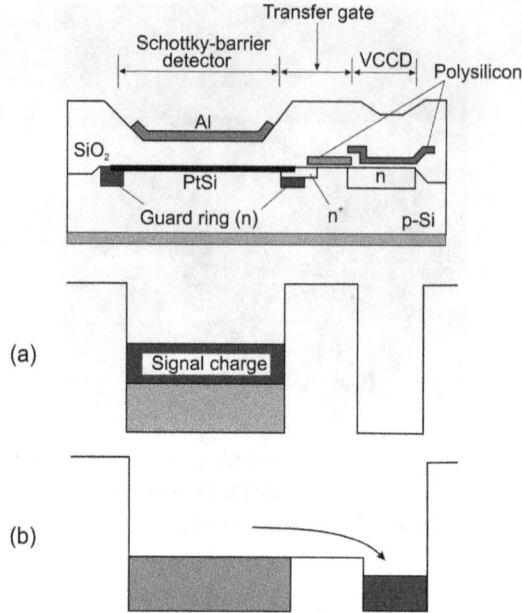

FIGURE 6.20 Typical construction and operation of PtSi Schottky-barrier IR FPA designed with interline transfer CCD readout architecture (a) and (b) show the potential diagrams in the integration and readout operations, respectively (after Reference 27).

cavity". The optical cavity structure consists of the metal reflector and the dielectric film between the reflector and metal electrode of the Schottky-barrier diode. The conventional 1/4 wavelength design for the optical cavity thickness is a good first approximation for optimising the responsivity.

Schottky photoemission is independent of such factors as semiconductor doping, minority carrier lifetime, and alloy composition, and, as a result of this, has spatial uniformity characteristics that are far superior to those of other detector technologies. Uniformity is only limited by the geometric definition of the detectors. Most of the reported Schottky-barrier FPAs have the interline transfer CCD architecture.

The typical cross-section view of the pixel and its operation in interline transfer CCD architecture is shown in the next figure (Figure 6.20). The pixel consists of a Schottky-barrier detector with an optical cavity, a transfer gate, and a stage of vertical CCD. The n-type guard ring on the periphery of the Schottky-barrier diode reduces the edge electric field and suppresses dark current. The effective detector area is determined by the inner edge of the guard ring. The transfer gate is an enhancement MOS transistor. The connection between detector and the transfer gate is made by an n^+ diffusion. A buried-channel CCD is used for the vertical transfer.

During the optical integration time the surface-channel transfer gate is biased into accumulation. The Schottky-barrier detector is isolated from the CCD register in this condition. The infrared radiation generates hot holes in the PtSi film and some of the excited hot holes are emitted into the silicon substrate leaving excess electrons in the PtSi electrode. This lowers the electrical potential of the PtSi electrode. At the end of the integration time, the transfer gate is pulsed-on to read out the signal electrons from the detector to the CCD register. At the same time, the electrical potential of the PtSi electrode is reset to the channel level of the transfer gate.

For improving the fill factor, a readout architecture called the charge sweep device (CSD) developed by Mitsubishi Corporation is also used. Kimata and co-workers [27, 28] have developed a series of IR image sensors with the CSD readout architecture with array sizes from 256×256 to 1040×1040 elements. The effectiveness of this readout architecture is enhanced, as the design rule becomes finer. Using a 1.2 μm CSD technology, a large fill factor of 71 per cent was achieved with a 26×20 μm^2 pixel in the 512×512 monolithic structure. The noise equivalent difference temperature (*NEDT*) was estimated as 0.033 K with f/1.2 optics at 300 K. The 1040×1040 element CSD FPA had the smallest pixel size (17×17 μm^2) among 2-dimensional IR FPAs. However, the performance of monolithic PtSi Schottky-barrier FPAs has reached a plateau, and a slow progress from now on is expected. Development of PtSi Schottky-barrier detectors was stopped in late 2010s. Both dark current and quantum efficiency have reached theoretical limits, and no further improvement is expected by refining the material and/or process technologies [30].

Various far infrared photoemissive detector approaches based on a high-low homojunctions have been discussed by Perera [31].

PROBLEMS

Example 6.1

A metal has a work function of 4.3 V. What is the minimum photon energy in Joule to emit an electron from this metal through the photoelectric effect? What is the photon frequency in the terahertz region and the photon wavelength in micrometres? What is the corresponding photon momentum? What is the velocity of a free electron with the same momentum?

Example 6.2

A photocathode (GaAsP) has a quantum efficiency of $\eta = 45$ per cent at $\lambda = 550$ nm. It receives a luminous power of 10^{-3} lumen from a 550-nm laser. What is the photocurrent generated by the photocathode?

Example 6.3

$N = 25 \times 10^9$ photons/s at $\lambda = 500$ nm fall on the photocathode surface. Calculate the current generated by the photocathode if the current sensitivity is 40 mA/W.

Example 6.4

A photocathode with a diameter of $\phi = 6$ mm and a responsivity of $R_i = 20$ mA/W was placed at the distance of 10 cm from the source with a temperature of $T_s = 6000$ K. The source area is $A_s = 2$ cm^2. Calculate the current obtained from the photocathode, assuming that radiation in the range of 200–300 nm reaches the surface of the photocathode.

Example 6.5

Calculate the photomultiplier gain if the collection efficiency of the first dynode $\eta_{d1} = 0.8$ and the gain of the i-th dynode is $g_i = 4$.

Example 6.6

For the data from Example 6.4 and a radiant flux of $\Phi_s = 1$ nW, calculate the output current I_{out} of the photomultiplier if the S20 photocathode is used, which for λ_m has a current sensitivity R_i of 70 mA/W and an efficiency of $\eta = 20$ per cent.

Example 6.7

For a dynode working with a gain $g = 5$, we wish to double the gain. Shall we double the voltage difference at which it works?

Example 6.8

A PMT is closed on an anode load $R = 10$ kΩ. What is the bandwidth we can expect for the PMT?

Example 6.9

A photomultiplier has six stages with dynode gains all equal to $g = 3.5$. If the single-electron response has a duration of $\Delta\tau = 3$ ns, what is the amplitude of the single electron response (SER) current pulse I_{SER}?

REFERENCES

1. J. Elster and H. Geitel, "Ueber die Entladung negativ electrischer Körper durch das Sonnen-und Tageslicht", *Ann. Physik* 38, 497 (1889).
2. L. Koller, "Photoelectric emission from thin films of caesium", *Phys. Rev.* 36, 1639–1647 (1930).
3. N.R. Campbell, "Photoelectric emission of thin films", *Phil. Mag.* 12, 173–185 (1931).
4. A.H. Sommer, *Photoemissive Materials: Preparation Properties and Uses*, Wiley, New York, 1968.
5. *Photomultiplier Tubes. Principles and Applications*, re-edited by S.-O. Flyckt and C. Marmonier, Photonics, Brive, 2002. www2.pv.infn.it/~debari/doc/Flyckt_Marmonier.pdf.
6. P.R. Norton, "Photodetectors", in *Handbook of Optics*, Vol. 1, 15.3–15.10, eds. M. Bass, E.W. Van Stryland, D.R. Williams, and W.L. Wolfe, McGraw Hill, New York, 1995.
7. P.N.J. Dennis, *Photodetectors*, Plenum Press, New York, 1986.
8. H.R. Zwieker, "Photoemissive detectors", in *Optical and Infrared Detectors*, pp. 149–228, edited by R.J. Keyes, Springer-Verlag, Berlin, 1977.
9. C. Ghosh, "Photoemissive materials", *Proc. SPIE* 62, 346 (1982).
10. *Characteristics of Photomultiplier Tubes*. Hamamatsu Handbook, chapter 4. www.hamamatsu.com/resources/pdf/etd/PMT_handbook_v3aE-Chapter4.pdf.
11. W.E. Spicer, "Photoemission and related properties of alkali antimonides", *J. Appl. Phys.* 31, 2077–2084 (1960).
12. R.L. Bell, *Negative Electron Affinity Devices*, Oxford University Press, Oxford, 1973.
13. R.L. Bell and W.E. Spicer, "3–5 compound photocathodes: A new family of photoemitters with greatly improved performance", *Proc. IEEE* 58, 1788–1802 (1970).
14. W.E. Spicer, "Negative affinity 3–5 photocathodes: Their physics and technology", *Appl. Phys.* 12, 115–130 (1977).

15. J.J. Scheer and J. Van Laar, "Fermi level stabilization at cesiated semiconductor surfaces", *Solid-State Commun.,* 5, 303–306 (1967).

16. B.F. Williams and R.E. Simon, "Direct measurement of hot electron-phonon interactions in GaP", *Phys. Rev. Lett.* 18, 485 (1967).

17. C.M. Thomas, "Photocathodes", *Proc. SPIE* 42, 71 (1973).

18. *Super-Kamiokande Official Website,* www-sk.icrr.u-tokyo.ac.jp/sk/index-e.html.

19. F. Yokozawa, "Technology trend on the photomultipliers", *JEE* 19, 94 (1982).

20. J. Wallance, "Photomultiplier tubes do what other photon counters can't", *Laser Focus World,* November 17, 2020, www.laserfocusworld.com/detectors-imaging/article/14185918/photomultiplier-tubes-do-what-other-photon-counters-cant.

21. J.L. Wiza, "Microchannel plate detectors", *Nucl. Instrum. Methods* 162, 587–601 (1979).

22. I.P. Csorba, *Image Tubes;* Howard Sams, Indianapolis, 1985.

23. K. Chrzanowski, "Review of night vision technology", *Opto-Electron. Rev.* 21, 153–182 (2013).

24. A.A. Cameron, "The development of the combiner eyepiece night vision goggle", *Proc. SPIE* 1290 16–19 (1990).

25. *TopOwl®. Designed by Pilots, for Pilots. Helmet Mounted Sight Display for Helicopters,* http://optronique.net/defense/wp-content/uploads/2012/07/TopOwl-Datasheet.pdf.

26. F.D. Shepherd and A.C. Yang, "Silicon Schottky retinas for infrared imaging", *Tech. Digest of IEDM,* 310–313 (1973).

27. M. Kimata and N. Tsubouchi, "Schottky barrier photoemissive detectors", in *Infrared Photon Detectors,* pp. 299–349, edited by A. Rogalski, SPIE Optical Engineering Press, Bellingham, WA, 1995.

28. M. Kimata, "Metal silicide Schottky infrared detector arrays", in *Infrared Detectors and Emitters: Materials and Devices,* pp. 77–98, edited by P. Capper and C.T. Elliott, Kluwer Academic Publishers: Boston, 2000.

29. W.F. Kosonocky, "Infrared image sensors with Schottky–barrier detectors", *Proc. SPIE* 869, 90–106 (1988).

30. M. Kimata, "My life in IRFPA R&D", *Proc. SPIE* 10177, 1017727-1-11 (2017).

31. A.G.U. Perera, "Homo- and heterojunction interfacial work function internal photo-emission detectors from UV to IR", in *Semiconductors and Semimetals,* Vol. 84, pp. 243–302, edited by S.D. Gunapala, D.R. Rhiger, and C. Jagadish, Elsevier, Amsterdam, 2011.

7 Photon Detectors

The operation of photon detectors is based on the photoeffect, in which the radiation is absorbed within the material by interaction directly with electrons, which are transited to a higher energy level. Under the effect of an electric field these carriers move and produce a measurable electric current. A general photon detector has basically three processes: carrier generation by incident radiation, carrier transport and/or multiplication by whatever current-gain mechanism may be present, and interaction of current with the external circuit to provide the output signal.

The photon detectors show a selective wavelength dependence of the response per unit incident radiation power. These detectors having long-wavelength limits above about 3 μm are generally cooled. This is necessary to prevent the thermal generation of charge carriers. The thermal transitions compete with the optical ones, making non-cooled devices very noisy.

7.1 INTRODUCTION

Developments in source and detection of electromagnetic radiation have a very long history. The first humans relied on the radiation from the Sun. Cave men used torches (approximately half a million years ago). Candles appeared around 1000 BC, followed by gas lighting (1772) and incandescent bulbs (Edison, 1897). Radio (1886–1895), X-rays (1895), UV radiation (1901), and radar (1936) were invented at the end of the nineteenth and the beginning of the twentieth centuries. The terahertz (THz) region of the electromagnetic spectrum (see Figure 7.1) is often described as the final unexplored area of spectrum and still presents a challenge for both electronic and photonic technologies.

Looking back over the past several hundreds of years we notice that following the invention and evolution of optical systems (telescopes, microscopes, eyeglasses, cameras, etc.), the optical image was formed on the human retina, photographic plate, or films. The birth of photodetectors can be dated back to 1873 when Smith discovered photoconductivity in selenium [1]. Progress was slow until 1905, when Einstein explained the newly observed photoelectric effect in metals, and Planck solved the blackbody emission puzzle by introducing the quanta hypothesis. Applications and new devices soon flourished, pushed by the dawning technology of vacuum tube sensors developed in the 1920s and 1930s, culminating in the advent of television. Zworykin and Morton, the celebrated fathers of videonics, concluded on the last page of their legendary book, *Television* (1940), that [2] "when rockets will fly to the moon and to other celestial bodies, the first images we will see of them will be those taken by camera tubes, which will open to mankind new horizons". Their foresight became a reality with the Apollo and Explorer missions. Beginning in the early 1960s, photolithography enabled the fabrication of silicon monolithic imaging focal planes for the visible spectrum. Some of these early developments were intended for a picturephone, other efforts were for television

DOI: 10.1201/9781003263098-7

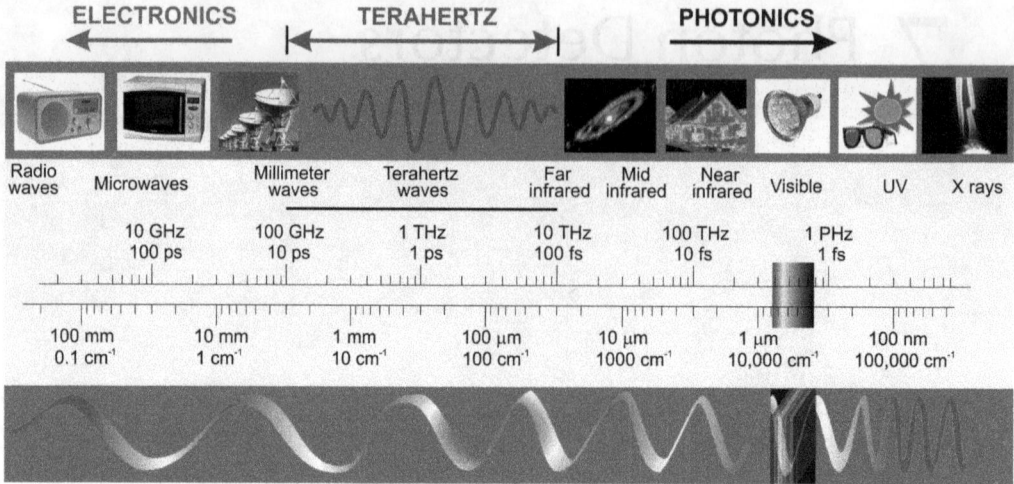

FIGURE 7.1 The electromagnetic spectrum.

cameras, satellite surveillance, and digital imaging. Infrared imaging has been vigorously pursed in parallel with visible imaging because of its utility in military applications. More recently (1997), the CCD camera aboard the Hubble space telescope delivered a deep-space picture, a result of ten days' integration, featuring galaxies of the 30th magnitude – an unimaginable figure even for astronomers of our generation. Probably, the next effort will be in the big-band age. Thus, photodetectors continue to open to mankind the most amazing new horizons.

This chapter is a guide for the photon detectors sensing optical radiation. Optical radiation is considered as a radiation over the range from vacuum ultraviolet to the far-infrared or submillimetre wavelength (25 nm to 1000 μm):

25–200 nm	vacuum ultraviolet	VUV
200–400 nm	ultraviolet	UV
400–700 nm	visible	VIS
700–1000 nm	near infrared	NIR
1–3 μm	short wavelength infrared	SWIR
3–5 μm	medium wavelength infrared	MWIR
5–14 μm	long wavelength infrared	LWIR
14–30 μm	very long wavelength infrared	VLWIR
30–100 μm	far infrared	FIR
100–3000 μm	submillimetre	SubMM

THz radiation is frequently treated as the spectral region within frequency range $\upsilon \approx 0.1\text{–}10$ THz ($\lambda \approx 3$ mm – 30 μm), and it is partly overlapping with the loosely treated submillimetre (sub-mm) wavelength band $\upsilon \approx 0.1\text{–}3$ THz ($\lambda \approx 3$ mm – 100 μm)

Both ultraviolet (UV) and visible, as well as infrared (IR) detectors technologies have undergone significant maturation, and high-performance detectors are available across most spectral bands from 0.2- to 100-μm. Significant improvements were possible for sensor systems by adding functionality, such as multi- and hyper-spectral responses, polarimetric sensitivity, dynamic resolution and sensitivity adaptation, as well as reductions in size, weight, power and cost. The increase in digital processing capabilities, fuelled by the semiconductor industry, is a trend that will continue to have a major effect on sensor systems.

Table 7.1 presents some physical properties of semiconducting families, including narrow-gap semiconductors used in fabrication of infrared photodetectors. All compounds have diamond (D) or

TABLE 7.1
Selected Properties of Common Families of Semiconductors Used in Fabrication of Photodetectors

	Si	Ge	GaN	GaAs	AlAs	InP	InGaAs	InAs	GaSb	AlSb	InSb	HgTe	CdTe
Group	IV	IV	III-V	III-V	III-V	III-V	III-V	III-V	III-V	III-V	III-V	II-VI	II-VI
Lattice constant (Å)/	5.431	5.658	3.189(a)/	5.653	5.661	5.870	5.870	6.058	6.096	6.136	6.479	6.453	6.476
structure	(D)	(D)	5.186(c)	(ZB)	(ZB)	(ZB)	(ZB)	(ZB)	(ZB)	(ZB)	(ZB)	(ZB)	(ZB)
			Wurtzite										
Bulk moduls (Gpa)	98	75	172	75	74	71	69	58	56	55	47	43	42
Bandgap (eV)	1.124	0.660	3.39	1.426	2.153	1.350	0.735	0.354	0.730	1.615	0.175	-0.141	1.475
	(id)	(id)		(d)	(id)	(d)	(d)	(d)	(d)	(id)	(d)	(d)	(d)
Electron effective mass	0.26	0.39	0.20	0.067	0.29	0.077	0.041	0.024	0.042	0.14	0.014	0.028	0.090
Hole effective mass	0.19	0.12	0.80(H)	0.082(L)	0.11(L)	0.12(L)	0.05(L)	0.025(L)	0.4	0.98	0.018(L)	0.40	0.66
				0.45(H)	0.40(H)	0.55(H)	0.60(H)	0.37(H)			0.4(H)		
Electron mobility (cm²/Vs)	1450	3900	1400	8500	294	5400	13800	3×10^4	5000	200	8×10^4	26500	1050
Hole mobility (cm²/Vs)	505	1900	300	400	105	180		500	880	420	800	320	104
Electron saturation velocity (10⁷ cm/s)	1.0	0.70	2.7	1.0	0.85	1.0		4.0			4.0		
Thermal cond. (W/cmK)	1.31	0.31	1.3	0.5		0.7		0.27	0.4	0.7	0.15		0.06
Relative dielectric constant	11.9	16.0	8.9	12.8	10.0	12.5		15.1	15.7	12.0	17.9	21	10.2

D – diamond, ZB – zincblende, id – indirect, d – direct, L – light hole, H – heavy hole.

zincblende (ZB) crystal structure apart from GaN – it has both ZB and wurtzite structures. Moving across the table from the left to the right, there is a trend in the change of chemical bonds, from the covalent group IV-semiconductors to more ionic II-VI semiconductors with increasing of the lattice constant. The chemical bonds become weaker, and the materials become softer, which is reflected by the values of the bulk. The materials with the larger contribution of covalent bound are more mechanically robust, which leads to better manufacturability. This is evidenced in the dominant position of silicon in electronic materials and GaAs in optoelectronics ones. On the other hand, the band-gap energy of semiconductors on the right side of the table tends to have smaller values. Due to their direct bandgap structure, strong band-to-band absorption leading to high-quantum efficiency is observed (e.g., in InSb and HgCdTe).

The properties of narrow-gap semiconductors that are used as the material systems for IR detectors result from the direct energy bandgap structure: a high density of states in the valence and conduction bands, which results in strong absorption of IR radiation and a relatively low rate of thermal generation. From the viewpoint of producibility, III-V materials offer much stronger chemical bonds and thus higher chemical stability compared to HgCdTe.

7.2   X-RAY AND γ-RAY DETECTORS

The first X-ray image was taken on December 22, 1895, by Wilhelm Röntgen. It was taken on a film, showing the finger bones and ring of his wife. X-ray imaging was established as the first medical imaging technique and has continuously evolved while new techniques such as magnetic resonance, positron emission tomography and ultrasound were introduced. Most applications of X rays are based on their ability to pass through matter. The more penetrating X-rays, known as hard X-rays, are of higher frequency and are thus more energetic, while the less penetrating X-rays, called soft X-rays, have lower energies. Photographs made with X-rays are known as radiographs. Radiography applied both in medicine and industry is valuable diagnostics and nondestructive testing of products. Also, derivative techniques collectively referred to as X-ray microscopy are also used in the quantitative analysis of many materials.

In the course of the past hundred years X-ray detection has migrated from film to digital cameras for dental and medical applications. Several classes of X-ray sensor arrays have been developed, including [3]

- phosphors;
- scintillators;
- microchannel plates;
- silicon detector arrays (CCD and CMOS devices, hybrid p-i-n structures, thin film silicon panels); and
- CdZnTe hybrid detector arrays.

Phosphors absorb X-ray photons and emit visible photons as a result of the returning to their ground state of the excited electrons in the material. Phosphors are generally used in a thin film layer of polycrystalline material and, hence, provide excellent spatial resolution, but they absorb X-rays relatively weakly. Usually, phosphors were combined with photographic films, but today they can be combined with a visible detector array to improve an X-ray detective system.

Also, scintillator crystals convert X-ray photons to visible light. To maximise the density of available electrons to interact with X-rays, large and optically transparent single crystals of high-atomic number materials are used. Examples include the alkali halide materials (NaI and CsI is doped with small amounts of Tl) and are more dense, with higher stopping power BGO ($Bi_4Ge_3O_{12}$) crystals [4]. The alkali halide are typically 5-mm thick to absorb incident energies from 20 to 100 keV with conversation efficiency (the fraction of X-ray energy converted to visible light) around 10 per cent. Scintillators are combined with a visible detector array.

MCP arrays are used in the UV and visible spectral regions as well as for X-rays. An X-ray-sensitive MCP is illustrated in Figure 7.2(a), which is used in the high-resolution camera on board the Advanced X-ray Astrophysics Facility (AXAF) satellite renamed Chandra after its 1999 launch. It is the most sophisticated X-ray observatory built to date. As we can see in the figure, two MCP stages amplify the electron stream, which is collected by a crossed grid of wires connected to charge-sensitive amplifiers. Each of two MCPs consist of a 10-cm square cluster of 69 million tiny lead-oxide glass tubes that are about 10 micrometres in diameter (1/8 the thickness of a human hair) and 1.2 millimetres long. Figure 7.2(b) shows another instrument installed in the Chandra satellite – the advanced CCD imaging spectrometer (ACIS) used for studying the temperature variation across X-ray sources, such as vast clouds of hot gas in intergalactic space.

The Auger cameras, named after their inventor since 1952, are generally used in nuclear medicine for gamma ray (γ–ray) imaging [6]. They have been used more than fifty years in improved versions. The basic design shown in Figure 7.3 consists of a large-area, continuous NaI(Tl) scintillator crystal coupled to an array of PMTs – generally with a light guide between the crystal and the PMTs. The original Auger's camera consisted of a NaI(Tl) crystal 0.25''-thick and 5'' in diameter,

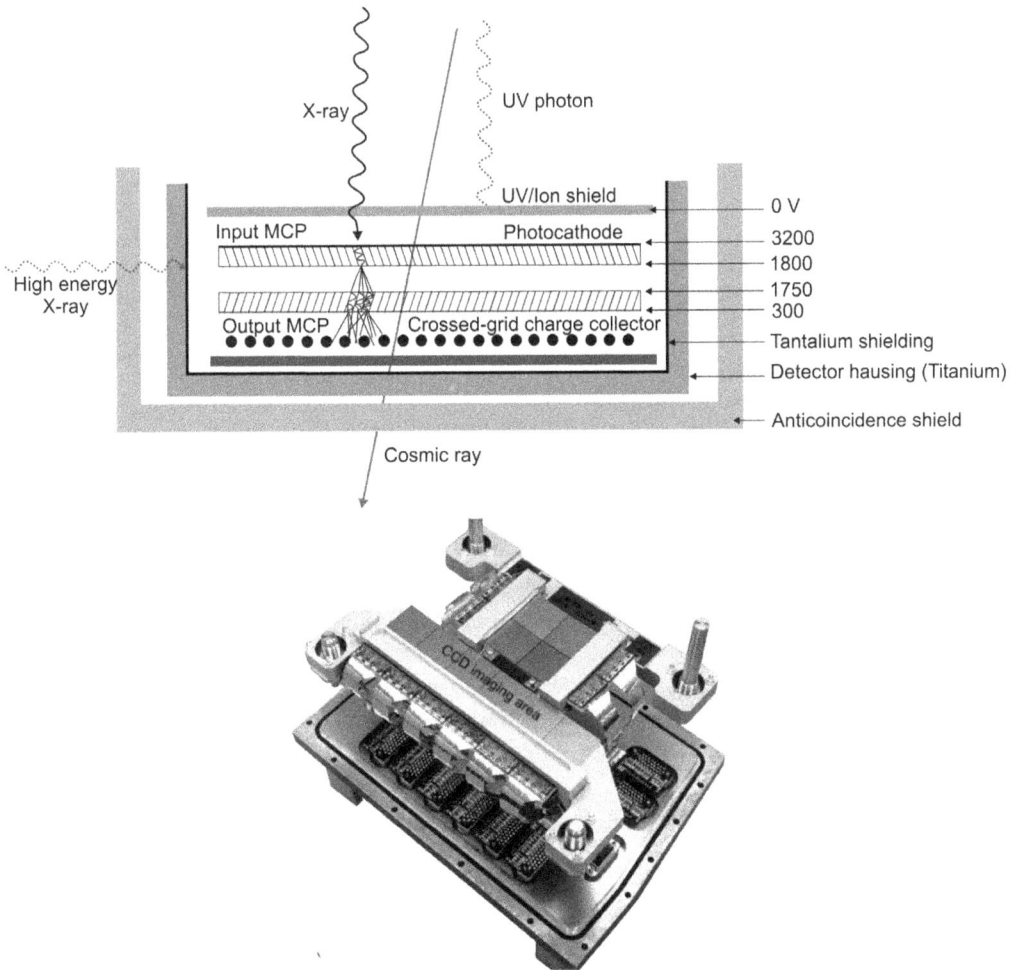

FIGURE 7.2 Science instruments on the Advanced X-ray Astrophysics Facility (AXAF) satellite renamed Chandra: (a) a diagram of MCP detector in the high-resolution camera (HRC) and (b) a diagram of the Chandra advanced CCD imaging spectrometer (ACIS) (after Reference 5).

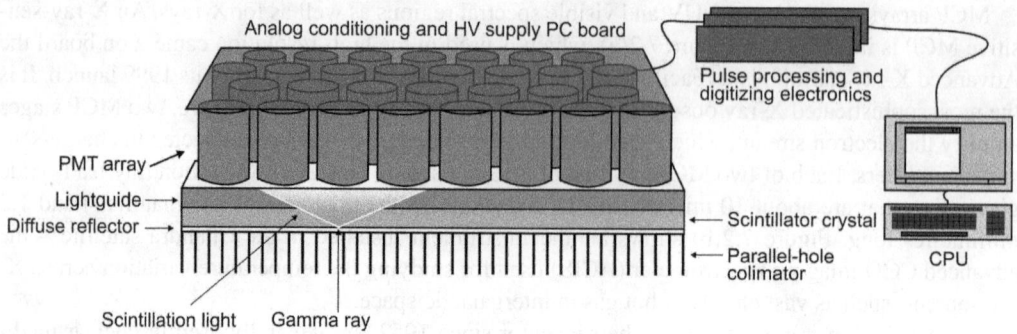

FIGURE 7.3   The basic structure of the Anger camera comprises a collimator, a monolithic scintillator crystal, a light guide that allows light to spread, and an array of photomultiplier tubes (PMTs) with related electronics. Position estimation was originally performed with analogue circuitry; in current systems PMT outputs are digitised and all processing is digital.

coupled to seven PMTs. Distribution of the energy deposited by a photon interaction is estimated by summing the signal amplitudes of all PMTs. The role of the PMTs is to measure the energy of each detected photon and the exact location of its interaction with the crystal material. The collimator consists of a thick sheet of lead (typically 1 to 3" thick), with thousands of adjacent hexagonal holes through it. A modern camera contains one large rectangular detector with an active surface of approximately 50×40 cm and a thickness of 0.9 cm [7]. Behind the crystal is an array of 50–90 PMTs, the associated electronics, and analogue-to-digital converters. Currently, the cameras used are optimised for photons in the 70–400 keV energy range and have relative energy resolution of approximately 9 per cent. Their important limitations are small spatial resolution of the order of 4 mm and small efficiency in photon counting – about 10^{-4}.

There are two primary X-ray imaging technologies in use today: direct and indirect detections. Their schematic designs are shown in Figure 7.4(a). The most common method, indirect detection, uses scintillators to convert X-rays to visible light. CCD devices were the first detectors introduced in radiology approximately forty years ago. CCDs are traditionally physically much smaller than the image area, so the light generated by the scintillator is imaged onto a CCD sensor using a bulky lens system which is some kind of optics reducing the size of the image. However, this optical system reduces the number of photons that reach the CCD and, moreover, geometric distortions and light scatter are other consequences of the use of optical reduction. As a result, the CCD-based indirect X-ray detectors are bulky and not flat-panel detectors, which is their most prominent inconvenience. This drawback of CCD-based indirect system is successively omitted due to development of large-format CCDs.

In indirect conversion thin-film transistor (TFT)-based detectors, X-ray photons are converted into visible light in the scintillator layer. A photodiode converts the visible light into electrical charges, which the TET array reads out row after row.

One potential inconvenience of transforming X-rays into visible light is that lateral diffusion of the light [see Figure 7.4(d)] reduces sharpness and spatial resolution of the image. To overcome this problem, some indirect conversion detectors use structured scintillators, consisting of CsI crystals that are grown perpendicularly to the detector surface with diameters of approximately 5–10 μm. A column-like structure significantly reduces lateral diffusion of the scintillator light, much like fibre optics. The reduction of light diffusion in turn allows the use of thicker scintillator layers, thus increasing the detective quantum efficiency of the detector system.

Direct conversion is used in flat-panel detectors and in recently developed hybrid arrays with CMOS readout. Flat-panel detectors usually use an amorphous selenium (a-Se) layer to convert

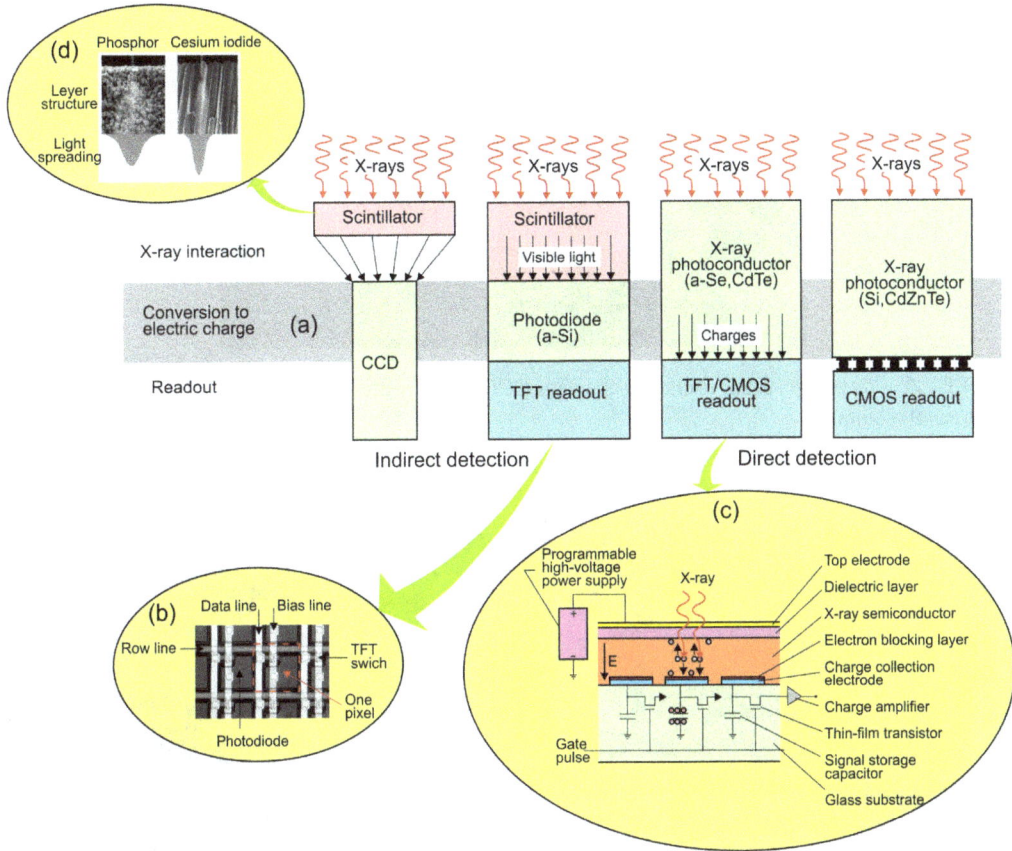

FIGURE 7.4 Direct and indirect X-ray detection: (a) different types of X-ray image systems, (b) pixel structure of indirect conversion imager, (c) operative design of direct conversion detector used in flat-panel imagers, and (d) light diffusion in phosphor and CsI.

X-ray photons directly to electrons for immediate image capture. The generated charge migrates to the pixel electrode in accordance with the polarity of the bias being applied to the X-ray photodetector and is stored in a storage capacitor within the TFT array [see Figure 7.4(c)]. By subsequently scanning the TFTs line by line, the charge information stored in the storage capacitors can be read out from the data bus lines. The data bus line terminations connect to charge amplifiers and A/D converters, and the scanned charge information is converted to digital image signals and output sequentially.

Selenium has relatively low X-ray absorption and requires about fifty electronvolts to produce a hole-electron pair. These restrict both the minimum dose needed and the size of the signal generated. In addition, an important drawback of selenium is the instability of the material over time and at elevated temperatures, as well as the environmental impact during production and repair or disposal. Other materials with lower energy requirements and higher x-ray absorption are under development.

Photolithographic techniques enable fabrication of large arrays with small pixels, which results in achieving high spatial resolution. Between different silicon detector arrays in the X-ray region the most important are CCD and CMOS devices. Many manufactures offer indirect detectors working with different scintillators and coupling fibre optics to CCD and CMOS imagers. Large, buttable CMOS tiles are assembled into panels of more than 30×24 cm in size, with less than one pixel

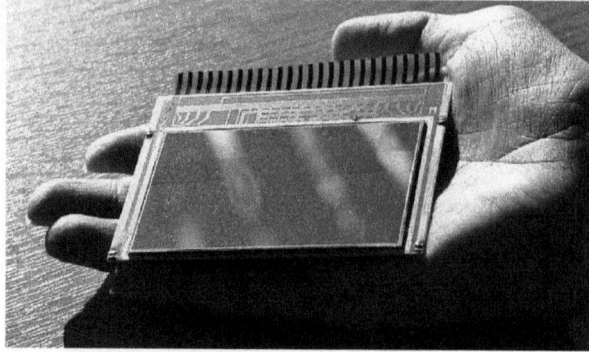

FIGURE 7.5 Very high spatial resolution Siemens CCD X-ray matrix with 4k×4k pixels, pixel size 12 μm, total area 49×86 mm.

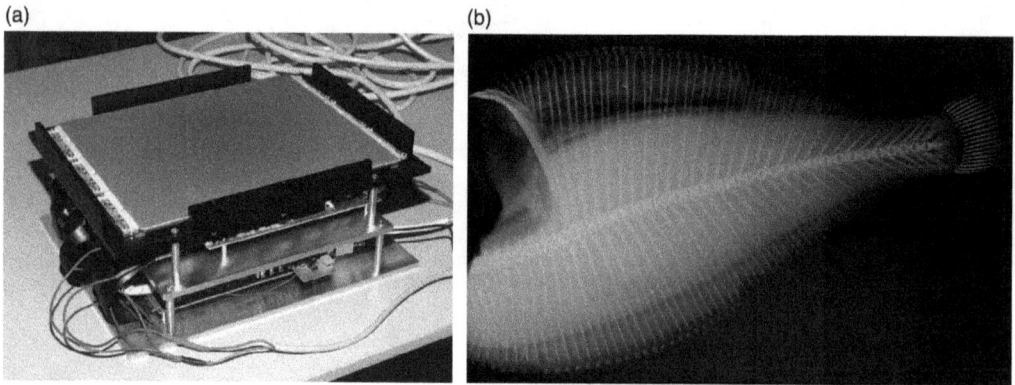

FIGURE 7.6 3-side buttable CMOS APS Dalsa mammography image sensor with the final 232×290 mm detector comprises 2×3 butted CMOS tiles with 33.55×33.55 μm pixel pitch, total 60 megapixels: (a) sensor assembly with a fibre optic plate + scintillator, and (b) "first patient result" obtained on a total detector.

spacing between individual sensors. For example, the next two figures (Figures 7.5 and 7.6) show large CCD and CMOS arrays fabricated by Siemens and Teledyne Dalsa [9].

CCD detectors are susceptible to radiation damage and failure when operated for extended periods in space environments. The main reason for that is CCD surface inversion from accumulated surface charge build-up. The advantages of CMOS in comparison to CCD include programmable readout modes, faster readout, lower power, radiation hardness, and the ability to put specialised processing within each pixel.

CMOS imagers are growing in popularity for many small-area imaging applications. These include medical imaging in the fields of dental, extremities imaging, and veterinary and industrial X-ray applications. The main advantage of CMOS imagers over a-Si flat-panel imagers is higher readout speed. The electron mobility in crystalline silicon is about 1400 cm^2/Vs, while it is less than 1 cm^2/Vs in amorphous silicon, which limits readout speed of imaging pixels. For comparison a 2000×3000 pixel a-Si based array can be read out about three times in a second, while the same size CMOS array can be read out about thirty times [10]. The ten times faster speed is especially useful for the high-resolution computer tomography (CT). The second advantage of CMOS imagers is their low noise, especially in comparison with large flat-panel detectors. CMOS circuitry eliminates

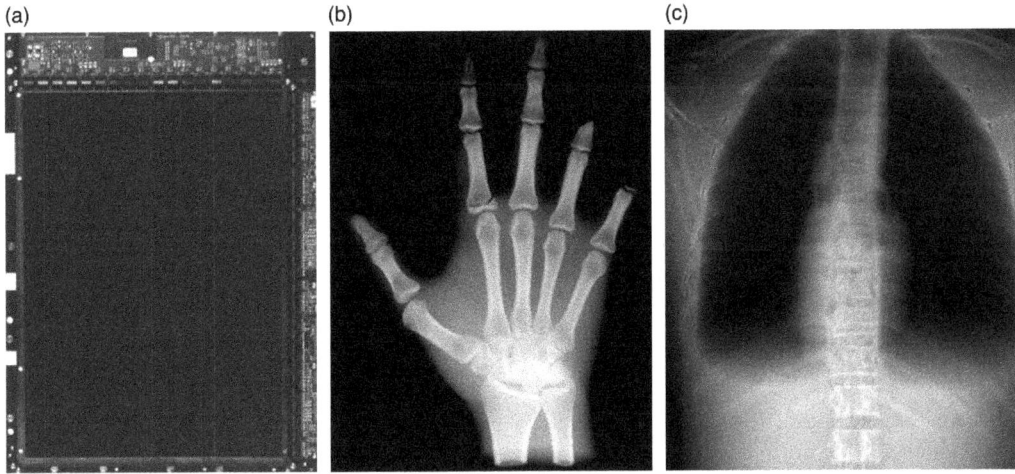

FIGURE 7.7 High-resolution a-Si X-ray medical image sensor: (a) a view of 2304×3200 pixel array module with a 30×40 cm active area (127-μm pixel size, fill factor 57%) connected to gate and data boards bonded to the glass, which is mounted on an aluminium backing plate, (b) a digital X-ray image of a human hand phantom, and (c) a digital X-ray image of a human chest phantom (after Reference 12).

the influence of noise because each pixel contains an active circuit. This low noise provides a huge advantage at low X-ray dose imaging, such as low dose CT application.

Thin-film silicon panels are usually used for medical imaging when a very large area and high-resolution arrays are needed. Usually, as an active material the thin-film of amorphous silicon is deposited on a substrate using the chemical vapour deposition (CVD) method. Each pixel of the array, photolithographically processed, consists of a photodiode and an addressable switch to read out the photocurrent [see Figure 7.4(a,b)].

In modern flat-panel detectors, the scintillator output is captured by either an amorphous silicon TFT panel or a CMOS sensor that converts the image to digital format. For example, this second solution is used by Dexela. The Dexela CMOS image sensor consists of a photodiode array with a pixel size of 75-μm. The detector is capable of multi-resolution readout with pixels binned 1×2, 2×2, 1×4, 2×4 and 4×4. A highly modular technology platform allows produce detectors of different dimensions with sizes up to 35×29 cm [11].

To convert incident X-rays to visible light, a scintillating material such as Gd_2O_2S:Tb is deposited in proximity over the amorphous silicon array [12]. Figure 7.7 shows X-ray images taken with this panel. Typical X-ray sensitivity converts the 40- to 150-keV range.

Unfortunately, the X-ray absorption of a-Si is very low, so the photodiode needs to be 10 to 20 mm thick. Fabricating such devices of amorphous silicon is not feasible. Photoconductive materials with higher X-ray absorption than silicon can be coated on an array of conductive charge collection plates, each supplied with a storage capacitor.

Crystalline silicon is an excellent material for direct detection of photons from soft X-ray to the silicon cut-off wavelength in the near infrared (NIR). Due to different absorption mechanisms (see Figure 7.8), 5–10 keV X-rays and 850–1000 nm NIR light have a long absorption length in silicon (20–200 μm); while low-energy X-rays and UV light are absorbed within 10 to 40 nm of the silicon surface. So, a low-loss surface region is required to provide a good response to low energy X-ray photons (< 500 eV).

It appears that hybrid structures with readouts compatible with silicon p-i-n diodes can be hardened to very high radiation doses, and the p-i-n devices itself is also quite resistant to radiation damage [3]. Figure 7.9(a) shows silicon p-i-n diodes fabricated in a lightly doped silicon wafer with

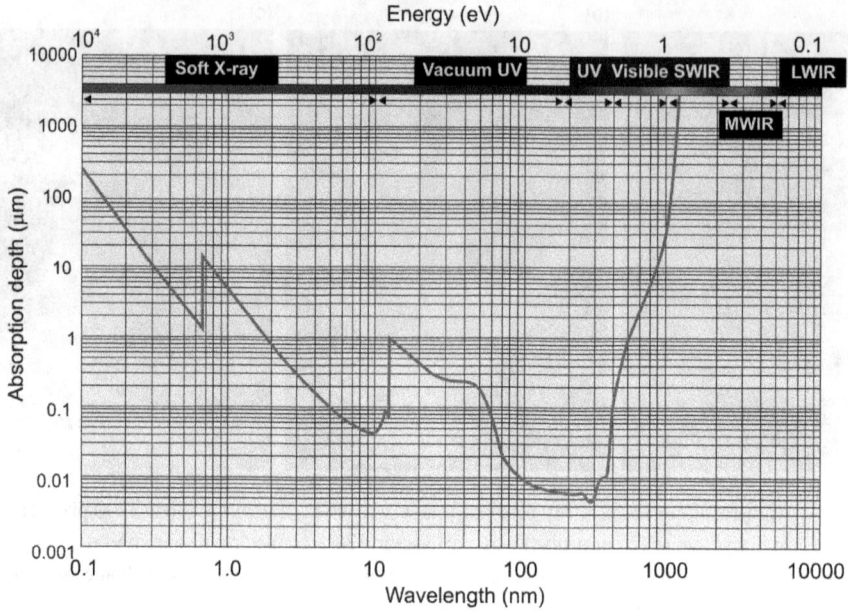

FIGURE 7.8 Absorption depth of photons in silicon as a function of the wavelengths and energy from UV to NIR.

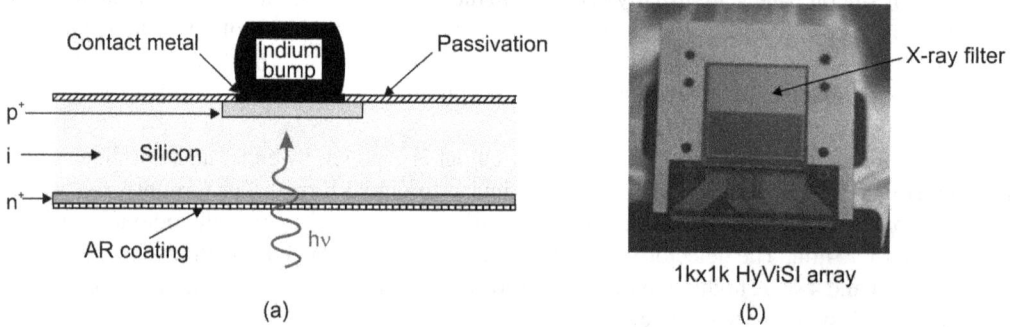

FIGURE 7.9 Hybrid silicon p-i-n photodiode X-ray arrays: (a) cross-section of p-i-n photodiode, and (b) photo of a 1024×1024 pixel HyViSI array with 50-nm Al blocking filter covering half of the active area of the detector surface (after Reference 13).

a common back electrode and an array of the opposite doping type on the front side. Metal contacts are made to the front-side p+-doped regions. These devices give relatively good energy resolution since the total thickness of i-region is fully depleted, and all the absorbed charge in the active region is efficiently collected.

Teledyne Imaging Sensors have produced large-array hybrid silicon p-i-n CMOS sensors with > 99.9 per cent operability, called HyViSI, which provide high quantum efficiency for the X-ray through NIR spectral range. The thickness of detectors is between 50 to 250 μm. For X-ray astronomy applications, a 50-nm thick Al optical blocking filter with nearly 100 per cent transmission of X-rays is typically used to decrease the influence of optical light on a noise level. Figure 7.9(b) shows a 1024×1024 18-μm pixel array with a 50-nm thick Al blocking filter covering half of the active area of the detector surface.

A wide range of detectors are currently in use at imaging facilities, and the overwhelming majority of these are semiconductor detectors. Semiconductor detectors can provide an outstanding combination of high speed, spatial resolution, and sensitivity, as compared to other types of detectors such as image plates.

The most popular semiconductor detectors are germanium and silicon doped lithium [Ge(Li) and Si(Li)], CdTe and HgI_2. Despite the excellent energy resolution and charge-transport properties of Si and Ge detectors, their low stopping power for high-energy photons limits their application to hard X-ray and gamma-ray detection. Improvements in crystal growth and device processing are keys to developing "high-Z" (high atomic number) semiconductors for hard X-ray detection. Germanium is the most mature high-Z semiconductor and is widely used in X-ray detectors, but it has the drawback of needing to be cooled during operation. Compound semiconductors with wide bandgaps can be used at room temperature, but crystal defects can degrade their performance.

Room-temperature semiconductors with high atomic numbers and wide bandgaps have long been under development. The great potential of these compounds has not been exploited for many decades due mainly to the limited commercial availability of high-quality crystals [14–16]. This situation changed dramatically during the last decade of the twentieth century with the emergence of a few companies committed to the advancement and commercialisation of these materials [17]. Table 7.2 reports the physical properties of the most common compound semiconductors typically used for radiation detection.

Over the last two decades, cadmium telluride (CdTe) and cadmium zinc telluride (CdZnTe) wide-bandgap semiconductors have become established as perhaps the most suitable materials for the detection of X-rays and gamma-rays. Discrete detectors and arrays fabricated from $Cd_{1-x}Zn_xTe$ (where x = 0.08–0.3) are becoming more widely used to detect nuclear radiation in medicine, industry and scientific research. Although NaI(Tl) scintillators do not require cooling, they suffer from low resolution compared to CdZnTe, and are bulky. NaI(Tl) relies on secondary detection; photons hit the scintillator, producing light, which is in turn detected by visible detector array. In contrast, photons reaching the CdZnTe detector are directly converted into an electrical signal, which is then amplified by standard electronic circuitry. The relatively high density (5.78 g/cm^3) of CdZnTe provides good absorption efficiency. As shown in Figure 7.10 [18], CdTe has a high photoelectric attenuation coefficient. Photoelectric absorption is the main process up to 300 keV for CdTe, as compared to 60 keV for Si and 150 keV for Ge. The higher resistivity of CdZnTe (around 3×10^{10} Ωcm)

TABLE 7.2
Properties of Semiconductors at Room Temperature (after Reference 16).

Material	Si	Ge	GaAs	CdTe	$Cd_{0.9}Zn_{0.1}Te$	HgI_2	TlBr
Crystal structure	Cubic	Cubic	Cubic(ZnS)	Cubic(ZnS)	Cubic(ZnS)	Tetragonal	Cubic(CsCl)
Growth method*	C	C	CVD	THM	HPB, THM	VAM	BM
Atomic number	14	32	31, 33	48, 52	48, 30, 52	80, 53	81, 35
Density (g/cm^3)	2.33	5.33	5.32	6.20	5.78	6.4	7.56
Bandgap (eV)	1.12	0.67	1.43	1.44	1.57	2.13	2.68
Pair creation energy (eV)	3.62	2.96	4.2	4.43	4.6	4.2	6.5
Resistivity	10^4	50	10^7	10^9	10^{10}	10^{13}	10^{12}
$\mu_e\tau_e$ (cm^2/V)	>1	>1	10^{-5}	10^{-3}	10^{-3}–10^{-2}	10^{-4}	10^{-5}
$\mu_h\tau_h$ (cm^2/V)	~1	>1	10^{-6}	10^{-4}	10^{-5}	10^{-5}	10^{-6}

*The more common growth methods: C = Czochralski, CVD = chemical vapor deposition, THM = travelling heater method, BM = Bridgman method, HPB = high-pressure Bridgman, and VAM = vertical ampoule method.

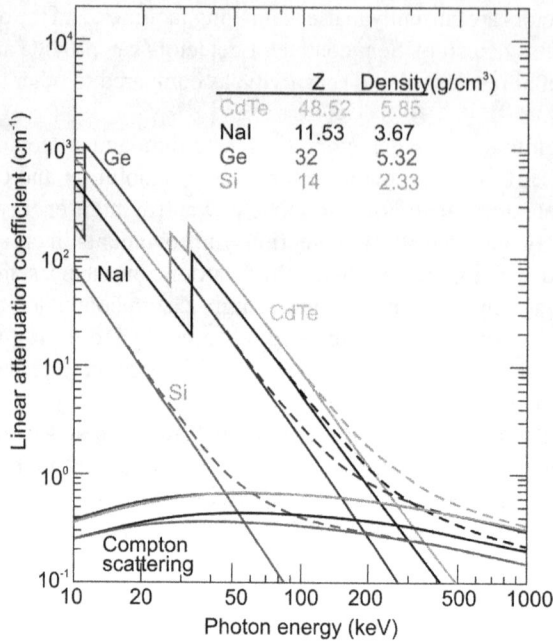

FIGURE 7.10   Linear attenuation coefficients for photoabsorption and Compton scattering in CdTe, Si, Ge, and NaI(Tl) (after Reference 18).

results in low leakage currents in photovoltaic devices (MSM devices and p-n junctions), and also allows the use of higher bias voltage. In turn, this improves the charge-collection efficiency and allows the fabrication of large-volume detectors.

The current developments in large-area/volume CdZnTe detectors and the common constraints on their design are summarised in References 14–17. The CdZnTe crystals used in the fabrication of hybrid focal plane arrays are grown using modified standard or vertical furnaces by the high pressure of inert gas inside the crucible. Generally, compound semiconductors are characterised by poor charge transport properties due to charge trapping – the hole and electron mobility life-time products ($\mu_e \tau_e$ and $\mu_h \tau_h$) are key parameters in the development of radiation detectors (see Table 7.2). However, the relatively high mobility and lifetime of the charge carriers in CdZnTe crystals, particularly those of electrons, allows the transport of the carriers through the whole depleted volume of mm- and cm-thick devices with minimum trapping loss.

An example of a CdZnTe X-ray detector structure is shown in Figure 7.11 [3]. This radiation-imaging digital technology combines a dedicated direct conversion detector substrate connected via micro bumps to a dedicated CMOS readout substrate. As an active material, lightly doped, high-resistivity material is used. To solve the problem of forming ohmic contacts to CdZnTe wide-bandgap material, the narrower-band-gap, both p- and n-type HgCdTe epitaxial layers, are used.

Different pixel sizes are used in hybrid CdZnTe/CMOS imaging sensors. For high spatial-image resolution the pixel size is typically 50 μm – see Figure 7.12(a) [19]. Such arrays can yield very high quality digital X-ray images of small objects. In Ajat solution [see Figure 7.12(b)], many hundreds of megabytes of image information at a high frame rate (up to 300 images per second) is reconstructed to the panoramic layer by intensive post acquisition computing like a computed tomography [20].

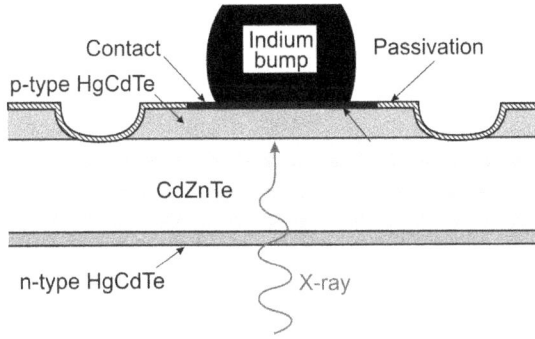

FIGURE 7.11 CdZnTe X-ray detector structure.

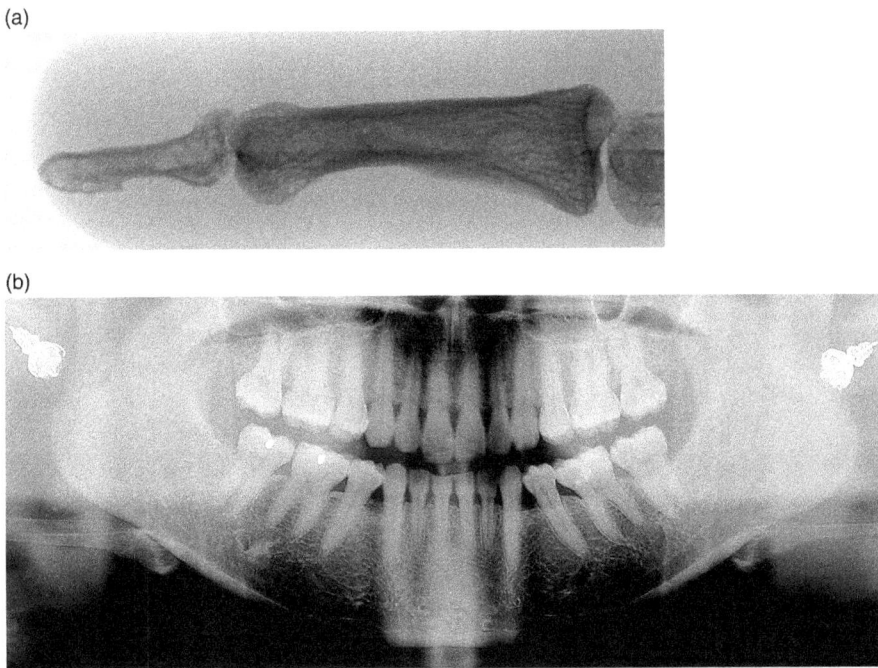

FIGURE 7.12 Digital CdZnTe/CMOS X-ray images: (a) of a human finger phantom taken with a CdZnTe array (192×340 pixels with 50-μm size and 0.15-mm thick CdZnTe detector) and (b) dental panoramic image.

7.3 ULTRAVIOLET DETECTORS

Ultraviolet (UV) detection technology is classified into two major categories. In the first group, a photoemissive device (photocathode) is combined with a gain component, usually with microchannel plate (MCP) [21–23]. The second group consists of solid-state devices based on silicon (CCD and CMOS) or hybrid structure wide bandgap semiconductor-based detectors such as AlGaN and SiC. Table 7.3 provides physical properties of important semiconductors used in fabrication of UV photodetectors.

Ternary AlGaN alloys are excellent photocathode materials due to their low electron affinity, chemical stability and direct bandgap. The quantum efficiency of planar cesiated p-type opaque

TABLE 7.3

Physical Properties of Semiconductors Used in Manufacture of UV Photodetectors

Parameters	Si	Diamond	4H-SiC	6H-SiC	GaN	AlN	ZnO	MgO	TiO$_2$	ZnSe
Energy gap (eV)	1.12	5.5	3.2	2.86	3.4	6.2	3.37	7.83	3.2 Anatase	2.82
Thermal conductivity (W/cmK)	1.5	20	3.7	4.9	1.3	3.19	5.4	4.82	1.17	0.18
Melting point (K)	1683	3773	>2800	>2800	>2500	>2400	2242	3073	1570	1100
Electron saturation velocity (10^5 m/s)	1	2.7	2	2	2.5	1.4				
Electron mobility (cm^2/Vs)	1400	2200	950	400	1000	135	170	10	10 Anatase	
Hole mobility (cm^2/Vs)	600	1600	120	75	30	14		2		
Dielectric constant	11.8	5.5	9.7	9.7	8.9	8.1	9.1	9.8	3.2 Anatase	
Breakdown field (10^5 V/cm)	3	100	20	24	26	20				

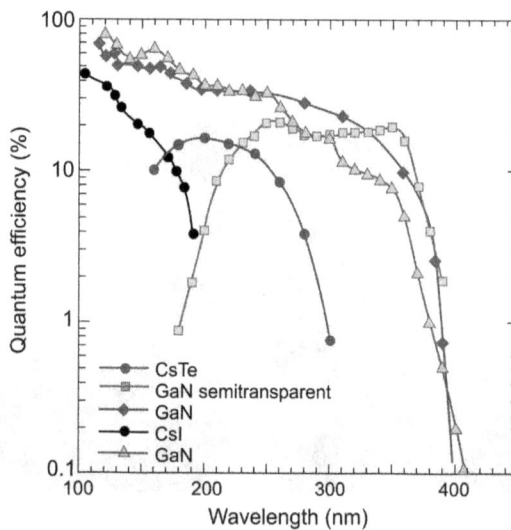

FIGURE 7.13 Quantum efficiencies as a function of wavelength for several photocathodes.

photocathodes reach 70–80 per cent at 122 nm and steadily decline to 10–20 per cent near 360 nm, which represents significant improvements over conventional CsI and CsTe photocathodes – see Figure 7.13 [24]. Cesiated photocathodes are limited to windowed detectors with wavelengths > 105 nm and require sealed tubes to retain the Cs.

Improvements of MCP devices have been made in spatial resolution, dynamic range, detector size, quantum efficiency and background together with decreasing the power and mass required to achieve these goals. Especially, there are significant challenges in the implementation of detectors on astrophysics instruments. For example, the Cosmic Origins Spectrograph (COS) installed on the Hubble Space Telescope (HST) in May 2009 contains two segments of far-UV MCP detector, each 85×10 mm active area, separated by 9 mm, and curved to a focal plane of 0.6 m radius for the Rowland circle [see Figure 7.14(a)]. The COS detector has a spatial resolution of ~25 μm with

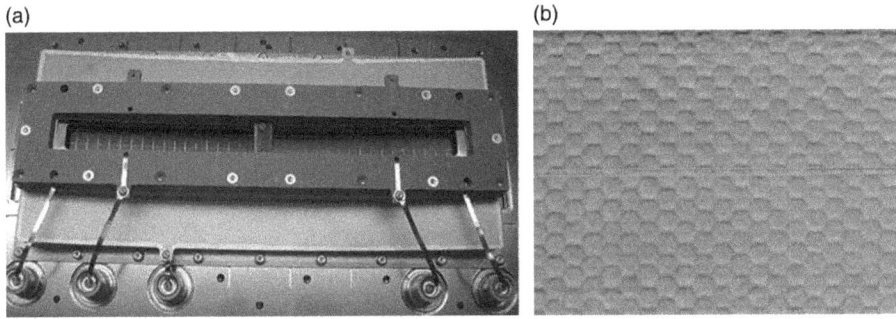

FIGURE 7.14 COS-HST detector: (a) head of detector with two abutting MCP detector segments (each 85×10 mm) curved to the focal plane of the spectrograph (after Reference 23); (b) flat field image of a 10×13 mm area of the MCP detector; the fibre bundles imprint an obvious fixed-pattern noise features in the image (after Reference 24).

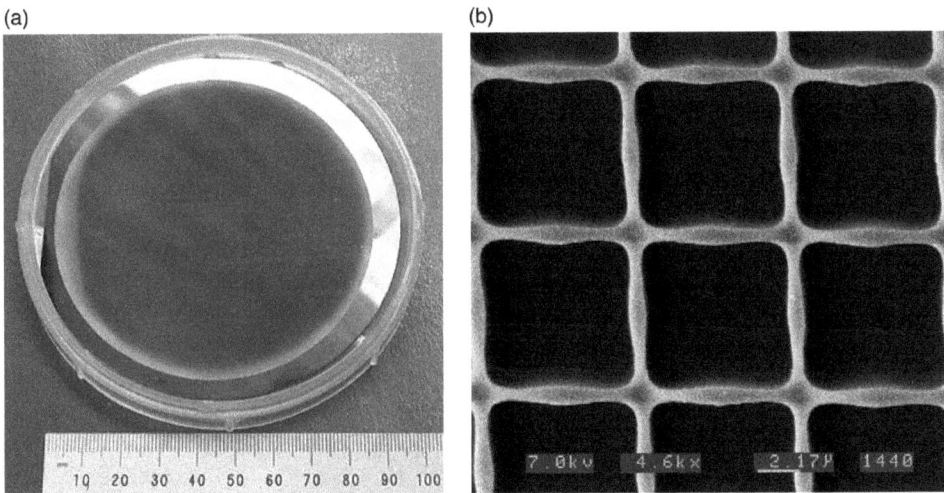

FIGURE 7.15 Silicon MCP detector: (a) produced on 10-cm wafer, and (b) square pore 7-μm pores (after Reference 21).

electronic sub-resolution sampling using a cross-delay line readout anode. Encouraging progress has been made on reduction of fixed-pattern noise introduced at the "dead zones" at the boundaries of the MCP fibre bundles [see Figure 7.14(b)].

With the emergence of photolithographic silicon-based microchannel plates and large-format high-resolution position sensing readouts, considerable progress has been made towards the next generation of microchannel plate detectors. Silicon-based MCPs have qualities that make them preferable to glass MCPs (very low intrinsic background, low fixed-pattern noise). Fabrication has been scaled to 6" wafers (Figure 7.15), so larger MCPs are possible.

Ultraviolet (UV) solid-state imagers are most commonly built with a hybrid structure. An example is $Al_xGa_{1-x}N$ (AlGaN) material sensitive to UV radiation while being insensitive to longer wavelength radiation [25–29]. Such devices have applications where there is a need to detect or control the source of UV radiation in an existing background of visible or infrared radiation. Examples of such applications include flame detection, furnace and engine monitoring for the automotive, aerospace and petroleum industry, undersea communications, UV astronomy, space-to-space communications secure from Earth, early missile threat warning and airborne UV countermeasures

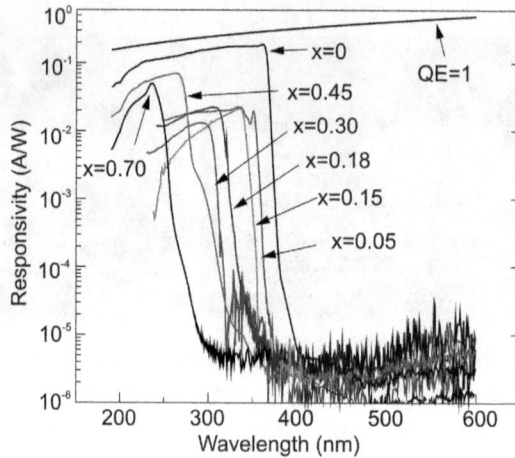

FIGURE 7.16 Responsivity of $Al_xGa_{1-x}N$ p-i-n photodiodes showing a cut-off wavelength continuously tuneable from 227 to 365 nm, corresponding to an Al concentration in the range 0–70 per cent (after Reference 27).

and portable battlefield reagent/chemical analysis systems. Because of their theoretical intrinsic solar blindness and low dark currents, III-Nitride based devices are expected to work without optical filters and complex electronics, thus significantly reducing the launch weight for space and airborne applications. The goal of this development is to achieve "solar blind" spectral response of 280 nm because ozone in the atmosphere absorbs nearly all sunlight shorter than this wavelength.

There are different types of AlGaN detectors, including photoconductors, MSM diodes, Schottky barrier and p-i-n photodiodes. Most of the research on UV photodetectors has been directed toward the demonstration of AlGaN based p-i-n junction photodiodes, which present the capability of tailoring the cut-off wavelength by controlling the alloy composition and thus the bandgap energy of the active layer. A full range of $Al_xGa_{1-x}N$ p-i-n photodiodes has been demonstrated with a cut-off wavelength continuously tuneable from 227 to 365 nm, corresponding to an Al concentration in the range 0–70 per cent. This can be seen in Figure 7.16, where the current responsivity of these detectors at room temperature is shown. Their internal quantum efficiencies were up to 86 per cent when operated in photovoltaic mode (i.e., at zero bias) and they exhibited a UV-to-visible rejection ratio as high as six orders of magnitude. At shorter wavelengths, the penetration depth decreases, and the detection of charge carriers is reduced by processes such as surface recombination and photo-emission losses. In addition to these front-side illuminated devices, backside illuminated AlGaN UV photodiodes have also recently been reported using sapphire substrates, which are UV transparent. Sapphire has only a moderate thermal coefficient of expansion mismatch with silicon readouts.

Hybrid AlGaN FPAs have been produced by several groups, for example, with 256×256 pixels [30–32] and 320×256 pixels [33–36]. These devices employ deposition of the array structure on a transparent substrate and illumination from the back side (back-illumination) through the substrate. However, for shorter wavelengths than the transmission cut-off of the substrate material, for example, in the vacuum UV (VUV) front-side illumination of the device is required. Further, in the extreme UV (EUV) below $\approx$ 30 nm, the back-side illumination is again possible with a device that is back-side thinned (e.g., removing the Si substrate [37]; sapphire absorbs the low wavelengths below approximately 170 nm) making it transparent to the EUV and X-ray radiation ranges.

Figure 7.17(a) shows a cross-section of the back-illuminated AlGaN p-i-n photodiodes [30]. The first Si-doped n-type AlGaN window bottom layer serves as the common n-side contact to all elements in the array. Its alloy composition determines the cut-on wavelength. Next, the absorber layer is an unintentionally doped (uid) n-type AlGaN with a smaller bandgap that forms an isotype n-N

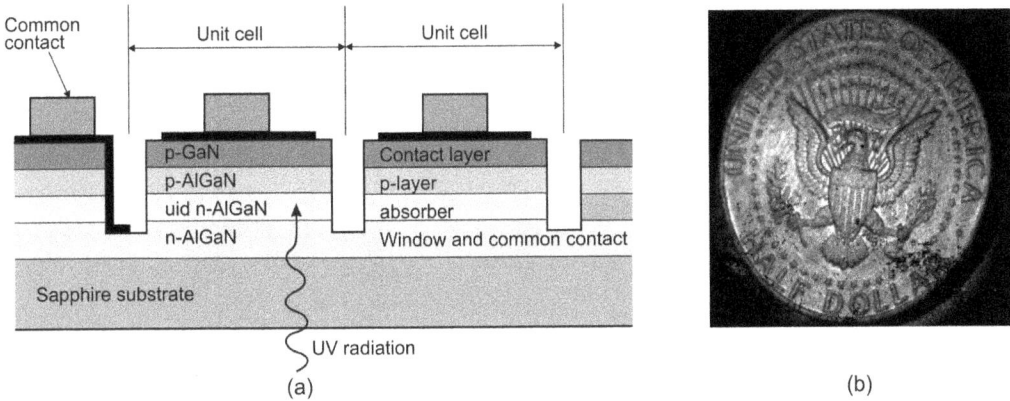

FIGURE 7.17   Hybrid 256×256 AlGaN p-i-n photodiode FPA with 30×30-μm unit pixels: (a) cross section of the back-illuminated photodiode array, and (b) UV reflection image of a U.S. half-dollar coin taken with this array (after Reference 30).

heterojunction with the window layer. The alloy composition of the absorber layer determines the cut-off wavelength. Next layer, a Mg-doped AlGaN p-type layer forms a p-n homojunction with the n-type absorber layer. The final layer is a thin, heavily doped, Mg-doped GaN cap layer that facilitates the p-side contact.

Figure 7.17(b) shows a UV reflection image of a United States half-dollar coin (3-cm diameter) taken with a 256×256 AlGaN FPA with 30×30-μm unit pixels. The UV detector array was hybridised to a BAE Systems 256×256 silicon CMOS ROIC chip with CTIA input circuits.

It should be marked that silicon photodiodes can be also used as UV detectors after proper technological modification [38]. The high absorption coefficient of silicon in the blue and UV spectral regions causes the generation of carriers within the heavily doped p^+ (or n^+) contact surface of p-n and p-i-n photodiodes, where the lifetime is short due to the high and/or surface recombination. As a result, quantum efficiency degrades rapidly in these regions. Blue- and UV-enhanced photodiodes optimise the response at short wavelengths by minimising near-surface carrier recombination using delta doping and antireflection coating. This is achieved by using very thin and highly graded p^+ (or n^+ or metal Schottky) contacts, by application of lateral collection to minimise the percentage of the surface area, which is heavily doped, and/or passivating the surface with a fixed surface charge to repeal minority carriers from the surface. For example, using molecular beam epitaxy, fully processed thinned CCDs are modified for UV enhancement by growing 2.5-nm thick boron-doped silicon on the back surface. The sharply-spiked dopant profile in the thin epitaxial layer improves device stability and external quantum efficiency to 50–90 per cent at wavelengths of 200–300 nm [38]. Figure 7.18 shows typical spectral characteristics of silicon planar diffusion photodiodes.

Figure 7.19(a) shows the 4k×4k CCD array, installed in Wide Field Camera 3 (WFC3) on the Hubble Space Telescope (HST), that covers the near-UV and near-IR wavelength ranges. This array has read noise level of $< 3e^-$ and quantum efficiency of 30–60 per cent between 200 and 300 nm [39]. WFC3 was installed by NASA astronauts in May 2009, during the Servicing Mission to upgrade and repair the 19-year-old Hubble. An image taken by the WFC3 is shown in Figure 7.19(b).

In comparison with existing siliconbased technology, the wide-bandgap semiconductors are significantly more radiation tolerant. Apart from AlGaN, other material systems such as SiC, MgZnO and diamond are good candidates to compete with silicon. Photodetectors based on diamond material have progressed due to success in producing high-quality thin films with sufficiently low defects and concentrations of n-type and p-type dopants [40]. The first two types of diamond detectors showing high

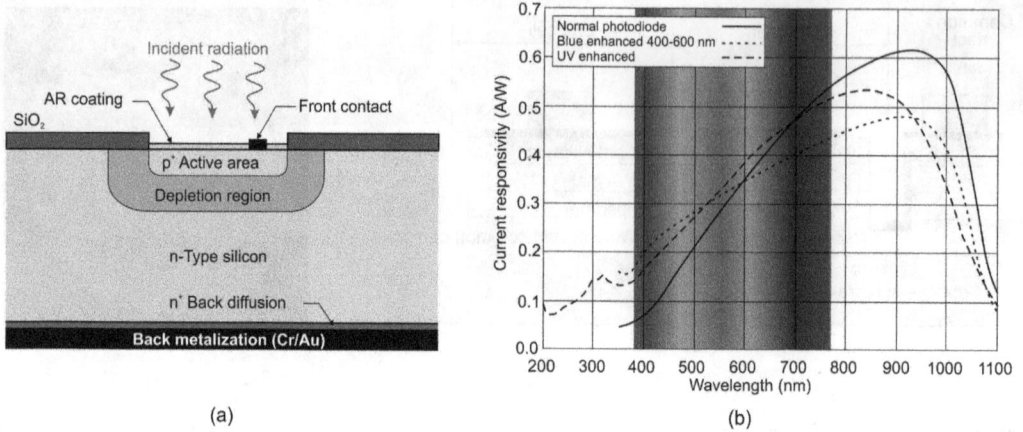

(a)   (b)

FIGURE 7.18   Planar diffused silicon photodiode: (a) cross section of p-n junction and (b) typical current responsivities of several different types of photodiodes.

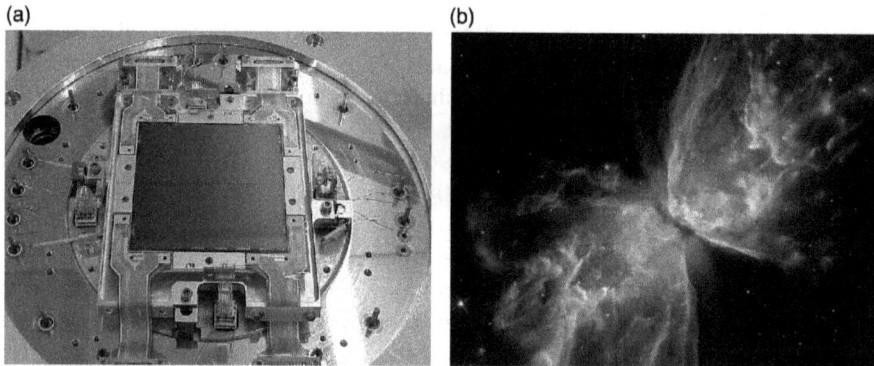

FIGURE 7.19   The WFC3 CCD, developed by e2v (formerly Marconi): (a) mounted on its TEC cooler, (b) WFC3 butterfly emerge snapped from stellar demise in planetary Nebula NG C 6302, more popularly called the Bug Nebula or the Butterfly Nebula.

responsivity around 200 nm, p-i-n photodiode and MSM detector [41], are flown on a space mission in the solar XUV-VUV radiometer LYRA (Large Yield Radiometer) aboard the PROBA-2 satellite.

7.4   VISIBLE DETECTORS

Silicon is the semiconductor that has dominated the electronic industry for over 60 years. While the first transistor fabricated in Ge and III-V semiconductor material compounds may have higher mobilities, higher saturation velocities, or larger bandgaps, silicon devices account for over 97 per cent of all microelectronics [42]. The main reason is that silicon is the cheapest microelectronic technology for integrated circuits. The reason for the dominance of silicon can be traced to a number of silicon's natural properties but, more importantly, two insulators of silicon, SiO_2 and Si_3N_4, allow deposition and selective etching processes to be developed with exceptionally high uniformity and yield.

Photodetectors are perhaps the oldest and best understood silicon photonic devices [43]. Silicon photodiodes are widely applied in spectral range below 1.1 μm and even are used for X-ray and gamma ray detectors. The main types are as follows:

- p-n junctions generally formed by diffusion (ion implantation is also used);
- p-i-n junctions (because of thicker active region, they have enhanced near-IR spectral response);
- UV- and blue-enhanced photodiodes; and
- avalanche photodiodes.

In the planar photodiode structure (diffused or implanted); cross section is shown in Figure 7.18(a), the highly doped p^+-region is very thin (typically about 1 μm) and is coated with the thin dielectric film (SiO_2 or Si_3N_4) that serves as an antireflection layer. The diffused junction can be formed either by a p-type impurity such as born into a n-type bulk silicon wafer, or the n-type impurity, such as phosphorous, into a p-type bulk silicon wafer. To form an ohmic contact another impurity diffusion (often coupled with implanting techniques) into the back side of the wafer is necessary. The contact pads are deposited on the front defined active area, and on the back side, completely covering the surface. An antireflection coating reduces the reflection of the light for specific predefined wavelength. The nonactive region on the top is covered with a thick layer of SiO_2. In dependence of the photodiode application, different design structures are used. By controlling the thickness of bulk substrate, both speed response and sensitivity of the photodiode can be controlled.

The main photodiode parameters of interest are spectral response, time constant and zero-bias resistance or reverse-bias leakage current. Silicon material has an indirect bandgap and, hence, the spectral cut-off is not very sharp near its long-wavelength cut-off – see Figure 7.18(b). The effective response time of p-n Si photodiodes is limited by resistance-capacitance (RC) time constant (τ_{RC}) rather than by the inherent speed of the detection mechanism (drift and/or diffusion). High reverse bias generally reduces cell capacitance, and therefore the RC product, which results in faster response. From the other side, increased reverse bias causes increased noise, so that a trade-off exists between speed and sensitivity. For high-frequency applications, load resistance should be made small (see Section 4.6), although this makes Johnson (thermal) noise comparatively greater, which limits sensitivity (see Figure 7.20). At high-frequency operation, high sensitivity is maintained using operational (current-mode) amplifiers, which are usually built into the detector package.

Note that the photodiodes can be operated as unbiased (photovoltaic) or reverse biased (photoconductive) modes (Figure 7.21). The amplifiers function is a simple current-to-voltage conversion (photodiode operates in a short circuit mode). Mode selection depends upon the speed requirements of the application, and the amount of dark current that is tolerable. The unbiased mode of operation

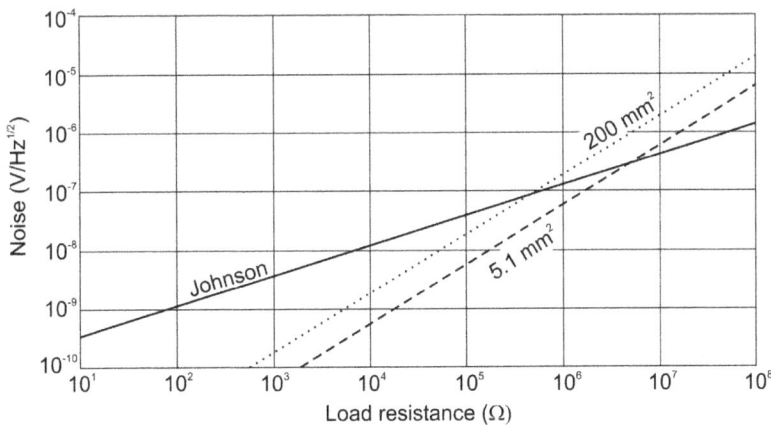

FIGURE 7.20 Output noise as a function of circuit load resistance for p-i-n Si photodiode with areas of 5.1 mm² and 200 mm², compared with the Johnson noise of the load resistor. Dark currents at 10 V reverse bias are 10 nA and 100 nA for the detectors with are of 5.1 mm² and 200 mm², respectively.

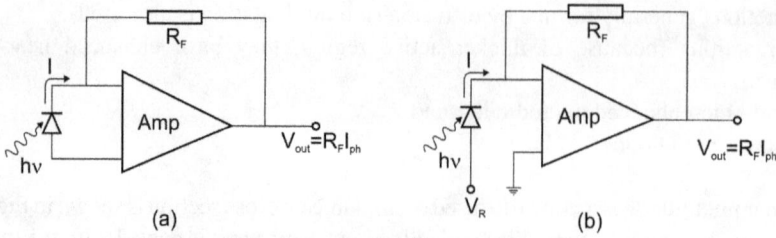

FIGURE 7.21   Modes of photodiode operation: (a) photovoltaic mode, and (b) photoconductive mode.

is preferred when a photodiode is used in low-frequency applications (up to 350 kHz) as well as ultra-low light applications. Application of a reverse bias can greatly improve the speed of response and linearity of the devices. This is due to an increase in the depletion region width and consequently a decrease in junction capacitance. The drawback of applying a reverse bias is an increase in the dark and noise currents.

The p-i-n detector is faster but is also less sensitive than conventional p-n junction detector and has slightly extended red response. This is a consequence of the extension of the depletion layer width, since longer wavelength photons will be absorbed in the active device region. Incorporation of a very lightly doped region between the p and n regions and a modest reverse bias form a depletion region the full thickness of the material ($\approx$ 500 μm for a typical silicon wafer). Higher dark current collected from generation within the wider depletion layer results in lower sensitivity.

Typical spectral characteristics of planar diffusion photodiodes are shown in Figure 7.18(b). The time constant of p-n junction silicon photodiodes is on the order of microseconds. Detectivity is typically between mid-10^{12} to 10^{13} cmHz$^{1/2}$/W usually amplifier-limited for small-area detectors.

The avalanche photodiodes (APDs) are especially useful where both fast response and high sensitivity are required (see section 4.8). An optimum gain exists below which the system is limited by receiver noise and above which shot noise dominates receiver noise and the overall noise increases faster than the signal. Noise is a function of detector area and increases as gain increases. Avalanche photodiodes require very careful regulation of the detector bias to support their stable operation. Typical detectivity if Si APDs is $(3–5)\times10^{14}$ cmHz$^{1/2}$/W.

Different semiconductor compounds have been used to fabricate photodetectors with responses in visible spectral band. Spectral detectivity curves for a number of commercially available detectors are shown in Figure 4.6.

Wide-bandgap photoconductors such as CdS and CdSe are mainly used in the near ultraviolet to visible spectral region. Both detectors have a spectral responsivity similar to that of the human eye [see Figure 7.22(c)]. CdS cells can be divided by the manufacturing process of the photoconductive layers into the sintered type, single crystal type and evaporated type. The sintered type offers high sensitivity and easy fabrication of large sensitive areas, a large mass production effect and relatively superior production profitability. The devices are typically made in a linear or serpentine configuration consisting of 2 to 500 squares to maximise the length-to-width ratio – see Figure 7.22(a). CdS cells are typically slow detectors with response times of 5 to 100 ms, with speed improving at higher light level. These devices exhibit "memory" or "history" effects – their resistance depends on the history of illumination.

Peak conductivity for a CdS cell is 515 nm, but by controlling the composition ratio of CdS to CdSe in CdSSe, the maximum sensitivity can be optimised at a wavelength between 515 and 730 nm; that is to say in spectral range close to the human eye.

Figure 7.22(b) explains the basic principles of the photoconductive effect. As is shown, both donor and acceptor levels are located near band edges. In darkness the photoconductor high resistance is a consequence of carriers cram in crystal lattice. During light illumination the electrons in

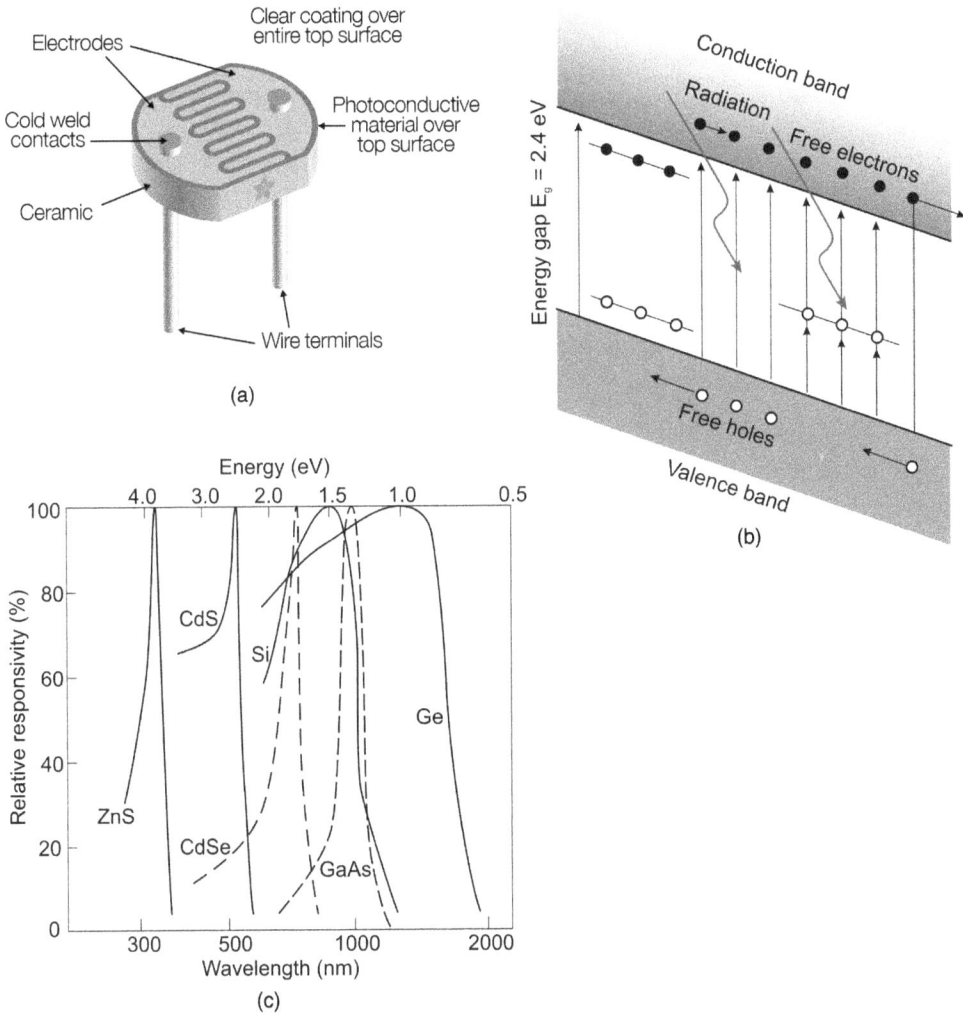

FIGURE 7.22 Photocells: (a) photocell structure, (b) photoconductivity mechanism in CdS photocell, (c) spectral response characteristics of CdS and other photoconductors.

the valence band are excited into the conduction band, which creates free holes in the valence band and free electrons in the conduction band, increasing the conductance. Furthermore, capture of free electrons by a separate acceptor level (in mid gap) is less effective than free holes. In this situation, the recombination probability of the electrons and holes is lower, which increases the number of electrons in the conduction band.

CdS and CdSe photoconductors are used in a variety of commercial applications, both analogue and digital (such as camera exposure control, automatic focus and brightness controls, densitometers, night light control, etc.). They are small, inexpensive, low-power, easy to use and do not wear out. For that reason, they often appear in toys, gadgets and appliances.

$GaAs_{1-x}P_x$ ternary alloys provide photodiodes operated in the spectral range between UV and near-infrared. The bandgap of GaP is 2.26 eV and is indirect, while that of GaAs is 1.43 eV and is direct. The ternary alloys with x-composition from 0 to ~ 0.50 are direct bandgap while alloys with x > 0.50 are indirect. Figure 7.23 shows spectral characteristics of different GaAsP photovoltaic detectors.

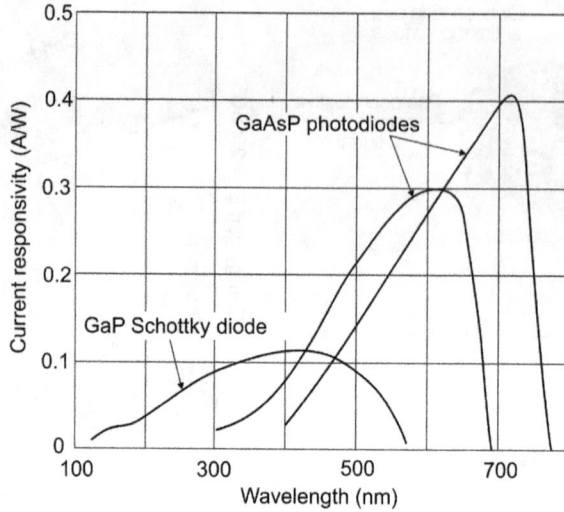

FIGURE 7.23 Spectral responses of GaAsP photodiodes.

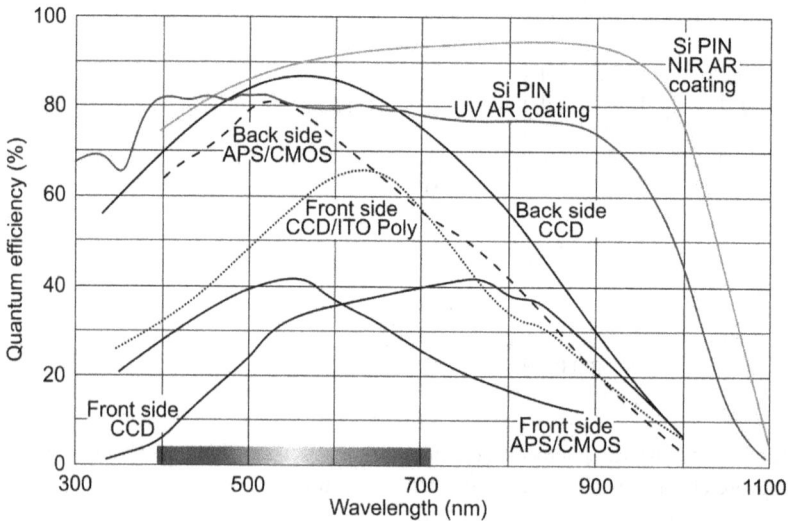

FIGURE 7.24 Comparison of quantum efficiency of different silicon photodetector technologies.

The detectors described above operate primarily as single-element detectors. Multi-element arrays can be fabricated by a simple solution – adding a number of individual detectors together. This unfruitful solution was applied in early stage of thermal imaging (in the 1960s). In the early 1970s, a new concept for creating images was introduced with the discovery of charge-transfer devices like charge-coupled devices (CCDs) and next (more recently) complementary metal-oxide-semiconductor (CMOS) devices. Both types of devices are described in detail in chapter 12. Figure 7.24 compares spectral characteristics of various front and back side illuminated imagers offered in the imaging market.

7.5 INFRARED PHOTODETECTORS

Different material families are used in fabrication of infrared detectors. A suitable detector material for near-IR (1.0–1.7-µm) spectral range is InGaAs lattice matched to the InP. InSb can respond to

5.5 µm at 80 K. Various HgCdTe alloys, in both photovoltaic and photoconductive configurations cover from 0.7 µm to over 20 µm. InAs/GaSb strained layer superlattices have emerged as an alternative to the HgCdTe. Impurity-doped (Sb, As and Ga) silicon-blocked impurity band (BIB) detectors operating at 10 K have a spectral response cut-off in the range of 16 to 30 µm. Impurity-doped Ge detectors can extend the response out to 100–200 µm.

7.5.1 GERMANIUM PHOTODIODES

Germanium photodiodes are usually fabricated by diffusion of arsenide into a p-type germanium (gallium doped to a 10^{15} cm^{-3} concentration and resistivity of 0.8 Ωcm). After creation of 1 µm thick n-type region, an oxide passivation film is deposited to reduce surface conductivity in the vicinity of the p-n junction. Finally, an antireflection coating is deposited (germanium has a high refractive index, $n \sim 4$, and a useful transmission range of 2–23 µm). Germanium is an excellent candidate material for the immersion lens because of its high refractive index.

Germanium does not form a stable oxide. GeO$_2$ is soluble in water, which leads to two process challenges: device passivation and stability. The lack of a high-quality passivation layer makes it difficult to achieve a low dark current. Interestingly, by scaling the device to smaller dimensions, a higher dark current can be tolerated.

Three germanium photodiode types are available: p-n junction, p-i-n junction and APD [44]. They are readily made in areas ranging from 0.05 to 3 mm^2, and the capability exists to make the area as small as 10×10 µm^2 or as large as 500 mm^2. The upper limit is imposed by raw material uniformity.

The previous discussion on silicon detectors applies in general to germanium ones, with the exception that blue- and UV-enhanced devices are not relevant to germanium detectors. Because of narrower bandgap, the germanium photodiodes have higher leakage currents, compared to silicon detectors. They offer submicrosecond response or high sensitivity from the visible to 1.8 µm. Zero bias is generally used for high sensitivity and large reverse bias for high speed. The peak of detectivity at room temperature is above 2×10^{11} cmHz$^{1/2}$W^{-1}. The performance can be improved significantly with thermoelectric cooling or cooling to liquid nitrogen temperature, which is shown in Figure 7.25 (detector impedance increases about the order of magnitude by cooling 20°C below room temperature) [45].

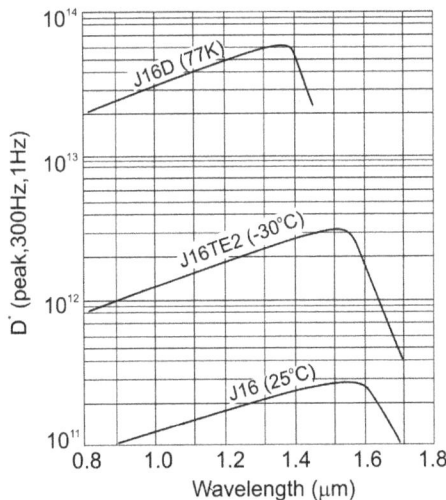

FIGURE 7.25 Detectivity as a function of wavelength for germanium photodiode at three temperatures.

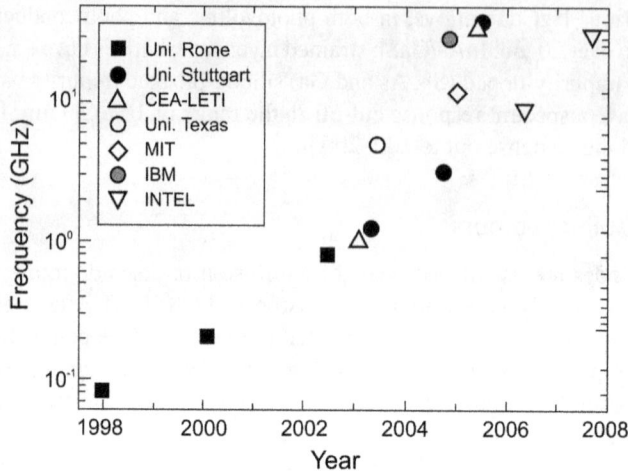

FIGURE 7.26   Speed evolution of Ge photodetectors (after Reference 47).

Usually, the performance of germanium photodiodes are Johnson-noise limited, and then we can improve detector performance by immersion in a hemispherical lens. The effective area of the detector increases by n^2, where n is the refractive index of the medium.

At the present stage of development, the research efforts are directed to integrate Ge detectors on silicon (Ge/Si) substrates into a CMOS-compatible process. It is an attractive goal for making arrays of on-chip detectors that can be used in an electronic-photonic chip [46]. The recent research activities on Ge photodiodes on Si (Figure 7.26) have shown a dramatic increase in speed to 40 GHz with prospects to 100 GHz and more [47].

7.5.2   InGaAs Photodiodes

The need for high-speed, low-noise $In_xGa_{1-x}As$ (InGaAs) photodetectors for use in light wave communication systems operating in the 1–1.7 µm wavelength region (x = 0.53) is well established. $In_{0.53}Ga_{0.47}As$ alloy is lattice matched to the InP substrate. Having lower dark current and noise than indirect-bandgap germanium (the competing near-IR material), the material is addressing both entrenched applications, including low light level night vision and new applications such as remote sensing, eye-safe range finding and process control.

The InAs/GaAs ternary system bandgaps span 0.35 eV (3.5 µm) for InAs to 1.43 eV (0.87 µm) for GaAs. By changing the alloy composition of the InGaAs absorption layer, the photodetector responsivity can be maximised at the desired wavelength of the end user to enhance the signal to noise ratio. Figure 7.27 shows the spectral response of three such InGaAs detectors at room temperature, whose cut-off wavelength is optimised at 1.7 µm, 2.2 µm and 2.5 µm, respectively.

The spectral response of an $In_{0.53}Ga_{0.47}As$ photodiode to the night spectrum makes it a better choice for use in a night-vision camera in comparison with the current state-of-art technology for enhancing night vision – GaAs Gen III image-intensifier tubes. Figure 7.27 also marks the key laser wavelengths.

InGaAs detector-processing technology is similar to that used with silicon, but the detector fabrication is different. The InGaAs detector's active material is deposited onto a substrate using chloride VPE or MOCVD techniques adjusted for thickness, background doping and other requirements. Planar technology evolved from the older mesa technology and at present is widely used due to its simple structure and processing as well as the high reliability and low cost.

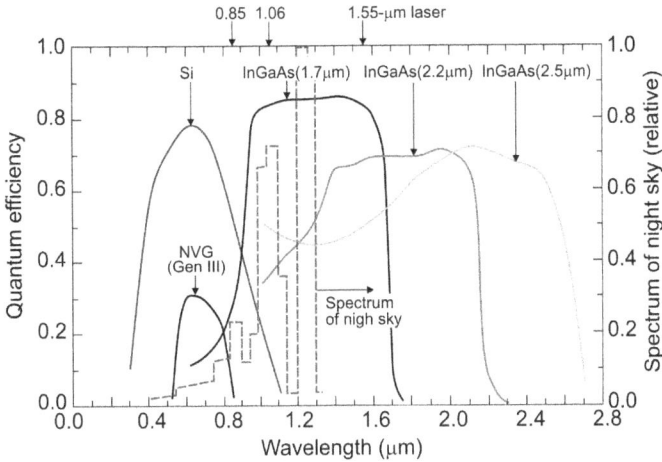

FIGURE 7.27 Quantum efficiency of silicon, InGaAs, and night vision tube detectors in the visible and SWIR. Key laser wavelengths are also noted. $In_{0.53}Ga_{0.47}As$ photodiode has nearly three times higher quantum efficiency than GaAs Gen III photocathodes; InGaAs also overlaps the illumination spectrum of the night sky more.

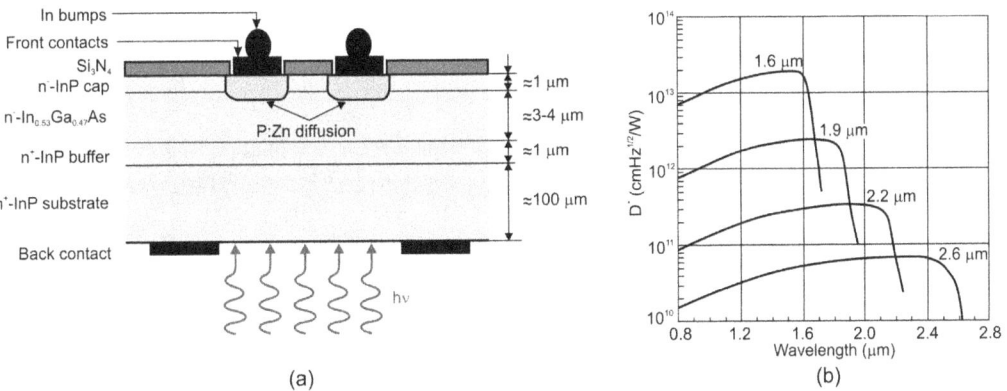

FIGURE 7.28 InGaAs photodiodes: (a) cross section of a planar back side illuminated p-i-n InGaAs photodiode (after Reference 48), (b) room-temperature spectral detectivity of photodiodes with different cut-off wavelength.

Figure 7.28(a) shows the structure of a InGaAs backside-illuminated p-i-n photodiode. The starting substrate is n+-InP on which is deposited approximately 1 μm of n+-InP as a buffer layer. 3–4 μm of the n−-InGaAs active layer is then deposited followed by a 1-μm n−-InP cap layer. The structure is covered with Si_3N_4. The p-on-n photodiodes are formed by the diffusion of zinc through the InP cap into the active layer. Ohmic contacts were formed by the sintering of a Au/Zn alloy. At this point, the substrate is thinned to approximately 100 μm and a sintered Au/Ge alloy is used as the back ohmic contact. The last step is the deposition of a 20 μm columns of indium on the front contacts.

Standard $In_{0.53}Ga_{0.47}As$ photodiodes have detector-limited room temperature detectivity of ~ 10^{13} cmHz$^{1/2}$W^{-1}. With increasing cut-off wavelength, detectivity decreases. Figure 7.28(b) shows the spectral response of three such InGaAs detectors at room temperature, whose peak responsivity is optimised at 1.7 μm, 2.0 μm, and 2.4 μm, respectively.

The arrays of InGaAs photodiodes are hybridised to CMOS readout integrated circuits (ROICs) and then integrated into cameras for video-rate output to a monitor or for use with a computer for quantitative measurements and machine vision (see Section 12.7.5.1). InGaAs photodetectors are also used in fibre-optic communications to take advantage of the dispersion and loss minima of silica fibres near 1310 and 1550 nm.

Attempting to obtain significant avalanche gain by increasing the electric field is not possible due to the onset of a tunnelling mechanism that causes very high leakage current. The small electron effective mass results in rapidly increasing the tunnelling current at low fields above 150 kV/cm [49, 50]. These problems were overcome by the combination of an InGaAs region capable of absorbing photons under a low electric field, and a lattice-matched wider bandgap InP region producing avalanche multiplication. The resulting structure is known as a separate absorption multiplication APD (SAM-APD).

An example of SAM-APD is shown in Figure 7.29 together with the band diagram of the entire heterostructure [51]. Light is absorbed in the InGaAs and holes (with a higher impact ionisation coefficient than electrons; this ensures low-noise operation) are swept to an InP junction, where the avalanche multiplication take place. This structure combines low leakage, due to the junction being placed in the high bandgap material (InP), which sensitivity at a longer wavelength is provided by the lower-bandgap InGaAs absorption region. Dark currents of the order pA can be obtained. However, there is a potential problem with the operation of a SAM-APD. Holes can accumulate at the valence band discontinuity at the InGaAs/InP heterojunction and thereby increase the response time. To alleviate this problem, a graded bandgap InGaAsP layer can be inserted between the InP and InGaAs. This modified structure is known as a separate absorption graded multiplication APD (SAGM-APD). The APD can achieve 5–10 dB better sensitivity than p-i-n, provided that the multiplication noise is low and the gain bandwidth product is sufficiently high.

In practical devices, the 1–2 μm thick absorption region is undoped. The graded layer (0.1–0.3 μm) and the avalanching layer (1–2 μm) are doped to 1×10^{16} cm^{-3}. The p$^+$-layer can be thin and doped to 10^{17}–10^{18} cm^{-3}. The junction is usually fabricated by zinc p$^+$-type diffusion in the InP for multiplication and Cd diffusion (or implantation) for guard-ring into the top InP layer through structures SiO$_2$ masks. The excellent stability of the device was demonstrated by long-term aging measurements (after 30,000 hours at 150°C and a 100 μA reverse current) [52].

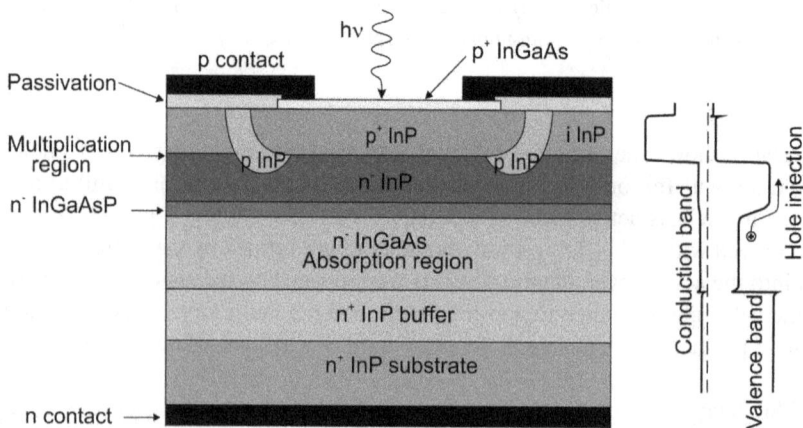

FIGURE 7.29 Cross section of SAGM-APD InP-based photodiode.

7.5.3 INSB-BASED PHOTODIODES

In the middle and late 1950s it was discovered that InSb had the smallest energy gap of any semiconductor known at that time, and its applications as a middle wavelength infrared detector became obvious. InSb is an intrinsic $A^{III}B^{V}$ semiconductor with zinc-blende cubic lattice structure and a direct-energy bandgap. At room temperature the energy gap of 0.17 eV corresponds to a long-wavelength response cut-off of around 7 μm. Cooling to a liquid-nitrogen temperature (77 K) causes increasing of energy gap to 0.23 eV and shifting the cut-off wavelength to 5.5 μm.

III-V photodiodes are generally fabricated by impurity diffusion, ion implantation, LPE, MBE and MOCVD. Initially p-n junctions in InSb were made by diffusing Zn or Cd into n-type substrates with net donor concentration in the range of 10^{14}–10^{15} cm^{-3} at 77 K [53].

At present, in InSb photodiode fabrication processes the standard manufacturing technique begins with bulk n-type single-crystal wafers with donor concentration about 10^{15} cm^{-3}. Relatively large bulk-grown crystals (InSb and GaSb) with 6-in. diameters are available on the market. Manufacturing of large hybrid arrays is possible because the InSb detector material is thinned to less than 10 μm (after surface passivation and hybridisation to a readout chip) which allows it to accommodate the InSb/silicon thermal mismatch. As shown in Figure 7.30(a), the backside illuminated InSb p-on-n detector is a planar structure with an ion-implanted junction. After hybridisation, epoxy is wicked between the detector and the Si ROIC and the detector is thinned to 10 μm or less by diamond-point-turning. One important advantage of a thinned InSb detector is that no substrate is needed; these detectors also respond in the visible portion of the spectrum.

The best quality InSb photodiodes are generation-recombination limited. In this limit, SRH traps created by imperfections in the semiconductor crystal lattice provide energy states located in the semiconductor bandgap. In a standard planar technology, p-on-n junctions are created by ion implantation into n-type substrates. A new approach involving MBE growth has been adopted for reducing the dark current. Because *in situ* MBE epilayer growth of p-n structures avoids implantation damage, the diodes have a much lower concentration of G-R centres than in standard planar p-n junctions [55]. The dark current is thus reduced according to the ratio of concentrations of G-R

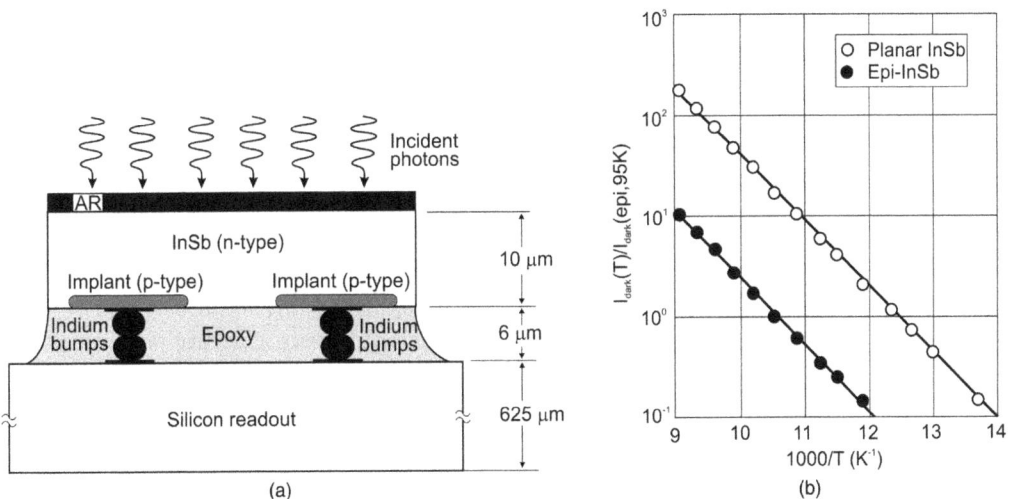

FIGURE 7.30 InSb planar photodiode: (a) architecture of an InSb sensor chip assembly (after Reference 54), (b) temperature dependence of the dark currents of 15-μm pitch InSb diodes fabricated using planar (open points) and MBE technology. Fitting lines are calculated assuming G-R formula (after Reference 55).

centres in the standard and MBE-grown structures. An example of improvement in dark-current characteristics is shown in Figure 7.30(b), where the temperature dependence of the dark current in planar implanted InSb and epi-InSb 15-μm pitches is compared. The dark current is normalised to that at the epi-InSb photodiode operated at 95 K. The solid lines are fitted assuming G-R limited behaviour with activation energy of 0.12 eV, which corresponds to approximately half the bandgap of InSb at low temperatures. Note that the same dark current is achieved at 80 K in planar InSb and 95 K in epi-InSb. The dark current has been decreased about 17× by going to the MBE-based technology.

The detectivity versus wavelength for a typical InSb photodiode is shown in Figure 7.31 [56]. Detectivity increases with reduced background flux (narrow FOV and/or cold filtering) as illustrated in the figure. InSb photodiodes can also be operated in the temperature range above 77 K. Of course, the RA products degrade in this region. The quantum efficiency in InSb photodiodes optimised for this temperature range remains unaffected up to 160 K.

The InSb photovoltaic detectors are widely used for ground- and space-based infrared astronomy. For applications in astrophysics, these devices are very often operated at 4–7 K with a resistive or capacitive transimpedance amplifier to achieve the lowest noise performance. At these low temperatures, the InSb photodiode resistance is so high that the detector Johnson noise is negligible, and the dominant noise sources are either the feedback resistance or input amplifier noise. Since the latter scales directly with the combined detector and input circuit capacitance, it becomes important to minimise them.

The $A^{III}B^V$ ternary alloy, $InAs_{1-x}Sb_x$, is potentially a very important material for the fabrication of photodetectors designed for mid-wavelength infrared (MWIR) applications. The dependence $E_g(x,T)$ for $InAs_{1-x}Sb_x$ has been experimentally investigated by many research groups since 1964 [57]. It indicates that this ternary alloy has a sufficiently small gap at 77 K for operation in the 8–14-μm wavelength range. $E_g(x,T)$ is generally a square function of the composition and indicates a fairly weak dependence of the band edge on composition in comparison with HgCdTe. Ten different relations $E_g(x,T)$ obtained from measurements over a different x-composition values performed in a wide range of temperatures are presented in Reference 58. The minimum of E_g appears at composition x ≈ 0.60–0.64. The bandgap expressions at room temperature are plotted in Figure 7.32. Discrepancies in the $E_g(x,T)$-dependence may result from several factors among others: strains, carrier concentrations, structural quality of samples and CuPt-type ordering effect.

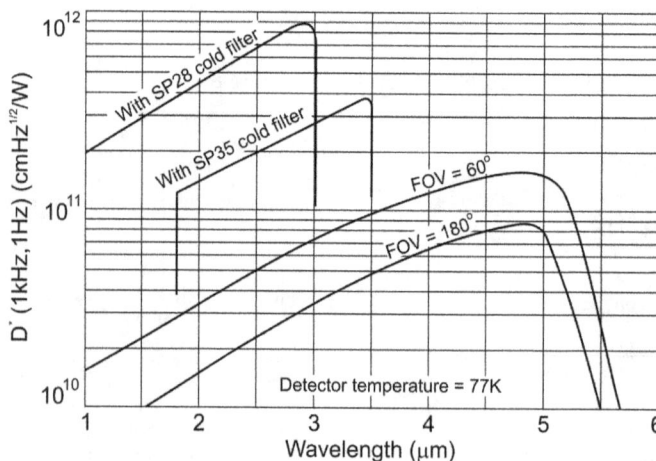

FIGURE 7.31   Detectivity as a function of wavelength for a InSb photodiode operating at 77 K.

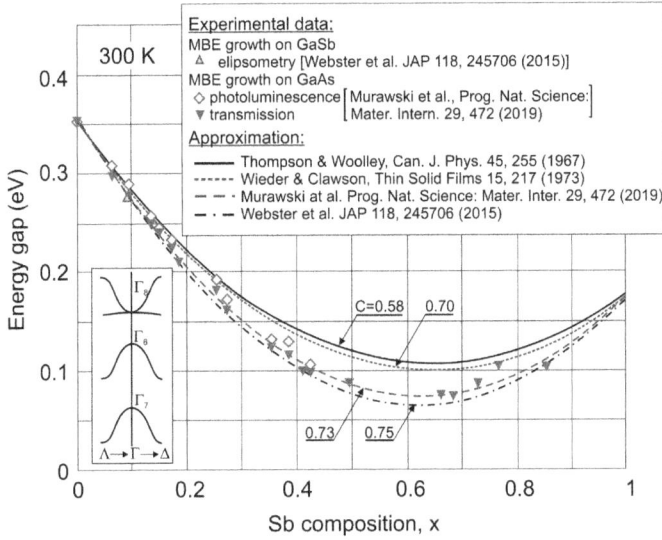

FIGURE 7.32 InAs$_{1-x}$Sb$_x$ bandgap energy versus the Sb composition at room temperature. The experimental data is taken with different papers as indicated in the legend (after Reference 57).

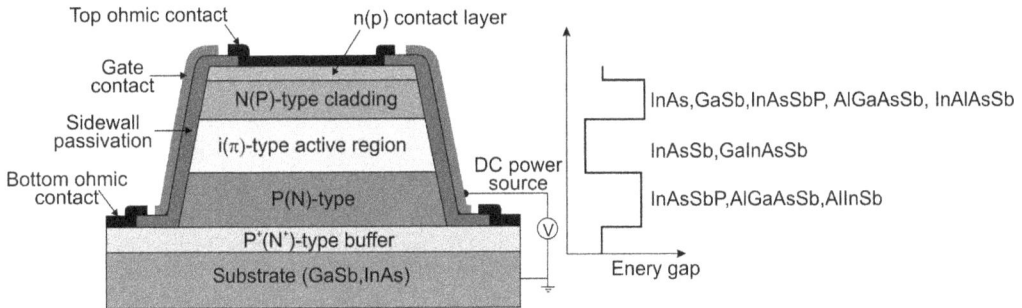

FIGURE 7.33 Schematic band diagram of the N-i-P double heterostructure antimonide based III-V photodiodes. Different combinations of active and cladding layers are also shown.

A recently published paper by Rogalski *et al.* [57] reports the latest achievements in fabrication of InSb-based heterostructure and barrier architectures operating in high temperature conditions. In order to improve device performance (lower dark current and higher detectivity), several groups have developed P-i-N heterostructure devices of an unintentionally doped InAsSb active layer sandwiched between P and N layers of larger bandgap materials. The lower minority carrier concentration in the high bandgap layers resulted in a lower diffusion dark and higher R_oA product and detectivity. Figure 7.33 shows schematic band diagram of the N-i-P double heterostructure (DH) antimonide based III-V photodiodes together with the different combinations of active and cladding layers in the device structure. In dependence on contact configurations and transparency of substrates, both backside and frontside illumination can be used. Usually p-type GaSb and n-type InAs are used, rarely GaAs. Despite the relatively low absorption coefficients, substrates required thinning to small thicknesses, even less than 10 μm.

Figure 7.34 summarises experimental data of R_oA product versus photon energy for n$^+$-InAs/ n-InAsSb/p-InAsSbP DH photodiodes in wide wavelength spectral range to 9 μm. The experimental

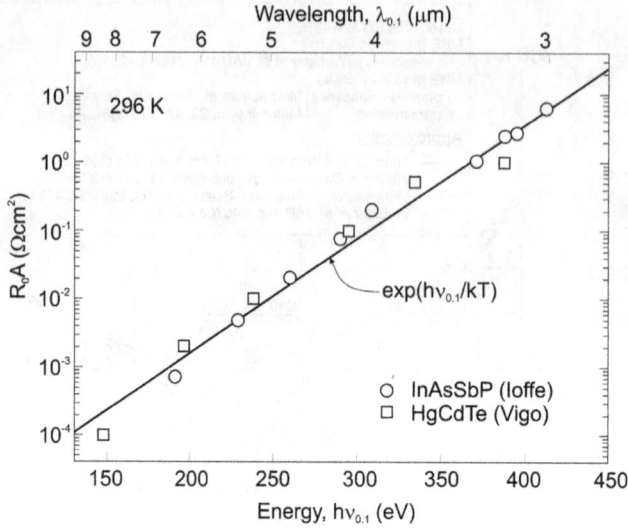

FIGURE 7.34 R_oA product in series of InAsSb DH at room temperature (after Reference 59).

data for InAsSb photodiodes are comparable with those of HgCdTe photodiodes produced by the VIGO System. It is assumed that the photon energy in the region of 90 per cent photocurrent drop is close to the energy gap of the photodiode active region. An exponential dependence of R_oA product, approximated by $\exp(h\nu_{0.1}/kT)$, shows that the transport properties are determined by the diffusion current, and the leakage current flow mechanism is negligible.

Figure 7.35 presents spectral detectivity curves of commercially available photovoltaic (PV) detectors at different temperatures, including InAsSb photodiodes manufactured by Hamamatsu [60]. The experimental data are compared with theoretical predictions for HgCdTe photodiodes. At the present stage of HgCdTe technology, the "Rule 07" metric (specified in 2007 [61]) is not a proper approach for prediction of the HgCdTe detector and system performance and as a reference benchmark for alternative technologies. For sufficiently long SRH carrier lifetime in HgCdTe, which is experimentally supported at a doping level below 5×10^{13} cm^{-3}, the internal P-i-N HgCdTe photodiode current is suppressed, and performance is limited by the background radiation. In a recently published paper [62], it was suggested to replace "Rule 07" with "Law 19". The "Law 19" corresponds exactly with the BLIP curve for room temperature. The internal photodiode current can be several orders of magnitude below "Rule 07" versus $\lambda_{cut-off}$ and operating temperature. In this context the alternative technologies should be considered and evaluated. Figure 7.35 shows that the potential properties of high operating temperature (HOT) HgCdTe photodiodes operating in longer wavelength IR range (above 3 μm) guarantee achieving more than an order of magnitude higher detectivity (above 10^{10} Jones) in comparison with value predicted by "Rule 07" [61]. The above estimates provide further mobilisation for achieving high performance MWIR and LWIR HgCdTe FPAs operating in HOT conditions, at a low production cost. In the most optimistic scenario, antimonide/arsenide-based photodetectors can totally supplant the $Hg_{1-x}Cd_xTe$ devices for each spectral range and operating temperature. Particular fabrication efforts provide Hamamatsu with a variety of IR detectors with different spectra response characteristics, which is presented in Figure 7.35.

7.5.4 HgCdTe Photodetectors

In 1959, a Lawson and co-workers publication [63] triggered development of variable bandgap $Hg_{1-x}Cd_xTe$ (HgCdTe) alloys providing an unprecedented degree of freedom in infrared detector

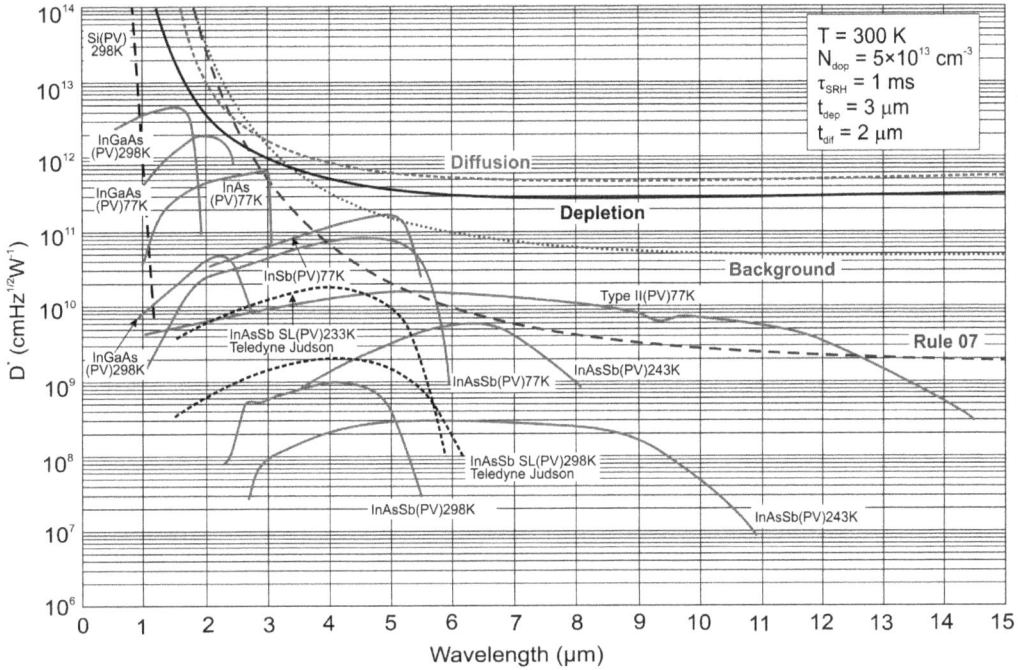

FIGURE 7.35 Spectral detectivity curves of commercially available photovoltaic (PV) detectors at different temperatures (after Reference 60). The theoretical curves are calculated for P-i-N HOT HgCdTe photodiodes assuming the value of $\tau_{SRH} = 1$ ms, the absorber doping level of 5×10^{13} cm^{-3} and the thickness of active region $t = 5$ μm (after Reference 57).

design. HgCdTe is a pseudo-binary alloy semiconductor that crystallises in the zinc blende structure. Because of its bandgap tunability with x, $Hg_{1-x}Cd_xTe$ has evolved to become the most important/versatile material for detector applications over the entire infrared (IR) range. As the Cd composition increases, the energy gap for $Hg_{1-x}Cd_xTe$ gradually increases from the negative value for HgTe to the positive value for CdTe. The bandgap energy tunability results in IR detector applications that span the short wavelength IR (SWIR: 1–3 μm), middle wavelength (MWIR: 3–5 μm), long wavelength (LWIR: 8–14 μm) and very long wavelength (VLWIR: 14–30 μm) ranges.

HgCdTe ternary alloy is nearly ideal infrared detector material system. Its position is conditioned by three key features [64]:

- tailorable energy bandgap over the 1–30-μm range;
- large optical coefficients that enable high quantum efficiency; and
- favourable inherent recombination mechanisms that lead to high operating temperature.

These properties are a direct consequence of the energy band structure of this zinc-blende semiconductor. In addition, the specific advantages of HgCdTe are the direct energy gap, ability to obtain both low and high carrier concentrations, high mobility of electrons and low dielectric constant. The extremely small change of lattice constant with composition makes it possible to grow high quality layers and heterostructures. HgCdTe can be used for detectors operated at various modes and can be optimised for operation at the extremely wide range of the IR spectrum (1–30 μm) and at temperatures ranging from that of liquid helium to room temperature.

Table 7.4 summarises various material properties of $Hg_{1-x}Cd_xTe$ [64]. A more detailed review of HgCdTe physical properties is presented, for example, in Rogalski's monographs [49].

TABLE 7.4

Summary of the Material Properties for the $Hg_{1-x}Cd_xTe$ Ternary Alloy, Listed for the Binary Components HgTe and CdTe, and for Several Technologically Important Alloy Compositions

Property	HgTe	$Hg_{1-x}Cd_xTe$						CdTe
x	0	0.194	0.205	0.225	0.31	0.44	0.62	1.0
a (Å)	6.461	6.464	6.464	6.464	6.465	6.468	6.472	6.481
	77 K	77 K	77 K	77 K	140 K	200 K	250 K	300 K
E_g (eV)	-0.261	0.073	0.091	0.123	0.272	0.474	0.749	1.490
λ_c (μm)	–	16.9	13.6	10.1	4.6	2.6	1.7	0.8
n_i (cm^{-3})	–	1.9×10^{14}	5.8×10^{13}	6.3×10^{12}	3.7×10^{12}	7.1×10^{11}	3.1×10^{10}	4.1×10^5
m^*_c/m_o	–	0.006	0.007	0.010	0.021	0.035	0.053	0.102
g_c	–	-150	-118	-84	-33	-15	-7	-1.2
$\varepsilon_s/\varepsilon_o$	20.0	18.2	18.1	17.9	17.1	15.9	14.2	10.6
$\varepsilon_\infty/\varepsilon_o$	14.4	12.8	12.7	12.5	11.9	10.8	9.3	6.2
n_r	3.79	3.58	3.57	3.54	3.44	3.29	3.06	2.50
μ_e (cm^2/Vs)	–	4.5×10^5	3.0×10^5	1.0×10^5	–	–	–	–
μ_{hh} (cm^2/Vs)	–	450	450	450	–	–	–	–
$b = \mu_e/\mu_\eta$	–	1000	667	222	–	–	–	–
τ_R (μs)	–	16.5	13.9	10.4	11.3	11.2	10.6	2
τ_{A1} (μs)	–	0.45	0.85	1.8	39.6	453	4.75×10^3	
$\tau_{typical}$ (μs)	–	0.4	0.8	1	7	–	–	–
E_p (eV)						19		
Δ (eV)						0.93		
m_{hh}/m_o						0.40–0.53		
ΔE_v (eV)						0.35–0.55		

τ_R and τ_{A1} calculated for n-type HgCdTe with $N_d = 1 \times 10^{15}$ cm^{-3} the last four material properties are independent of or relatively insensitive to alloy composition.

The first report of the synthesis of the semimetal HgTe and wide band-gap semiconductor CdTe to form HgCdTe ternary alloy system concerns both photoconductive and photovoltaic response at wavelengths extending out to 12 μm [63] and made the understated observation that this material showed promise for intrinsic infrared detectors. In that time the importance of the 8–12-μm atmospheric transmission window was well known for thermal imaging, which enables night vision by imaging the emitted IR radiation from the scene. Since 1954 the Cu-doped extrinsic photoconductive detector has been known [65], but its spectral response extended to 30 μm (far longer than required for the 8–12-μm window), and to achieve background-limited performance the Ge:Cu detector had to to cool down to liquid helium temperature. In 1962, it was discovered that the Hg acceptor level in Ge has an activation energy of about 0.1 eV [66], and detector arrays were soon made from this material; however, the Ge:Hg detectors were cooled to 30 K to achieve maximum sensitivity. It was also clear from theory that an intrinsic HgCdTe detector (where the optical transitions were direct transitions between the valence band and the conduction band) could achieve the same sensitivity at a much higher operating temperature (as high as 77 K). Early recognition of the significance of this fact led to intensive development of HgCdTe detectors in a number of countries, including England, France, Germany, Poland, the former Soviet Union and the United States [67]. However, little has been written about the early development years; for example, the existence of work going on in the United States was classified until the late 1960s.

Photoconductive devices had been built in the United States at Texas Instruments as early as 1964 after development of a modified Bridgman crystal growth technique. The high performance MWIR

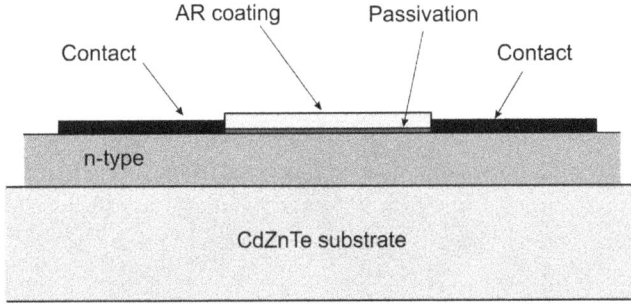

FIGURE 7.36 Cross-section of a basic HgCdTe photoconductor.

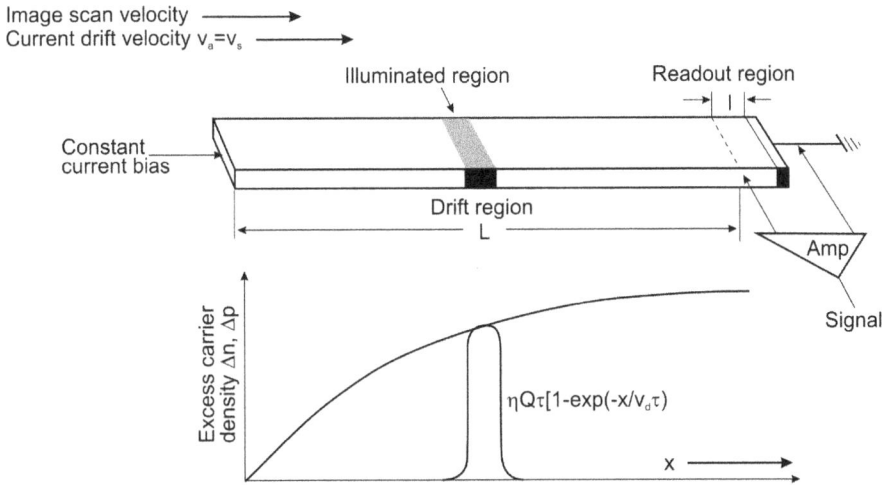

FIGURE 7.37 The operating principle of a SPRITE detector. The upper part of the figure shows a HgCdTe filament with three ohmic contacts. The lower part shows the build-up of excess carrier density in the device as a point in the image is scanned along it.

and LWIR linear arrays developed and manufactured in the 1970s were n-type photoconductors used in the first-generation scanning systems. In 1969, Bartlett *et al.* [68] reported background limited performance of photoconductors operated at 77 K in the LWIR spectral region. The basic photoconductive device structure is illustrated in Figure 7.36, where metal electrodes are applied to pure n-type material thinned to approximately 10 μm. Typical photoconductors are passivated with anodic oxide and antireflection coated with zinc sulphide. The photoconductors required far more simple materials growth and device-processing technologies than p-n junctions. The highly doped n⁺ layer for the contact windows fabricated by ion milling provides an excellent ohmic contact for electron flow and a blocking contact to minority carrier holes (so-called excluding contact). This leads to nonequilibrium effects when the bias voltage is applied – no holes are injected into the material (the flow of holes is sustained in the bulk away from the contact) and in consequence, both hole and electron densities drop to maintain space-charge neutrality.

A novel variation of the standard photoconductive device, the SPRITE detector (the acronym of Signal PRocessing In The Element), was invented in England [69, 70]. A family of thermal imaging systems has utilised this device, however, a decline in its usage is observed. The SPRITE detector provides signal averaging of a scanned image spot, which is accomplished by synchronisation between the drift velocity of minority carriers along the length of photoconductive bar of material and the scan velocity of the imaging system (see Figure 7.37). Then the image signal builds

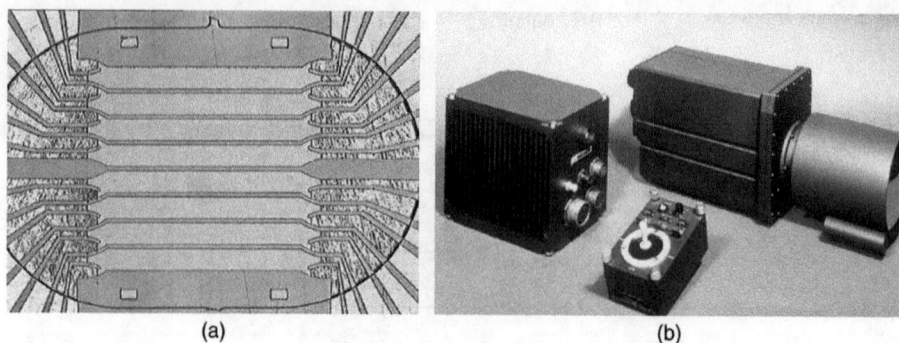

FIGURE 7.38 The UK Class II Common Modules imager: (a) eight-element SPRITE array with horn readout zones (the devices are 800-μm long on 75-μm pitch); (b) Horned OctoSPRITE camera modules. Production began in 1981 (after Reference 71).

up a bundle of minority charge which is collected at the end of the photoconductive bar, effectively integrating the signal for a significant length of time and thereby improving the signal-to-noise ratio.

The SPRITE detectors are fabricated from lightly doped ($\approx 5 \times 10^{14}$ cm^{-3}) $Hg_{1-x}Cd_xTe$. Both bulk material and epilayers are being used. Single and 2, 4, 8, 16 and 24 element arrays have been demonstrated; the 8-element arrays are the most commonly used (Figure 7.38a). Large SPRITE arrays are limited by Joule heating in the elements, which increases the heat load of the cooler to impractical levels. Figure 7.38(b) shows the UK Class II Common Modules imager, which has seen service in the Falklands conflict and in two Gulf wars.

The simplest scanning linear FPA consists of a row of detectors [see Figure 12.5(a)]. An image is generated by scanning the scene across the strip using, as a rule, a mechanical scanner. These types of arrays can provide enhanced sensitivity and gain in camera weight. In a general sense, the signal-to-noise ratio of a sensor will improve with the square root of the number of detector elements in an array – to the extent that they can collect proportionally more signal from the scene. The scanning system, which does not include multiplexing functions in the focal plane, belongs to the first-generation systems. A typical example of this kind of detector is a linear photoconductive array in which an electrical contact for each element of a multielement array is brought off the cryogenically cooled focal plane to the outside, where there is one electronic channel at ambient temperature for each detector element. The United States' common module HgCdTe arrays employ 60, 120 or 180 photoconductive elements, depending on the application [see Figure 12.5(a) at right].

The low impedance of the photoconductor makes it unsuitable for signal injecting into a silicon readout integrated circuit (ROIC); therefore, each element requires a lead-out through the vacuum encapsulation to an off-focal plane amplifier. The complexity of the dewar limits the size of the array, and the photoconductor technology is not suitable for two-dimensional (2-D) arrays.

After the invention of charge-coupled devices (CCDs) by Boyle and Smith [72], the idea of an all-solid-state electronically scanned two-dimensional (2D) IR detector array turned attention to HgCdTe photodiodes. These include p-n junctions, heterojunctions and MIS photo-capacitors. Each of these different types of devices has certain advantages for IR detection, depending on the particular application. More interest has been focused on the first two structures, so further considerations are restricted to p-n junctions and heterostructures. Photodiodes with their very low power dissipation, inherently high impedance, negligible $1/f$ noise and easy multiplexing on focal plane silicon chip, can be assembled in 2D arrays containing a very large number of elements, limited only by existing technologies. They can be reverse-biased for even-higher impedance and can therefore match electrically with compact low-noise silicon readout preamplifier circuits. The response of photodiodes remains linear to significantly higher photon flux levels than that of photoconductors (because of higher doping levels in the photodiode absorber layer and because the photogenerated carriers are collected rapidly by the junction). At the end of the 1970s, emphasis was directed toward large photovoltaic HgCdTe arrays in the MW and LW spectral bands for thermal imaging. Recent efforts have been extended to short wavelengths – for example, for starlight imaging in the short wavelength (SW) range, as well as to very LWIR (VLWIR) space-borne remote sensing beyond 15 μm.

Epitaxy is the preferable technique to obtain device-quality HgCdTe epilayers for IR devices. Epitaxial techniques offer the possibility to grow large area epilayers and sophisticated layered structures with abrupt and complex composition and doping profiles.

Among the various epitaxial techniques, liquid phase epitaxy (LPE) is the most matured method. The recent efforts are mostly on low-growth temperature techniques, MBE and MOCVD. MBE offers unique capabilities in material and device engineering, including the lowest growth temperature, superlattice growth and potential for the most sophisticated composition and doping profiles. The growth temperature is less than 200°C for MBE but around 350°C for MOCVD, making it more difficult to control the p-type doping in the MOCVD due to the formation of Hg vacancies.

Different HgCdTe photodiode architectures have been fabricated that are compatible with backside and frontside illuminated hybrid FPA technology [49]. Figure 7.39 shows the schematic band profiles of the most commonly used unbiased homo- (n^+-on-p) and heterojunction (p-on-n) photodiodes. To avoid contribution of the tunnelling current, doping concentration in the base region below 10^{16} cm^{-3} is required. In both photodiodes, the lightly doped narrow gap absorbing region ["base" of the photodiode: p(n)-type carrier concentration of about 5×10^{15} cm^{-3} (10^{14} cm^{-3})] determines the dark current and photocurrent. The internal electric fields at interfaces are "blocking" for minority carriers and the influence of surface recombination is eliminated. Also, suitable passivation minimises the influence of surface recombination. Indium is most frequently used as a well-controlled dopant for n-type doping due to its high solubility and moderately high diffusion. Elements of the VB group are acceptors substituting Te sites. They are very useful for fabrication of stable junctions due to very low diffusivity. Arsenic has proved to be the most successful p-type dopant to date. Its main advantages are stability in the lattice, low activation energy and possibility to control concentration over the 10^{14}–10^{18} cm^{-3} range. Intensive efforts are currently underway to reduce the high temperature (400°C) required to activate As as an acceptor.

N-on-p junctions are fabricated in two different manners using Hg vacancy doping and extrinsic doping. Hg vacancies (V_{Hg}) provide intrinsic p-type doping in HgCdTe. In this case, the doping level depends on only one annealing temperature. However, the use of Hg vacancy as p-type doping is known to greatly decrease the electron lifetime, and the resulting detector exhibits a higher dark current than in the case of extrinsic doping. However, for very low doping (< 10^{15} cm^{-3}), the hole lifetime becomes Shockley-Read (SR) limited and does not depend on doping anymore. V_{Hg}

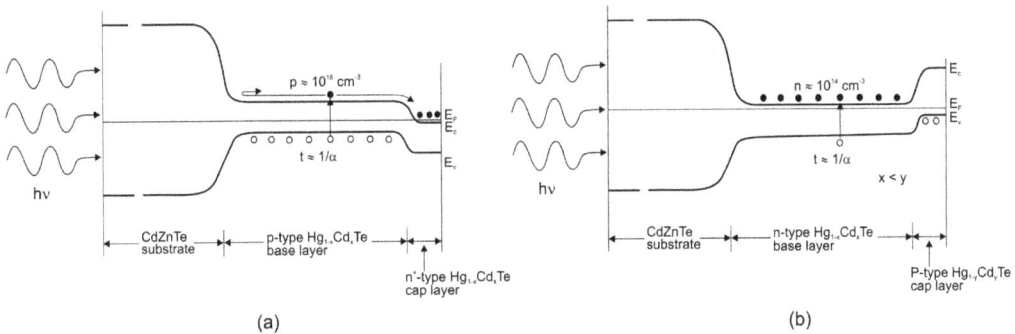

FIGURE 7.39 Schematic band diagrams of n^+-on-p (a) and p-on-n (b) HgCdTe photodiodes.

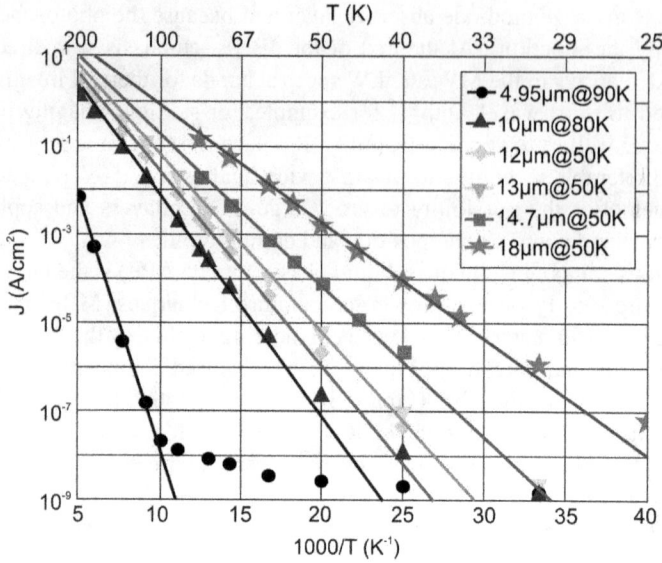

FIGURE 7.40 Mercury vacancy dark current modelling for n-on-p HgCdTe photodiodes with different cut-off wavelengths (after Reference 73).

technology leads to low minority diffusion length of the order of 10–15 μm, depending on doping level. Generally, n-on-p vacancy doped diodes give rather high diffusion currents but lead to a robust technology as its performance weakly depends on doping level and absorbing layer thickness. Simple modelling manages to describe dark current behaviour of V_{Hg} doped n-on-p junctions over a range of at least eight orders of magnitude (see Figure 7.40). In the case of extrinsic doping, Cu, Au and As are often used [73]. Due to higher minority carrier lifetime, extrinsic doping is used for low dark current (low flux) applications. The extrinsic doping usually leads to larger diffusion length and allows lower diffusion current but might exhibit performance fluctuations, thus affecting yield and uniformity.

In high-quality $Hg_{1-x}Cd_xTe$ photodiodes with x ≈ 0.20, the diffusion current in the zero-bias, and the low-bias region is usually the dominant dark current down to 40 K [49]. At medium values of reverse bias, the dark current is mostly due to trap-assisted tunnelling. Trap-assisted tunnelling dominates the dark current also at zero bias and very low temperature (below 30 K). At high values of reverse bias, bulk band-to-band tunnelling dominates. At very low temperatures, below 30 K, significant spreads in the dark current distributions are typically observed due to the onset of tunnelling currents associated with localised defects. Moreover, HgCdTe photodiodes often have an additional surface-related component of the dark current, particularly at low temperatures.

Tennant et al. [61] have developed a simple empirical relationship that describes the dark current behaviour with temperature and wavelengths for the better Teledyne HgCdTe diodes and arrays – primarily double layer planar heterojunction (DLPH) structure devices. Called "Rule 07", it coincides well with the theoretically predicted curve for Auger-suppressed p-on-n photodiode with electron concentration in active region ~10^{15} cm^{-3}.

The formula for "Rule 07" is approximately (exact formula given in the reference)

$$J_{dark} = 8367 \exp\left(-\frac{1.44212q}{k\lambda_c T}\right) \text{ for } \lambda_c \geq 4.635 \text{ μm} \tag{7.1}$$

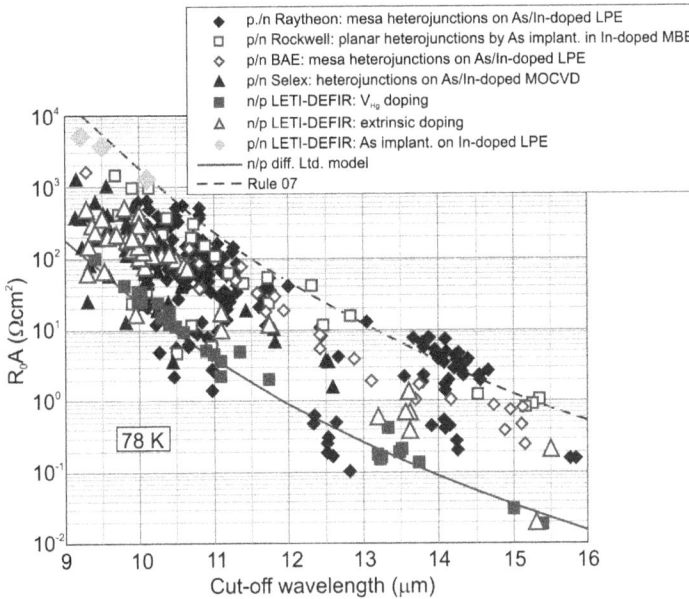

FIGURE 7.41 R_oA product versus cut-off wavelength at 78 K, summarised with bibliographic data (after Reference 73).

and

$$J_{dark} = 8367\exp\left\{-\frac{1.44212q}{k\lambda_c T}\left[1 - 0.2008\left(\frac{4.635 - \lambda_c}{4.635\lambda_c}\right)^{0.544}\right]\right\} \text{for } \lambda_c < 4.635 \text{ μm} \quad (7.2)$$

where λ_c is the cut-off wavelength in μm, T is the operating temperature in K, q is the electron charge, and k is the Boltzmann's constant (both of the latter in SI units). Rule 07 was developed for operating temperature–cut-off wavelength products between 400 μmK and ~1700 μmK, and for operating temperatures above 77 K.

Figure 7.41 is an accumulation of R_oA-data with different cut-off wavelength, taken from LETI LIR using both V_{Hg} and extrinsic doping n-on-p HgCdTe photodiodes compared with P-on-n data from other laboratories, extracted from various recent literature reports, using various techniques and different diode structures. It is clearly shown that extrinsic doping of n-on-p photodiodes leads to higher R_oA product (lower dark current), whereas mercury vacancy doping remains on the bottom part of the plot. P-on-n structures are characterised by the lowest dark current (highest R_oA product) – see trend line calculated with Teledyne empirical model [61].

At the present stage of HgCdTe technology, the "Rule 07" metric is not a proper approach for prediction of the HgCdTe detector and system performance. It is shown that the uncooled depletion-limited HgCdTe photovoltaic detector can achieve background limited detectivity in long wavelength infrared spectral range at room temperature. "Rule 07" should be replaced by "Law 19" [62]. The internal photodiode current can be several orders of magnitude below "Rule 07" in dependence on specific cut-off wavelength and operating temperature.

The experimental data published in literature for p-on-n HgCdTe photodiodes (Teledyne) and for an alternative to HgCdTe material systems like III-V barrier detectors (Raytheon and SCD) operated at about 80 K, and room temperature interband quantum cascade infrared photodetectors (IB QCIPs)

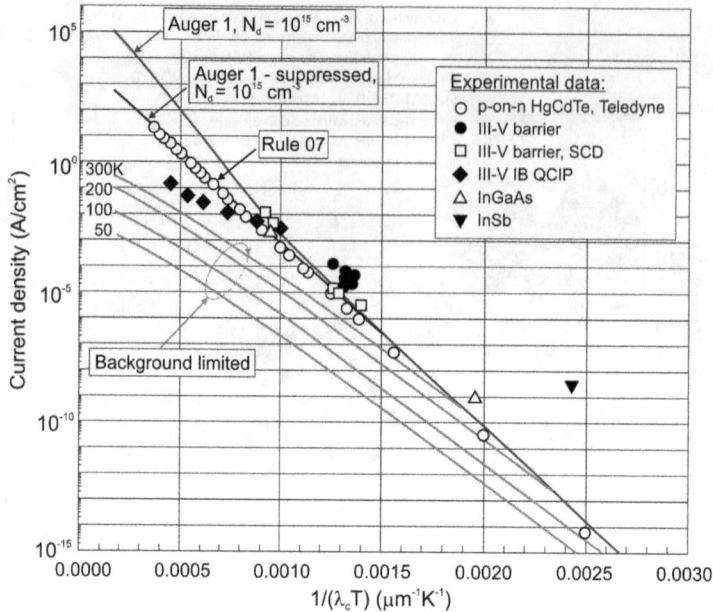

FIGURE 7.42 Current density of p-on-n HgCdTe photodiodes versus $1/(\lambda_c T)$ product (after Reference 74). Experimental data is gathered for Teledyne and alternative technologies.

are presented in 7.42 [74]. It is easy to notice that experimental data for III-V barrier detectors are slightly worse in comparison with the p-on-n HgCdTe photodiodes, but III-V IB QCIPs operated at 300 K are even better in LWIR spectral region. Figure 7.42 shows also representative data for both InSb ($\lambda_c = 5.3$ μm, $T = 78$ K) and InGaAs ($\lambda_c = 1.7$ and 3.6 μm, $T = 300$ K) photodiodes. InSb detector is characterised by several orders higher dark current density than the HgCdTe one; however, for optimal InGaAs photodiodes the dark current density is close to HgCdTe data.

Figure 7.43 gathers the highest detectivity values published in literature for different types of single element photodetectors operating at room temperature. This fact should be clearly emphasised, since detectivity data marked for commercial photodetectors are typical for pixels of infrared focal plane arrays. Figure 7.43 also indicates on the fundamental indicator for future trend in development of HOT IR photodetectors. It is shown that the detectivity of low-doping P-i-N HgCdTe (5×10^{13} cm^{-3}) photodiodes, operating at room-temperature in spectral band above 3 μm, is limited by background radiation (with D^* level above 10^{10} Jones, not limited by detector itself) and can be improved more than one order of magnitude in comparison with predicted by "Rule 07". Between different material systems used in fabrication of HOT LWIR photodetectors, only the HgCdTe ternary alloy can fulfil required expectations: low doping concentration – 10^{13} cm^{-3} and high SRH carrier lifetime – above 1 ms [62]. In this context it will be rather difficult to rival two-dimensional (2D) material photodetectors and colloidal quantum dot (CQD) photodetectors with HgCdTe photodiodes. The above estimations provide further encouragement for achieving low-cost and high-performance MWIR and LWIR HgCdTe focal plane arrays operating in HOT conditions. The performance of type-II superlattice (T2SL) IB QCIPs is close to HgCdTe photodiodes, and quantum cascade photodetectors can operate in temperatures above 300 K; however their disadvantages are challenging technology and higher cost of fabrication.

Since HgCdTe ternary alloy is a direct bandgap semiconductor; it is a very efficient absorber of radiation due to a high absorption coefficient. To achieve high quantum efficiency, the thickness of active detector layer should be equal to at least the cut-off wavelength. Typical quantum efficiency with antireflection coating is about 90 per cent. Substrate removal of backside illuminated

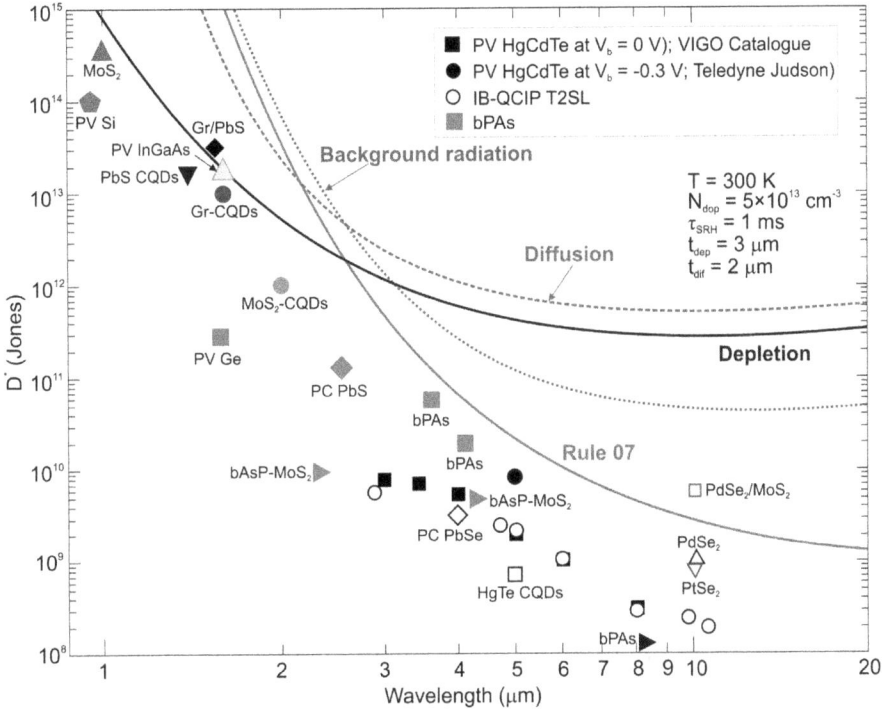

FIGURE 7.43 Detectivity versus wavelength for the commercially available room-temperature IR photodetectors (PV Si and Ge, PV InGaAs, PC PbS and PbSe, PV HgCdTe). There are also included experimental data for IB QCIP T2SLs, different type of 2D material and colloidal quantum dot (CQD) photodetectors taken from literature as marked. The theoretical curves are calculated for P-i-N HOT HgCdTe photodiodes assuming the value of τ_{SRH} = 1 ms, the absorber doping level of 5×10^{13} cm^{-3} and the thickness of active region t = 5 μm. PC – photoconductor, PV – photodiode (after Reference 74).

photodiode results in increasing of quantum efficiency in the short wavelength spectral range. Figure 4.7 illustrates the representative spectral detectivities of HgCdTe photodetectors.

HgCdTe ternary alloy is also attractive material for room temperature avalanche photodiodes (APDs). Its operation at 1.3–1.6 μm wavelengths for fibre optical communication applications was recognised in the 1980s. The resonant enhancement occurs when the spin-orbit splitting energy in the valence band, Δ, is equal to the fundamental energy gap, E_g. This has the beneficial effect, first pointed out by Verie *et al.* of making the electron and hole impact ionisation rates quite different, which is highly desirable for low-noise APDs [75].

E-APDs are proving to be vital components in many future infrared systems with low photon counts. Although their concept dates back to the 1980s, the first e-APD arrays were produced in the early 2000s [76], and at present a number of manufacturers developed e-APDs for laser-gating imaging and burst-illumination LIDAR for long-range target identification.

As shown in Figure 7.44, the avalanche properties of $Hg_{1-x}Cd_xTe$ vary dramatically with bandgap. Leveque *et al.* [77] described two regimes in which the ratio $k = \alpha_h/\alpha_e$ of the hole ionisation coefficient to the electron ionisation coefficient is either much greater or much less than unity. For cut-off wavelengths shorter than approximately 1.9 μm (x = 0.65 at 300 K), they predict $\alpha_h \gg \alpha_e$ because of resonant enhancement of the hole ionisation coefficient when $E_g \cong \Delta$ = 0.938 eV. The situation, when $k = \alpha_h/\alpha_e \gg 1$, is favourable for low-noise APDs with hole-initiated avalanche.

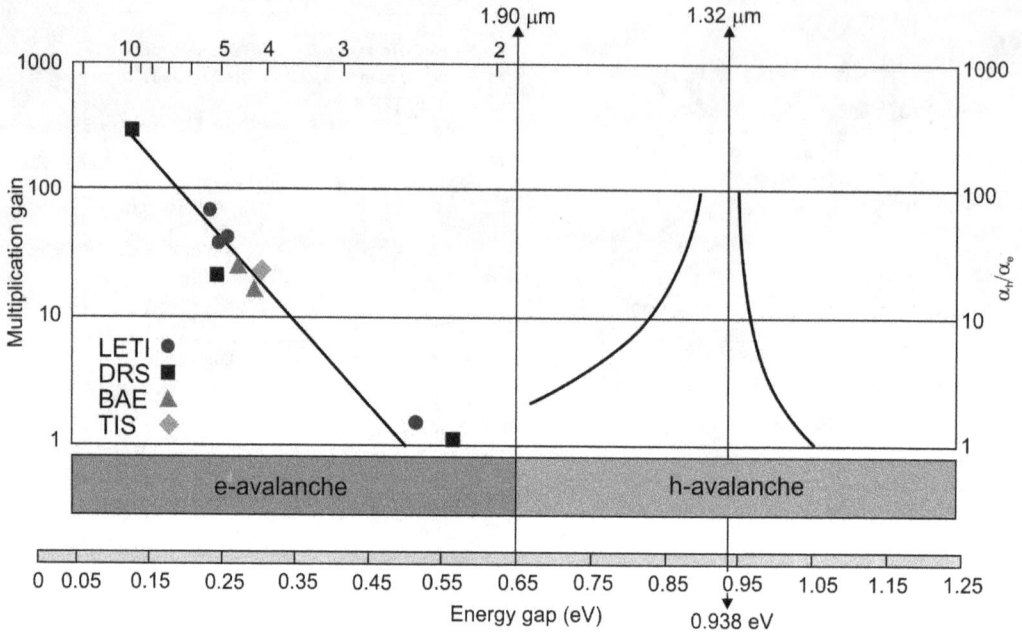

FIGURE 7.44 The distinct e-APD and h-APD regimes of $Hg_{1-x}Cd_xTe$ cross over at $E_g \approx 0.65$ eV ($\lambda_c = 1.9$ μm). At lower bandgaps the e-APD gain increases exponentially (material for four manufacturers shows remarkably consistent results).

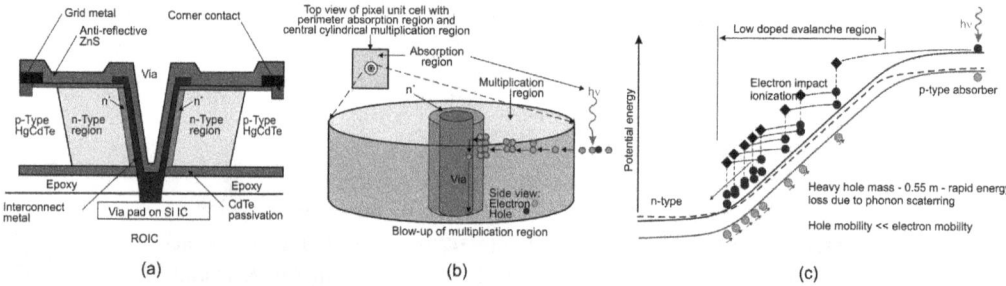

FIGURE 7.45 Electron avalanche process in HgCdTe HDVIP: (a) n⁺-n⁻p photodiode design, (b) cross-section view and operation of photodiode, (c) avalanche mechanism.

In 1999 DRS researchers proposed an APD based on their cylindrical p-around-n HDVIP (high-density vertically integrated photodiode). This architecture is shown in Figure 7.45 and is used also in production of avalanche photodiode FPAs [78]. As the figure shows, this is an electron-gain mechanism, so the p-type absorber dictates an n-on-p structure. Theoretical studies indicate that there is an optimum width for the depletion region (gain zone) of 1.5–2.5 μm. If the reverse bias increases from typical 50 mV to several volts, the centralised n-region becomes fully depleted and produces the high field region in which multiplication occurs. The hole-electron pairs are optically generated in the surrounding p-type absorption region and next diffuse to the multiplication region and thus comprise the injection species. DRS's APD is a front side illuminated photodiode with high quantum efficiency response from visible region to IR cut-off. APDs fabricated by Leti and Selex are backside illuminated. Typical gain values for MWIR photodiodes are above 100.

7.5.5 Lead Salt Photoconductors

Lead salt thin film photoconductors were first produced in Germany and next in the United States at Northwestern University in 1944 and, in 1945 at the Admiralty Research Laboratory in England. During the Second World War the Germans produced systems using PbS detectors which were able to detect hot aircraft engines. Immediately after the war, communications, fire-control and search systems began to stimulate a strong development effort that has extended to the present day. The Sidewinder heat-seeking infrared-guided missiles received a great deal of public attention. After 70 years, low-cost, versatile PbS and PbSe polycrystalline thin films remain the photoconductive detectors of choice for many applications in the 1–3 μm and 3–5 μm spectral range.

The PbSe and PbS films used in commercial IR detectors are made by chemical bath deposition (CBD), the oldest and most-studied PbSe and PbS thin-film deposition method. The basis of CBD is a precipitation reaction between a slowly produced anion (S^{2-} or Se^{2-}) and a complexed metal cation. The commonly used precursors are lead salts, $Pb(CH_3COO)_2$ or $Pb(NO_3)_2$, thiourea [$(NH_2)_2CS$] for PbS and selenourea [$(NH_2)_2CSe$] for PbSe, all in alkaline solutions. Lead may be complexed with citrate, ammonia, triethanolnamine, or with selenosulfate itself. Most often, however, the deposition is carried out in a highly alkaline solution where OH⁻ acts as the complexing agent for Pb^{2+}.

As-deposited PbS films exhibit significant photoconductivity. However, a post-deposition baking process is used to achieve final sensitisation. In order to obtain high-performance detectors, lead chalcogenide films need to be sensitised by oxidation. The oxidation may be carried out by using additives in the deposition bath, by postdeposition heat treatment in the presence of oxygen, or by chemical oxidation of the film. The effect of the oxidant is to introduce sensitising centres and additional states into the bandgap and thereby increase the lifetime of the photoexcited holes in the p-type material.

The films are deposited, either over or under plated gold electrodes, and on fused quartz, crystal quartz, single crystal sapphire, glass, various ceramics, single crystal strontium titanate, Irtran II (ZnS), Si and Ge. Different shapes of substrates are used: flat, cylindrical, or spherical. To obtain higher collection efficiency, detectors may be deposited directly by immersion onto optical materials with high indices of refraction (e.g., into strontium titanate). Lead salts cannot be immersed directly; special optical cements must be used between the film and the optical element. Standard active area sizes are typically 1, 2, or 3 mm squares. However, most manufacturers offer sizes ranging from 0.08×0.08 to 10×10 mm² for PbSe detectors, and 0.025×0.025 to 10×10 mm² for PbS detectors.

The spectral distribution of detectivity of lead salt detectors is presented in Figure 7.46 [79]. Usually, the operating temperatures of detectors are between −196 and 100°C; it is possible to operate at a temperature higher than recommended, but 150°C should never be exceeded.

7.5.6 Extrinsic Photoconductors

Extrinsic photoresistors are used in a wide range of the IR spectrum extending from a few μm to approximately 300 μm. They are the principal detectors operating in the range $\lambda > 20$ μm [80]. The basic operation of extrinsic photoconductors is similar to that of intrinsic ones except that the excitation energy required to free a charge carrier from an impurity atom must be substituted for the bandgap energy. The absorption coefficient is

$$\alpha(\lambda) = \sigma_i(\lambda) N_i, \tag{7.3}$$

where $\sigma_i(\lambda)$ is the photoionisation cross section and N_i is the neutral impurity concentration. The N_i is limited by the solubility of the impurity atoms in the semiconductor. In addition, the conductivity mode cannot be adequately controlled by operating the detector at low temperature to freeze them out or by other means, for example, hopping. Typical impurity concentration is around 10^{15} to 10^{16} cm⁻³ for silicon and somewhat lower for germanium, which causes the absorption coefficients to be

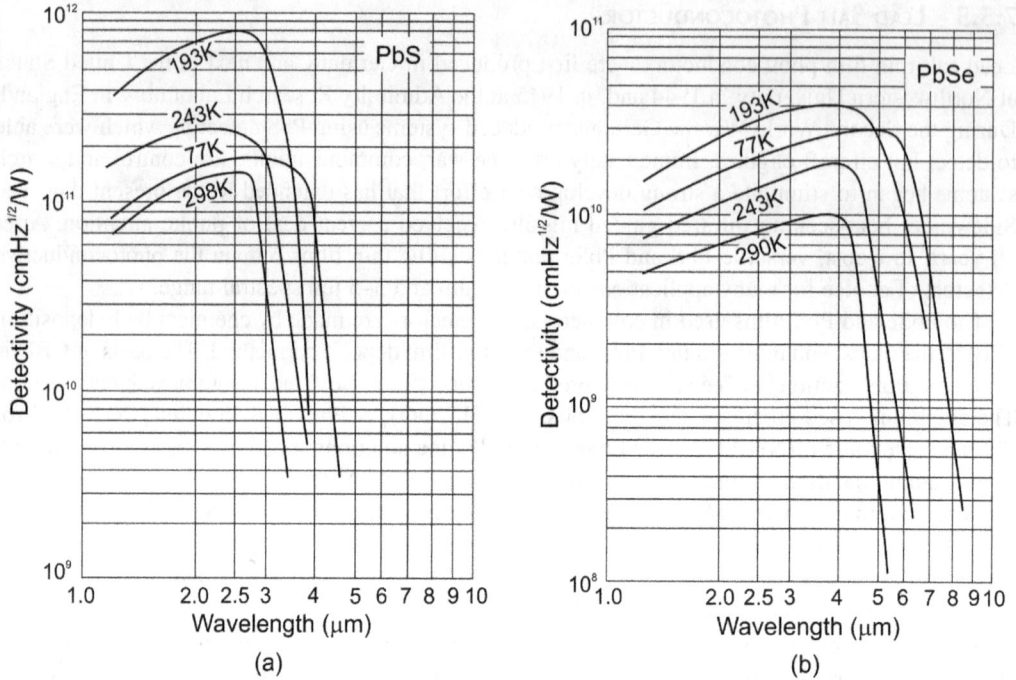

FIGURE 7.46 Typical spectral detectivity for (a) PbS, and (b) PbSe photoconductors.

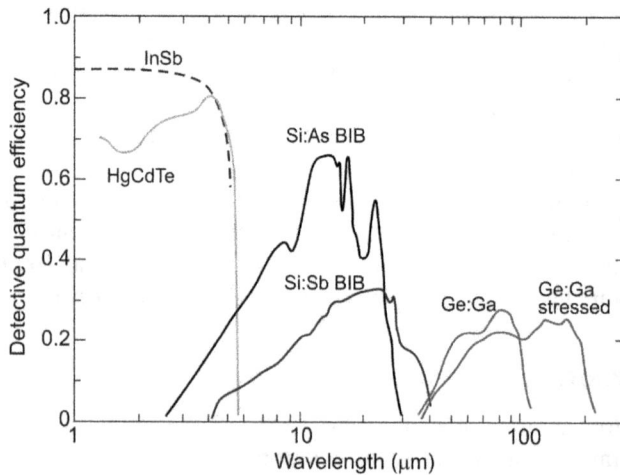

FIGURE 7.47 Typical quantum efficiency of semiconductors used in the wavelength range between 1 and 300 μm.

about three orders of magnitude less than those for direct absorption in intrinsic semiconductors. Practical values of α for optimised photoconductors are in the range 1–10 cm^{-1} for Ge and 10–50 cm^{-1} for Si. Thus, to maximise quantum efficiency, the thickness of the detector crystal should be not less than about 0.5 cm for doped Ge and about 0.1 cm for doped Si. There is a limit in thickness of extrinsic detectors, because photocarriers generated beyond the drift length $L_d = \mu\tau E$ recombine before being collected. Fortunately, for the most extrinsic detectors the drift length is sufficiently long that quantum efficiencies approaching 30–50 per cent can be obtained, which is shown in Figure 7.47.

A key difference between intrinsic and extrinsic detectors is that extrinsic detectors require much more cooling to achieve high sensitivity at a given spectral response cut-off in comparison with intrinsic detectors. Low-temperature operation is associated with longer-wavelength sensitivity in order to suppress noise due to thermally induced transitions between close-lying energy levels – see Figure 4.5.

Detectors based on silicon and germanium have found the widest application as compared with extrinsic photodetectors on other materials. Si has several advantages over Ge; for example, three orders of magnitude higher impurity solubilities are attainable, hence, thinner detectors with better spatial resolution can be fabricated from silicon. Si has lower dielectric constant than Ge, and the related device technology of Si has now been more thoroughly developed, including contacting methods, surface passivation and mature MOS and CCD technologies. Moreover, Si detectors are characterised by superior hardness in nuclear radiation environments. Figure 7.48 illustrates the spectral response for several extrinsic detectors.

Germanium photoconductors have been used in a variety of infrared astronomical experiments, both airborne and space-based at wavelengths ranging from 3 to more than 200 μm. Very shallow

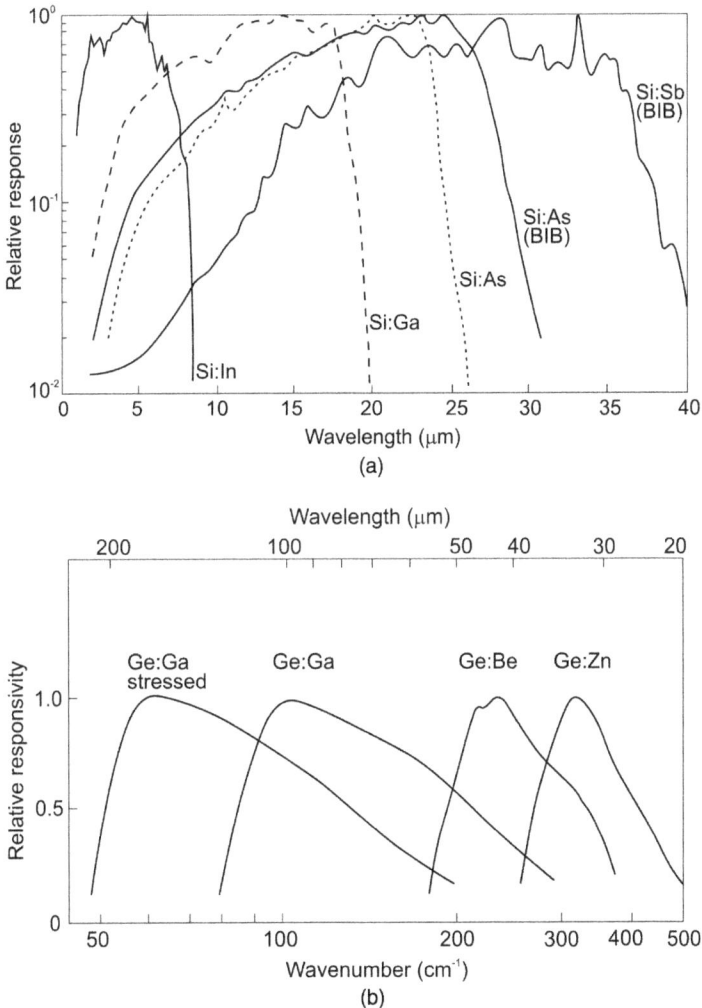

FIGURE 7.48 Examples of extrinsic silicon (a) and germanium (b) detector spectral response (after References 81 and 82).

donors, such as Sb, and acceptors, such as B, In or Ga, provide cut-off wavelengths in the region of 100 μm. Application of uniaxial stress along the [100] axis of Ge:Ga crystals reduces the Ga acceptor binding energy, extending the cut-off wavelength to ≈ 240 μm. At the same time, the operating temperature must be reduced to less than 2 K.

The availability of a highly developed silicon CMOS technology facilities the integration of large detector arrays with devices for readout and signal processing. The well-established technology also helps in the manufacturing of uniform detector arrays and the formation of low-noise contacts. Although the potential of large extrinsic silicon focal plane arrays for terrestrial applications has been examined, interest has declined in favour of HgCdTe and InSb with their more convenient operating temperatures. Strong interest in doped silicon continues for space applications, particularly in low background flux and for wavelengths from 14 to 30 μm, where compositional control is difficult for HgCdTe.

To maximise the quantum efficiency and detectivity of extrinsic photoconductors, the doping level should be as high as possible. This is particularly important when the devices are required to be radiation hard and are made as thin as possible to minimise the absorbing volume for ionising radiation. The limit to useful doping possible in conventional extrinsic detectors is set by the onset of impurity banding. This occurs when the doping level is sufficiently high that the wavefunctions of neighbouring impurities overlap, and their energy level is broadened to a band, which can support hopping conduction.

Blocked impurity band (BIB) detectors overcome the limitation of the doping density present in a standard extrinsic photoconductor by placing a thin intrinsic (undoped) silicon blocking layer between a heavily doped IR active layer and a planar contact (see Figure 7.49) [83]. The active region of detector structure, usually based on epitaxially grown n-type material, is sandwiched between a higher doped degenerate substrate electrode and an undoped blocking layer. Doping of active layer is high enough for the onset of an impurity band in order to display a high quantum efficiency for impurity ionisation (in the case of Si:As BIB, the active layer is doped to ≈ 5×10^{17} cm^{-3}). The device exhibits a diode-like characteristic, except that photoexcitation of electrons takes place between the donor impurity and the conduction band. The heavily doped n-type IR-active layer has a small concentration of negatively charged compensating acceptor impurities. In the absence of an applied bias, charge neutrality requires an equal concentration of ionised donors. Whereas the negative charges are fixed at acceptor sites, the positive charges associated with ionised donor sites (D$^+$ charges) are mobile and can propagate through the IR-active layer via the mechanism of hopping between occupied (D^0) and vacant (D$^+$) neighbouring sites. A positive bias to the contact creates a field that drives the pre-existing D$^+$ charges towards the substrate, while the undoped blocking layer prevents the injection of new D$^+$ charges. A region depleted of D$^+$ charges is therefore created, with a width depending on the applied bias and on the compensating acceptor concentration.

BIB detectors effectively use the hopping conductivity associated with "impurity banding" in relatively heavily doped semiconductors. Because of the presence of the blocking layer, BIB detectors do not follow the usual photoconductor model. The gap between the impurity band and the conduction band is narrow; therefore, the response of a BIB detector extends to the VLWIR region of the spectrum. BIB detectors have demonstrated other significant advantages, such as freedom from the irregular behaviour typical of photoconductive detectors (spiking, anomalous transient response), increased frequency range for constant responsivity and superior uniformity of response over the detector area and from detector to detector.

The main application of BIB arrays today is for ground- and space-based far-infrared astronomy. The details of the arrangement of steps in detector preparation depend on whether the detector is to be front illuminated through the first contact and blocking layer or back illuminated through the second contact. These two geometries are illustrated in Figure 7.50 and are described in detail in Rieke's monograph [84]. Fabrication of a back-illuminated BIB detector begins with an ion-implanted buried electrical contact. The relatively highly doped IR-active layer and undoped

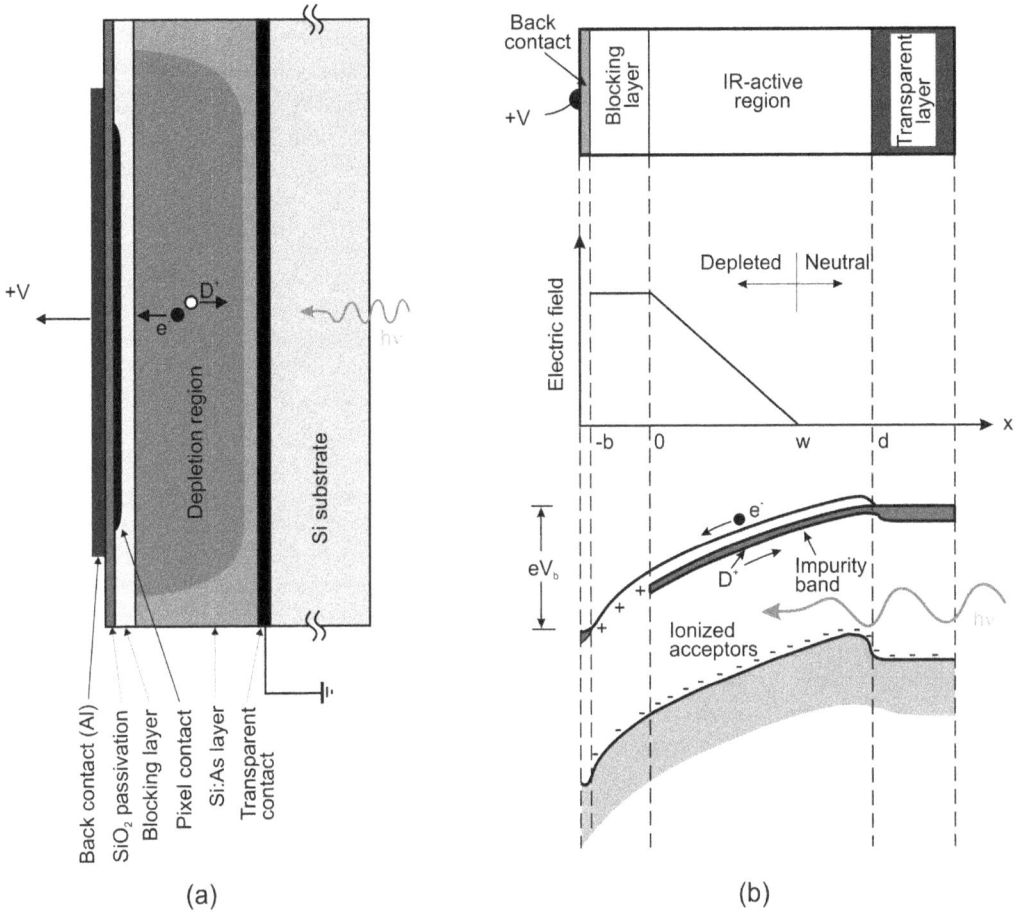

FIGURE 7.49 Si:As BIB detector: (a) layer structure of Si:As BIB detector, and (b) energy band structure of a positively biased detector.

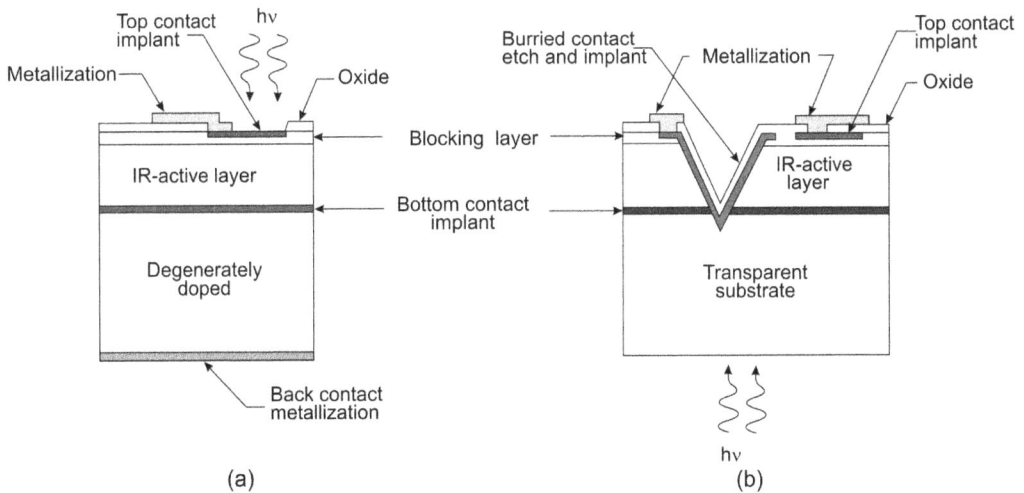

FIGURE 7.50 (a) Front illuminated BIB detector compared with (b) a back illuminated detector.

blocking layer are grown epitaxially over the buried contact. In the front illuminated detector, a transparent contact is implanted into the blocking layer, and the second contact is made by growing the detector on an extremely heavily doped, electrically conducting (degenerate) substrate. In the latter case, a thin degenerate but transparent contact layer is grown underneath the active layer on a high-purity, transparent substrate. The bias voltage on the buried contact is established through a V-shaped etched trough, metal-coated to make it conductive and placed to one side of the detector.

PROBLEMS

Example 7.1

Illumination of the SiC detector resulted in a voltage of 1 V across the 50-Ω R_L resistor. Calculate the radiant flux on the detector surface, assuming that the energy gap $E_g = 3.1$ eV and the quantum efficiency is 95 per cent.

Example 7.2

In a p-i-n photodiode, one electron-hole pair is produced by three photons with a wavelength of 800 nm. Assume that all electrons are counted at the detector output. Calculate the quantum efficiency, the maximum value of the semiconductor energy gap at which the photodiode will detect radiation and the average value of the photocurrent when $\Phi_e = 10^{-7}$ W.

Example 7.3 (Adapted after S.O. Kasap, Optoelectronics and Photonics: Principles and Practices, 2nd edition, Pearson, Essex, 2013)

Show that a photodiode has maximum quantum efficiency when $dR / d\lambda = R / \lambda$, that is, when the tangent of current responsivity, R, (see Figure 4.4) passes through the origin ($R = 0$ at wavelength $\lambda = 0$).

Example 7.4

Calculate the photocurrent density of a p-i-n Si photodiode with a 8 μm i-region when 0.87 μm light of power density 0.5 W/cm^2 is incident upon it. The absorption coefficient is equal to 600 cm^{-1}. It is assumed that the top-illuminated surface is coated with antireflection coating.

Example 7.5 (Adapted after S.O. Kasap, Optoelectronics and Photonics: Principles and Practices, 2nd edition, Pearson, Essex, 2013)

A p-i-n Si photodiode has an i-Si layer of width 20 μm. The p$^+$-layer on the illumination side is very thin (0.1 μm). The p-i-n is reverse-biased by a voltage of 100 V and then illuminated with a very short optical pulse of wavelength 900 nm. The absorption coefficient at 900 nm is 3×10^4 m^{-1}. What is the duration of the photocurrent if absorption occurs over the whole i-Si layer?

Example 7.6 (Adapted after S.O. Kasap, Optoelectronics and Photonics: Principles and Practices, 2nd edition, Pearson, Essex, 2013)

A Si p-i-n photodiode has an active light-receiving area of diameter 0.4 mm. When radiation of wavelength 700 nm (red light) and intensity 0.1 mW/cm² is incident, it generates a photocurrent of 56.6 nA. What is the responsivity and external quantum efficiency of the photodiode at 700 nm?

Example 7.7 (Adapted after S.O. Kasap, Optoelectronics and Photonics: Principles and Practices, 2nd edition, Pearson, Essex, 2013)

An InGaAs APD has a quantum efficiency of 60 per cent at 1.55 μm in the absence of multiplication ($M = 1$). It is biased to operate with a multiplication of 12. Calculate the photocurrent if the incident optical power is 20 nW. What is the responsivity when the multiplication is 12?

Example 7.8

Illumination of n-type Si ($N_d = 10^{16}$ cm^{-3}) generates 10^{21} cm^{-3}/s electron-hole pairs. Si has $N_t = 10^{15}$ cm^{-3} generation-recombination centres with capture cross section $\sigma_n = \sigma_p = 10^{-16}$ cm^2. Calculate equilibrium concentration of electrons and holes if $E_t = E_i$, where E_i is the Fermi level of intrinsic Si, and $v_t = 10^7$ cm/s.

Example 7.9 (Adapted after S.O. Kasap, Optoelectronics and Photonics: Principles and Practices, 2nd edition, Pearson, Essex, 2013)

A Si p-i-n photodiode has a quoted *NEP* of 1×10^{-13} W/Hz$^{1/2}$. What is the optical signal power it needs for a signal to noise ratio (SNR) of 1 if the bandwidth of operation is 1 GHz?

Example 7.10 (Adapted after S.O. Kasap, Optoelectronics and Photonics: Principles and Practices, 2nd edition, Pearson, Essex, 2013).

Consider an ideal photodiode with quantum efficiency equal 1 (100%) and no dark current, $I_d = 0$. Show that the minimum optical power required for a signal to noise ratio (SNR) of 1 is

$$P = \frac{2hc}{\lambda} \Delta f$$

Calculate the minimum optical power for a SNR = 1 for an ideal photodetector operating at 1300 nm with a bandwidth of 1 GHz. What is the corresponding photocurrent?

REFERENCES

1. W. Smith, "Effect of light on selenium during the passage of an electric current", *Nature* 7, 303 (1973).
2. V.K. Zworykin and G.A. Morton, *Television*, 1st edition, John Wiley, New York, 1940.

3. P. Norton, "Detector focal plane array technology", in *Encyclopedia of Optical Engineering*, edited by R. Driggers, pp. 320–348, Marcel Dekker, New York, 2003.

4. B.D. Milbrath, A.J. Peurrung, M. Bliss, and W.J. Weber, "Radiation detector materials: An overview", *J. Mater. Res.* 23, 2561–2581 (2008).

5. http://chandra.harvard.edu/about/science_instruments.html.

6. T.E. Peterson and L.R. Furenlid, "SPECT detectors: the Anger Camera and beyond", *Phys. Med. Biol.* 56, R145–R182 (2011).

7. A. Celler, "Single photon imaging and instrumentation", in *Encyclopedia of Spectroscopy and Spectrometry*, 2nd edition, pp. 2531–2538, edited by J.C. Lindon, G.E. Tranter, and D.W. Koppenaal, Elsevier, Oxford, 2010.

8. B.G. Lowe and R.A. Sareen, *Semiconductor X-Ray Detectors*, CRC Press, Boca Raton, 2017.

9. L. Korthout, D. Verbugt, J. Timpert, A. Mierop, W. de Haan, W. Maes, L.J. de Meulmeester, W. Muhammad, B. Dillen, H. Stoldt, I. Peters, E. Fox, "A wafer-scale CMOS APS imager for medical X-ray applications", www.teledynedalsa.com/download/9702540b-5a05-4b11-a463-add8131a9845/.

10. G. Zentai, "Comparison of CMOS and a-Si flat panel imagers for X-ray imaging", *IEEE Int. Conf. Imaging Syst. Tech.* 194–200 (2011).

11. www.dexela.com/cmos.aspx.

12. R.L. Weisfield, "Amorphous silicon TFT X-ray image sensors", *Electron Devices Meeting, 1998. Technical Digest*, January 1999. doi: 10.1109/IEDM.1998.746237.

13. Y. Bai, J. Bajaj, J.W. Beletic, and M.C. Farris, "Teledyne imaging sensors: silicon CMOS imaging technologies for x-ray, UV, visible and near infrared", *Proc. SPIE* 7021, 702102-1–16 (2008).

14. C. Szeles, "CdZnTe and CdTe materials for X-ray and gamma ray radiation detector applications", *Phys. Stat. Sol. (b)* 241, 783–790 (2004).

15. A.E. Bolotnikov, G.S. Camarda, G.A. Carini, G.W. Wright, L.Li, A. Burger, M. Groza, and R.B. James, "Large area/volume CZT nuclear detectors", *Phys. Stat. Sol. (c)* 2, 1495–1503 (2005).

16. S. Del Sordo, L. Abbene, E. Caroli, A.M. Mancini, A. Zappettini, and P. Ubertini, "Progress in the development of CdTe and CdZnTe semiconductor radiation detectors for astrophysical and medical applications", *Sensors* 9, 3491–3526 (2009).

17. D. Pennicard, B. Pirard, O. Tolbanov, and K. Iniewski, "Semiconductor materials for x-ray detectors", *MRS Bulletin* 42(6), 445–450 (2017).

18. T. Takahashi and S. Watanabe, "Recent progress in CdTe and CdZnTe detectors", *IEEE Trans. Nuclear Science* 48, 950–959 (2001).

19. T.O. Tümer, S. Yin, V. Cajipe, H. Flores, J. Mainprize, G. Mawdsleyb, J.A. Rowlands, M.J. Yaffe, E.E. Gordon, W.J. Hamilton, D. Rhiger, S.O. Kasap, P. Selline, and K.S. Shah, "High-resolution pixel detectors for second generation digital mammography", *Nucl. Instrum. Methods Phys. Res. A* 497, 21–29 (2003).

20. www.autoklaw.com/produkty/rtg-i-obrazowanie/rtg-pantomograficzne-2/ajat-pantomografy-cdte/ajat-art-plus-ceph-rtg.pdf.

21. O.H.W. Siegmund, J.V. Vallerga, J. McPhate, and A.S. Tremsin, "Next generation microchannel plate detector technologies for UV astronomy", *Proc. SPIE* 5488, 789–800 (2004).

22. O.H.W. Siegmund, A.S. Tremsin, J.V. Vallerga, J.B. McPhate, J.S. Hull, J. Malloy, and A.M. Dabiran, "Gallium nitride photocathode development for imaging detectors", *Proc. SPIE* 7021, 70211B-1-1–9 (2008).

23. J.V. Vallerga, J.B. McPhate, A.S. Tremsin, and O.H.W. Siegmund, "The current and future capabilities of MCP based UV detectors", *Astrophys. Space Sci.* 320, 247–250 (2009).

24. K. Sembach, "Technology investments to meet the needs of astronomy at ultraviolet wavelengths in the 21st century", www.astro.princeton.edu/~dns/Theia/Sembach_UVtechnology_EOS.pdf.

25. M. Razeghi and A. Rogalski, "Semiconductor ultraviolet detectors", *J. Appl. Phys.* 79, 7433–7473 (1996).

26. D. Walker and M. Razeghi, "The development of nitride-based UV photodetectors", *Opto-Electron. Rev.* 8, 25–42 (2000).

27. Y.S. Park, "Wide bandgap III-Nitride semiconductors: Opportunities for future optoelectronics", *Opto-Electron. Rev.* 9, 117–124 (2001).

28. F. Monroy, F. Omnes, and F. Calle, "Wide-bandgap semiconductor ultraviolet photodetectors", *Semicon. Sci. Technol.* 18, R33–R51 (2003).

29. Z. Alaie, S.M. Nejad, and M.H. Yousefi, "Recent advances in ultraviolet photodetectors", *Mater. Sci. Semicond. Process.* 29, 16–55 (2015).

30. P. Lamarre, A. Hairston, S.P. Tobin, K.K. Wong, A.K. Sood, M.B. Reine, M. Pophristic, R. Birkham, I.T. Ferguson, R. Singh, C.R. Eddy, Jr., U. Chowdhury, M.M. Wong, R.D. Dupuis, P. Kozodoy, and E. J. Tarsa, "AlGaN p-i-n photodiode arrays for solar-blind applications", *Phys. Stat. Sol. (a)* 188, 289–292 (2001).

31. S. Aslam, F. Yan, D.E. Pugel, D. Franz, L. Miko, F. Herrero, M. Matsumara, S. Babu, and C.M. Stahle, "Development of ultra-high sensitivity wide-bandgap UV-EUV detectors at NASA Goddard Space Flight Center", *Proc. SPIE* 5901, 59011J-1–12 (2005).

32. P.E. Malinowski, J.Y. Duboz, P. De Moor, J. John, K. Minoglou, P. Srivastava, Y. Creten, T. Torfs, J. Putzeys, F. Semond, E. Frayssinet, B. Giordanengo, A. BenMoussa, J.F. Hochedez, R. Mertens, and C. Van Hoof, "10 μm pixel-to-pixel pitch hybrid backside illuminated AlGaN-on-Si imagers for solar blind EUV radiation detection", *2010 International Electron Devices Meeting*, doi: 10.1109/IEDM.2010.5703362

33. J.P. Long, S. Varadaraajan, J. Matthews, and J.F. Schetzina, "UV detectors and focal plane array imagers based on AlGaN p-i-n photodiodes", *Opto-Electron. Rev.* 10, 251–260 (2002).

34. R. McClintock, K. Mayes, A. Yasan, D. Shiell, P. Kung, and M. Razeghi, "320×256 solar-blind focal plane arrays based on $Al_xGa_{1-x}N$", *Appl. Phys. Lett.* 86, 011117-1–3 (2005).

35. J.-L. Reverchon, S. Bansropun, J.-P. Truffer, E. Costard, E. Frayssinet, J. Brault, and J.-Y. Dubom, "Performances of AlGaN based focal plane arrays from 10 nm to 200 nm", *Proc. SPIE* 7691, 769109-1–9 (2010).

36. E. Cicek, Z. Vashaei, R. McClintock, and M. Razeghi, "Deep ultraviolet (254 nm) focal plane array", *Proc. SPIE* 8155, 81551O-1–9 (2011).

37. P.E. Malinowski, J.-Y. Duboz, P. De Moor, J. John, K. Minoglou, P. Srivastava, H. Abdul, M. Patel, H. Osman, F. Semond, E. Frayssinet, J.-F. Hochedez, B. Giordanengo, C. Van Hoof, and R. Mertens, "Backside illuminated AlGaN-on-Si UV detectors integrated by high density flip-chip bonding", *Phys. Stat. Sol. (c)* 8, 2476–2478 (2011).

38. S. Nikzad, T.J. Jones, S.T. Elliott, T.J. Cunningham, P.W. Deelman, A.B.C. Walker II, and H.M. Oluseyi, "Ultrastable and uniform EUV and UV detectors", *Proc. SPIE* 4139, 250–207 (2000).

39. www.stsci.edu/hst/wfc3/documents/handbooks/currentIHB/wfc3_cover.html.

40. M. Nesladek, "Conventional n-type doping in diamond: state of the art and recent progress", *Semicond. Sci. Technol.* 20, R19–R27 (2005).

41. A. BenMoussa, J.F. Hochedez, U. Schühle, W. Schmutz, K. Haenen, Y. Stockman, A. Soltani, F. Scholze, U. Kroth, V. Mortet, A. Theissen, C. Laubis, M. Richter, S. Koller, J.-M. Defise, S. Koizumi, "Diamond detectors for LYRA, the solar VUV radiometer on board PROBA2", *Diam. Relat. Mater.* 15, 802–806 (2006).

42. D.J. Paul, "Si/SiGe heterostructures: from material and physics to devices and circuits", *Semicond. Sci. Technol.* 19, R75–R108 (2004).

43. L. Pavesi, "Will silicon be the photonic material of the third millenium?", *J. Phys. Condens. Matter* 15, R1169–R1196 (2003).

44. A. Bandyopadhyay and M. J. Deen, "Photodetectors for optical fiber communications", in *Photodetectors and Fiber Optics*, ed. H. S. Nalwa, 307–368, Academic Press, San Diego, 2001.

45. Teledyne Judson Technologies, www.teledynejudson.com/products/germanium-detectors.

46. A.K. Sood, J.W. Zeller, R.A. Richwine, Y.R. Puri, H. Efstathiadis, P. Haldar, N.K. Dhar, and D.L. Polla, "SiGe based visible-NIR photodetector technology for optoelectronic applications", Chapter 10 in *Advances in Optical Fiber Technology: Fundamental Optical Phenomena and Applications*, edited by M. Yasin, H. Arof and S.W. Harun, InTech, 2015.

47. E. Kasper and M. Oehme, "High speed germanium detectors on Si", *Physica Status Solidi (c)* 5, 3144–3149, 2008.

48. M.J. Cohen and G. H. Olsen, "Room-temperature InGaAs camera for NIR imaging", *Proc. SPIE* 1946, 436–443, 1993.

49. A. Rogalski, *Infrared and Terahertz Detectors*, CRC Press, Boca Raton, 2019.

50. J.S. Ng, J.P.R. David, G.J. Rees, and J. Allam, "Avalanche breakdown voltage of $In_{0.53}Ga_{0.47}As$", *J. Appl. Phys.* 91, 5200–5202 (2002).

51. A.S. Huntington, *InGaAs Avalanche Photodiodes for Ranging and Lidar*, Elsevier, Duxford, 2020.

52. I. Gyuro, "MOVPE for InP-based optoelectronic device application", *III-Vs Rev.* 9(2), 30–35 (1996).

53. T.S. Moss, G.J. Burrel, and B. Ellis, *Semiconductor Optoelectronics*, Butterworths, London, 1973.

54. P.J. Love, K.J. Ando, R.E. Bornfreund, E. Corrales, R.E. Mills, J.R. Cripe, N.A. Lum, J.P. Rosbeck, and M.S. Smith, "Large-format infrared arrays for future space and ground-based astronomy applications", *Proc. SPIE* 4486, 373–384 (2002).

55. I. Shtrichman, D. Aronov, M Ben Ezra, I. Barkai, E. Berkowicz, M. Brumer, R. Fraenkel, A. Glozman, S. Grossman, E. Jacobsohn, O. Klin, P. Klipstein, I. Lukomsky, L. Shkedy, N. Snapi, M. Yassen, and E. Weiss, "High operating temperature epi-InSb and XBn-InAsSb photodetectors", *Proc. SPIE* 8353, 83532Y (2012).

56. Teledyne Judson Technologies, www.teledynejudson.com/products/indium-antimonide-detectors.

57. A. Rogalski, P. Martyniuk, M. Kopytko, and P. Madejczyk, "InAsSb-based infrared photodetectors: Thirty years later on", *Sensors* 20, 7047 (2020).

58. E.H. Steenbergen, "InAsSb-based photodetectors", in *Mid-Infrared Optoelectronics. Materials, Devices, and Applications*, pp. 415–453, edited by E. Tournie and L. Cerutti, Elsevier, Duxford, 2020.

59. N.D. Il'inskaya, S.A. Karandashev, A.A. Lavrova, B.A. Matveev, M.A. Remennyi, N.M. Stus', and A.A. Usikova, "InAsSbP photodiodes for 2.6–2.8-μm wavelengths", *Tech. Phys.* 63(2), 226–229 (2018).

60. www.hamamatsu.com/resources/pdf/ssd/infrared_kird0001e.pdf.

61. W.E. Tennant, D. Lee, M. Zandian, E. Piquette, and M. Carmody, "MBE HgCdTe technology: A very general solution to IR detection, described by 'Rule 07', a very convenient heuristic", *J. Electron. Materials* 37, 1406–1410 (2008).

62. D. Lee, P. Dreiske J. Ellsworth. R. Cottier, A. Chen, S. Tallaricao, A. Yulius, M. Carmody, E. Piquette, M. Zandian, and S. Douglas, "Law 19: The ultimate photodiode performance metric", *Proc. SPIE* 11407, 114070X (2020).

63. W.D. Lawson, S. Nielson, E.H. Putley, and A.S. Young, "Preparation and properties of HgTe and mixed crystals of HgTe-CdTe", *J. Phys. Chem. Solids* 9, 325–329 (1959).

64. M.B. Reine, "Fundamental properties of mercury cadmium telluride", in *Encyclopedia of Modern Optics*, Academic Press, London, 2004.

65. E. Burstein, J.W. Davisson, E.E. Bell, W.J. Turner, and H.G. Lipson, "Infrared photoconductivity due to neutral impurities in germanium", *Phys. Rev.* 93, 65–68 (1954).

66. S. Borrello and H. Levinstein, "Preparation and properties of mercury-doped germanium", *J. Appl. Phys.* 33, 2947–2950 (1962).

67. D. Long and J.L. Schmit, "Mercury-cadmium telluride and closely related alloys", in *Semiconductors and Semimetals,* Vol. 5, pp. 175–255, edited by R. K. Willardson and A. C. Beer, Academic Press, New York, 1970.

68. B.E. Bartlett, D.E. Charlton, W.E. Dunn, P.C. Ellen, M.D. Jenner, and M.H. Jervis, "Background limited photoconductive detectors for use in the 8–14 micron atmospheric window", *Infrared Phys.* 9, 35–36 (1969).

69. C.T Elliott, D. Day, and B.J. Wilson, "An integrating detector for serial scan thermal imaging", *Infrared Phys.* 22, 31–42 (1982).

70. A. Blackburn, M.V. Blackman, D.E. Charlton, W.A.E. Dunn, M.D. Jenner, K.J. Oliver, and J.T.M. Wotherspoon, "The practical realization and performance of SPRITE detectors", *Infrared Phys.* 22, 57–64 (1982).

71. T. Elliott, "Recollections of MCT work in the UK at Malvern and Southampton", *Proc. SPIE* 7298, 72982M-2-23 (2009).

72. W.S. Boyle and G.E. Smith, "Charge-coupled semiconductor devices", *Bell Syst. Tech. J.* 49, 587–593 (1970).

73. O. Gravrand, L. Mollard, C. Largeron, N. Baier, E. Deborniol, and Ph. Chorier, "Study of LWIR and VLWIR focal plane array developments: comparison between p-on-n and different n-on-p technologies on LPE HgCdTe", *J. Electron. Mater.* 38, 1733–1740 (2009).

74. A. Rogalski, P. Martyniuk, M. Kopytko, and W. Hu, "Trends in performance limits of the HOT infrared photodetectors", *Appl. Sci.* 11, 501 (2021).

75. C. Verie, F. Raymond, J. Besson, and T. Nquyen Duy, "Bandgap spin-orbit splitting resonance effects in $Hg_{1-x}Cd_xTe$ alloys", *J. Cryst. Growth* 59, 342–346 (1982).

76. J. D. Beck, C.-F. Wan, M. A. Kinch, and J. E. Robinson, "MWIR HgCdTe avalanche photodiodes", *Proc. SPIE* 4454, 188–197 (2001).

77. G. Leveque, M. Nasser, D. Bertho, B. Orsal, and R. Alabedra, "Ionization energies in $Cd_xHg_{1-x}Te$ avalanche photodiodes", *Semicond. Sci. Technol.* 8, 1317–1323 (1993).

78. J. Beck, C. Wan, M. Kinch, J. Robinson, P. Mitra, R. Scritchfield, F. Ma, and J. Campbell, "The HgCdTe electron avalanche photodiode", *IEEE LEOS Newsletter*, October 8–12, 2006.

79. New England Photoconductor data sheet, www.nepcorp.com.

80. N. Sclar, "Properties of doped silicon and germanium infrared detectors", *Prog. Quant. Electr.* 9, 149–257 (1984).

81. P.R. Norton, "Infrared image sensors", *Opt. Eng.* 30, 1649–1663 (1991).

82. J. Leotin and C. Meny "Far infrared photoconductors", *Proc. SPIE* 1341, 193–201 (1990).

83. M.D. Petroff and M.G. Stapelbroek, "Blocked impurity band detectors", *U.S. Patent*, No. 4 568 960, filed October 23, 1980, granted February 4, 1986.

84. G.H. Rieke, *Detection of Light: From the Ultraviolet to the Submillimeter*, 2nd ed., Cambridge University Press, Cambridge, 2003.

8 Quantum Well, Superlattice and Quantum Dot Photodetectors

Since the initial proposal by Esaki and Tsu [1] and the advent of MBE, the interest in semiconductor quantum well (QW) and superlattices (SLs) structures has increased continuously over the years, driven by technological challenges, new physical concepts and phenomena as well as promising applications. A new class of materials and heterojunctions with unique electronic and optical properties has been developed. Here we focus on devices that involve excitation of carriers in low dimensional solids (quantum wells, quantum dots, and superlattices). A distinguishing feature of these photodetectors is that they can be implemented in chemically stable wide bandgap materials, as a result of the use of intraband processes. On account of this, it is possible to use such material systems as GaAs/Al$_x$Ga$_{1-x}$As (GaAs/AlGaAs), In$_x$Ga$_{1-x}$As/In$_x$Al$_{1-x}$As (InGaAs/InAlAs), InSb/InAs$_{1-x}$Sb$_x$ (InSb/InAsSb), InAs/Ga$_{1-x}$In$_x$Sb (InAs/GaInSb), and Si$_{1-x}$Ge$_x$/Si (SiGe/Si), as well as other systems, although most of the experimental works have been carried out with AlGaAs. Some devices are sufficiently advanced that there exists the possibility of their incorporating in high-performance integrated circuits. High uniformity of epitaxial growth over large areas shows promise for the production of large- area two-dimensional arrays. In addition, flexibility associated with control over composition during epitaxial growth can be used to tailor the response of quantum photodetectors to particular spectral bands or multiple bands.

8.1 LOW DIMENSIONAL SOLIDS: BACKGROUND

In addition to the quantum well case, where energy barriers for electron motion exist in one direction of propagation, one can also imagine electron confinement in two directions and, as the ultimate case, in all three directions. The structures of these kinds are now known as quantum wires (QWs) and quantum dots (QDs). Thus, the family of dimensionalities of the device structures involves a bulky semiconductor epilayer [three-dimensional (3D)], a thin epitaxial layer of quantum well [two-dimensional (2D)], an elongated tube or quantum wire [one-dimensional (1D)] and, finally, an isolated island of QD [zero-dimensional (0D)]. These three cases are shown in Figure 8.1.

In a crystalline semiconductor, the electrons and holes that determine the transport and optical properties are considered as "quasi free" with the effective mass m^* taking account of the periodic crystal potential. The dimensions of a bulk semiconductor crystal are macroscopic on the scale of the de Broglie wavelength

$$\lambda = \frac{h}{\left(2m^*E\right)^{1/2}}, \tag{8.1}$$

DOI: 10.1201/9781003263098-8

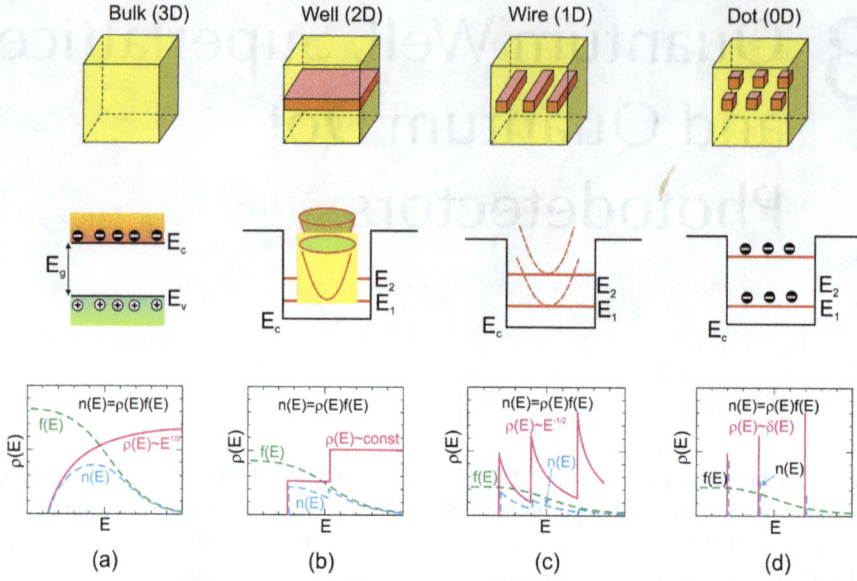

FIGURE 8.1 Schematics of density of states and carrier distribution for (a) bulk, (b) quantum wells, (c) quantum wires, and (d) quantum dots. Quantum dot density of states is independent of temperature.

and, thus, so-called size quantisation is negligible. The quasi-free electron wave functions are given by the Bloch functions

$$\Psi_{jk}^{3D}(r) = \frac{1}{V} u_{j\vec{k}}(\vec{r}) \exp(i\vec{k}\vec{r}), \tag{8.2}$$

where V is the macroscopic volume, $k = 2\pi/\lambda$, is the electron wave vector, and j is the band index. The Bloch-functions have the free particle wave function $\exp(i\vec{k}\vec{r})$ as the envelope, instead, allowed k-values as defined by the crystal boundaries are quasi continuous. The energy dispersion of quasi-free electrons (holes) at the bottom of the conduction band (at the top of the valence band) is given by

$$E^{3D} = \frac{\hbar^2 k^2}{2m^*}, \tag{8.3}$$

where $\hbar$ is Planck's constant. This quadratic dispersion results in a parabolic density of states function

$$\rho^{3D} = \frac{1}{2\pi^2}\left(\frac{2m^*}{\hbar^2}\right)^{3/2} E^{1/2}. \tag{8.4}$$

While the density of states characterises the energy distribution of allowed states, the Fermi function, f, gives the probability of electron occupation at certain energy even if no allowed state exists at all at that energy. Thus, the product of ρ and the Fermi function describe the total concentration of the charge carriers of the given type in a crystal:

$$n = \int \rho(E) f(E) dE. \tag{8.5}$$

The transport and optical properties of semiconductors are basically determined by the upper-most valence band and lowest conduction band, which are separated in energy by the bandgap E_g. The bandgap structure of GaAs consists of a heavy hole, light hole, and split-off valence band and the lowest conduction band. GaAs is a direct gap semiconductor with the maximum of the valence band and minimum of the conduction band at the same position in the Brillouin zone at $k = 0$ (Γ-point). AlAs is an indirect-gap semiconductor with the lowest conduction band minimum close to the boundary of the Brillouin zone in (100) direction at the X-point. In addition, the conduction band minimum in AlAs is highly unisotrop with a longitudinal and transverse electron mass $m_l^* = 1.1m_o$ and $m_t^* = 0.2m_o$, respectively.

Confinement of electrons in one or more dimensions modifies the wave functions, dispersion and density of states (see Figure 8.1). The effective potential associated with spatial variation of the conduction and valence band edges is spatially modulated in so-called compositional superlattices that consist of alternating layers of two different semiconductors. Figure 8.2 illustrates the electronic states associated with planar quantum wells and superlattices. Widths of minibands in superlattices are related by the uncertainty principle to well-to-well tunnelling times. In a typical case, barrier regions would be AlGaAs layers, and wells would be GaAs. Typical distance scales (≈ 50 Å) over which composition is varied is small compared with distances over which ballistic electron propagation has been observed. This supports the notion that wave functions can be coherent throughout structures that have spatially modulated composition. The wave functions just referred to are the envelope wave functions of effective mass theory. Spatial variation of the host composition introduces a number of sublattices, but the basic picture of potentials and wave functions guides much of the effort in the field of quantum devices.

Each quantum well can be considered to be a three-dimensional rectangular potential well. When the thickness of the well is much less than the transverse dimensions ($L_z << L_x, L_y$), and the thickness is comparable to the de Broglie wavelength of the carriers in the well, quantisation of the carrier motion in the z-direction must be taken into account in the dispersion carrier dynamics. Motion in the x and y directions is not quantised, so that each state of the system corresponds to a subband. Electrons (or holes) in such a well can be regarded as a two-dimensional (2D) electron (or hole) gas. When the well is infinitely deep, the Schrödinger equation energy eigenvalues are

$$E^{2D} = E_{n_z} + \frac{\hbar^2 \left(k_x^2 + k_y^2 \right)}{2m^*}, \tag{8.6}$$

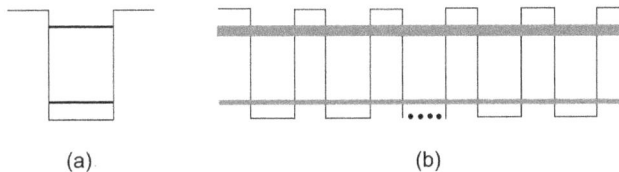

(a)   (b)

FIGURE 8.2   (a) Electron bound states in a quantum well, and (b) the formation of minibands in a superlattice. The confining potentials are associated with the conduction band edge.

with the confinement energy

$$E_{n_z} = \frac{\hbar^2}{2m}\left(\frac{n_z \pi}{L_z}\right)^2,$$ (8.7)

where k_x and k_y are momentum vectors along the x and y axes, and n_z is the quantum number ($n_z = 1, 2, ...$). The electron wave functions are represented by plane waves in x and y direction and by even or odd harmonic functions in z direction:

$$\Psi_{n_z}^{2D} = \left(\frac{2}{L}\right)\exp\left(ik_x x\right)\exp\left(ik_y y\right)\left(\frac{2}{L_z}\right)^{1/2}\sin\left(k_{n_z} z\right).$$ (8.8)

Confinement of electrons by potential wells with finite height [see Figure 8.2(a)] does not affect the principal features of size quantisation as described above; however, it modifies the results in three important respects:

- The confinement energy for a given quantum state characterised by the quantum number n_z is lower for a finite barrier height.
- Only a finite number of quantised states is bound in a well with finite barrier height (for an infinitely high barrier an infinite number of quantised states exists); when the width of a single quantum well is decreased, the first excited state merges from the well and becomes a virtual state (Figure 8.3).
- The electron wave functions do not vanish at the boundary but penetrate into the barrier where the amplitude drops exponentially.

In a crystalline semiconductor, the electrons and holes that determine the transport and optical properties are considered as "quasi free" with the effective mass m^* taking account of the periodic crystal potential. The transport/optical properties are basically determined by the uppermost valence band and lowest conduction band, which are separated in energy by the bandgap, E_g. Farther confinement in two or finally three dimensions results in size quantisation in the corresponding directions and stronger discretisation of the energy spectrum and density of state distribution approaching atomic behaviour for three-dimensional confinement.

An ideal quantum dot, also known as a quantum box, is a structure capable of confining electrons in all three directions, thus allowing zero dimensions in their degree of freedom. The energy spectrum is completely discrete, similar to that in an atom. The total energy is the sum of three discrete components:

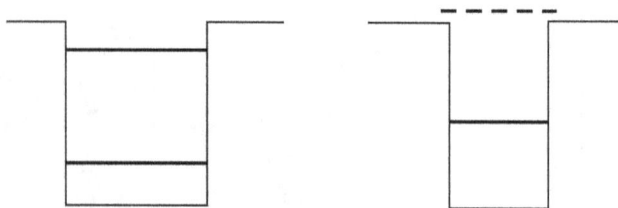

FIGURE 8.3   Illustration of the formation of a virtual state as the width of the quantum well is decreased.

$$E^{0D} = E_{nx} + E_{my} + E_{lz} = \frac{h^2 k_{nx}^2}{2m^*} + \frac{h^2 k_{my}^2}{2m^*} + \frac{h^2 k_{lz}^2}{2m^*}, \tag{8.9}$$

where n, m, and l are integers (1, 2, …) used to index the quantised energy levels and quantised wave numbers, which result from the confinement of the electron motion in the x, y, and z-directions, respectively.

As for the bulk material, the most important characteristic of a QD is its electron density of states in the conduction band given by

$$\rho^{0D}(E) = 2 \sum_{n,m,l} \delta\left[E_{nx} + E_{my} + E_{lz} - E\right], \tag{8.10}$$

where $\delta(E)$ is the Heaviside step function with $\delta(E \geq E_{nx}) = 1$ and $\delta(E < E_{nx}) = 0$. Each QD level can accommodate two electrons with different spin orientation.

The density of states of zero-dimensional electrons consists of Dirac functions, occurring at the discrete energy levels $E(n,m,l)$, as shown in Figure 8.1. The divergences in the density of states shown in Figure 8.1 are for ideal electrons in a QD and are smeared out in reality by a finite electron lifetime ($\Delta E \geq \hbar/\tau$). Since QDs have a discrete, atom-like energy spectrum, they can be visualised and described as "artificial atoms". This discreteness is expected to render the carrier dynamics very different from that in higher-dimensional structures where the density of states is continuous over a range of values of energy.

8.2 TYPES OF SUPERLATTICES

Early attempts to realise superlattices with properties suitable for infrared detection were unsuccessful, largely because of the difficulties associated with epitaxial deposition of HgTe/CdTe superlattices. More recently, significant interest has been shown in multiple quantum well AlGaAs/GaAs photoconductors. However, these detectors are extrinsic in nature, and have been predicted to be limited to performance inferior to that of intrinsic HgCdTe detectors. On account of this – in addition to the use of intersubband absorption and absorption in doping superlattice – two additional intrinsic intersubband transitions are utilised to directly shift bandgaps into the infrared spectral range:

- superlattice quantum confinement without strain: HgTe/HgCdTe;,
- strained type-II superlattices: InAs/GaSb and InAs/InAsSb.

Figure 8.4 shows schematics the band gap diagrams of three basic types of superlattices used in infrared detector fabrications [2].

Type I superlattices consist of alternating thin wider-bandgap layers of AlGaAs and GaAs. Their bandgaps are approximately aligned – the valence band (with symmetry of Γ_8) of one does not overlap the conduction band (with symmetry of Γ_6) of the other. Various forms exist, but generally the device is a majority photoconductor with infrared absorption achieved by transitions between the energy levels induced in the conduction band by dimensional quantisation. The AlGaAs layers are very thick barriers that inhibit excess current, such as tunnelling through the superlattice. Absorption coefficients of quantum well infrared photodetectors (QWIPs) are typically very small, and, due to selection rules for the optical transitions, ingenious tricks must be employed to couple efficiently incident-normal radiation into the structure efficiently due to selection rules for the optical transitions. The advantages of AlGaAs/GaAs QWIP architecture are: foundry materials technology,

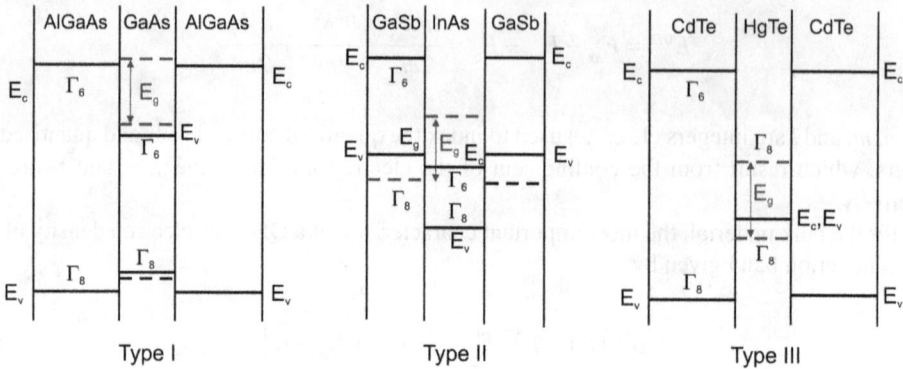

FIGURE 8.4 Bandgap diagrams of three basic types of superlattices designated for infrared detector applications.

design complexity capability, and low $1/f$ noise. The disadvantages are: high dark current, low quantum efficiency, and low operating temperatures.

Type II superlattice, representative of which is InAs/GaSb superlattice, is similar to type I with the exception of overlapping conduction and valence bands in adjacent bands. It utilises the quantised levels associated with the conduction band of one layer and the valence band of the adjacent layer. The electron and hole levels are separated in real space and transitions only occur in spatial regions in which the wave functions of the carriers overlap. To provide a suitable absorption, the extremely thin layers are used. The enhancement of absorption can be achieved by the additional introduction of lattice misfit and strain between alternating layers.

In a type III superlattice the alternating layers are of different conduction and valence band symmetry. The architecture is essentially that of the type I except for the use of a semimetal instead of a semiconductor alternated with a semiconductor barrier layer. However, in this case the thickness of the semimetal layer determines a system of 2D quantised levels in both the conduction and valence bands. Conduction of electrons and holes occurs via tunnelling through the thin barrier layers of the superlattice.

Type II and type III superlattices are essentially minority carrier intrinsic semiconductor materials. Their absorption coefficients of IR radiation are similar to direct-bandgap alloys, and the effective masses are larger than those associated with a direct-bandgap alloy of the same bandgap.

Summarising, the advantages of type II and type III superlattices are: direct-bandgap absorption, large effective masses, and reduced Auger generation (especially to type-II InAs/GaSb superlattices due to space charge separation). The disadvantages of type III are surface passivation and layer interdiffusion at typical processing temperatures. Also, for type II superlattices, the surface passivation is serious issue. However, the main drawback of type II superlattices is short SRH (Shockley-Read-Hall) lifetimes.

8.3 SUPERLATTICE AVALANCHE PHOTODIODES

In most compound semiconductor avalanche photodiodes (APDs) the electron and hole ionisation rates are comparable. In this situation, as results from Section 4.8, the bandwidth of the device is limited. The response time of APD is specified by the carrier-multiplication process and transit time, and generally the response time is greater than the transit time because of the avalanche buildup time. In turn, the avalanche buildup time depends upon the electron and hole impact ionisation rates. Taking into account the GaAs/AlGaAs system with different conduction and valence

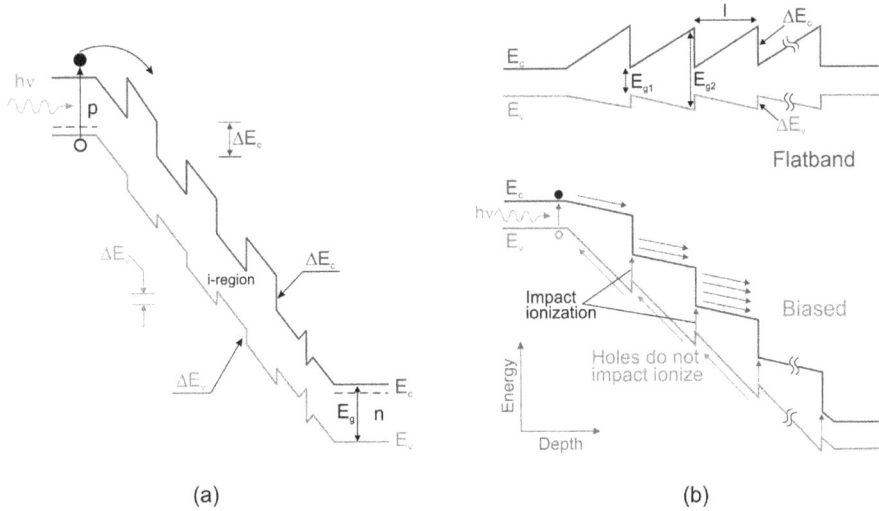

FIGURE 8.5 Multiquantum well APDs: (a) sketch of the energy band diagram of a multiquantum well p-i-n APD, highlighting the intrinsic region (i) of the device; (b) band diagrams of a staircase APD unbiased (top) and under reverse bias (bottom).

band edge discontinuities, the electron ionisation rate can be enhanced. This idea was examined for the first time by Capasso *et al.* [3] in the multiquantum well AlGaAs/GaAs APD shown in Figure 8.5(a). Since the conduction band edge discontinuity is larger than the valence band edge discontinuity, the local electron ionisation coefficient should be larger than that of the holes near the heterointerface. In a simple theoretical estimation, Chin *et al.* estimated that the hole-phonon scattering rate is substantially higher than that for electrons in GaAs quantum wells and predicted enhancement of the electron to hole ionisation rate coefficients in a GaAs/AlGaAs a multiquantum well structure [4]. However, the above design is not restricted to the GaAs/AlGaAs system. Further studies have shown that GaAs/AlGaAs did not offer sufficiently large conduction band offsets and energy separations between the direct and indirect valleys to realise the full potential of the staircase gain mechanism. Other material systems have been extensively employed, as is discussed in Reference [5]. More recently published paper [6] has demonstrated that AlInAsSb/GaSb staircase APD with near-ideal gain of 1.8 ± 0.2 per step, resulting in highly deterministic and low-noise operations.

In fact, the novel APD model described above mimics the functionality of a photomultiplier tube (PMT) – see section 6. As is shown in Figure 8.5(b), a series of discontinuities within the band structure ("steps") reflect the functionality of the PMT dynodes. At sufficient reverse bias, the graded bandgap regions flatten, allowing photogenerated carriers to drift across the discontinuities. Thus, the staircase APD is a solid-state replacement for the PMT [7], offering the lower-bias gain of a traditional APD with greatly reduced excess noise due to spatially-deterministic single-carrier impact ionisation.

Figure 8.6 shows the design of MBE-fabricated InGaAs/InAlAs superlattice APD with separated absorption and multiplication layers. The avalanche region consists of undoped n-type 1-μm thick InGaAs/InAlAs superlattice grown on high-doped n^+-InAlAs. The electric field between the absorption and multiplication layers is adjusted by thin Be-sheet-doped InGaAs layer. The electric field in p-type lightly doped InGaAs photoabsorption layer is controlled by Be doping concentration profile. Top three thin layers are deposited to eliminate the electric field (p^+-InGaAs layer), create a window (p^+-InAlAs layer), and prepare ohmic contact (p^+-InGaAs layer).

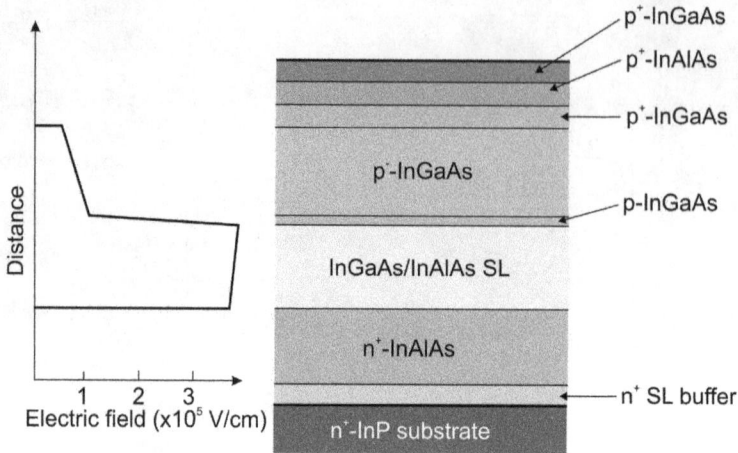

FIGURE 8.6 Design of InGaAs/InAlAs superlattice APD. Distribution of the electric field is shown in left figure (after Reference 8).

8.4 GaAS/ALGaAs QUANTUM WELL INFRARED PHOTODETECTORS

Among the different types of quantum well infrared photodetectors (QWIPs), the technology of the GaAs/AlGaAs multiple quantum well detectors is the most mature. Rapid progress has been made in the performance of these detectors. Detectivities have improved dramatically, and they are now high enough so that large megapixel FPAs with LWIR imaging performance comparable to state of the art of HgCdTe are fabricated [9,10]. Despite major research and development efforts, large photovoltaic HgCdTe FPAs remain expensive, primarily because of the low yield of operable arrays. This low yield is due to sensitivity of LWIR HgCdTe devices to defects and surface leakage, which is a consequence of basic material properties. With respect to HgCdTe detectors, GaAs/AlGaAs quantum well devices have a number of potential advantages, including the use of standard manufacturing techniques based on mature GaAs growth and processing technologies, highly uniform and well-controlled molecular beam epitaxy (MBE) growth on greater than 6-inch GaAs wafers, high yield and thus low cost, more thermal stability, and extrinsic radiation hardness. To cover the MWIR range, a strained-layer InGaAs/AlGaAs material system is used. InGaAs in the MWIR stack produces high in-plane compressive strain, which enhances the responsivity.

Figure 8.7 shows two detector configurations used in fabrication of QWIP FPAs. The major advantage of the bound-to-continuum QWIP [Figure 8.7(a)] is that the photoelectron can escape from the quantum well to the continuum transport states without being required to tunnel through the barrier. As a result, the voltage bias required to efficiently collect the photoelectrons can be reduced dramatically, thereby lowering the dark current. The multilayer structure consists of a periodic array of Si-doped ($N_d \approx 10^{18}$ cm^{-3}) GaAs quantum wells of thickness L_w separated by undoped Al$_x$Ga$_{1-x}$As barriers of thickness L_b. The heavy n-type doping in the wells is required to ensure that freezeout does occur at low temperatures and that a sufficient number of electrons are available to absorb the IR radiation. For operation at $\lambda = 7$–11 μm, typically $L_w = 40$ Å, $L_b = 500$ Å, $x = 0.25$–0.30, and 50 periods are grown. It appears that the dark current decreases significantly when the first excited state is decreased in energy from the continuum to the well top in a bound-to-quasi-bound QWIP (Figure 8.8 [12]), without sacrificing responsivity. In comparison with the narrow response of bound-to-bound transitions, the bound-to-continuum transitions are characterised by a broader response.

A miniband transport QWIP contains two bound states, the higher-energy one being in resonance with the ground state miniband in the superlattice barrier [see Figure 8.7(b)]. In this

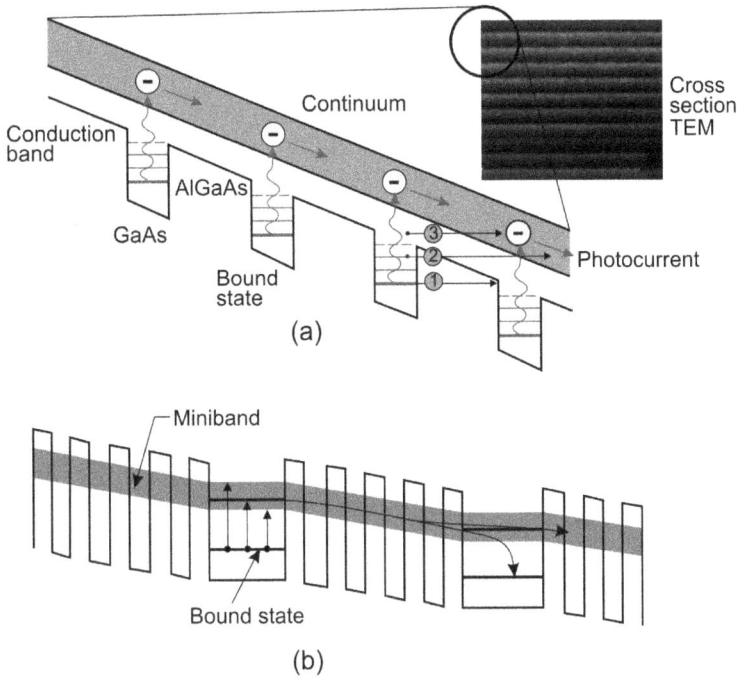

FIGURE 8.7   Band diagram of demonstrated QWIP structures: (a) bound-to-extended (after Reference 11) and (b) bound-to-miniband. Three mechanisms creating dark current are also shown in Figure (a): ground-state sequential tunnelling (1), intermediate thermally assisted tunnelling (2), and thermionic emission (3).

approach, IR radiation is absorbed in the doped quantum wells, exciting an electron into the miniband, which provides the transport mechanism, until it is collected or recaptured into another quantum well.

A distinct feature of n-type QWIPs is that the optical absorption strength is proportional to the electric-field polarisation component of an incident photon in a direction normal to the plane of the quantum wells. For imaging, it is necessary to couple light uniformly to 2D arrays of these detectors, so a diffraction grating is incorporated on one side of the detectors to redirect a normally incident photon into propagation angles more favourable for absorption. Figure 8.9 presents four popular light-coupling mechanisms: 2D gratings with optical cavity, random scatterer reflector, corrugated quantum wells, and resonator detector.

Rogalski [13] used simple analytical expressions for detector parameters described by Andersson [14]. Figure 8.10 shows the dependence of detectivity on the long wavelength cut-off for GaAs/AlGaAs QWIPs at different temperatures. The satisfactory agreement with experimental data in a wide range of cut-off wavelength $8 \leq \lambda_c \leq 19$ μm and temperature $35 \leq T \leq 77$ K has been obtained, considering the samples have different doping, different methods of crystal growth (MBE, MOCVD, and gas source MBE), different spectral widths, different excited states (continuum, bound, and quasicontinuum), and even in one case a different materials system (InGaAs).

Even though QWIPs are photoconductors, several of their properties such as high impedance, fast response time, and low power consumption comply well with the requirements for large FPAs fabrication. However, LWIR QWIP cannot compete with HgCdTe photodiode as the single device, especially at higher temperature operation (>70 K) due to fundamental limitations associated with intersubband transitions. QWIP detectors have relatively low quantum efficiencies, typically less than 10 per cent. The spectral response band is also narrow for this detector, with a full-width, half-maximum of about per cent. The typical value of the absorption coefficient in 77 K in LWIR region

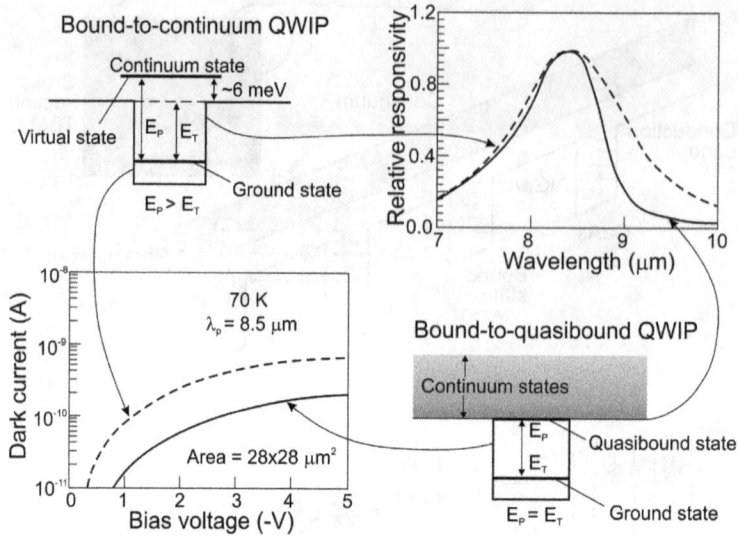

FIGURE 8.8 In typical photoresponse curves of bound-to-quasibound and bound-to-continuum 8.5 μm QWIPs at a temperature of 77 K the dark current (lower left) decreases significantly when the first excited state is dropped from the continuum to the well top, bound-to-quasibound QWIP, without sacrificing the responsivity (upper right). The first excited state now resonating with barrier top produces sharper absorption and photoresponse (after Reference 12).

is between 600–800 cm^{-1} (see Figure 4.24). All the QWIP data with cut-off wavelength about 9 μm is clustered between 10^{10} and 10^{11} cm Hz$^{1/2}$W^{-1} at about 77 K operating temperature. However, the advantage of HgCdTe is less distinct in temperature range below 50 K due to the problems involved in an HgCdTe material (p-type doping, Shockley-Read recombination, trap-assisted tunnelling, surface and interface instabilities). Table 8.1 compares the essential properties of three types of devices at 77 K used in fabrication of LWIR focal plane arrays.

QWIPs are ideal detectors for the fabrication of pixel co-registered simultaneously readable two-colour IR FPAs because a QWIP absorbs IR radiation only in a narrow spectral band and is transparent outside of that absorption band. Thus, it provides zero spectral cross-talk when two spectral bands are more than a few microns apart. Devices capable of simultaneously detecting two separate wavelengths can be fabricated by vertical stacking of the different QWIP layers during epitaxial growth. Separate bias voltages can be applied to each QWIP simultaneously via doped contact layers that separate the MQW detector heterostructures. Figure 8.11(a) shows schematically the structure of a two-colour stacked QWIP with contacts to all three ohmic-contact layers [15]. The device epilayers are grown by MBE on up to 6 six inches semi-insulating GaAs substrates. An undoped GaAs layer, called an isolator, is grown between two AlGaAs etch stop layers, followed by a 0.5 μm thick doped GaAs layer. Next, the two QWIP heterostructures are grown, separated by another ohmic contact. The long wavelength sensitive stack (red QWIP) is grown above the shorter wavelength sensitive stack (blue QWIP). Typical responsivity spectra at 77 K using a common bias of 1.5 V, recorded simultaneously for two QWIPs at the same pixel are shown in Figure 8.11(b). The gaps between FPA detectors and the readout multiplexer are backfilled with epoxy. The epoxy backfilling provides the necessary mechanical strength to the detector array and readout hybrid prior to array thinning. The initial GaAs substrate of dual-band FPAs are completely removed, leaving only a 50 nm thick GaAs membrane. This allows the array to accommodate any thermal expansion by eliminating the thermal mismatch between the silicon readout and the detector array.

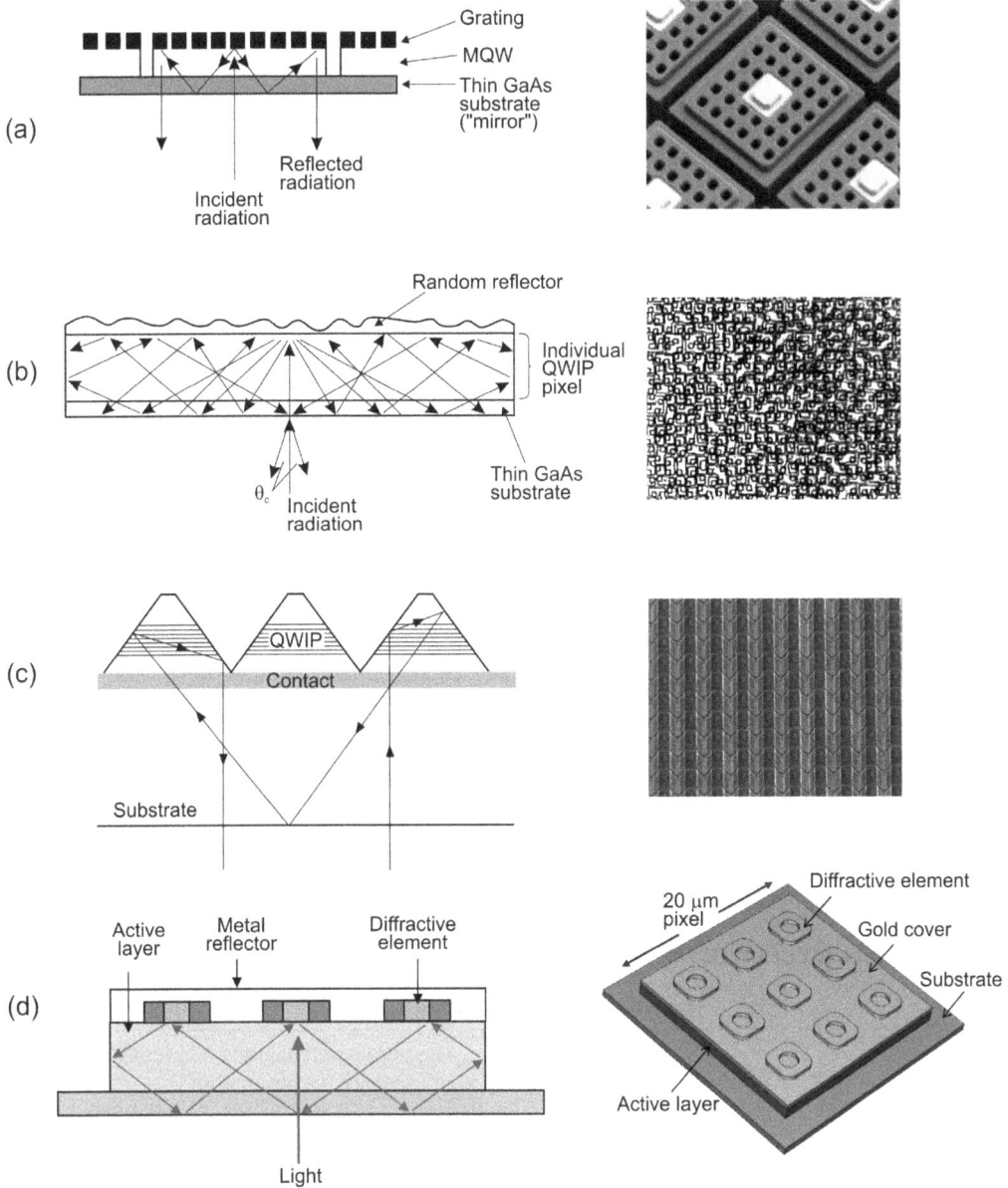

FIGURE 8.9   Gratings light-coupling mechanisms used in QWIPs: (a) gratings with optical cavity, (b) random scatterer reflector, (c) corrugated quantum wells and (d) resonator detector.

8.5   TYPE-II SUPERLATTICE PHOTODETECTORS

Currently, the III-V antimonide-based detector technology is under strong development as a possible alternative to HgCdTe detector material [16]. The apparent rapid success of the type-II superlattices (T2SLs) depends not only on the previous five decades of III-V materials, but mainly on novel ideas coming recently in design of infrared photodetectors. During the last decade, antimonide-based FPA technology has achieved a level close to HgCdTe after a shorter period of time. However, the modern version of the technology is as yet in its infancy. The advent of bandgap engineering has

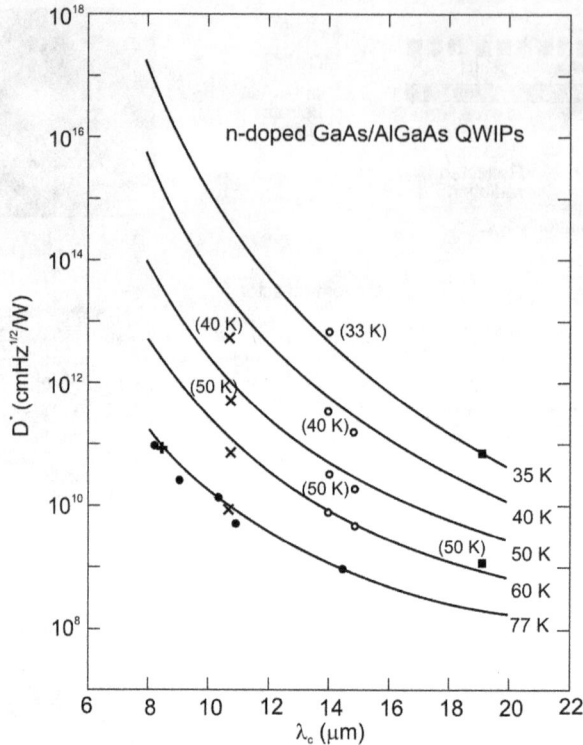

FIGURE 8.10 Detectivity versus cut-off wavelength for n-doped GaAs/AlGaAs QWIPs at temperatures ≤ 77 K. The solid lines are theoretically calculated. The experimental data are taken from different papers (after Reference 13).

TABLE 8.1
Essential Properties of LWIR HgCdTe, Type II SL Photodiodes, and QWIPs at 77 K

Parameter	HgCdTe	QWIP (n-type)	InAs/GaSb SL
IR absorption	Normal incidence	$E_{optical} \perp$ plane of well required Normal incidence: no absorption	Normal incidence
Quantum efficiency	$\geq 70\%$	$\leq 10\%$	≈ 50–60%
Spectral sensitivity	Wide-band	Narrow-band (FWHM ≈ 1 µm)	Wide-band
Optical gain	1	0.2–0.4 (30–50 wells)	1
Thermal generation lifetime	≈ 1µs	≈ 10 ps	≈ 0.1µs
$R_o A$ product ($\lambda_c = 10$ µm)	10^3 Ωcm^2	10^4 Ωcm^2	500 Ωcm^2
Detectivity ($\lambda_c = 10$ µm, FOV= 0)	2×10^{12} cmHz$^{1/2}$W^{-1}	2×10^{10} cmHz$^{1/2}$W^{-1}	1×10^{12} cmHz$^{1/2}$W^{-1}

given III-Vs a new lease on life. III-Vs offer similar performance to HgCdTe at an equivalent cut-off wavelength, but with a sizeable penalty in operating temperature, due to the inherent difference in SRH lifetimes. Important advantage of T2SLs is the high quality, high uniformity and stable nature of the material. In general, III-V semiconductors are more robust than their II-VI counterparts due to stronger, less ionic chemical bonding. As a result, III-V-based FPAs excel in operability, spatial uniformity, temporal stability, scalability, producibility, and affordability – the so-called "ibility" advantages.

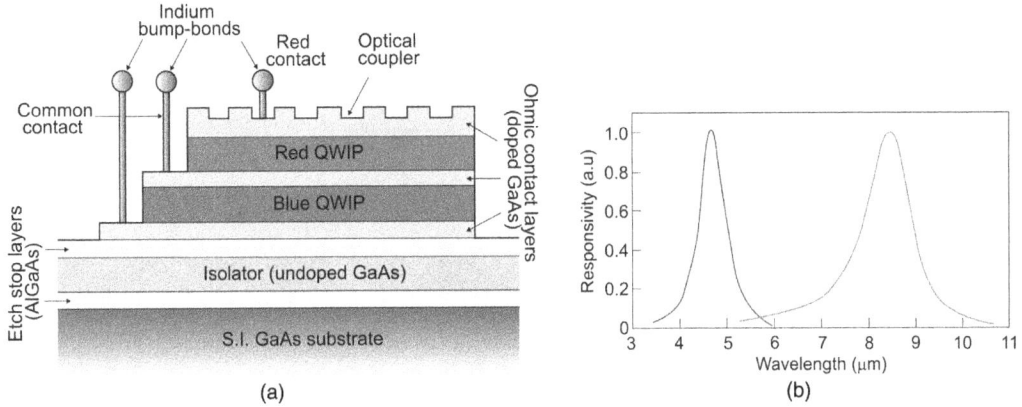

FIGURE 8.11 Schematic representation of the (a) dual-band QWIP detector structure and (b) typical responsivity spectra at 77 K and a common bias of 1 V, recorded simultaneously for two QWIPs at the same pixel (after Reference 15).

8.5.1   6.1 Å III-V Semiconductor Family

As is shown in Figure 8.12, T2SL materials belong to 6.1 Å III-V semiconductor family. They are the most important in proposing new solutions of high- performance IR detectors exhibiting direct energy gaps, high optical absorption and high design flexibility. This group consists of three alloys having approximately matched lattice constant about 6.1 Å: InAs, GaSb, and AlSb. Their energy gaps are varying in the range starting from 0.417 eV (InAs) to 1.696 eV (AlSb) at lower temperatures. Similarly to other semiconductor compounds, they are chosen as the subject of research due to their heterostructures, in particular combining InAs with the three antimonides (InSb, AlSb and GaSb) and their alloys. This combination provides a band alignment that is fundamentally different from that of the more thoroughly researched AlGaAs, and that band alignment flexibility draws the attention of scientists on the 6.1 Å materials. InAs/GaSb heterojunctions reveal the most unique band alignment, which is defined as the broken gap. The top of the VB of GaSb is located above the bottom of CB of InAs by ~150 meV at the interface. On both sides of the heterointerface, electrons and holes are separated and located in self-consistent QWs what is related to partial overlapping of the InAs CB with the GaSb VB. Consequently, exceptional tunnelling-assisted radiative recombination transitions and novel transport properties are observed. A wide range of different alloys and SLs can be designed due to high versatility of these compounds, with the accessibility of type-I (nested, or straddling), type-II staggered, and type-II broken gap (misaligned) band offsets between the GaSb/AlSb, InAs/AlSb, and InAs/GaSb material pairs, respectively, as illustrated in Figure 8.12.

The basic difference in profiles of the CB and VB in the InAs/GaSb and InAs/InAsSb T2SLs is presented in Figure 8.13. The band alignment of T2SL is causing a state in which the energy bandgap of the SLs can be adjusted to the configuration either a semimetal or a narrow bandgap semiconductor material. Because of only two common elements (In and As) in SL layers and rather uncomplicated interface structure with Sb-shifting elements, the InAs/InAsSb SLs growth follows with a better controllability and is more easily manufactured.

Transitions between electron and hole bands are spatially indirect. The first electron miniband (C_1) is more sensitive to layer thickness than first heavy hole state (HH_1) because of the large value of the heavy-hole mass.

Below, distinctions in the fundamental properties of InAs/GaSb and InAs/InAsSb SLs are emphasised:

InSb	InAs	GaSb	AlSb	InAs
0.235 eV	0.417 eV	0.812 eV	1.696 eV	0.417 eV
6.479 C	6.058 C	6.095 C	6.136 C	6.058 C

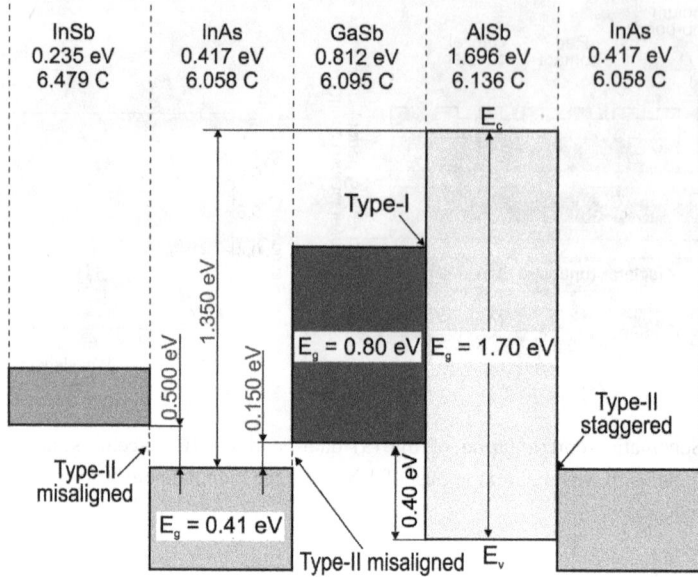

FIGURE 8.12 Schematic diagram of the low-temperature energy band alignment in the nearly 6.1 Å lattice matched InAs/GaSb/AlSb compounds. In this material system three types of band alignment are possible: type-I (nested) band alignment between GaSb and AlSb, type-II staggered alignment between InAs and AlSb, and type-II misaligned (or broken gap) alignment between InAs and GaSb. The approximate values of band offsets are marked in red.

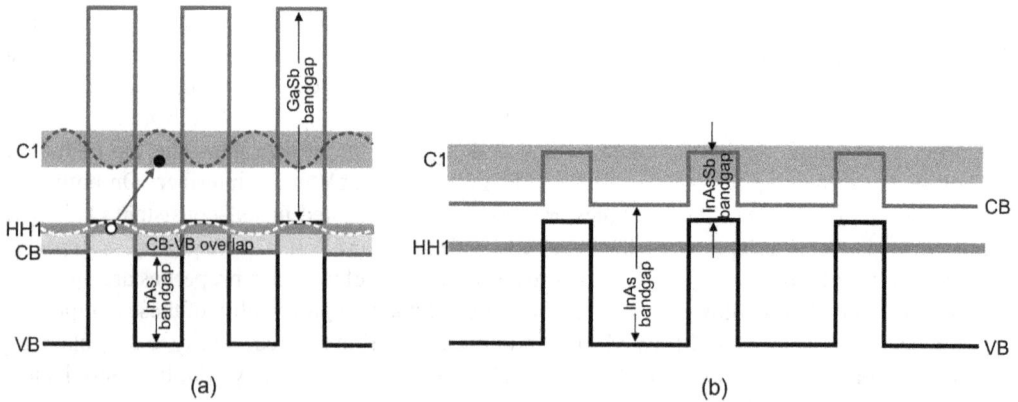

FIGURE 8.13 Bandgap diagram for (a) InAs/GaSb and (b) InAs/InAsSb T2SLs.

- both types of T2SLs are based on nearly lattice-matched III-V semiconductors and provide a large range of tunability in $\lambda_{cut-off}$;
- in T2SLs the electron and hole wave functions are located in separate layers;
- the resulting energy gap is determined by the transition energy between the HH_1 and the C_1 and depends upon the layer thicknesses and interface compositions;
- the band offsets in conduction (ΔE_c) and valence (ΔE_v) bands in the InAs/InAsSb SL (ΔE_c ~ 142 meV, ΔE_v ~226 meV) are much smaller as compared to InAs/GaSb SL (ΔE_c ~ 930 meV, ΔE_v ~510 meV);
- a much larger broken gap of the InAs/GaSb SLs makes it easier to achieve small SL bandgaps;

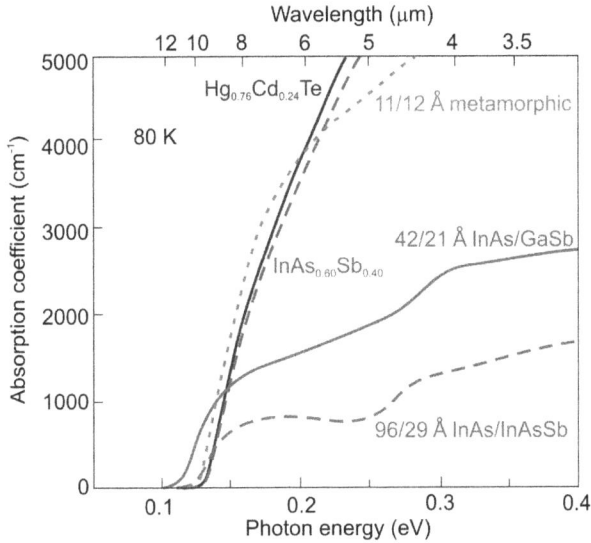

FIGURE 8.14 Calculated interband absorption coefficients for bulk $InAs_{0.60}Sb_{0.4}$, $Hg_{0.76}Cd_{0.24}Te$, and T2SLs: 42Å InAs/21Å GaSb, 96Å InAs/29Å $InAs_{0.61}Sb_{0.39}$ and 11Å $InAs_{0.66}Sb_{0.34}$/12Å $InAs_{0.36}Sb_{0.64}$ metamorphic.

- as the period increases, the $\lambda_{cut\text{-}off}$ of the InAs/GaSb SL increases much faster than in the case of the InAs/InAsSb SL. The shorter period of InAs/GaSb SL gives the same $\lambda_{cut\text{-}off}$ as for InAs/InAsSb SL.

Figure 8.14 demonstrates that the absorption coefficient near $\lambda_{cut\text{-}off}$ is weaker for the InAs/InAsSb SL than for the InAs/GaSb SL. From the other side, the absorption coefficient of HgCdTe is stronger than those for both T2SLs. In addition, these estimates show that only for the small period metamorphic $InAs_{1-x}Sb_x/InAs_{1-y}Sb_y$ SLs is its value of absorption coefficient comparable with bulk materials.

Theoretical estimations show that the carrier lifetime is enhanced in T2SLs due to suppression of Auger mechanisms resulting from the separation of electrons and holes. However, these theoretical considerations have not yet been experimentally confirmed. In practical devices based on III-V material systems, more active SRH centres are observed, compared to those of HgCdTe ternary alloys, resulting in lower carrier lifetime.

The next two figures (8.15 and 8.16) summarise carrier lifetimes data for bulk HgCdTe and both types of T2SLs (InAs/GaSb and InAs/InAsSb) operating in MWIR ($\lambda_c \approx 5$ µm), and LWIR ($\lambda_c \approx 10$ µm). The trend lines HgCdTe carrier lifetimes are given after Kinch *et al.* [17]. InAs/InAsSb SL system shows a significantly longer minority carrier lifetime (1 µs for MWIR material at 77 K) in comparison to the InAs/GaSb SL operating at the same wavelength range and temperature (~100 ns).

In lightly doped n- and p-type HgCdTe, the SRH mechanism determines the carrier lifetime. Generally, values of τ_{SRH} are approximately more than two orders of magnitude larger for HgCdTe than those reported for the III-V semiconductors with similar bandgaps. At lower temperatures and doping level below 10^{14} cm^{-3}, the HgCdTe P-i-N photodiodes become depletion limited due to SRH centres having lifetimes in the range to 10 ms [18]. As a consequence, the potential properties of room-temperature HgCdTe photodiodes operating above 3 µm guarantee achieving more than order of magnitude higher detectivity (above 10^{10} Jones) in comparison with value predicted by Rule 07 [19], and this detectivity is limited by the background flux [20]. Up till now, the long SRH lifetime

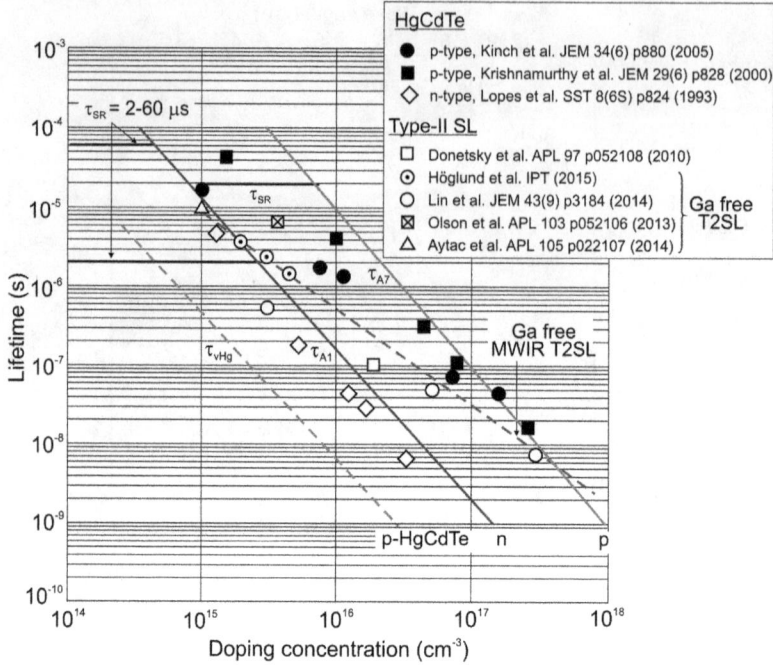

FIGURE 8.15 Minority carrier lifetimes versus doing concentration for MWIR HgCdTe and T2SLs at 77 K. Theoretical trend lines for n-type and p-type HgCdTe ternary alloys are taken from Reference 17. The dashed line for Ga-free T2SLs follows experimental data.

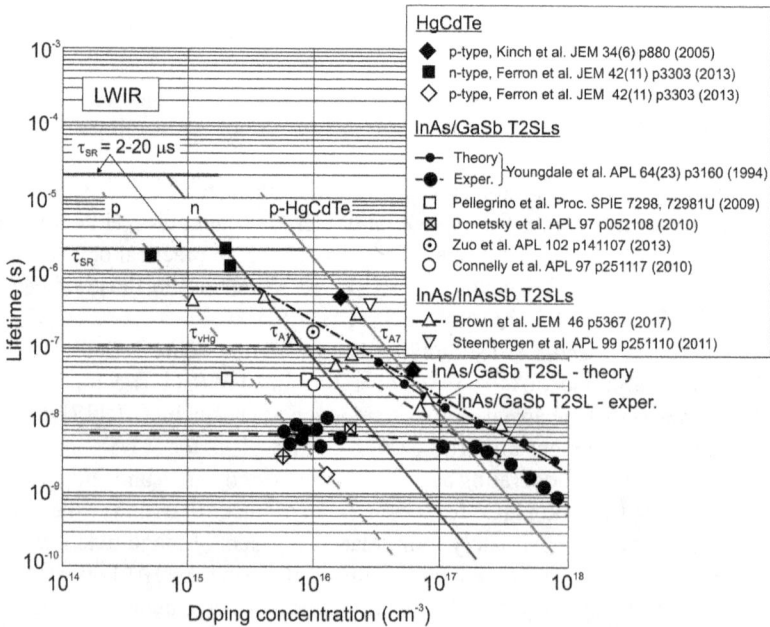

FIGURE 8.16 Minority carrier lifetimes versus doing concentration for LWIR HgCdTe and T2SLs at 77 K. Theoretical trend lines for n-type and p-type HgCdTe ternary alloys are taken from Reference 17. The dashed line for T2SLs follows experimental data.

of HgCdTe offers the potential to use this material system for background limited performance (BLIP) at room-temperature operation – see also Section 7.5.4.

8.5.2 P-I-N PHOTODIODES

T2SL photodiodes are typically based on p-i-n double heterostructures with an unintentionally doped, intrinsic region (v or π) sandwiched between heavily doped p and n lattice-matched layers of larger bandgap materials. The lower minority carrier concentration in the high bandgap layers resulted in a lower diffusion dark and higher R_oA product and detectivity. The main technological challenge for the fabrication of photodiodes is the growth of thick enough high-quality active region to achieve acceptable quantum efficiency. High quantum efficiency above 50 per cent is obtained thanks to a thick absorption region (> 5 μm) for both LWIR p-i-n phtotodiodes.

Figure 8.17 shows the schematic photodiode structure and its design. The device structure was grown on Te-doped epiready (100) GaSb substrates [21]. It consists of 100 periods of ten monolayers (10 MLs) of InAs:Si ($n = 4 \times 10^{18}$ cm^{-3})/10 MLs of GaSb as the bottom contact layer. This was followed by 50 periods of graded n-doped 10 MLs of InAs:Si/10 MLs of GaSb, 350 periods of absorber, 25 periods of 10 MLs of InAs:Be ($p = 1 \times 10^{18}$ cm^{-3})/10 MLs of GaSb and, finally, 17 periods of 10 MLs InAs:Be (p = 4×10^{18} cm^{-3})/10 MLs GaSb, which formed a p-type contact layer. Twenty-five periods of the SL structure with graded doping layers were added between the absorber and the contact layer in order to improve transport of minority carriers in detector structure. A normal-incidence, single-pixel mesa photodiode, with a 450×450 μm^2 electrical area, was fabricated by photolithography and inductively coupled plasma etching. The rest of the fabricated devices were dipped in a phosphoric acid-based solution to remove the native oxide film on the etched mesa sidewalls, then covered with SU-8 (~1.5-μm thickness) to act as the passivation layer.

Figure 4.37 presents the comparisons of experimental and theoretically predicted characteristics of the dark current density, J-V, and the resistance area product, $RA(V)$, versus bias voltage for the MWIR p-i-n InAs/GaSb superlattice photodiodes at temperature 160 K. As we can see, in a wide region of bias voltages between +0.1 V up to –1.6 V and temperatures (also bellow 160 K), the

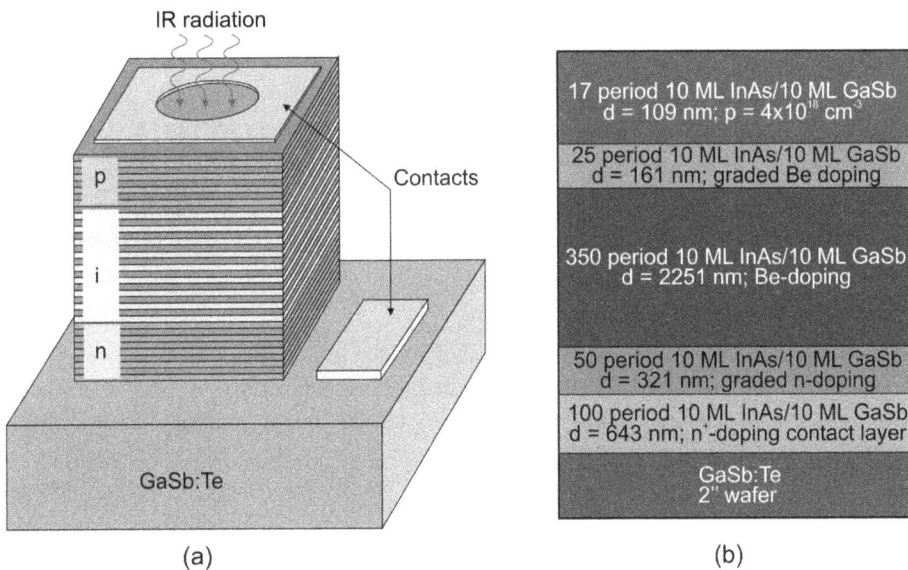

FIGURE 8.17 MWIR InAs/GaSb type-II superlattice photodiode: schematic device structure (a) and photodiode design (b).

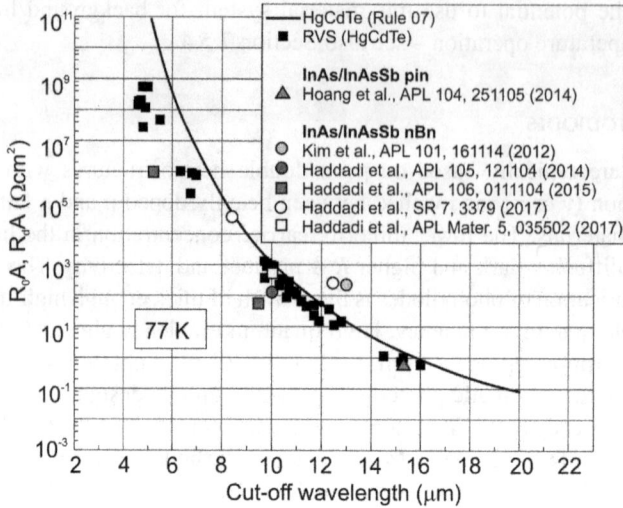

FIGURE 8.18 Dependence of the R_0A product of InAs/GaSb SLS photodiodes on cut-off wavelength compared to theoretical and experimental trendlines for comparable HgCdTe photodiodes at 77 K (adapted after Reference 22).

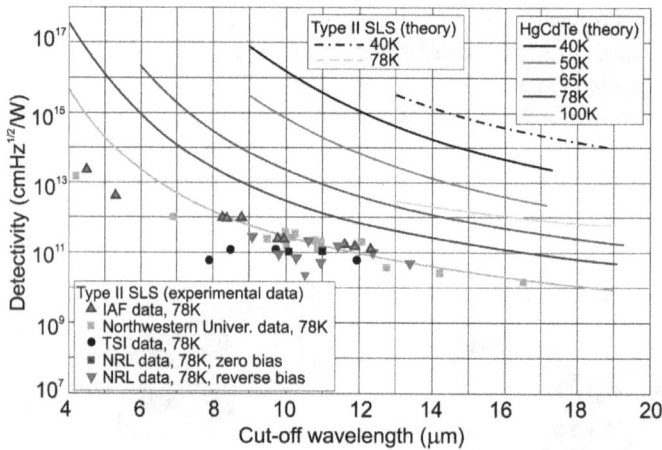

FIGURE 8.19 The predicted detectivity of type-II and P-on-n HgCdTe photodiodes as a function of wavelength and temperature. The experimental data are taken with several sources (adapted after Reference 23).

excellent agreement between both types of results has been obtained. Instead, Figure 8.18 compares the R_0A values of InAs/GaSb SL and HgCdTe photodiodes in the long wavelength spectral range. The solid line denotes the theoretical diffusion limited performance of p-type HgCdTe material. As can be seen in the figure, the recent photodiode results for SL devices rival that of practical HgCdTe devices, indicating substantial improvement has been achieved in SL detector development.

Figure 8.19 compares the calculated detectivity of type-II and P-on-n HgCdTe photodiodes as a function of wavelength and temperature of operation with the experimental data of type II SL detectors operated at 78 K [23]. The solid lines are theoretical thermal limited detectivities for HgCdTe photodiodes, calculated using one-dimensional (1D) model that assumes diffusion current from narrower bandgap n-side is dominant, and a minority carrier recombination via Auger and radiative process. In calculations typical values for the n-side donor concentration ($N_d = 1 \times 10^{15}$

cm^{-3}), the narrow bandgap active layer thickness (10 μm), and quantum efficiency (60%) have been used. The predicted thermally limited detectivities of the T2SL are larger than those for HgCdTe.

From Figure 8.19, results that the measured thermally limited detectivities of T2SL photodiodes are as yet inferior to current HgCdTe photodiode performance. Their performance has not achieved theoretical values. This limitation appears to be due to two main factors: relatively high background concentrations (about 5×10^{15} cm^{-3}, although values below 10^{15} cm^{-3} have been reported) and a short minority carrier lifetime (typically tens of nanoseconds in lightly doped p-type material). Up till now non-optimised carrier lifetimes have been observed and at desirably low carrier concentrations is limited by an SRH recombination mechanism. The minority carrier diffusion length is in the range of several micrometres. Improving these fundamental parameters is essential to realise the predicted performance of type-II photodiodes.

8.5.3 Barrier Photodetectors

The sophisticated physics associated with the antimonide-based bandgap engineering concept started at the beginning of the 1990s gave a new impact and interest in development of infrared detector structures within academic and national laboratories. In addition, implementation of barrier in photoconductor structure, in a so-called barrier detector (see Section 4.11), prevents current flow in the majority carrier band of the detector's absorber but allows unimpeded flow in the minority carrier band. As a result, this concept resurrects the performance of antimonide-based focal plane arrays and gives a new perspective in their applications. New emerging strategies include especially antimonide-based T2SLs, barrier structures such as nBn detector with lower generation-recombination leakage mechanisms and multi-stage/cascade infrared devices.

Klipstein et al. [24] proposed the division of the barrier detectors into two groups: XB$_n$n and XB$_p$p, where X is a contact layer where doping, material, or both can be varied. Usually however, the most popular are four types of SLs barrier detectors schematically described in Table 8.2.

The main activity in development of the T2SLs barrier detectors is directed to nBn devices operating in MWIR spectral range. Figure 8.20 shows an example of such an nBn structure that was considered theoretically by Martyniuk and Rogalski [28], along with the *J-V* characteristics as a function of temperature that were taken from Reference 29. The alloy composition of $x = 0.09$ of the InAs$_{1-x}$Sb$_x$ absorber layer provided a cut-off wavelength of ~ 4.9 μm at 150 K. J_{dark} was 1.0×10^{-3} A/cm^2 at 200 K and 3.0×10^{-6} A/cm^2 at 150 K. The detectors are dominated by diffusion currents at −1.0 V bias where the quantum efficiency peaks.

An interesting difference in dark-current density versus temperature is shown in Figure 8.21 for two nominally identical devices with opposite barrier polarities, each operating at a bias of -0.1 V [30]. The nB$_n$n device exhibits a single straight line, characteristic of diffusion limited behaviour, while the nB$_p$n device exhibits two-slope behaviour characteristic of a crossover from diffusion limited behaviour at high temperatures to GR limited behaviour at low temperatures. As is shown, the dark current density at 150 K is more than two orders of magnitude greater for the detector with the p-type barrier because it is already GR limited. It appears, for a typical quantum efficiency of 70 per cent at *f*/3 optics, the BLIP temperature is about 140 K, compared with ~175 K for the detector with the n-type barrier.

Considerable progress also has been achieved in development of LWIR pB$_p$p T2SL barrier detectors. These detectors enable diffusion-limited behaviour with dark currents comparable with HgCdTe "Rule 07" and with high quantum efficiency. The active and contact layers of these devices are both made from InAs/GaSb T2SLs with approximately 13 ML InAs/7 ML GaSb, while the barrier layer is based on an 15 ML InAs/4 ML AlSb T2SL. As is shown in Figure 8.22(a), the dark current in standard LWIR n-on-p diode based solely on InAs/GaSb T2SLs is higher in the lower temperature region in comparison with pB$_p$p T2SL barrier detector, whose schematic profile of band edges is shown in the inset figure [30]. The barrier device is diffusion limited down to 77 K, while

TABLE 8.2

T2SLs Barrier Detectors

	Flat-band energy diagrams	Example of detector structure	Description	Reference
nBn	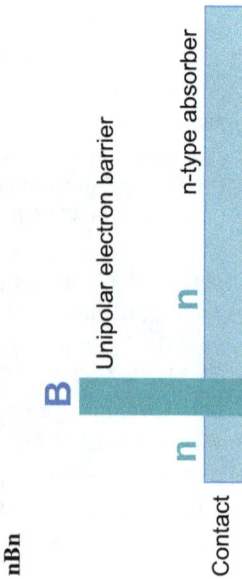 Unipolar electron barrier; B; n; n-type absorber; Contact	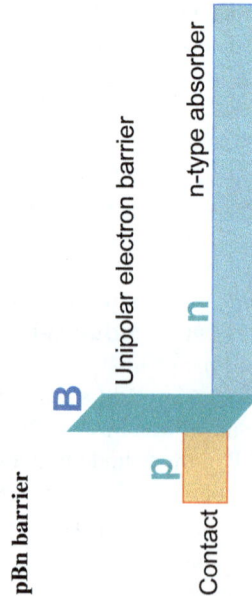 Top contact; InAs/InAsSb SL; $N_D=10^{15}$ cm^{-3} d~100 nm; AlAsSb barrier; d~100 nm; Absorber InAs/InAsSb SL; $N_D=10^{15}$ cm^{-3} d~3 μm; InAs/InAsSb SL; $N_D=10^{17}$ cm^{-3} d~100 nm; Te-doped GaSb(100) substrate; Bottom contact	The top contact, absorber, and bottom contact layers are built of T2SLs InAs/InAsSb. As a unipolar barrier located between the top contact and absorber, about 100-nm thick AlAsSb Be-doped to 10^{15} cm^{-3} is used. The top contact and absorber layers are n.i.d while the bottom contact is Te-doped to 10^{17} cm^{-3}.	25
pBn barrier	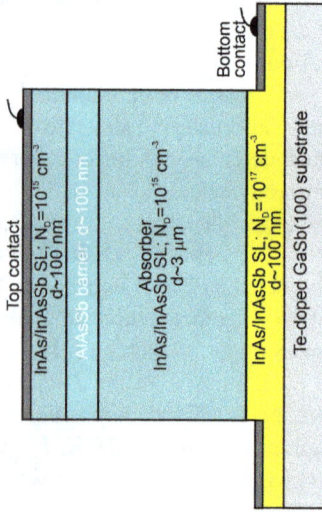 Unipolar electron barrier; B; n; n-type absorber; p; Contact	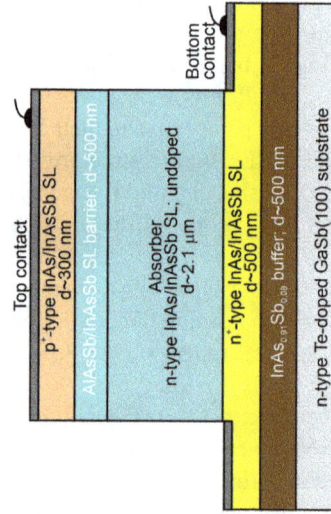 Top contact; p$^+$-type InAs/InAsSb SL; d~300 nm; AlAsSb/InAsSb SL barrier; d~500 nm; Absorber n-type InAs/InAsSb SL; undoped d~2.1 μm; n$^+$-type InAs/InAsSb SL d~500 nm; InAs$_{0.91}$Sb$_{0.09}$ buffer; d~500 nm; n-type Te-doped GaSb(100) substrate; Bottom contact	The epitaxial growth starts with a 700 nm thick n$^+$-doped GaSb/InAs$_{0.91}$Sb$_{0.09}$ buffer layer, next a 500 nm thick n$^+$-doped bottom contact layer, a 2.1 μm n.i.d active layer, a 500 nm electron barrier, and a 300 nm thick p-type top contact. The top/bottom contacts and active layer are built of T2SLs InAs/InAsSb. Si and Be are used for n-type and p-type dopants, respectively.	26

pBp

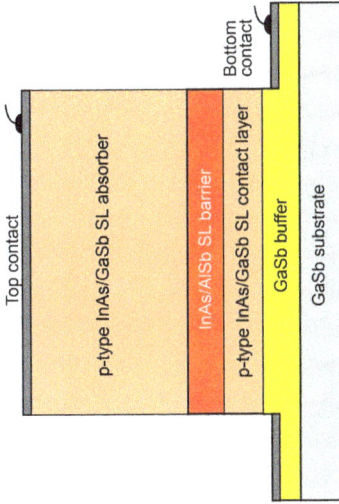

Contact | p | p | p-type absorber
B | Unipolar hole barrier

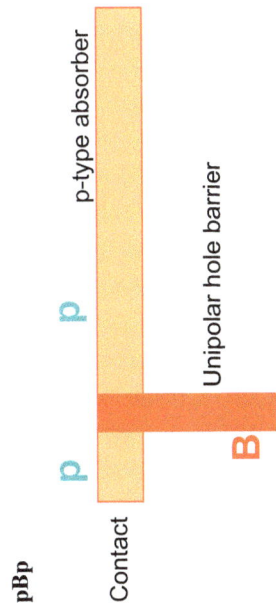

Top contact
p-type InAs/GaSb SL absorber
InAs/AlSb SL barrier
p-type InAs/GaSb SL contact layer
Bottom contact
GaSb buffer
GaSb substrate

24

The contact layers and absorber are built of T2SLs InAs/GaSb. The barrier layer is based on a T2SLs InAs/AlSb. The proper lattice match to the GaSb substrate is ensured by InSb-like interfaces.

CBIRD (Complementary barrier infrared detector)

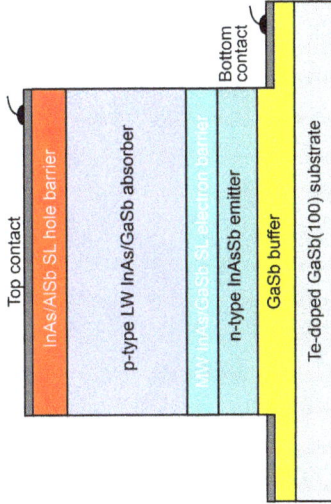

Contact | n | n- or p-type absorber
B | Unipolar hole barrier
B | Unipolar electron barrier | p

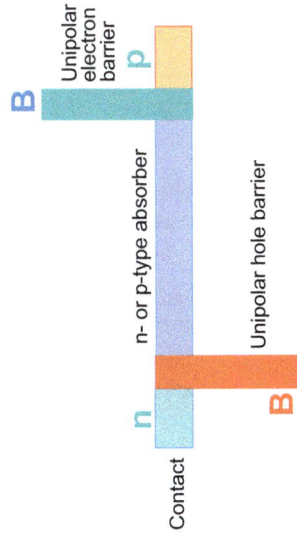

Top contact
InAs/AlSb SL hole barrier
p-type LW InAs/GaSb absorber
MW InAs/GaSb SL electron barrier
n-type InAsSb emitter
Bottom contact
GaSb buffer
Te-doped GaSb(100) substrate

27

The detector is built of a lightly p-type T2SLs InAs/GaSb active layer being sandwiched between n-type T2SLs InAs/AlSb hole barrier (hB) and wider T2SLs InAs/GaSb electron barrier (eB). The barriers are designed to exhibit zero CBO and VBO in relation to the active layer. A heavily doped n-type InAsSb layer adjacent to the eB plays the role of the bottom contact. The SRH and trap-assisted tunnelling (TAT) are reduced by the N-p heterojunction between the hB and active layer.

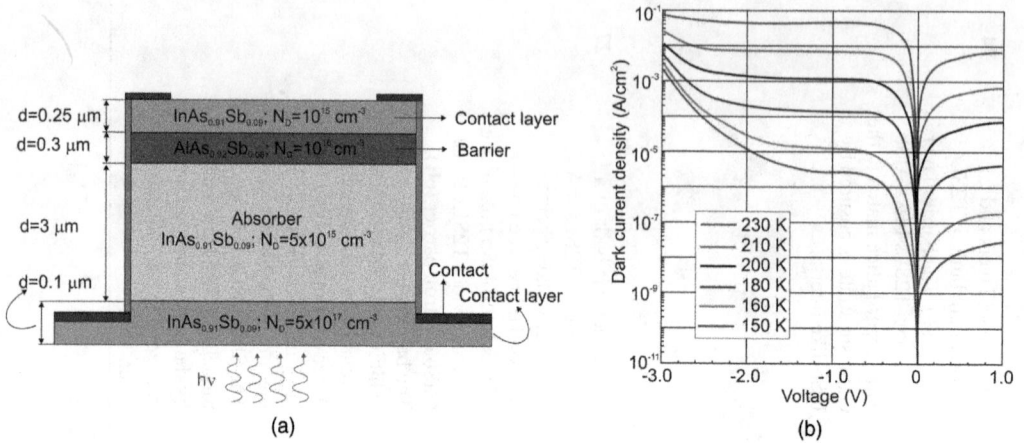

FIGURE 8.20 InAsSb/AlAsSb nBn MWIR detector: (a) the device structure and (b) dark current density versus bias voltage as a function of temperature for 4096 (18 μm pitch) detectors ($\lambda_c \approx 4.9$ μm at 150 K) tied together in parallel (after Reference 29).

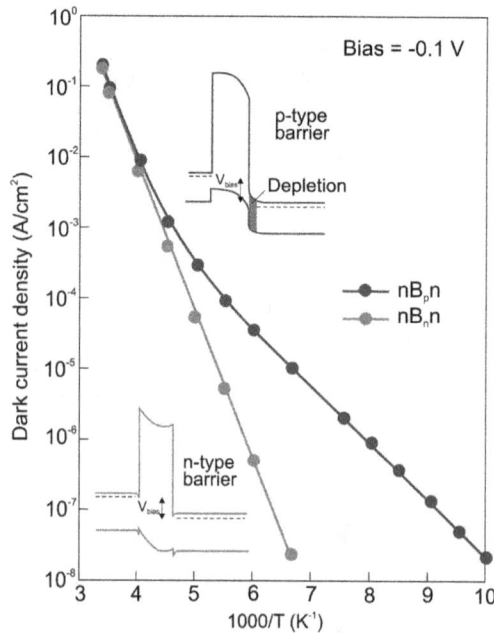

FIGURE 8.21 Dark current density vs. temperature for two identical InAsSb/AlSbAs nBn devices with opposite barrier doping polarities. Active layer bandgap wavelength is 4.1-μm at 150 K (adapted after Reference 30).

the p-n diode is generation-recombination limited at this temperature, with a dark current over 20× larger. The dark current in pB_pp devices, with thickness of active layers between 1.5 and 6.0 μm, is within one order of magnitude of HgCdTe "Rule 07" [see Figure 8.22(b)].

Figure 8.23 collects values of dark current density for non-barrier (homojunction) and barrier (heterojunction) LWIR T2SLs devices operating at 78 K gathered by Rhiger [32]. The non-barrier dark currents are generally higher, with the best approaching "Rule 07" to within a factor of about

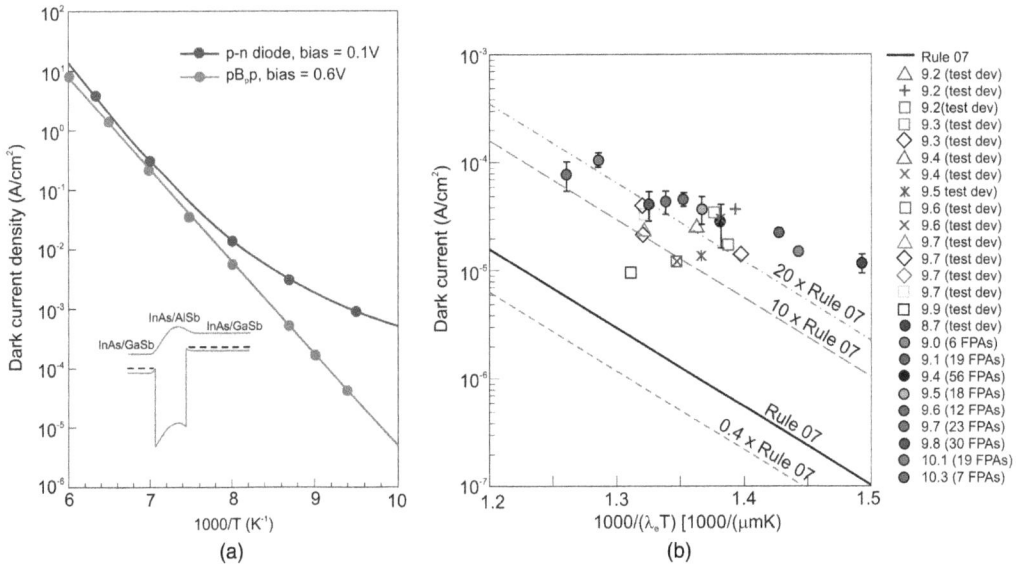

FIGURE 8.22 Dark current density of pB$_p$p T2SL barrier detector (area = 100×100 μm^2): (a) in comparison with p-n diode (after Reference 30), (b) Rule 07 plot for barrier structures with different thicknesses of active layers. Range of bandgap wavelengths: $9.0 < \lambda_e < 10.3$ μm. Solid line shows HgCdTe Rule 07 with uncertainty factors of 0.4, 10 and 20 (dashed lines) (after Reference 31).

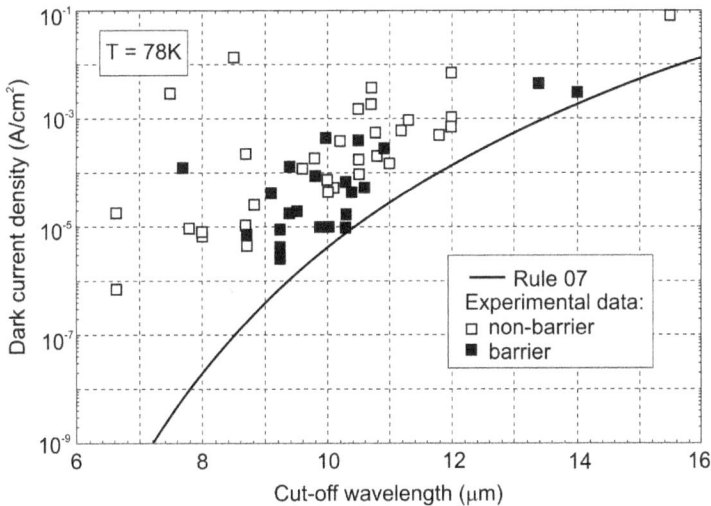

FIGURE 8.23 The 78 K dark current densities plotted against cut-off wavelength for T2SL non-barrier and barrier detectors reported in the literature since late 2010. The solid line indicates the dark current density calculated using the empirical "Rule 07" model (after Reference 32).

8. The barrier devices clearly show lower dark currents on average, and some are close to the curve Rule 07 for a cut-off wavelength of ≥ 9 μm. It can be concluded that although the minority carrier lifetime in the SL detector active region is not limited by an Auger mechanism, the diffusion current does not differ so greatly from "Rule 07".

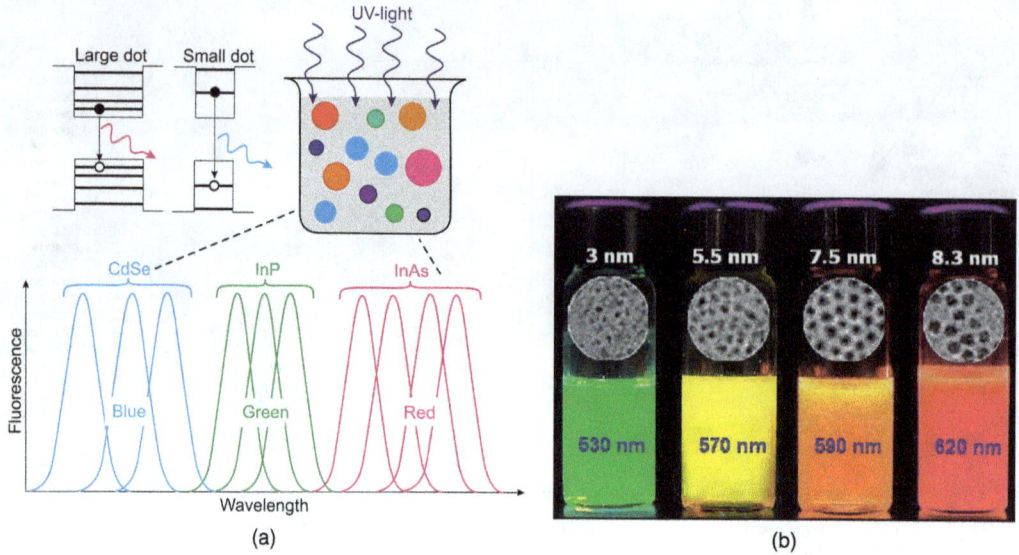

FIGURE 8.24 Emission spectra of nanocrystal QDs: (a) fluorescence of QDs illuminated by UV-light, (b) emission of the QDs suspended in toluene and contained a core of CdSe and a shell of ZnS. Emission spectra depends both on the material composition and the size of the QDs.

8.6   QUANTUM DOT PHOTODETECTORS

Progress in epitaxial growth and advances in patterning and other processing techniques have made it possible to fabricate "artificial" dedicated materials for microelectronics and microphotonics. The electronic structure can be tailored by changing the local material composition and by confining the electrons in nanometer-size grains. As is marked in section 8.1, due to quantisation of electron energies, these systems are called quantum structures. For example, Figure 8.24(a) shows the dependence of the fluorescence wavelength on the dimensions and material composition of the nanocrystals. The differences between the blue, green and red emissions result from using materials having different bandgaps: CdSe (blue), InP (green), and InAs (red). The fine-tuning of the fluorescence emission within each colour is controlled by the size of the quantum dots (QDs). The spectral absorption intensity of QDs depends on the specific transitions between discrete energy levels. Figure 8.24(b) shows the size-dependent colour in the visible spectrum for QDs comprising a core of CdSe and a shell of ZnS.

The success of quantum well (QW) structures for infrared detection applications has stimulated the development of quantum dot infrared photodetectors (QDIPs). There are two primary types of quantum dots: self-assembled (also called epitaxial) quantum dots and colloidal quantum dots (CQDs). At the beginning most QD photodetector structures were grown by MBE as self-assembled QDs in the Stranski–Krastanov (SK) growth mode [33]. Recently, more activity is directed toward colloidal quantum dot photodetectors as a better alternative to SK QDs. They are fabricated using solution-based chemistry techniques [34], where a nanocrystal colloidal suspension is created.

8.6.1   Self-assembled Quantum Dots

The self-assembling method for fabricating QDs has been recognised as one of the most promising methods for forming QDs that can be practically incorporated into photodetectors. In the crystal growth of highly lattice-mismatched materials system, self-assembling formation of nanometer-scale 3-D islands has been reported [35]. The lattice mismatch between a QD and the matrix is

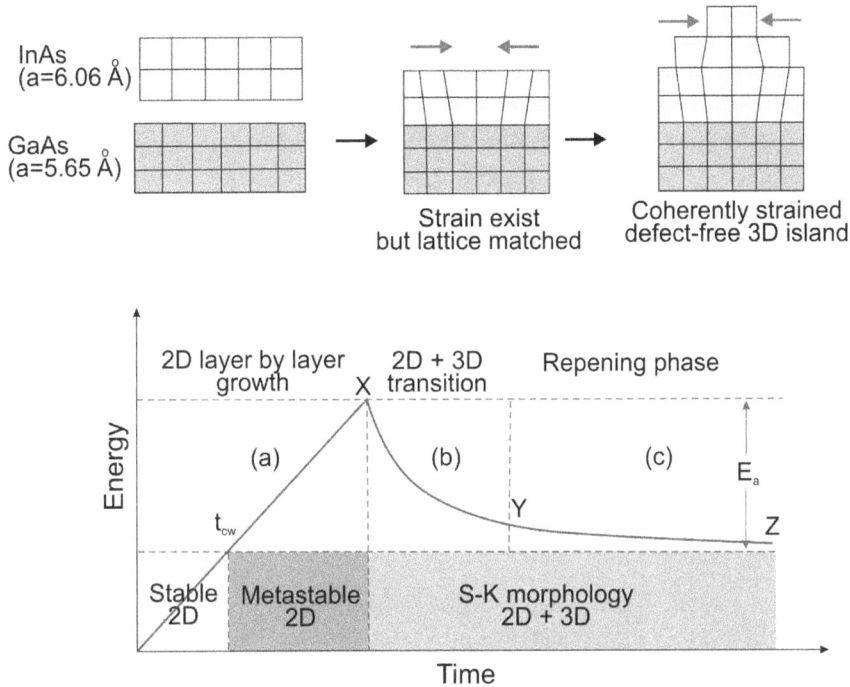

InAs
(a=6.06 Å)

GaAs
(a=5.65 Å)

Strain exist
but lattice matched

Coherently strained
defect-free 3D island

2D layer by layer
growth

2D + 3D
X transition

Repening phase

Energy

(a)

(b)

(c)

E_a

t_{cw}

Y

Z

Stable
2D

Metastable
2D

S-K morphology
2D + 3D

Time

FIGURE 8.25 Schematics of total energy versus time for the 2D-3D morphology transition. t_{cw} is the critical wetting layer thickness, E_a is the barrier for formation of 3D islands, X is the point where a pure strain-induced transition becomes. Between Y and Z a slow ripening process continues (after Reference 35).

the fundamental driving force of self-assembling. In(Ga)As on GaAs is the most commonly used material system because lattice mismatched can be controlled by the In alloy ratio up to about 7 per cent.

Under certain growth conditions, when the film with the larger lattice constant exceeds a certain critical thickness, the compressive strain within the film is relieved by the formation of islands. Figure 8.25 qualitatively shows the changes in the total energy of a mismatched system versus time [35]. The plot can be divided into three sections: period (a) (2D deposition), period (b) (2D-3D transition) and period (c) (ripening of islands). In the beginning of the deposition a 2D layer by layer mechanism leads to a perfect wetting of the substrate. At point t_{cw} (the critical wetting layer thickness) stable 2D growth enters into an area of the metastable growth. A supercritically thick wetting layer builds up, and the epilayer is potentially ready to undergo a transition toward a Stranski–Krastanow morphology [33]. This transition starts around point X in Figure 8.25, and its dynamic depends primarily on the height of the transition barrier E_a. It is presumed that further growth continues without materials supply simply by consuming the excess material accumulated in the supercritically thick wetting layer. Between points Y and Z (ripening: period c) the process has lost most of the excess energy; the mobile material is consumed as a result of the potential differences between smaller and larger islands. These islands may be QDs.

The 2D-3D transition typically occurs after the deposition of a certain number of monolayers. For InAs on GaAs, this transition occurs after about 1.7 monolayers of InAs have been grown; this is the onset of islanding and, hence, quantum-dot formation. Noncoherent islands are typically produced by too-high materials supply and contain misfit dislocations at the interface.

The detection mechanism of QDIP is based on the intraband photoexcitation of electrons from confined states in the conduction band wells or dots into the continuum. The emitted electrons drift

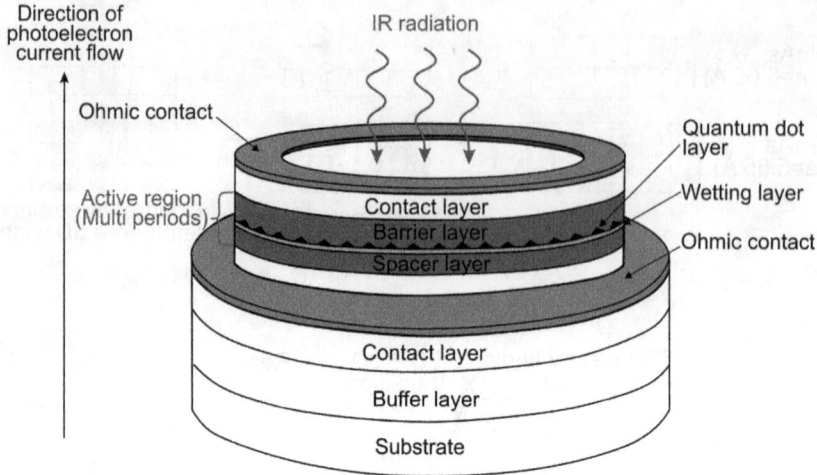

FIGURE 8.26 Schematic diagram of conventional quantum dot detector structure.

toward the collector in the electric field provided by the applied bias, and photocurrent is created. In practice, since the dots are spontaneously self-assembled during growth, they are not correlated between multilayers in the active region.

Two types of QDIP structures have been proposed: conventional structure (vertical, see Figure 8.26) and lateral structure. In a vertical QDIP, the photocurrent is collected through the vertical transport of carriers between top and bottom contacts. The device heterostructure comprises repeated InAs QD layers buried between GaAs barriers with top and bottom contact layers at active region boundaries. The mesa height can vary from 1 to 4 μm depending on the device heterostructure. The QDs are directly doped (usually with silicon) in order to provide free carriers during photoexcitation, and an AlGaAs barrier can be included in the vertical device heterostructure in order to block dark current created by thermionic emission [36].

Lateral QDIPs have demonstrated lower dark currents and higher operating temperatures than vertical QDIPs, since the major components of the dark current arise from interdot tunnelling and hopping conduction [37]. However, these devices will be difficult to incorporate into a FPA hybrid-bump bonded to a silicon readout circuit. Because of this, more effort is directed to improving the performance of vertical QDIPs, which are more compatible with commercially available readout circuits.

Both quantum QW and QD structures are used in fabrication of infrared detectors. In general, quantum dot infrared photodetectors (QDIPs) are similar to quantum well infrared photodetectors (QWIPs) but with the quantum wells replaced by QDs, which have size confinement in all spatial directions. Figure 8.27(a) shows the schematic layers of a QDIP. The detection mechanism is based on the intraband photoexcitation of electrons from confined states in the conduction dots into the continuum [Figure 8.27(b)]. The emitted electrons drift toward the collector in the electric field provided by the applied bias, and photocurrent is created. It is assumed that the potential profile at the conduction band edge along the growth direction has a similar shape, as shown in the figure. The image of an InGaAs quantum dot buried in GaAs is shown in Figure 8.27(c). Self-assembled quantum dots are typically between 5 and 50 nm in size.

In addition to the standard InAs/GaAs QDIP, several other heterostructure designs have been investigated for use as IR photodetectors. An example is InAs QDs embedded in a strain-relieving InGaAs quantum well, which are known as dot-in-a-wall (DWELL) heterostructures (see Figure 8.28) [38, 39]. This device offers two advantages: challenges in wavelength tuning through dot-size control can be compensated in part by engineering the quantum well sizes, which can be

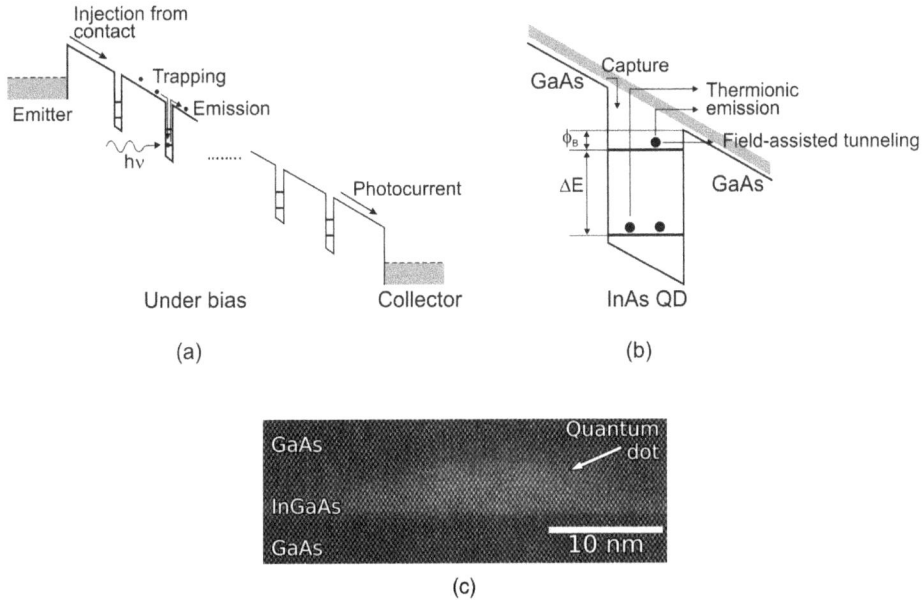

FIGURE 8.27 Schematic design of QDIP: (a) potential profile structure under bias; influence of wetting layer is neglected, (b) conduction band structure of the dot, and (c) atomic resolution scanning transmission electron microscopy image of an InGaAs quantum dot buried in GaAs.

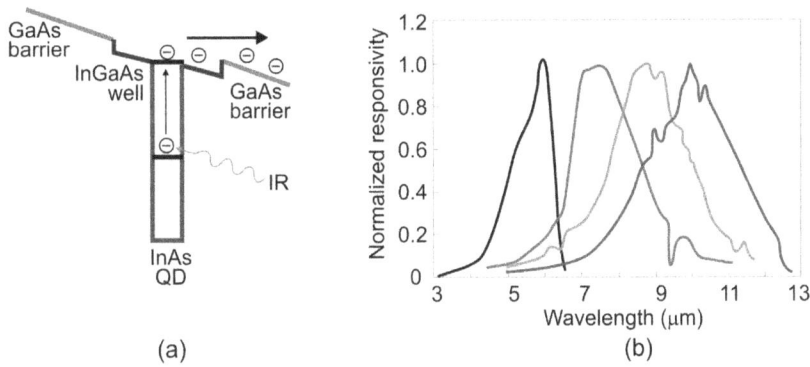

FIGURE 8.28 DWELL infrared detector: (a) the operation mechanism, and (b) experimentally measured spectral tunability by varying well width from 55 to 100 Å (after Reference 39).

controlled precisely, and quantum wells can trap electrons and aid in carrier capture by QDs, thereby facilitating ground state refilling. Figure 8.28(b) shows DWELL spectral tuning by varying well geometry.

The potential advantages in using QDIPs over quantum wells are as follows:

- Intersubband absorption may be allowed at normal incidence (for n-type material). In QWIPs, only transitions polarised perpendicularly to the growth direction are allowed, due to absorption selection rules. The selection rules in QDIPs are inherently different, and normal incidence absorption is observed.
- Thermal generation of electrons is significantly reduced due to the energy quantisation in all three dimensions. As a result, the electron relaxation time from excited states increases due

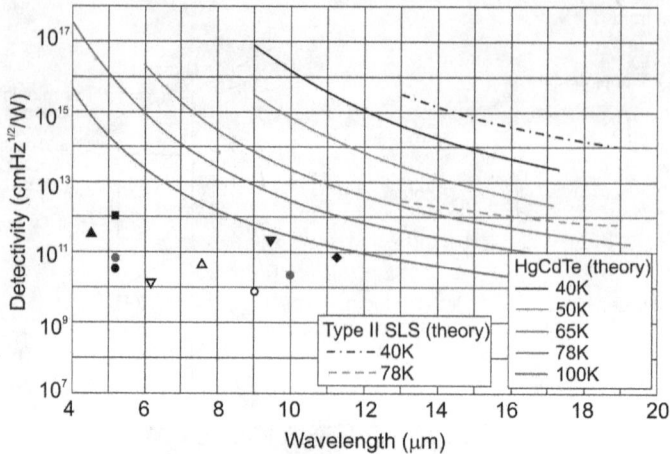

FIGURE 8.29 The predicted detectivity of P-on-n HgCdTe and type II InAs/GaInSb SLS photodiodes, compared with measured QDIP detectivities at 77 K.

to phonon bottleneck. Generation by LO phonons is prohibited unless the gap between the discrete energy levels equals exactly that of the phonon. This prohibition does not apply to quantum wells, since the levels are quantised only in the growth direction, and a continuum exists in the other two directions (hence, generation-recombination by LO phonons with capture time of a few picoseconds). Thus, it is expected that signal-to-noise (S/N) ratio in QDIPs will be significantly higher than that of QWIPs.

• Lower dark current of QDIPs is expected than of QWIPs due to 3D quantum confinement of the electron wavefunction.

Figure 8.29 compares the highest measurable detectivities at 77 K of QDIPs found in literature with the predicted detectivities of P-on-n HgCdTe and type II InAs/GaSb superllattice (SL) photodiodes. The solid lines are theoretical thermal-limited detectivities for HgCdTe photodiodes, calculated using a 1-D model that assumes diffusion current from narrower bandgap n-side is dominant, and minority carrier recombination via Auger and radiative processes. In calculations of typical values for the p-side donor concentration ($N_d = 1 \times 10^{15}$ cm^{-3}), the narrow bandgap active layer thickness (10 μm) and quantum efficiency (60%) have been used. It should be insisted that for HgCdTe photodiodes theoretically predicted curves for temperature range between 50 and 100 K coincide very well with experimental data (not shown in the figure). The predicted thermally limited detectivities of the type II SL are larger than those for HgCdTe [40].

The measured values of QDIPs' detectivities at 77 K gathered in Figure 8.29 indicate that QD device detectivities are considerably inferior to current HgCdTe detector performance. In the LWIR region, the upper experimental QDIP data at 77 K coincide with HgCdTe ones at temperature 100 K.

Both the increased electron lifetime and the reduced dark current indicate that QDIPs should be able to provide high-temperature operation. Until now, however, most of the QDIP devices reported in the literature have been working in the temperature range of 77–200 K. An interesting insight on achievable QDIP performance in temperature ranges above 200 K in comparison with other type of detectors is given in Reference [41]. In practice, however, it has been a challenge to meet all of the above expectations.

Carrier relaxation times in QDs are longer than the typical 1–10 ps measured for quantum wells. It is predicted that the carrier relaxation time in QDs is limited by electron hole scattering, rather than phonon scattering. For QDIPs, the lifetime is expected to be even larger, greater than 1 ns, since the QDIPs are majority carrier devices due to the absence of holes.

The main disadvantage of the QDIP is the large inhomogeneous linewidth of the quantum-dot ensemble variation of dot size in the Stranski–Krastanow growth mode [42]. As a result, the absorption coefficient is reduced, since it is inversely proportional to the ensemble linewidth. Large, inhomogeneously broadened linewidth has a deleterious effect on QDIP performance. Subsequently, the quantum efficiency QD devices tend to be lower than what is predicted theoretically. Vertical coupling of quantum-dot layers also reduces the inhomogeneous linewidth of the quantum-dot ensemble; however, it may also increase the dark current of the device, since carriers can tunnel through adjacent dot layers more easily. As in other types of detectors, nonuniform dopant incorporation adversely affects the performance of the QDIP. Therefore, improving QD uniformity is a key issue in the increasing absorption coefficient and in improving performance. Thus, the growth and design of unique QD heterostructure is one of the most important issues related to achievement of state-of-the art QDIP performance.

8.6.2 COLLOIDAL QUANTUM DOTS

In the past decade, a significant technological progress in the development of colloidal quantum dot (CQD) photodetectors has been made. In comparison with self-assembled QDs, CQDs have several potential advantages such as: size tunability across wide spectral range, cheaper fabrication and the possibility of direct coating of QD structures on silicon electronics for imaging.

CQDs are synthesised by liquid-phase chemistry using inexpensive reagents. Many experiences are transferred from visible display companies regarding how to scale up CQDs synthesis to reduce unit costs. The most common approach to fabricate colloidal infrared QDs is a colloidal solution-phase synthesis [43].

Colloidal QD photodetectors typically comprise a single nanocomposite layer deposited on a substrate and large-area, two-terminal, vertical devices are fabricated using p-(indiumtin-oxide) and n-type (aluminum) contacts, as shown schematically in Figure 8.30(a). Figure 8.30(b) illustrates the capture and transport mechanism of a colloidal dot film.

The charge transport mechanisms in colloidal QD nanocomposites exhibit differences compared to epitaxial QDIPs. As is shown in Figure 8.31 for the interband device, the bipolar, interband (or excitonic) transitions across the colloidal QD bandgap contribute to the photoresponse of the detector. In addition, since CQDs are electron acceptors and the polymers are typically hole conductors, the photogenerated excitons are dissociated at the QD/polymer interface. Thus, photoconduction through the nanocomposite occurs as electrons hop among QDs and holes transport through the polymer [44]. This incoherent hopping between nanocrystals results in carrier mobilities four to six orders of magnitude lower in QDs than in bulk crystals [45].

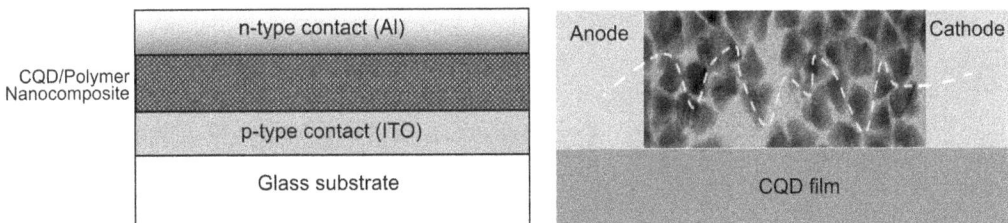

FIGURE 8.30 Colloidal quantum dot photodetector: (a) schematic diagram of device heterostructure in CQD/conducting polymer nanocomposites; (b) an SEM image of a PV QD detector with transport illustration of photo-generated charge.

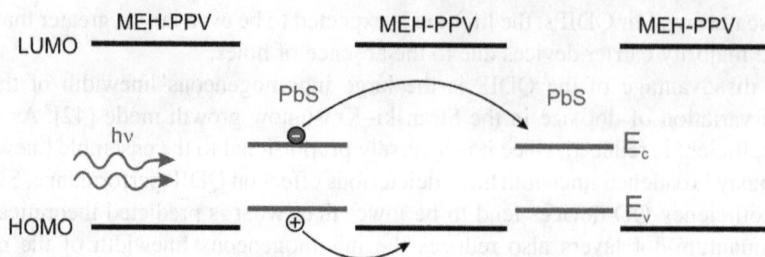

FIGURE 8.31 Schematic diagram of energy versus position for interband transitions in PbS/MEH-PPV colloidal QD-conducting polymer nanocomposites demonstrating photocurrent generation for IR photodetection (after Reference 46).

TABLE 8.3
Advantages and Disadvantages of CQD Photodetectors in Comparison with Single Crystal

QD photodetectors

Advantages	Disadvantages
• control of dot synthesis and absorption spectrum by ability of QD size-filtering, what leads to highly-uniform ensembles	• inferior chemical stability and electronic passivation of the nanomaterials in comparison with epitaxial materials
• much stronger absorption than in Stranski–Krastanov grown QD due to close-packed of CDs	• bipolar, interband (or excitonic) transitions across the CQD bandgap (e.g. electrons hopping among QDs and holes transport through the polymer) contrary to the intraband transitions in the epitaxial QDs
• considerable elimination of strains influencing the growth of epitaxial QDs by greater selection of active region materials	
• reduction of cost fabrication (using e.g. such solution as spin coating, inject printing, doctor blade or roll-to-roll printing) compared to epitaxial growth	• insulating behaviour due to slow electron transfer through many barrier interfaces in a nanomaterial
• deposition methods are compatible with a variety of flexible substrates and sensing technologies such as CMOS (e.g. direct coating on silicon electronics for imaging)	• problems with long term stability due to the large density of interfaces with atoms presenting different or weaker binding
	• high level of $1/f$ noise due to disordered granular systems

Progress in doping of nanoparticles has opened the way for the use of intraband absorption. However, the intraband devices still suffer from three main limitations: too large dark current, small thermal activation energy and slow photoresponse. Nevertheless, the intraband transitions are an attractive possibility for longer wavelength device availability.

CQDs offer a promising alternative to the single-crystal materials. These nanoparticles could improve CQD photodetector performance compared to epitaxial QDs due to many aspects gathered in Table 8.3. It is expected that the extension of application of CQD-based devices will be significant, especially in the area of near IR imaging which is currently dominated by epitaxial semiconductor and hybrid technologies.

CQDs belong to wider class of low-dimensional materials such as 2D materials, nanowires, and their hybrid structures. The effective active regions of photodetectors are fabricated also by hybridisation of 2D materials with CQDs [47].

The infrared QDs are found in different semiconductor groups, including group IV (Si, Ge, GeSn), IV-VI (PbS, PbSe, PbTe), III-V (InAs, InSb), II-VI (HgTe, HgSe), I-VI (Ag$_2$S, Ag$_2$Se), and ternary I-III-VI (CuInS$_2$, CuInSe$_2$) and their alloys [48]. To date, the majority of research has focused on lead salt [44, 49] and Hg-based CQDs [50, 51]. In the lead chalcogenide family, the most popular are lead sulfide (PbS) CQDs with absorption tunable in the NIR spectral range (1–3 μm). Their technology is compatible with CMOS readout technology used in fabrication of monolithic focal plane arrays (FPAs).

As is shown in Figure 8.32(a), the absorption peak depends on the nanocrystal size. Using a larger size (5.5 nm diameter), the peak absorption occurs at the wavelength of 1440 nm, but using a smaller size (3.4 nm), the peak is at 980 nm. This size-dependent tunability can be applied in hyperspectral visible image sensors. Despite strong progress in PbS CQD fabrication, their quantum efficiency is quite low with value to 20 per cent compared to 70 per cent for commercial InGaAs photodiodes. From a performance standpoint, short wavelength infrared (SWIR) PbS CQD have achieved detectivities above 10^{12} Jones at room temperature, which is comparable to commercial InGaAs photodiodes [see Figure 8.32(c)].

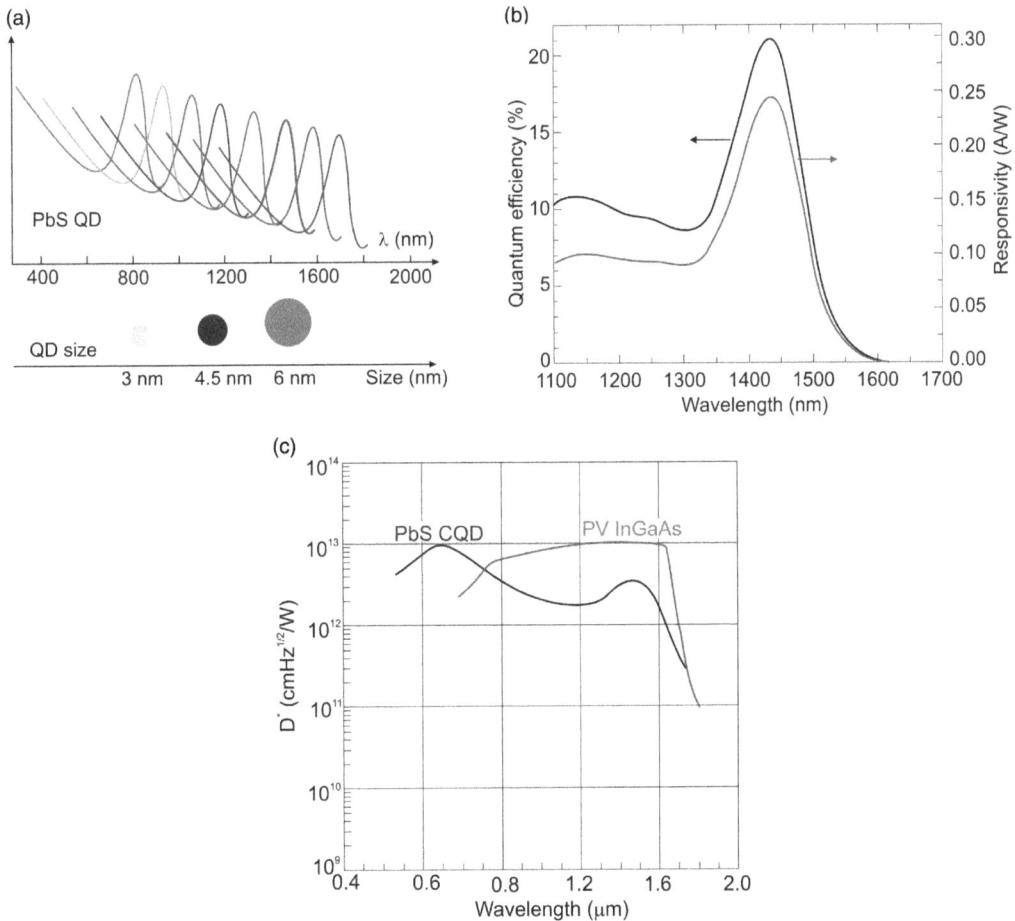

FIGURE 8.32 PbS CQD photodiode: (a) spectral tunability in dependence on dot size (after Reference 44), (b) quantum efficiency and responsivity, (c) detectivity comparison of PbS CQD photodiode with commercial InGaAs photodiode (after Reference 49).

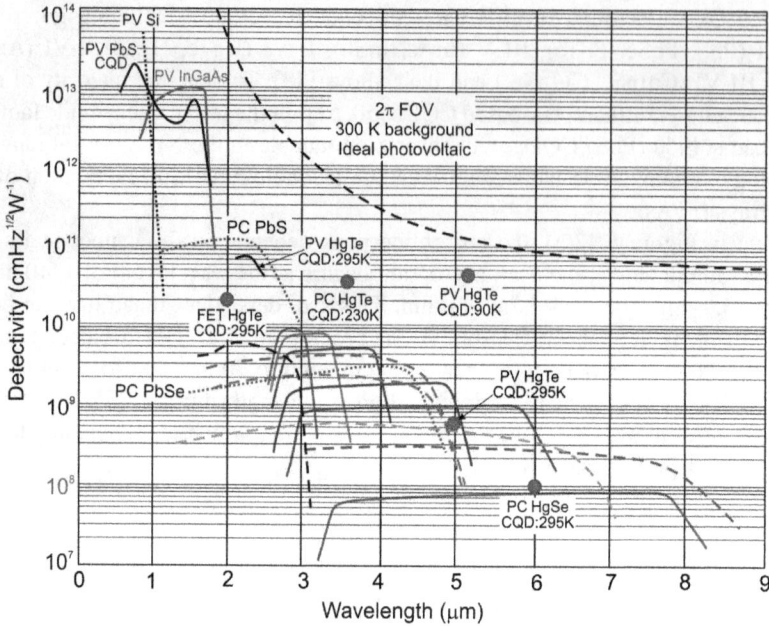

FIGURE 8.33 Room-temperature spectral detectivity curves of the commercially available photodetectors [PV Si and InGaAs, PC PbS and PbSe, HgCdTe photodiodes (solid lines – Vigo catalogue)]. The experimental data for different types of CQD photodetectors operated at 295 K and lower temperatures are marked by dot points (Reference 47). Also spectral detectivities of new emerging T2SL IB QCIPs (dashed lines) are included [52]. PC – photoconductor, PV – photodiode.

Figures 7.43 and 8.33 indicate on sub-BLIP photodetectors performance at room temperature. In addition, Figure 8.33 contains several detectivity data for CQDs photodetectors operated at temperatures below 295 K. Both figures clearly show that the detectivity values of CQD photodetectors are inferior in comparison with HgCdTe photodiodes.

Although the performance of IR focal plane arrays (FPAs) remains paramount, especially in defence and security applications, the ability to produce FPAs at low cost becomes an increasingly integral part of the implementation strategy for existing and emerging infrared imaging systems. It is expected that the extension of application of CQD-based devices will be significant, especially in the area of IR imaging which is currently dominated by epitaxial semiconductor and hybrid technologies. Hybrid technology, due to the complexity of production stages, reduces yield and increases overall cost. The IR CQD-based photodetectors are an alternative solution without these limitations.

IR FPAs are usually fabricated from two separate wafers [see Figure 8.34(a)], one bearing detector photodiodes and other containing silicon readout integrated circuit (ROIC), which are physical bonded (hybridised) together via indium bumps. The complexity of these multiple production steps (about 150) reduces yield and increases overall cost. The CQD-based vertical technology shown in Figure 8.34(b) permits fabrication of detector arrays directly onto ROIC substrates using solution process. Individual pixels are defined by the area of the metal pads arranged on the top of the ROIC surface. The traditional hybrid FPAs are typically limited to smaller arrays (1 megapixel range) due to a small detector wafer and low throughput. Pixel pitch with size up to 5 μm has been demonstrated [53]. With a thin-film active layer integrated monolithically directly on top of the ROIC, submicron pixel size below 1 μm can be achieved. At present the state-of-the-art for CMOS image sensors is 0.9 μm [54].

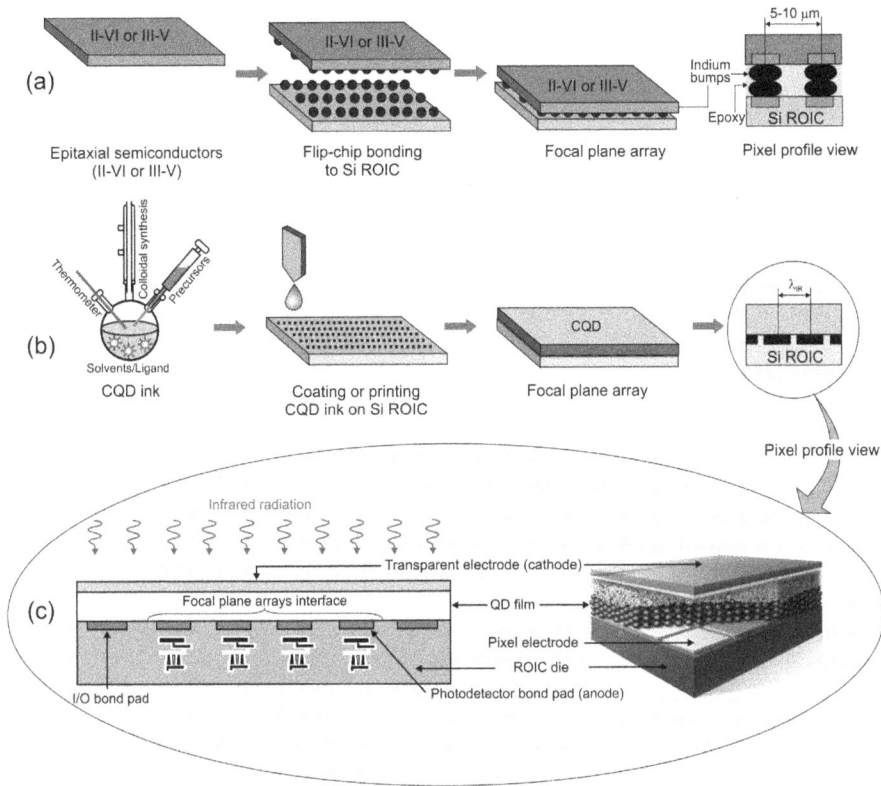

FIGURE 8.34 Comparison of the process flow for integrated hybrid II-VI and III-V compound semiconductor arrays (a) and colloidal quantum dot monolithic arrays (b). The smallest pixel pitch of hybrid arrays is 5 μm. Figure (c) shows the cross-section view on monolithic array structure based on CQDs with potentially pixel pitch below 1 μm.

8.7 QUANTUM CASCADE PHOTODETECTORS

In a conventional photodiode, the responsivity and diffusion length are closely coupled, and an increase in the absorber thickness much beyond the diffusion length may not result in the desired improvement in the signal-to-noise (S/N) ratio. This effect is particularly pronounced at high temperatures, where diffusion lengths are typically reduced. Only charge carriers that are photogenerated at distances shorter than the diffusion length from junction can be collected. In high operating temperature (HOT) photodetectors the absorption depth of LWIR radiation are longer than the diffusion length. Therefore, only a limited fraction of the photogenerated charge contributes to the quantum efficiency.

To avoid the limitation imposed by reduced diffusion length and effectively increase the absorption efficiency of standard photodiodes, novel detector designs, called intersubband (IS) quantum cascade photodetectors (IS QCPs) were introduced in the early 2000s from quantum well infrared photodetectors (QWIPs) and quantum cascade lasers (QCLs). A distinguishing feature of both types of photodetectors is that they can be implemented in chemically stable wide bandgap materials, as a result of the intraband processes used.

Both QWIP and IS QCP devices are characterised by three essential features:

- They are unipolar, majority carrier devices with small effective bandgaps are sandwiched in wider gap semiconductors. The interband activation energy, E_g^{IB}, is much bigger than the

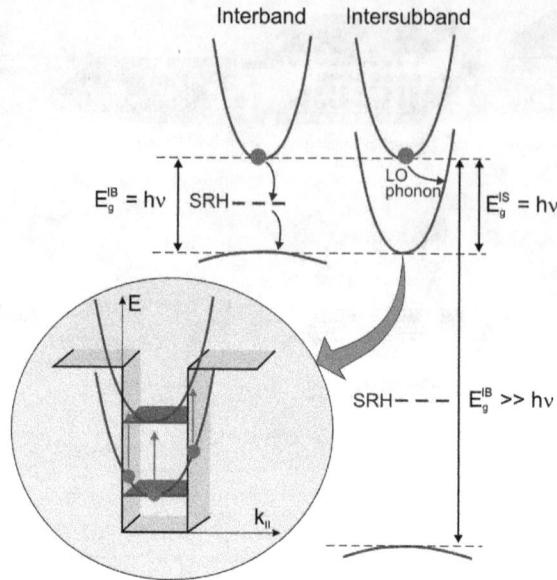

FIGURE 8.35 Comparison carrier recombination mechanisms in interband and intersubband photodetectors. In wide bandgap energy semiconductors, the extrinsic SRH defects have decisive influence on recombination mechanism. In the case of IS transitions, the main recombination mechanism is the LO phonon emission.

energy of detected photons, $h\nu = E_g^{IS}$. The dark current is determined mainly by the small energy gap, E_g^{IS} (see Figure 8.35). Due to large bandgap semiconductors used in fabrication of QW structures, IS devices are self-passivated, which is a valuable advantage in comparison with narrow gap semiconductor photodetectors;

- A key factor affecting IS device performance is the light-coupling scheme. The IS selection rule requires that only the z (TM)-component of the incident light polarisation scatters electrons between subbands (see Figure 8.9). In the case of normal light incidence, IS photodetectors are blind;

- The main recombination mechanism in the IS photodetectors is longitudinal (LO) phonon scattering with photocarrier lifetimes in picoseconds range. It means that QWIP and QCP devices are very fast with their transit-time cut-off frequency in the 100 GHz range.

The fundamental difference between interband (IB) quantum cascade detectors (IB QCPs) and IS QCPs results from the fact that in IB QCLs the injected carriers relax to the lower energy level at a considerably slower rate than in IS QCLs. IB QC devices are intrinsic in their character, instead IS QC devices are extrinsic (doped). Similar to common bulk semiconductors, the interband transitions in IB QCLs are characterised by radiative, Auger and SRH processes, in which carrier lifetimes are on the order of nanosecond. In contrast, the intersubband relaxation in QCLs is accompanied with LO phonon emission and has a picosecond time scale. From the other side, IB QCPs are more sensitive to surface leakage currents because of the presence of surface states in their bandgap.

Figure 8.36(a) shows the measured and fitted dark current-voltage characteristics of large-area ($400 \times 400 \ \mu m^2$) eight-stage IB QCL and fifty-stage IS QCP ($110 \times 110 \ \mu m^2$) with the same transition energy of 230 meV at 300 K [55]. The dark current is at least an order of magnitude lower in the IB device than in the IS one. The consequence of much longer carrier lifetime in the IB QCP is also visible in the saturation current density, which in IB quantum cascade

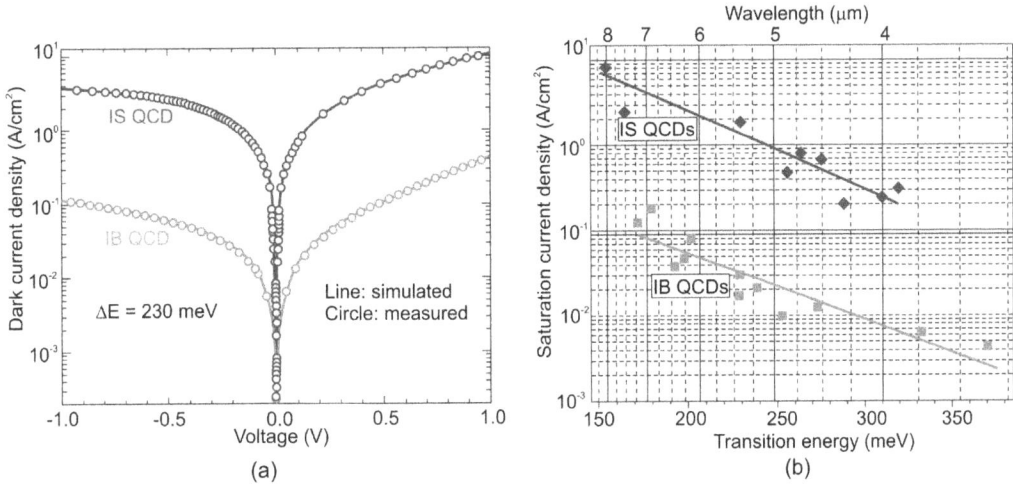

FIGURE 8.36 Differences in dark current characteristics between IS and IB quantum cascade devices at room temperature: (a) the measured and fitted dark current-voltage characteristics of a eight-stage IB QCL and fifty-stage IS QCP with the same transition energy of 230 meV, (b) saturation current density for IS and IB quantum cascade devices (after Reference 55).

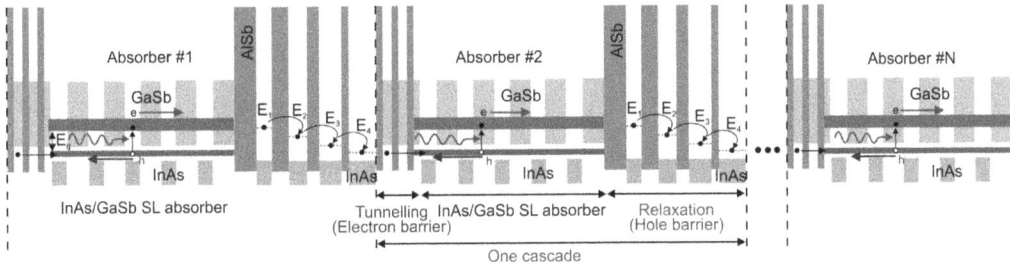

FIGURE 8.37 Schematic illustration of a regular IB QCIP configuration with T2SL InAs/GaSb absorbers, GaSb/AlSb tunnelling and InAs/AlSb relaxation layers.

devices (QCPs) is almost two orders of magnitude lower than values obtained for IS QCPs – see Figure 8.36(b) [55].

The IB QCPs contain very complex structures; in certain cases, even thousands of layers. This structure is not possible to fabricate using conventional growth techniques like chemical vapor deposition or physical vapor deposition of liquid-phase epitaxy. Only molecular beam epitaxy (MBE) is the reliable layered technique in fabrication of multistage devices. This sophisticated technique, due to atomic layer-by-layer growth, enables control of molecular (or atoms) beams onto a heated substrate in ultrahigh environments. Because the design of multistage devices is relatively complicated, involving many interfaces and strained thin layers, their growth by MBE is challenging.

The MBE systems used in fabrications of T2SLs IB QCP structures are equipped with Sb and As crackers, several effusion cells (In, Ga, Al) and doping cells (typically Si for donor doping and Be for acceptor doping). The new MBE systems contain about 10 cells.

A single stage of reverse configuration is similar to a CBIRD structure (see Table 8.2) in which absorber (InAs/GaSb T2SLs) is shorter than the diffusion length and is located between an engineered GaSb/AlSb quantum well (QW) electron barrier and a AlSb/ InAs QW hole barrier. The design of this structure is shown in details in Figure 8.37. The electron relaxation region and the interband-tunnelling region serve also as the hole and the electron barriers, respectively. The barriers act as a means for suppressing current leakage. The electron-relaxation region is precisely designed to facilitate the extraction of photogenerated carriers from the conduction miniband of the absorber and transport them, ideally (with little or no resistance) to the valence band of the absorber in the next stage. As is shown, the energy levels of coupled InAs/AlSb multi-QWs in the conduction band form several staircases, with energy-ladder separations comparable to the LO-phonon energy. The uppermost energy level of the relaxation region staircase is close to the conduction miniband in the InAs/GaSb SL, and the bottom energy-level is positioned below the valence-band edge of the adjacent GaSb layer, allowing the interband tunnelling of extracted carriers move to the next stage.

The total photocurrent is independent on the number of the detector's constituent stages and the photons absorbed in following stages do not enlarge photocurrent but only maintain the current continuity flowing through the device. Discrete absorber design imposes that the photogenerated electrons recombine with holes in the next stage within short transport distance, circumventing the diffusion length limitation in traditional detectors with thick absorbers. To suppress noise, multiple discrete short absorbers are configured in series, and the total thickness of the individual absorbers can be even longer than the absorption depth. The thermal and shot noises are suppressed for shorter individual absorbers and a larger number of cascade stages. The detectivity of quantum cascade infrared photodetector (QCIP), including Johnson noise and electrical shot noise components, is determined by [56]

$$D^* = \frac{\eta \lambda q}{hc} \left(\frac{4kT}{NR_0A} + \frac{2qI_{dark}}{N} \right)^{-1/2},$$

(8.11)

where R_0A is the resistance at zero bias times the detector area corresponding to one period of QCID, T is the detector temperature, N is the number of periods, and I_{dark} is the dark current. Equation (8.11) shows that the signal-to-noise ratio is $\propto \sqrt{N}$.

Figure 7.43 demonstrates that bipolar devices based on type-II InAs/GaSb IB supperlattice absorbers are good candidates for detectors operating near room temperature. The estimated Johnson-noise limited detectivities under zero bias for IB cascade photodetectors with T2SL InAs/GaSb absorbers (based on the measured R_0A product and responsivity) are comparable with those available for commercially HgCdTe photovoltaic detectors. We can see that performance of both type of detectors are similar in a short wavelength infrared region, but interband cascade detectors outperform commercially available uncooled HgCdTe detectors with a similar LW cut-off wavelength. In addition, due to strong covalent bonding of III-V semiconductors, IB QCIPs can be operated at temperatures up to 350°C, which is not possible to achieve for HgCdTe counterpart.

Considering that $D^* \sim \sqrt{R_0A}$, and $R_0A = kT / qJ_o$, the detectivity is inversely proportional to the square root of J_o. As is shown in Figure 8.38, the peak detectivity values of IS detectors at room temperature are at least one order of magnitude lower than T2SL IB detectors. For most IS photodetectors D^* are less than 3×10^7 cmHz$^{1/2}$/W, while IB that are above 1×10^8 cmHz$^{1/2}$/W but in the MWIR region even exceed 1×10^9 cmHz$^{1/2}$/W. These IB cascade detectors combine the advantages of IB optical transitions with the excellent carrier transport properties. The thermal generation rate at any specific temperature and cut-off wavelength in these devices is usually orders of magnitude smaller than that for corresponding IS QCIPs. In consequence, the operating temperature of IB cascade detectors is considerable higher in comparison with IS ones.

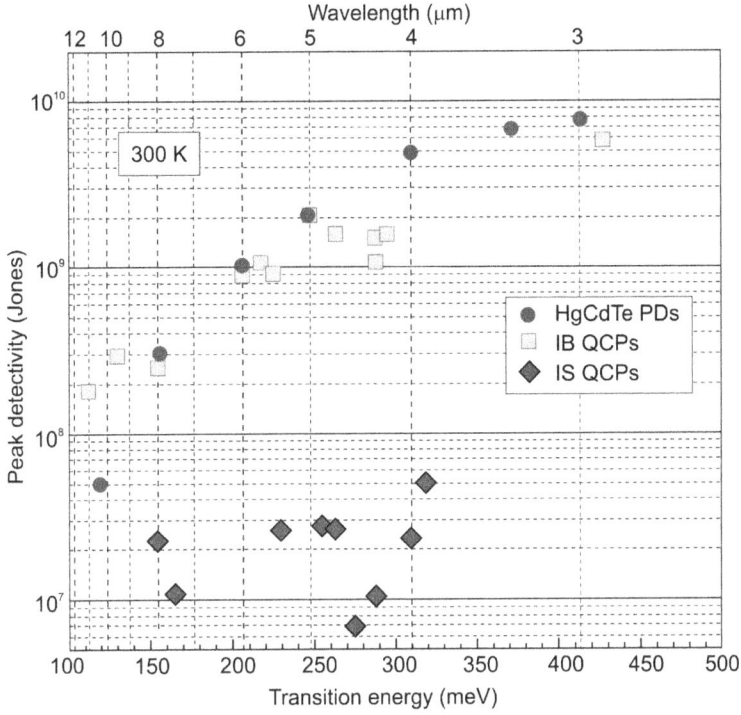

FIGURE 8.38 Peak detectivity at room temperature versus transition energy and wavelength for commercial HgCdTe photodiodes (Vigo catalogue) and IB and IS cascade photodetectors (after Reference 52).

PROBLEMS

Example 8.1

Calculate the wavelength of a photon with a photon energy of 2 eV. Also, calculate the wavelength of a free electron with a kinetic energy of 2 eV.

Example 8.2

Calculate the de Broglie wavelength for electrons with acceleration voltage $V_a = 1000$ V.

Example 8.3

Compare the density of states in 3 (3D), 2 (2D) and 1 (1D) dimension structures

Example 8.4

Determine the wave function $\psi(x)$ for the case when electrons are approaching a potential-energy barrier, as shown in figure below. Consider the case when the electron energy is smaller than the barrier height (tunnelling effect).

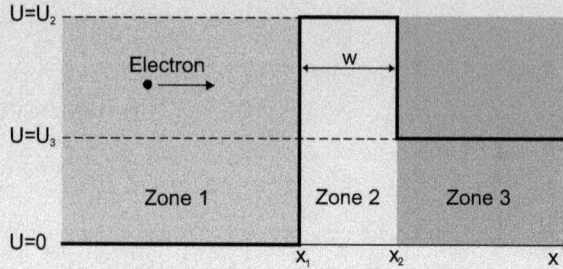

Example 8.5

A potential well has a hight of 0.05 eV. What should be the width of the well so that the binding energy of the electron ($m^* = 0.063m_o$) would be equal to 0.025 eV.

Example 8.6

Determine the band offset of a GaAs/Al$_{0.2}$Ga$_{0.8}$As heterojunction. The valence band position can be calculated as $E_v = E_{v,av} + \Delta/3$, where $E_{v,av}$ is the average valence band position that is obtained from theory and is referred to as the absolute energy level; E_v is the valence band position, and Δ is the spin-orbit splitting energy. The material parameters for GaAs and AlAs are listed below.

	$E_{v,av}$ (eV)	Δ(eV)	E_g (eV)
GaAs	-6.92	0.34	1.52
AlAs	-7.49	0.28	3.13

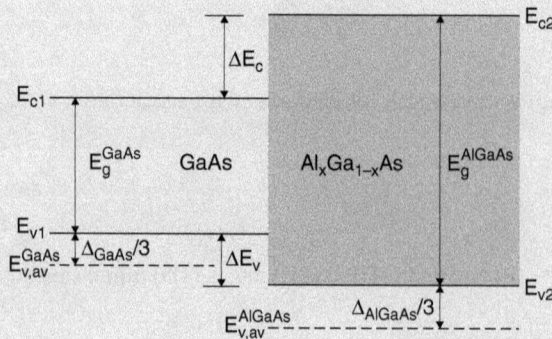

REFERENCES

1. L. Esaki and R. Tsu, "Superlattice and negative conductivity in semiconductors", *IBM J. Res. Dev.* 14, 61–65 (1970).

2. M.A. Kinch, *State-of-the-Art Infrared Detector Technology*, SPIE Press, Bellingham, 2014.

3. F. Capasso, W.T. Tsang, A.L. Hutchinson, and G.F. Williams, "Enhancement of electron impact ionization in a superlattice: A new avalanche photodiode with a large ionization rate ratio", *Appl. Phys. Lett.* 40, 38–40 (1982).

4. R. Chin, N. Holonyak, Jr, G.E. Stillman, J.Y. Tang, and K. Hess, "Impact ionization in multilayer heterojunction structures", *Electron Lett.* 16, 467 (1980).

5. K.F. Brennan and J. Haralson, "Superlattice and multiquantum well avalanche photodetectors: physics, concepts and performance", *Superlattices Microstruct.* 28, (2), 77–104 (2000).

6. M. Ren, S. Maddox, Y. Chen, M. Woodson, J.C. Campbell, and S. Bank, "AlInAsSb/GaSb staircase avalanche photodiode", *Appl. Phys. Lett.* 108, 081101 (2016).

7. F. Capasso, W.-T. Tsang, and G.F. Williams, "Staircase solid-state photomultipliers and avalanche photodiodes with enhanced ionization rates ratio", *IEEE Trans. Electron Devices* 30, 381–390 (1983).

8. T. Kagawa, Y. Kawamura, H. Asai, and M. Naganuma, "InGaAs/InAlAs superlattice avalanche photodiode with a separated photoabsorption layer", *Appl. Phys. Lett.* 57, 1895 (1990).

9. H. Schneider and H. C. Liu, *Quantum Well Infrared Photodetectors*, Springer, Berlin, 2007.

10. S.D. Gunapala, S.V. Bandara, S.B. Rafol, and D.Z. Ting, "Quantum well infrared photodetectors", in *Semiconductors and Semimetals*, Vol. 84, pp. 59–151, edited by S. D. Gunapala, D.R. Rhiger, and C. Jagadish, Elsevier, Amsterdam, 2011.

11. S.D. Gunapala and S.V. Bandara, "Quantum well infrared photodetectors (QWIP)", in *Handbook of Thin Devices*, Vol. 2, pp. 63–99, edited by M.H. Francombe, Academic Press, San Diego, 2000.

12. S. Gunapala, M. Sundaram, S. Bandara. "Sharp infrared eyes: the journey of QWIPs from concept to large inexpensive sensitive arrays in hand-held infrared cameras", *Opto-Electron. Rev.* 7, 271–283 (1999).

13. A. Rogalski, "Comparison of the performance of quantum well and conventional bulk infrared photodetectors", *Infrared Phys. & Technol.* 38, 295–310 (1997).

14. J.Y. Andersson, "Dark current mechanisms and conditions of background radiation limitation of n-doped AlGaAs/GaAs quantum-well infrared detectors", *J. Appl. Phys.* 78, 6298–6304 (1995).

15. S. D. Gunapala, S. V. Bandara, J. K. Liu, J. M. Mumolo, C. J. Hill, S. B. Rafol, D. Salazar, J. Woollaway, P. D. LeVan, and M. Z. Tidrow, "Towards dualband megapixel QWIP focal plane arrays", *Infrared Phys. & Technol.* 50, 217–226 (2007).

16. A. Rogalski, P. Martyniuk and M. Kopytko, *Antimonide-based Infrared Detectors – A New Perspective*, SPIE Press, Bellingham, 2017.

17. M.A. Kinch, F. Aqariden, D. Chandra, P-K Liao, H.F. Schaake, and H.D. Shih, "Minority carrier lifetime in p-HgCdTe", *J. Electron. Mater.* 34, 880–884 (2005).

18. D. Lee, M. Carmody, E. Piquette, P. Dreiske, A. Chen, A. Yulius, D. Edwall, S. Bhargava, M. Zandian, and W.E. Tennant, "High-operating temperature HgCdTe: A vision for the near future", *J. Electronic Mater.* 45(9), 4587–4595 (2016).

19. W.E. Tennant, D. Lee, M. Zandian, E. Piquette, and M. Carmody, "MBE HgCdTe technology: A very general solution to IR detection, described by 'Rule 07', a very convenient heuristic", *J. Electron. Materials* 37, 1406–1410 (2008).

20. D. Lee, P. Dreiske, J. Ellsworth, R. Cottier, A. Chen, S. Tallaricao, A. Yuliusb, M. Carmody, E. Piquette, M. Zandian, and S. Douglas, "Law 19 – the ultimate photodiode performance metric", *Proc. SPIE* 11407, 114070X (2020).

21. H.S. Kim, E. Plis, A. Khoshakhlagh, S. Myers, N. Gautam, Y.D. Sharma, L.R. Dawson, S. Krishna, S.J. Lee, S.K. Noh, "Performance improvement of InAs/GaSb strained layer superlattice detectors by reducing surface leakage currents with SU-8 passivation", *Appl. Phys. Lett*, 96, 033502-1–3 (2010).

22. C.L. Canedy, H. Aifer, I. Vurgaftman, J.G. Tischler, J.R. Meyer, J.H. Warner, and E.M. Jackson, "Antimonide type-II W photodiodes with long-wave infrared R_oA comparable to HgCdTe", *J. Electron. Mater.* 36, 852–856 (2007).

23. J. Bajaj, G. Sullivan, D. Lee, E. Aifer, and M. Razeghi, "Comparison of type-II superlattice and HgCdTe infrared detector technologies," *Proc. SPIE* 6542, 65420B (2007).

24. P.C. Klipstein, E. Avnon, Y. Benny, R. Fraenkel, A. Glozman, S. Grossman, O. Klin, L. Langoff, Y. Livneh, I. Lukomsky, M. Nitzani, L. Shkedy, I. Shtrichman, N. Snapi, A. Tuito, and E. Weiss, "InAs/GaSb type II superlattice barrier devices with a low dark current and a high quantum efficiency", *Proc. SPIE* 9070, 90700U-1-10 (2014).

25. D.Z. Ting, A. Soibel, A. Khoshakhlagh, Sir B. Rafol, S.A. Keo, L. Höglund, A.M. Fisher, E.M. Luong, and S.D. Gunapala, "Mid-wavelength high operating temperature barrier infrared detector and focal plane array", *Appl. Phys. Lett.* 113, 021101 (2018).

26. D. Wu, J. Li, A. Dehzangi, and M. Razeghi, "Mid-wavelength infrared high operating temperature pBn photodetectors based on type-II InAs/InAsSb superlattice", *AIP Adv.* 10, 025018 (2020).

27. D.Z.-Y. Ting, C.J. Hill, A. Soibel, S.A. Keo, J.M. Mumolo, J. Nguyen, and S.D. Gunapala, "A high-performance long wavelength superlattice complementary barrier infrared detector", *Appl. Phys. Lett.* 95, 023508 (2009).

28. P. Martyniuk and A. Rogalski, "Modeling of InAsSb/AlAsSb nBn HOT detector's performance limits", *Proc. SPIE* 8704, 87041X (2013).

29. A.I. D'Souza, E. Robinson, A.C. Ionescu, D. Okerlund, T.J. de Lyon, R.D. Rajavel, H. Sharifi, N.K. Dhar, P.S. Wijewarnasuriya, and C. Grein, "MWIR InAsSb barrier detector data and analysis", *Proc. SPIE* 8704, 87041U (2013).

30. P.C. Klipstein, "XB_nn and XB_pp infrared detectors", *J. Cryst. Growth* 425, 351–256 (2015).

31. P.C. Klipstein, E. Avnon, D. Azulai, Y. Benny, R. Fraenkel, A. Glozman, E. Hojman, O. Klin, L. Krasovitsky, L. Langof, I. Lukomsky, M. Nitzani, I. Shtrichman, N. Rappaport, N. Snapi, E. Weiss, and A. Tuito, "Type II superlattice technology for LWIR detectors", *Proc. SPIE* 9819, 98190T (2016).

32. D.R. Rhiger, "Performance comparison of long-wavelength infrared type II superlattice devices with HgCdTe", *J. Elect. Mater.* 40, 1815–1822 (2011).

33. I.N. Stranski and L. Krastanow, "Zur theorie der orientierten ausscheidung von lonenkristallen aufeinander," *Sitzungsberichte d. Akad. d. Wissenschaften in Wein. Abt. IIb*, 146, 797–810 (1937).

34. P. Guyot-Sionnest, "Colloidal quantum dots", *C. R. Physique* 9, 777–787 (2008).

35. W. Seifert, N. Carlsson, J. Johansson, M-E. Pistol, and L. Samuelson, "In situ growth of nano-structures by metal-organic vapour phase epitaxy", *J. Crystal Growth* 170, 39–46 (1997).

36. S.Y. Wang, S.D. Lin, W. Wu, and C.P. Lee, "Low dark current quantum-dot infrared photodetectors with an AlGaAs current blocking layer", *Appl. Phys. Lett.* 78, 1023–1025 (2001).

37. S. W. Lee, K. Hirakawa, and Y. Shimada, "Bound-to-continuum intersubband photoconductivity of self-assembled InAs quantum dots in modulation-doped heterostructures", *Appl. Phys. Lett.* 75, 1428–1430 (1999).

38. S. Krishna, "Quantum dots-in-a-well infrared photodetectors", *J. Phys. D: Appl. Phys.* 38, 2142–2150 (2005).

39. S.D. Gunapala, S.V. Bandara, C.J. Hill, D.Z. Ting, J.K. Liu, B. Rafol, E.R. Blazejewski, J.M. Mumolo, S.A. Keo, S. Krishna, Y.-C. Chang, and C.A. Shot, "640 × 512 pixels long-wavelength infrared (LWIR) quantum-dot infrared photoconductor (QDIP) imaging focal plane array", *IEEE J. Quant. Electron.* 43, 230–237 (2007).

40. A. Rogalski, *Infrared and Terahertz Detectors*, CRC Press, Boca Raton, 2019.

41. P. Martyniuk, S. Krishna, and A. Rogalski, "Assessment of quantum dot infrared photodetectors for high temperature operation", *J. Appl. Phys.* 104, 034314 (2008).

42. J. Phillips, "Evaluation of the fundamental properties of quantum dot infrared detectors", *J. Appl. Phys.* 91, 4590–4594 (2002).

43. F.P. Garcia de Arquer, A. Armin, P. Meredith, and E.H. Sargent, "Solution-processed semiconductors for next-generation photodetectors", *Nat. Rev. Mater.* 2, 16100 (2017).

44. P.E. Malinowski, E. Georgitzikis, J. Maes, I. Vamvaka, F. Frazzica, J. Van Olmen, P. De Moor, P. Heremans, Z. Hens, and D. Cheyns, "Thin-film quantum dot photodiode for monolithic infrared image sensors", *Sensors* 17, 2867 (2017).

45. M.M. Ackerman, "Bringing colloidal quantum dots to detector technologies", *Inf. Disp* 36(6), 19–23 (2020), https://doi.org/10.1002/msid.1165-.

46. D. Stiff-Roberts, "Quantum-dot infrared photodetectors: a review", *J. Nanophotonics* 3, 031607, 2009

47. A. Rogalski, *2D Materials for Infrared and Terahertz Detectors*, CRC Press, Boca Raton, 2020.

48. H. Lu, G.M. Carroll, N.R. Neale, and M.C. Beard, "Infrared quantum dots: Progress, challenges, and opportunities", *ACS Nano* 13, 939–953 (2019).

49. E.J.D. Klem, C. Gregory, D. Temple, and J. Lewis, "PbS colloidal quantum dot photodiodes for low-cost SWIR sensing", *Proc. SPIE* 9451, 945104-1-5 (2015).

50. X. Tang, M.M. Ackerman, and P. Guyot-Sionnest, "Thermal imaging with plasmon resonance enhanced HgTe colloidal quantum dot photovoltaic devices", *ACS Nano* 12, 7362–7370 (2018).

51. S.B. Hafiz, M. Scimeca, A. Sahu, and D.-K. Ko, "Colloidal quantum dots for thermal infrared sensing and imaging", *Nano Convergence* 6:7 (2019), https://doi.org/10.1186/s40580-019-0178-1.

52. A. Rogalski, P. Martyniuk, and M. Kopytko, "Type-II superlattice photodetectors versus HgCdTe photodiodes", *Prog. Quant. Electron.* 68, 100228 (2019).

53. A. Rogalski, P. Martyniuk, and M. Kopytko, "Challenges of small-pixel infrared detectors: A review", *Rep. Prog. Phys.* 79, 046501 (2016).

54. M. Takase, Y. Miyake, T. Yamada, T. Tamaki, M. Murakami, and Y. Inoue, "First demonstration of 0.9 μm piel global shutter operation by novel charge control in organic photoconductive film", *Proceedings of the 2015 IEEE International Electron Devices Meeting* (IEDM), Washington, DC, 7–9 December 2015.

55. W. Huang, S.M.S. Rassela, L. Li, J.A. Massengale, R.Q. Yang, T.D. Mishima, and M.B. Santos, "A unified figure of merit for interband and intersubband cascade devices", *Infrared Phys & Technol.* 96, 298–301 (2019).

56. A. Gomez, M. Carras, A. Nedelcu, E. Costard, X. Marcadet, V. Berger, "Advantages of quantum cascade detectors", *Proc. SPIE* 6900, 69000J-1–14 (2008).

9 2D Material Photodetectors

Since the discovery of graphene, its applications to electronic and optoelectronic devices have been intensively and thoroughly researched. Extraordinary and unusual electronic and optical properties allow graphene and other two-dimensional (2D) materials to be promising candidates for new class of photodetectors. The unique and distinctive optoelectronic properties of 2D materials create a new platform for a variety of photonic applications, including fast photodetectors, transparent electrodes in displays and photovoltaic modules, optical modulators, plasmonic devices and ultrafast lasers.

High-quality 2D materials are promising for next-generation alternative sensor platforms, however it will take several decades of research, development and, most importantly, billions of dollars of investment at the national and international levels to become the ultimate benchmark for standard electronic materials and devices. From the other side, the evolutionary path of Si technology, driven by Moore's Law of Scaling, seems to be narrowing and fast approaching an end simply due to the fundamental limitations of Si at the atomic scale [1]. In fact, it is unlikely that 2D technology will supplant Si, but instead may coexist with Si technology [2]. This, too, will require significant research and resource investment in large area growth of 2D materials at temperatures compatible with silicon-based technology. All these aspects are in the infancy stage of manufacturability.

9.1 RELEVANT PROPERTIES OF GRAPHENE AND RELATED 2D MATERIALS

2D materials are atomically thin films originally derived from layered crystals such as graphite, hexagonal boron nitride (h-BN), the family of transition metal dichalcogenides (TMDs, such as MoS_2, WSe_2, $MoTe_2$, and others) and black phosphorus (bP). The materials have attracted significant attention, especially in the last decade, owing to extraordinary physical and chemical properties:

- quantum confinement in the direction to the 2D plane, which leads to extraordinary electronic and optical properties that are beneficial for light absorption;
- a weak stack of atomic planes layered on each other by Van der Waals forces leave no dangling bonds, which makes it easy to construct vertical heterostructures and integrate 2D materials with silicon chips;
- the atomically thin characteristic enables scaling down to nanodevices without parasitic capacitance.

In this section we briefly discuss the fundamental properties of 2D crystals. As there are many comprehensive papers focusing on 2D material synthesis, this field will not be reviewed here.

Although 2D materials cover a wide range of compounds across the periodic table and a very wide range of the electromagnetic spectrum, only a handful of material groups have been explored

DOI: 10.1201/9781003263098-9

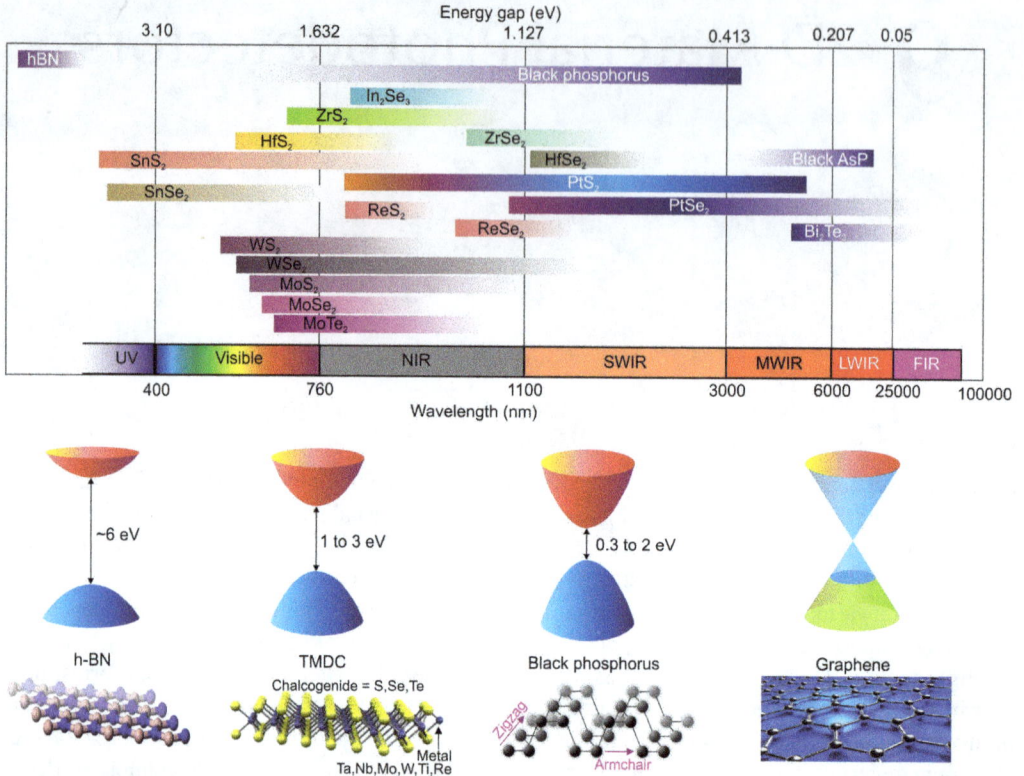

FIGURE 9.1 The bandgap of the different layered semiconductors and electromagnetic spectrum. The exact bandgap value depends on the number of layers, strain level and chemical doping. FIR: far infrared; LWIR: long wavelength infrared; MWIR: mid wavelength infrared; SWIR: short wavelength infrared; NIR: near infrared; UV: ultraviolet. The atomic structures of hexagonal born nitride (h-BN), TMDs, black phosphorus (bP) and graphene are shown at the bottom of the panel, left to right. The crystalline directions (x and y) of anisotropic bP are indicated.

for traditional optoelectronic applications. As is shown in Figure 9.1, the 2D materials range from graphene and its zero bandgap to small/mid-bandgap materials, such as phosphorene and the TMDs, and to wide bandgap hexagonal boron nitride (h-BN), which is used exclusively as a topologically smooth insulator. Table 9.1 lists the significant 2D materials used for fabricating optoelectronic devices and a few of their electronic properties [3].

9.1.1 GRAPHENE

Since its discovery in 2004, graphene has been extensively and comprehensively studied due to its unique and exceptional electronic and optical properties [4]. The most intriguing and fascinating electronic property of graphene is its linear dispersion relation between the energy and the wave vector where the mentioned relativistic-like energy dispersion is accompanied by electrons being transported at a Fermi velocity, only 100 times lower than light speed.

Graphene consists of sp^2 hybridised carbon atoms arranged as a honeycomb with lattice constant $a = 1.42$ Å. The valence and conduction bands drop at the Brillouin zone corners (Dirac points), making graphene a nearly zero bandgap semiconductor, as shown in Figure 9.2. Due to the zero density of states at the Dirac points (the Brillouin zone corners), the conductivity is reasonably low.

TABLE 9.1
Room Temperature Properties of Selected 2D Materials (after Reference 3)

2D material	Bandgap (eV)	Effective mass (m_o)	Device mobility (cm^2/Vs)	Saturation velocity (m/s)	Young's mod. (GPa)	Thermal conductivity (W/mK)	CTE* (10^6 K^{-1})
Graphene	0 (D)	< 0.01	$10^3 - 5 \times 10^4$	$(1-5) \times 10^5$	1000	600 – 5000	– 8
1L MoS$_2$	1.8 (D)	~0.5	10 – 130	4×10^4	270	40	NA
Bulk MoS$_2$	1.2 (I)		30 – 500	3×10^4	240	50(‖), 4(⊥)	1.9(‖)
1L WSe$_2$	1.7 (D)	0.31	140 – 250	4×10^4	195	NA	NA
Bulk WSe$_2$	1.2 (I)		500	NA	75 – 100	9.7(‖), 2(⊥)	11(‖)
h-BN	5.9 (D)		NA	NA	220 – 880	250 – 360(‖), 2 (⊥)	– 2.7
Phosphorene	0.3–2 (D)	0.17	50 – 1000	NA	35 – 164	10 – 35(‖)	NA

All listed values should be considered estimates. In some cases, experimental or theoretical values are not available (NA).
D, I; direct and indirect energy gap.
The ‖ symbol signifies the in-plane direction; ⊥ signifies the out of plane direction.
*CTE, coefficient of thermal expansion.

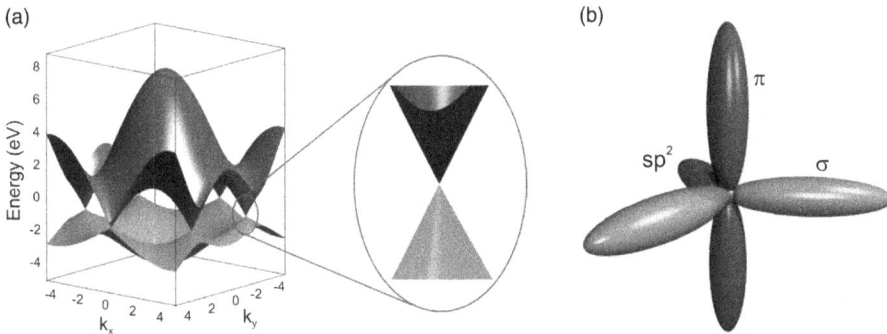

FIGURE 9.2 The band structure of graphene in the honeycomb lattice (a). The enlarged picture shows the energy bands close to one of the Dirac points. Schematic of electron σ- and π-orbitals of one carbon atom in graphene (b).

However, the Fermi level (E_F) position can be changed and modified by doping (with electrons or holes) to create a material that is potentially better in terms of conductivity than copper at room temperature. It is commonly known that carbon atoms have a total of 6 electrons; 2 in the inner shell and 4 in the outer shell. The 4 outer shell electrons in carbon atom are available for chemical bonding but, in graphene, each atom is connected to 3 other carbon atoms on the 2D plane, leaving 1 electron freely available in the third dimension for electrical conduction. These π-electrons exhibit high mobility and are located above and below the graphene sheet where π-orbitals overlap and enhance the carbon-to-carbon bonds in graphene. Fundamentally, the electronic properties of graphene are determined by the bonding and anti-bonding (the valence and conduction bands) π-orbitals.

Graphene exhibits the potential for ballistic carrier transport with the predicted and assessed mean free path > 2 μm at room temperature, where carriers were found to propagate via diffraction similarly to the light in a waveguide, rather than by carrier diffusion in comparison with conventional semiconductors.

As mentioned before, the graphene carrier mobility and saturation velocity show the potential for high-speed photonic devices [5]. A graphene-layered structure with long both electrons and holes relaxation times allow for a significant performance improvement of optoelectronic devices. Theoretically, graphene exhibits a room temperature electron mobility of 250000 cm²/Vs; however, the transport mechanism is extremely dependent on the local environment and material processing. Vacuum-suspended graphene fabricated by exfoliation is characterised by extremely high carrier mobilities > 200000 cm²/Vs at room temperature. Unfortunately, these films were reported to have a very small area (approx. 100 µm²), making it expensive for industrial applications. When placed on a substrate, graphene mobility is reduced by both the charged impurity and remote interfacial phonon-scattering effects (see Figure 9.3). On SiO_2, interfacial phonon scattering limits the graphene mobility to 40000 cm²/Vs [6]. Exposure to atmospheric conditions and processing contaminants that resist residue, water and metallic impurities also act as scattering sources limiting mobility.

Another feature making graphene interesting in terms of optoelectronic devices is its high thermal conductivity (approx. 10 times copper and 2 times diamond) and high conductivity (approx. 100 times copper). Graphene is also characterised by high tensile strength (130 GPa, compared to 400 MPa for A36 structural steel).

In comparison with metals that have a large quantity of free charges, graphene should be considered as a semimetal where carriers can be induced through chemical doping or electrical gating with great flexibility due to its 2D nature, where the doping concentration from 10^{12} to 10^{13} cm^{-2} can be easily reached. Therefore, the semimetal nature of graphene causes electrical tunability to be unfeasible for conventional metals.

In addition, optical properties of graphene are interesting [7] where graphene's optical conductivity is defined as $\pi\beta$, where β is equal $\left(1/4\pi\varepsilon_o\right)\left(e^2/\hbar c\right)$, e is the electron charge, $\hbar$ is Planck's constant, c is light speed providing graphene with broadband (visible and IR) linear absorption of 2.3 per cent per monolayer. The graphene 0.33 nm monolayer absorbs roughly 2.3 per cent of the incident light being 10–1000 times higher than for semiconductors like silicon and GaAs and covering a much broader spectral bandwidth.

Although pristine graphene is a zero-gap semiconductor, one can open a bandgap in graphene using different methods. It was found that the graphene's bandgap structure can be modified: by substitutional doping, by the addition of two layers and bilayer doping. The graphene's bandgap also can be opened by its patterning into nanoribbon shape or applying a perpendicular electric

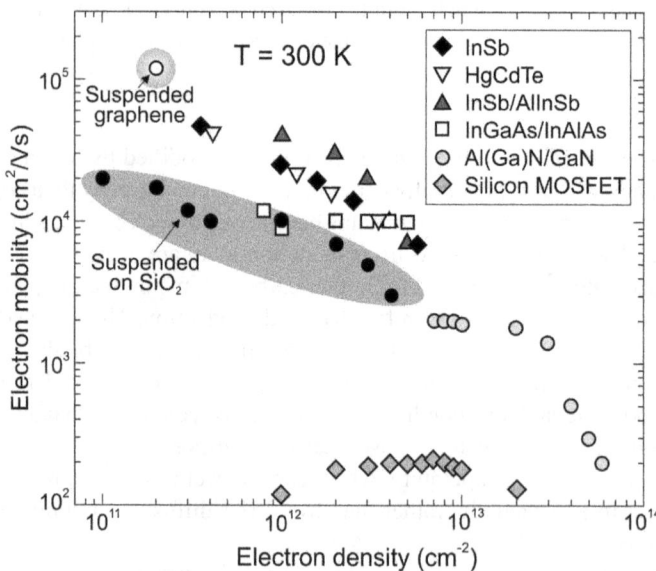

FIGURE 9.3 Electron mobility in graphene at room temperature in comparison with other material systems.

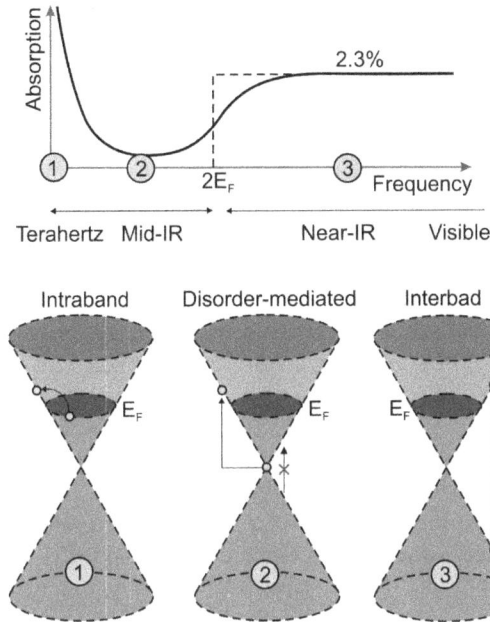

FIGURE 9.4 Characteristic absorption spectrum of doped graphene (adapted after Reference 9).

field to bilayer graphene. In fact, graphene can cover the range from 0 eV to 0.2 eV. The doping of graphene layers can move the E_F either up or down, decreasing both electrons and holes mobility. Graphene's thickness restriction creates large resistance and chemical inertness, making pure conductive applications less feasible.

Graphene was reported to exhibit the highest specific interaction strength (absorption per atom of material). Silicon has typically a 10 μm absorption depth, causing the 2.3 per cent light absorption in a 200 nm layer, while graphene reaches the same optical absorption in a much smaller 0.3 nm layer (interplane spacing).

The absorption spectrum of graphene covers an ultra-broadband range from visible to terahertz spectral range [8]. There are two photo-excitation modes: interband transition and intraband transition. Figure 9.4 presents a typical absorption spectrum of doped graphene [9]. For visible and near infrared light, electrons can be excited from the valence band to the conduction band though the interband transition. In the low frequency THz region, the photon energy is below $2E_F$ and interband transition is forbidden while the intraband transition dominates. The absorption is mainly due to the free-carrier (Drude) response. In doped graphene in the mid-IR region, the optical absorption is minimal, and the residual absorption is generally attributed to the disorder in imparting the momentum for the optical transition. A transition occurs close to $2E_F$, where direct interband processes lead to a universal 2.3 per cent absorption. In the THz band, the coupling of graphene and photons can be enhanced by intraband transition, and thus it is possible to achieve sensitive THz detection.

9.1.2 2D Crystalline Materials

The high dark current of conventional graphene materials arising from the gapless nature of graphene significantly reduces the sensitivity of photodetection and restricts further developments of graphene-based photodetectors. The discovery of new 2D materials with direct energy gaps in the infrared to the visible spectral regions has opened up a new window for photodetector fabrication. Even though the technology readiness levels are still low, and device manufacturability and reproducibility remain a challenge, the 2D materials technology can be found in research labs around the globe, including materials like silicene, germanene, stanene and phosphorene, transition metal dichalcogenides (TMDs), black phosphorus and, recently discovered, all inorganic perovskites.

2D materials are a class of materials derived from layered Van der Waals (vdW) solids. The in-plane atoms are held together by tight covalent or ionic bonds along 2D directions to form atomic layers, while the atomic layers are bonded together by weak vdW interactions along out-of-plane direction. Because of that, a large number of 2D atomic crystals could be mechanically exfoliated from bulk single crystals. Moreover, because of the week physical bonds between the layers, it is possible to mechanically stack arbitrary 2D materials, and this offers a freedom in fabricating the heterostructures based on 2D materials.

Nicolosi *et al.* [10] summarised different types of layered materials that can be grouped into diverse families (see Figure 9.1), and which can cover a broad range of electrical and optical properties:

- atomically thin hexagonal boron nitride (h-BN, similar to hexagonal sheets of graphene);
- transition metal dichalcogenides (TMDs);
- black phosphorus (bP), metal halides (e.g. PbI_2, $MgBr_2$), metal oxides (such as MnO_2 and MnO_3), double hydroxides, III-Vs (such as InSe and GaS), V-VIs (such as Bi_2Te_3 and Sb^2Se_3; and
- halide perovskites.

Layered TMDs are atomically thin materials with the chemical formula of MX_2, in which M is a transition metal atom (e.g., W, Mo, Re) and X is a chalcogen atom (e.g., S, Se, or Te). As is shown at the bottom of Figure 9.1, one layer of M atoms is sandwiched by two layers of X atoms. 2D TMDs exist in three polytypes (trigonal – 1T, hexagonal – 2H, and rhombohedral – 3R) which are characterised by different electronic properties, spanning from metallic to semiconducting or even superconducting [11]. The trigonal phase has only been reported in monolayer shape with a trigonal unit cell, while the 2H and 3R phases have two and three layers with hexagonal and rhombohedral unit cells, respectively.

Unlike graphene, where the optoelectronic properties are based on s and p hybridisation, the optoelectronic properties of TMDs depend on the d electron count, that is, filling of the d orbitals of transition metals and its coordination environment. The number of d electrons in transition metal varies between 0 and 6 for group 4 to group 10 TMDs, respectively. The completely filled d orbitals, as in the case of $2H\text{-}MoS_2$ (group 6) and $1T\text{-}PtS_2$ (group 10), give rise to semiconducting nature, while partially filled, as in the case of $2H\text{-}NbSe_2$ (group 5) and $1T\text{-}ReS_2$ (group 7), exhibit metallic conductivity.

In practical applications, the stability of materials is an important factor that affects the reliability and lifetime of a device. The electronic properties of TMD materials are mainly determined by the filling of metal atom d orbitals, while the lattice parameters and stability primarily depend on the chalcogen atom [12]. The bonding of the M–X is covalent: the metal (M) atom provides four electrons to fill the bonding states, while the lone-pair electrons of the chalcogen (X) atoms terminate the surfaces of the layers. The absence of dangling bonds reduces the chemical instability and protects the surface atoms from reacting with environmental species. Thus, notably, the more stable the lone pair of the chalcogen (X) atoms are, the more stable the 2D materials will be. This explains, for example, why monolayer MoS_2 is more stable than monolayer $MoTe_2$.

Due to the quantum confinement and surface effects, 2D TMDs exhibit many interesting layer-dependent properties that significantly differ from their bulk crystals. The bulk materials are indirect semiconductors having a bandgap typically of ~ 1 eV. In contrast, monolayer TDM is direct semiconductors with higher bandgap. As the material becomes thinner from the bulk to the monolayer, the band structure of TMDs transits from smaller indirect bandgap one to a larger direct bandgap one. In consequence, TMDs can detect light at different wavelengths by tuning the bandgap by varying the number of layers due to quantum confinement effects [8,13–16]. Moreover, the optical and electronic properties of these materials can be strongly affected by large strains. Compared to graphene, TMDs – like molybdenum disulfide (MoS_2), tungsten disulfide (WS_2) and molybdenum diselenide ($MoSe_2$) – exhibit even higher absorption in the visible and the near infrared range and cover a very broad portion of the spectrum from infrared to ultraviolet (see Figure 9.1).

The optical absorption of TMDs in visible to near-infrared (NIR) regions is dominated by carrier direct transitions between the valence and conduction band states around K and K' points of the 2D hexagonal Brillouin zone [17] with the contribution of strong excitonic effects. The light absorption can be extended to the mid-infrared spectral region because of the existence of defect- or edge-states inside the bandgap and the relatively high ratios of edge-to-surface area. The absorption coefficient is typically on the order of 10^4–10^6 cm^{-1} so more than 95 per cent of the sunlight is absorbed for TMD films with sub-micrometre thickness. This high optical absorption can be explained by dipole transitions between localised d-states and excitonic coupling of such transitions.

The carrier mobility of TMDs increases with the number of layers, in general, however, their mobility is low (typically less than 250 cm^2/Vs), and this disadvantage is hard to overcome. Similar to graphene, the carrier mobilities of TMDs are limited by ripples, phonon scattering, impurity scattering and interface scattering [18]. Figure 9.5 summarises the room-temperature carrier mobility of typical group-6 TMDCs with the comparison of different layers of noble TMDs ($PtSe_2$, PtS_2, and $PdSe_2$) and bP on back-gated SiO_2 substrates [19]. The charge-carrier density depends on the doping levels and recombination centres, and the typical value is 10^{12} cm^{-2} [20].

Recently, group-10 noble TMDs have been reintroduced as new 2D materials displaying widely tunable bandgap, moderate carrier mobility, anisotropy, and ultrahigh air stability. For long wavelength infrared (LWIR) detector applications the layered semiconductors with narrow bandgaps and high mobilities are required. Among the TMDs, noble metal dichalcogenides provide such opportunity. It has been theoretically predicted that at room temperature the carrier mobility of group X transition-metal dichalcogenides PtX_2 (X = Se, S) is over 1000 cm^2/Vs, and the bandgaps of their bilayers and bulks could be very small, between 0–0.25 eV [21, 22].

The band structure of MX_2 (M = Ni, Pt, Pd; X = S, Se) changes dramatically with the change of layer number. Monolayer MS_2 (M = Ni, Pt, Pd) are semiconductors with indirect bandgaps of 0.51, 1.11 and 1.75 eV for NiS_2, PdS_2 and PtS_2, respectively [23]. Furthermore, the bilayer NiS_2 and

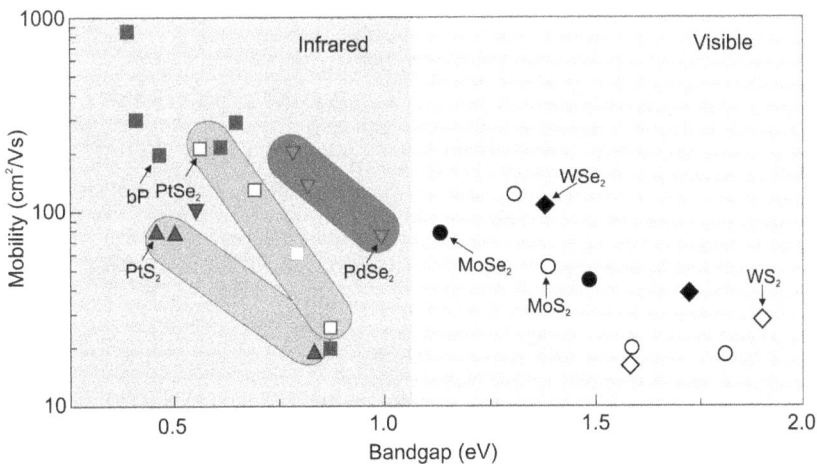

FIGURE 9.5 The layer-dependent room temperature mobility of group-6 TMDCs, bP, and typical noble TMDs on back-gated SiO_2 substrate (after Reference 19).

PdS$_2$ become metallic as predicted by first-principles calculation theory. Similar to PtS$_2$, monolayer PtSe$_2$ is also an indirect bandgap semiconductor. First-principles calculation shows that the bandgap of PtSe$_2$ becomes narrow in bilayer and turns to zero in trilayer which basically implies metallic character [24]. Optical absorption measurements confirm that PdSe$_2$ exhibits a gradual transition from a semiconductor (monolayer) to semimetal (bulk), which is consistent with theoretical simulation based on density functional theory. Specifically, when the layer number reaches 50 layers, the bandgap is close to 0.

Discovery of black phosphorus (bP), the most stable allotrope of phosphorus, can be dated back a century long ago. It was first synthesised from red phosphorus under high temperature and pressure [26]. Studies of black P as a bulk material did not receive much attention from the semiconductor research community up to 2014. At the beginning of 2014, a few research teams reintroduced bP from the perspective of a layered thin film material [27].

Bulk bP has an orthorhombic structure symmetry [15]. In the atomic layer, each phosphorous atom connects to three neighbouring atoms, leading to two special directions: armchair and zigzag directions along the x and y axis, respectively (see bottom of Figure 9.1). This highly anisotropic arrangement of phosphorous atoms leads to anisotropic electric band dispersion, further bringing the anisotropic optoelectronic properties. The effective mass of carriers of bP along the zigzag direction is about 10 times larger than that along the armchair direction [28], which induces strong in-plane anisotropy in its electronic, optical, and phonon properties. The strong anisotropic properties can be used to invent new electronic and optoelectronic device applications, such as plasmonic devices with intrinsic anisotropy in their resonance properties and high-efficiency thermoelectric using the orthogonality in the heat and electron transport directions [27].

The strong in-plane anisotropy results in a high hole mobility of 1000 cm^2/Vs along the light effective mass direction and about 500 cm^2/Vs along the heavy effective mass direction. bP at the same time exhibits considerable conductivity in samples with thickness from 2 to 5 μm.

The second feature of bP is its wide thickness-dependent bandgaps which come from the relatively strong interlayer interaction of buckled bP atomic sheets. The bandgap of bP varies with the number of layers [29], which has been demonstrated both in theory and in experiment as shown in Figure 9.6. Obviously, the bandgap of bP increases monotonically as the layer thickness decreases. It should be marked, that bP always keeps its direct-bandgap nature while changing its thickness. It is important to note that the bandgap of bP covers the range of 0.3–1.2 eV.

Besides thickness, the bandgap of bP can also be modulated by other strategies, including applying strain, electric field and composition alloying. Liu *et al.* [30] have demonstrated fully compositional

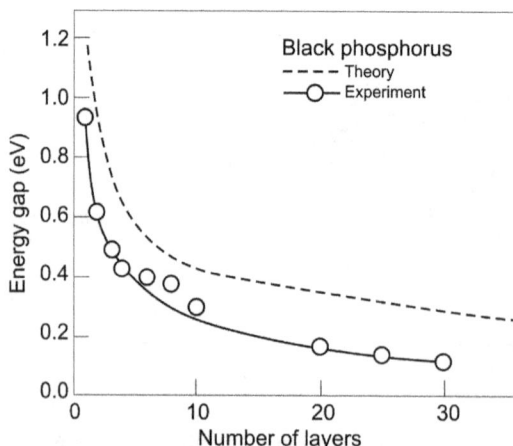

FIGURE 9.6 Thickness depends on bandgap of bP, both in theory and in experiment (after Reference 29).

tunability of layered bAs_xP_{1-x} that cover a long wavelength region down to around 0.15 eV (corresponds to a wavelength of 8.27 μm, LWIR regime). So, the bandgap of bP (and its compounds) itself covers an extremely wide range of energy ~0.15–2 eV corresponding to ~8–0.6 μm, which has not been achieved in any other 2D layered materials. Thus, bAsP bridges the gap between graphene (nearly zero bandgap semiconductor) and TMDs (wide bandgap semiconductors).

Also the transport properties of bP lie between that of graphene and most TMDs previously studied, which is shown in Figure 9.7. This figure demonstrates carrier mobilities versus current on/off ratio reported for field-effect transistors based on typical 2D materials [27]. Here, it should be explained that the on/off ratio represents the ratio between the channel currents when the transistor is in the conduction mode (I_{on}) and when it is switched off (I_{off}). Since the ideal I_{off} value is minimal (to avoid power consumption when not operating), I_{on}/I_{off} should be at the highest possible. Typical good values for on/off ratio are above 10^5–10^6. The onset voltage is defined as the gate voltage necessary for the transistor switch from the "off state" to the "on state".

Despite the possible variation of the mobility at different 2D material classes, they fall into three zones. Graphene with very high mobility is characterised by the on-off transistor ratio often less than 10 due to its zero bandgap (high dark current). TMDs materials are predisposed for ultra-low power nanoelectronics. Black phosphorus falls into a region on the plot of the mobility/on-off ratio not easily covered by graphene or TMDs. This region, where the mobility is in a range of a few hundred cm²/Vs and at the same time the on/off ratio is roughly around 10^4, is attractive for gigahertz thin film electronics.

The stability of 2D materials in ambient conditions remains a crucial issue for the nanodevices. The lack of good stability in ambient air conditions greatly restricted their practical application. With the rising research interest on bP, the study on the chemical stability of this material is most intensive, owing to its large reactivity and environmental instability in ambient conditions. Exfoliated flakes of bP are highly hydroscopic and tend to take up moisture from air. The long-term contact with the water condensed on the surface degrades the bP. Many researchers have been focused on the methods to improve its air-stability using materials and chemicals like Al_2O_3, TiO_2, HfO_2, titanium sulfonate ligand (TiL_4); and coating materials, such as graphene, MoS_2, or h-BN [12].

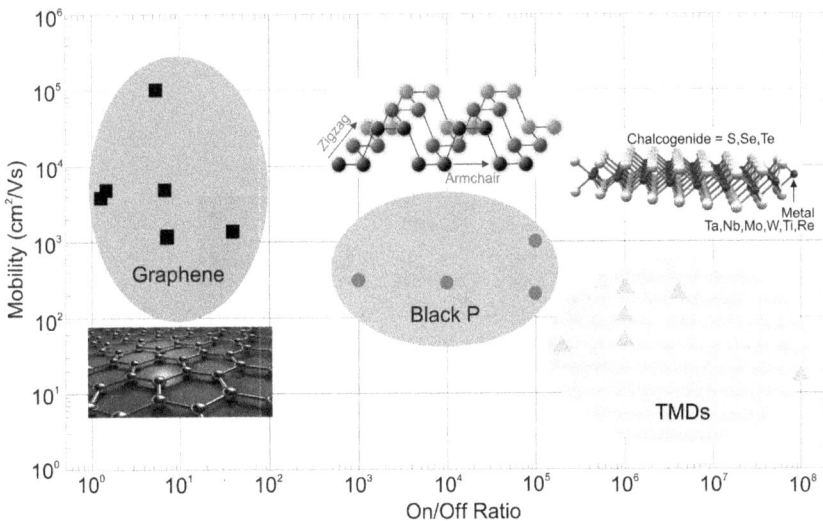

FIGURE 9.7 Carrier mobility versus current on/off ratio reported for typical 2D materials electronics.

9.2 2D MATERIAL-BASED DETECTORS

Generally, 2D material detectors can be divided into two categories: either photon or thermal detectors. Both categories of detectors are described in Chapter 4. One is related to the excitation of free carriers as a result of optical transition, including the photoconductive effect and photovoltaic effect. The other is attributed to the thermal effect, including for example the bolometric effect and the photothermoelectric (PTE) effect. In this section, additional general information is limited to specific types of 2D material detectors.

A particular example of the photoconductive effect is photogating. The photogating effect can be realised in two ways by

- generation of e-h pairs, when one type of carrier is trapped by the localised states (nanoparticles and defects), and
- generation of e-h pairs in trap-states, and one type of carrier is transferred to 2D materials, whereas the other resides at the same place to modulate the layered materials.

In both cases, due to long carrier lifetime, the enhancement of sensitivity is at the cost of photoresponse speed.

If holes/electrons are trapped in localised states (see Figure 9.8), they act as a local gate, effectively modulating the resistance of active materials. In this case, the photocarriers are only limited by the recombination lifetime of the localised trap states, leading to a large photoconductive gain, g. The trap states where carriers can reside for long times are usually located at defects or at the surface of the semiconducting material. This effect is of particular importance for nanostructured materials, like colloidal quantum dots, nanowires and 2D semiconductors, where the large surface and reduced screening play a major role in the electrical properties.

In the case of the photodiode, the photoelectric effect is usually equal to 1, due to separation of minority carriers by the electrical field of the depletion region. However, in a hybrid combination of 2D material photodetectors, photosensitisation and carrier transport take place in separately optimised regions: one for efficient light absorption, and the second to provide fast charge reticulation. In this way, ultra-high gain up to 10^8 electrons per photon and exceptional resposivities for short-wavelength infrared photodetectors have been demonstrated [31, 32].

The simple architecture of the hybrid phototransistor, very popular in design of 2D material photodetectors with the fast transfer channel for charge carriers, is shown in Figure 9.9(b). Since, for example, the graphene in these devices is not responsible for light absorption but only the sensing

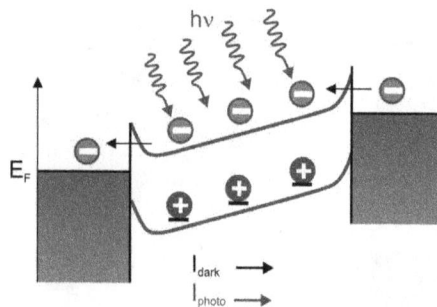

FIGURE 9.8 Band alignment under illumination with photon of energy higher than the bandgap generating e-h pairs. Holes are trapped at the band edge and act as a local gate. In consequence, the field-effect induces more electrons in the channel, generating a photocurrent that adds to the dark current. If the electron lifetime exceeds the time it takes for the electron to transit device, then the long time of the trapped holes ensures the electrons can circulate through an external circuit many times, resulting in gain.

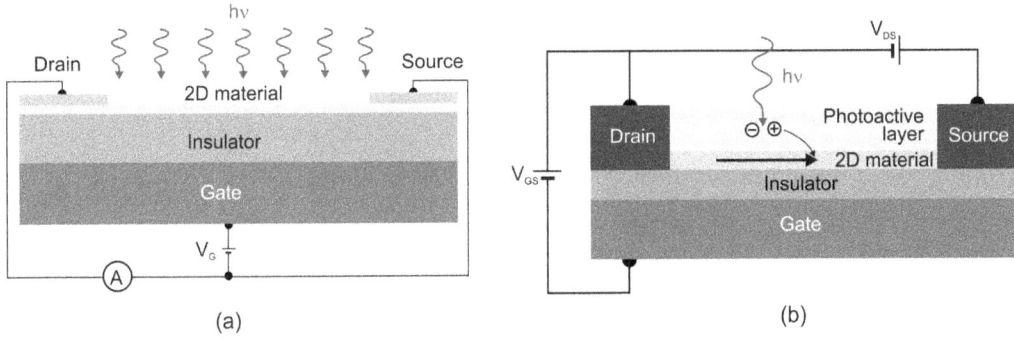

FIGURE 9.9   Operation of 2D material phototransisor (a) and hybrid phototransistor (b).

of charge, absorber choice determines the spectral response. Graphene's large ambipolar mobility ($\sim 10^3$–10^5 cm^2/Vs) acts as a built-in photogain mechanism (i.e., amplifier) enhancing the detector response.

2D materials with thickness down to the atomic layer are more susceptible to local electric fields than conventional bulk materials, and the photogating effect can strongly modulate the channel conductivity by external gate voltage. Improving the optical gain is particularly important since the quantum efficiency is limited because of the weak absorption in 2D materials.

Figure 9.9(a) shows graphene phototransistor architecture accompanied by the short-circuit photocurrent induced by light. Phototransistors basically have the same three-terminal configuration as field-effect transistors (FETs). While in the operational mode of a normal FET, the amount of current (the drain current) flowing in the accumulated channel is controlled by the magnitude of gate voltage (V_G) at a given source to drain bias (V_{DS}), for phototransistors, the control of channel conductance can be additionally enabled by the absorption of light. If there is no bias applied between the source and the drain, minimal photocurrent is collected when the light spot is focused on the middle of the graphene channel. Significant photocurrent is observed when the light is incident on the metal graphene interface area, which is attributed to the conventional PV effect. The built-in electric field in graphene (due to different work functions of the graphene and metal contacts) separates e-h pairs, creating photocurrent in the external circuit. In the middle of the channel, there is no built-in electric field and, as a result, no photocurrent is observed. The built-in electric field can be further adjusted by a gate bias influencing photocurrent.

In the case of a hybrid detector shown in Figure 9.9(b), the holes are injected into a transporting channel, whereas the electrons remain in the photoactive layer. The injected charges can reticulate as much as several thousand times before recombination, giving contribution in gain under illumination. The photocarrier's lifetime is enhanced through both the bandgap structure and defect engineering, and at the same time the trapping mechanisms limit the response time of the photodetector as much as several seconds. There is a trade-off between the enhancement of sensitivity and photoresponse speed.

The graphene p-n junctions can be feasibly obtained since the Fermi level can be easily tuned because of the limited density of states and easy formation of p-type or n-type doping. The electrical and optical properties of graphene p-n junctions are different from traditional silicon p-n junctions in terms of the response speed and physical mechanisms involved in photoconversion. Figure 9.10 illustrates the creation of junction between positively (p-type) and negatively (n-type) doped regions of graphene. The same effect can be achieved by applying a source-drain bias producing an external electric field. Since graphene is a semimetal generating a large dark current, that last approach is usually avoided. The built-in field can be introduced in different ways: either by local chemical doping and electrostatically using split gates, or by exploiting of the work-function

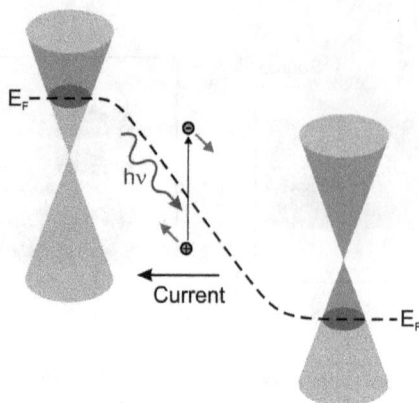

FIGURE 9.10   Schematic of photo-induced extraction of electron-hole pairs and its separation at graphene p-n junction.

difference between graphene and the contacts. Typically, p-type doping is reached for metals with a work function higher than that of intrinsic graphene (4.45 eV), whereas the graphene channel can be adjusted to p- or n-state by the gate.

Photodiodes are usually operated at zero bias (photovoltaic mode) or under reverse bias (photo-conductive mode). The absolute response of the photodiode is usually smaller than a photodetector working with the photoconducting or photogaiting mechanisms, since there is no internal gain. Under reverse-bias operation, the junction capacity is reduced, increasing the speed of the photodiode. Strong reverse bias can initiate impact ionisation multiplication of carriers, or avalanching (avalanche photodiode). The large internal gain results in detection of extremely low signal power. Electron-electron scattering in graphene can lead to the conversion of one high electron-hole pair (e-h) energy into multiple e-h pairs of lower energy potentially enhancing the photodetection efficiency [8].

Nonlinear properties of plasma wave excitations (the electron density waves) in nanoscale field effect transistor (FET) channels enable their response at frequencies appreciably higher than the device cut-off frequency, which is due to electron ballistic transport. In the ballistic regime of operation, the momentum relaxation time is longer than the electron transit time. The FETs can be used both for resonant (tuned to a certain wavelength) and non-resonant (broadband) THz detection and can be directly tunable by changing the gate voltage.

The graphene FET can be also used for detection of THz radiation, which was first proposed by Dyakonov and Shur in 1993 based on formal analogy between the equations of the electron transport in a gated 2D transistor channel and those describing the shallow-water behaviour or acoustic waves in musical instruments indicating that hydrodynamic-like effect should exist also in the carrier dynamics in the channel [33]. It must be stressed that instability of that flow in the form of plasma waves was predicted under certain boundary conditions.

The physical mechanism supporting the development of stable oscillations lies in the refection of plasma waves at the borders of a transistor with subsequent amplification of the wave's amplitude. Figure 9.11 schematically shows the resonant oscillation of plasma waves in FET's gated region. Even if there is no extra antenna in the system, the THz radiation is coupled to the FET by contact pads and bonding wires. An improvement in sensitivity can be reached by adding a proper antenna or a cavity coupling. Broadband detection occurs when plasma waves are overdamped – meaning when plasma waves launched at the source decay before reaching the drain.

The detection by FETs is due to nonlinear properties of the transistor leading to the rectification of the AC current induced by the radiation where photoresponse appears in the form of a DC voltage between source and drain and is proportional to the radiation intensity (PV effect). In the resonant

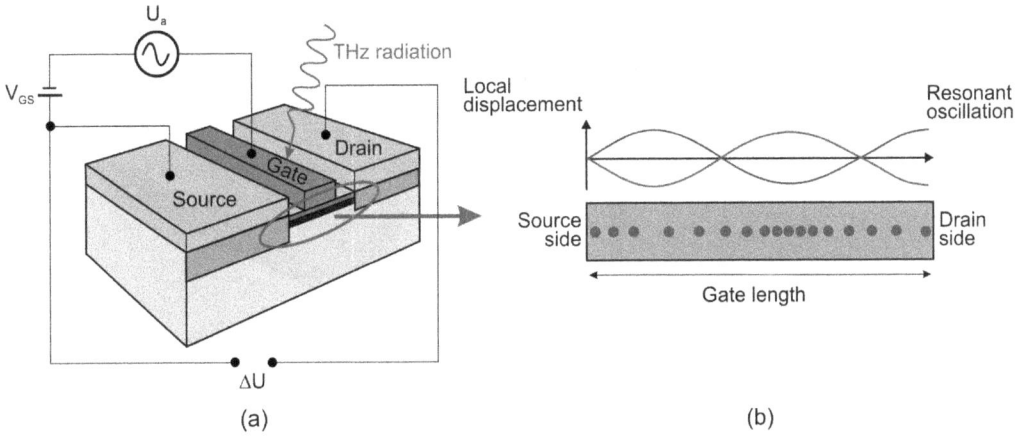

FIGURE 9.11 THz CMOS detector (a) and plasma oscillations in a transistor (b).

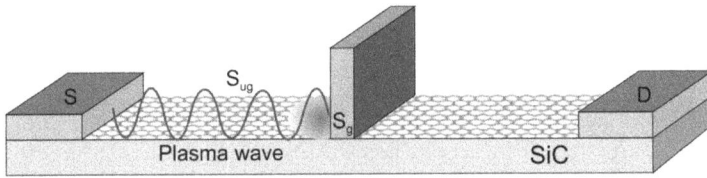

FIGURE 9.12 The detection mechanism in graphene FET THz photodetector.

regime, the plasma waves are dimly damped – when a plasma wave launched at the source can reach the drain in a time shorter than the momentum relaxation time – and the detection mechanism exploits interference of the plasma waves in the cavity, resulting in a resonantly enhanced response.

The photovoltage dependence on carrier density in the FET channel also shows photo-thermoelectric effect (PTE) contributions. Figure 9.12 presents and schematically explains two competitive independent detection effects: the plasmonic detection due to the nonlinearity of electron transport, and the thermoelectric effect due to the presence of both carrier density junctions and induced temperature gradient across the FET channel. The region near gate indicates the locally heated area at the interface of ungated and gated sections with thermopower S_{ug} and S_g, respectively. Even though strongly counterbalanced by the thermoelectric response, the plasma wave detection is the dominant mechanism.

9.3 2D MATERIAL-BASED DETECTOR PERFORMANCE

The majority of graphene pristine photodetectors exploit graphene metal junctions, graphene p-n junctions, and FET transistors. The development of the graphene high-responsivity photodetectors is determined by the two major challenges: the low optical absorption in the detector's active region (~100–200 nm), and the short photocarrier lifetime, meaning that graphene photodetectors are mainly limited by a trade-off between high responsivity, ultrafast time response and broadband operation.

9.3.1 Photon Detectors

Responsivity improvement in graphene detectors can be reached by increasing the photocarrier lifetime through both band structure and defect engineering, where carrier-trapping mechanisms and

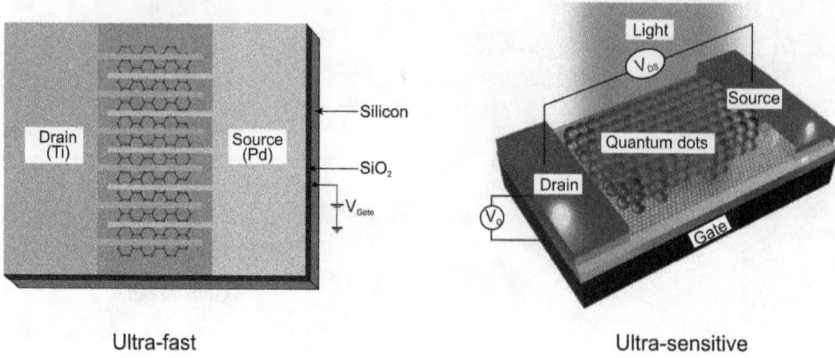

Ultra-fast   Ultra-sensitive

FIGURE 9.13 Ultrafast and ultrasensitive graphene photodetectors: structure of metal-graphene-metal photodetector (a) and hybrid graphene quantum dots photodetector (after Reference 31).

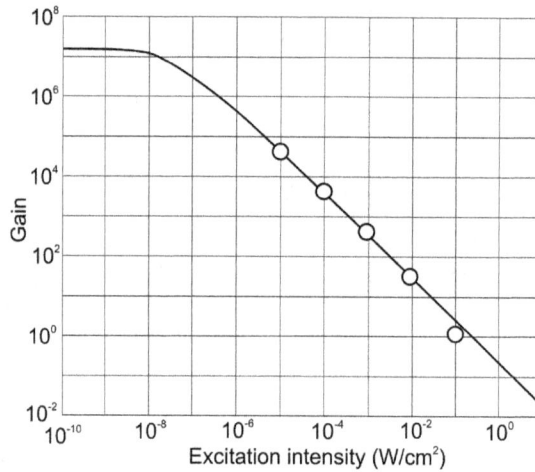

FIGURE 9.14 Gain as a function of excitation intensity for hybrid graphene/ZnO quantum dots detector. The circles are experimental data, and the solid curve is the theoretical plot with best fitting (after Reference 34).

patterned graphene nanostructures have been employed to introduce bandgap and mid-gap defect states while the response time is limited by long carrier-trapping time due to introduced defect states.

The built-in field formed by graphene and light absorption regions can separate the photoinduced carriers generated at the active layer and then inject holes/electrons into graphene. The photo-response beyond the light absorption region of semiconductors can also be detected contributing to the photo induced carriers provided by graphene. Unlike the pure graphene photoconductor, the built-in field at the interface can efficiently separate the photo induced carriers and extend their lifetime (photogating effect), resulting in the relatively high responsivity. Figure 9.13 shows schematically the differences between a pure graphene photoconductor (ultra-fast) and a hybrid photoconductor (ultra-sensitive).

Hybrid photodetectors offer improvements in responsivity, but the majority of these devices have a limited linear dynamic range due to the charge relaxation time, which quickly saturates the available states for photoexcitation, leading to a drop in responsivity with incident optical power. For example, Figure 9.14 shows the gain as a function of excitation intensity, as compared to the theory (solid line), for hybrid single layer graphene/ZnO quantum dots (QDs) detector. This ZnO QDs/graphene hybrid structure shows a photoconductive gain as high as 10^7.

TABLE 9.2

Performance of 2D Material Photodetectors at Room Temperature (after Reference 29)

Materials	Wavelength	Responsivity (A/W)	Bias (V)	Gain (%)	Time	Detectivity (Jones)
Graphene	1 mm (0.3 THz)	0.07–0.15 V/W	0			
Graphene	30–220 μm	$(5–10)\times10^{-9}$	0.1		10 ps, 50 ps	
Graphene	1550 nm	0.5×10^{-3}			0.26 s,	3.3×10^{13}
Graphene/Si waveguide	2750 nm	0.13	1.5			
PbSe/TiO$_2$/Graphene	350–1700 nm	0.506–0.13	-1		50 ns, 83 ns	3×10^{13}
Graphene/PbS	350–1700 nm	5×10^{7}	5	10^{8}	10–20 ms	7×10^{13}
Graphene/Ti$_2$O$_3$	3–13 μm	~ 100				
MoS$_2$	0.5–1.1	0.1	-10	25%	< 15 ms	
WS$_2$ (CVD)	0.5–0.9	3.5×10^{5}	2	1×10^{5}	23 ms	10^{14}
In$_2$Se$_3$	0.4–0.94	9.8×10^{4}	0.05		9 s	3.3×10^{13}
GeAs	1.6	6			3 s	
MoS$_2$/PbS	0.4–1.5	6×10^{5}	1		0.35 s	7×10^{14}
MoS$_2$/Si	0.4–1.0	0.9082	-2		56 ns; 825 ns	1.889×10^{13}
MoS$_2$/bP	0.5–1.6	22.3	3	50	15 μs; 70 μs	3.1×10^{13}
MoS$_2$/G/WS$_2$	0.4–2.4	1×10^{4}	1	10^{6}	53.6 μs; 30.3 μs	1×10^{15}
bP (gated-photocon.)	3.5	10	0.5	270		6×10^{10}
bP/MoS$_2$ (p-n hetero)	4.3		0.5		~ 1ms	2×10^{9}
bAsP (phototransitor)	2–8	$(30–10)\times10^{-3}$	0			3×10^{8}
PtSe$_2$ (phototransitor)	0.6–10	4.5			1.1, 1.2 ms	7×10^{8}
PdSe$_2$ (phototransitor)	1–10.6	~ 45	1	10^{3}-49	74.5, 93.1 ms	1×10^{9}
PdSe$_2$/MoS$_2$ (p-n hetero)	1–10.6	~ 4	1		65.3, 62.4 μs	8×10^{9}
Gr/Ti$_2$O$_3$	10	300	0.1		1.2, 2.6 ms	7×10^{8}
Bi$_2$Te$_3$/Si	UV-THz	1	-5		0.1 s	2.5×10^{11} (635 nm)

The performance of 2D-based material photodetectors is gathered in Table 9.2 [29].

The spectral responsivity of graphene photodetectors operating in visible and NIR spectral ranges is compared with commercially available silicon and InGaAs photodiodes in Figure 9.15. The highest current responsivity, above 10^{7} A/W, has been achieved for hybrid Gr/quantum dot (QD) photodetectors with enhancement of trapped-charge lifetimes. As is shown, graphene's high mobility, together with the enhance trapped-charge lifetimes in the quantum dots, produced a photo-detector responsivity up to seven orders of magnitude higher in comparison with standard bulk photodiodes, where $g \approx 1$. Higher responsivity of Si avalanche photodiode (APD), up to 100 A/W, is caused by the avalanche process. The high responsivity allows for fabrication of devices suitable for measuring low-level signals. However, due to the long lifetime of the traps, the demonstrated frequency response of 2D material photodetectors is very slow (< 10 Hz), which considerably limits real detector functions.

Similarly for graphene-based photodetectors, ultrahigh responsivity and ultrashort time response cannot be obtained at the same time in 2D-related material photodetectors. 2D layered materials show potential in photodetection covering UV, visible and IR ranges (see Figure 9.16). Generally, however, most of them cover visible and NIR spectral ranges, and only graphene-based, bPAs, bismuthene (like Bi$_2$Te$_3$ and Bi$_2$Se$_3$) and noble transition metal dichalcogenides, play a main role in the infrared region. In addition, as Figure 9.16 shows, the performance of graphene-based infrared photodetectors is inferior in comparison with alternative 2D material photodetectors.

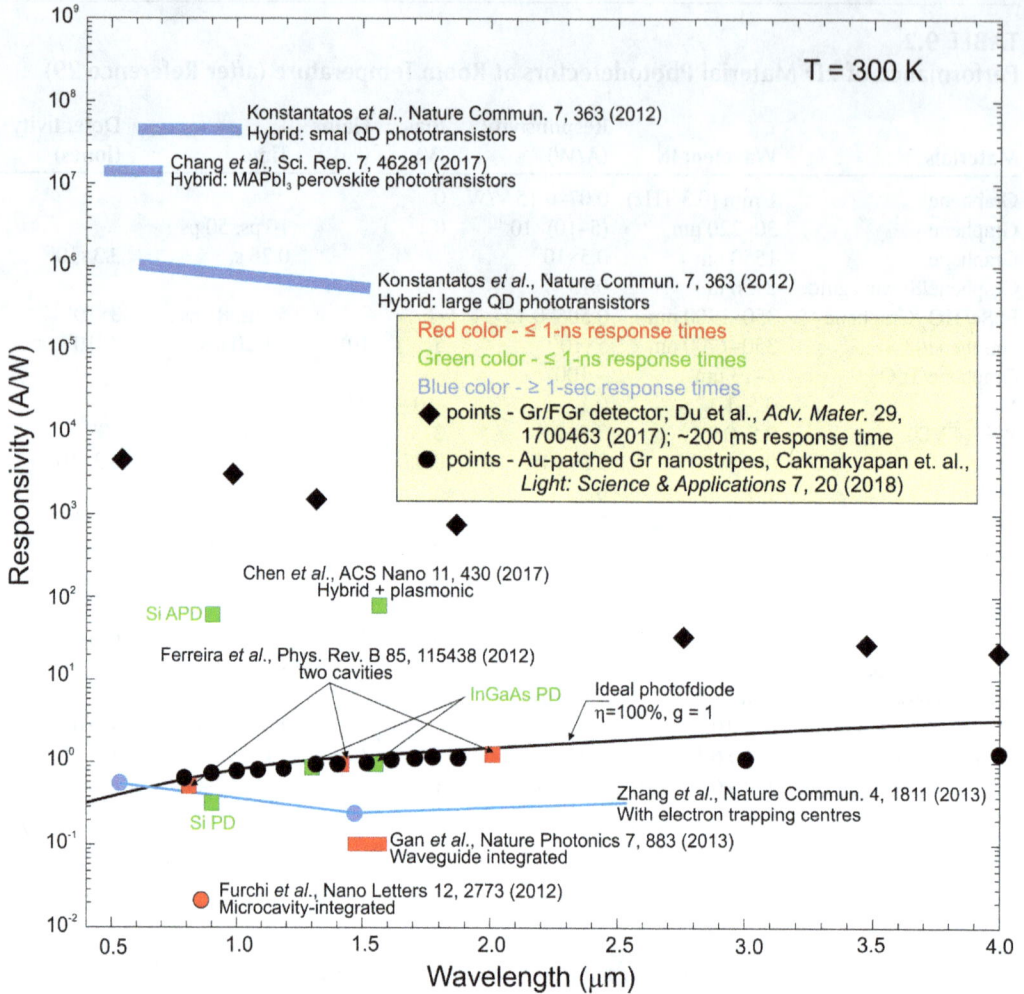

FIGURE 9.15 Spectral responsivity of graphene photodetectors compared with commercial ones. Dotted line shows 100 per cent quantum efficiency. Red and green colours denote ≤ 1 ns response times, while the blue colour denotes ≥ 1 second response times. The graphene photodetectors are labelled with their reference as well as a brief description of the photodetector style. The commercial photodiodes are shown in green.

At present, HgCdTe is the most widely used variable gap semiconductor for IR photodetectors, including uncooled operation, and provides a benchmark for alternative technologies. Literature data for longer wavelength infrared graphene-based photodetectors, with a cut-off wavelength above 3 μm, are limited. Figures 7.43 and 9.17 compare their detectivities with commercially available HgCdTe photodiodes operating at room temperature [35]. The upper detectivity of the Gr/FGr photodetector in SWIR range is close to HgCdTe photodiodes. This figure also shows experimental data for black phosphorus arsenic (bAsP) photodetectors and noble transition metal dichalcogenides entering the second atmospheric transmission window.

As is shown, the detectivity values for selected 2D material photodetectors are closed to data presented for commercial detectors ((PV Si and Ge, PV InGaAs, PC PbS and PbSe, PV HgCdTe), and in the case of black phosphorus and noble TMD, detectors are even higher. The enhanced sensitivity of 2D material photodetectors is introduced by band-gap engineering and photogating effect.

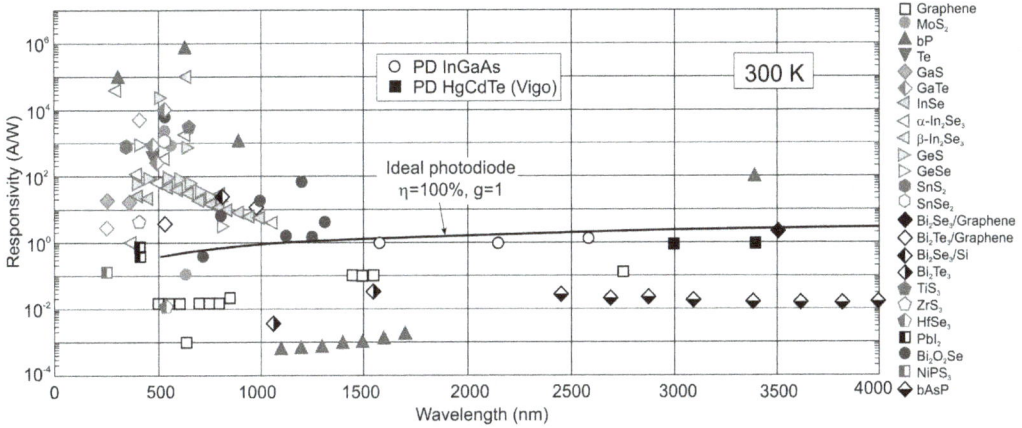

FIGURE 9.16 Summary of spectral responsivities to the layered 2D material photodetectors at room temperature (after Reference 29). Black line shows spectral responsivity for ideal photodiode with 100 per cent quantum efficiency and $g = 1$. For comparative goals, the responsivities of commercially available photodetectors (InGaAs and HgCdTe photodiodes) are marked.

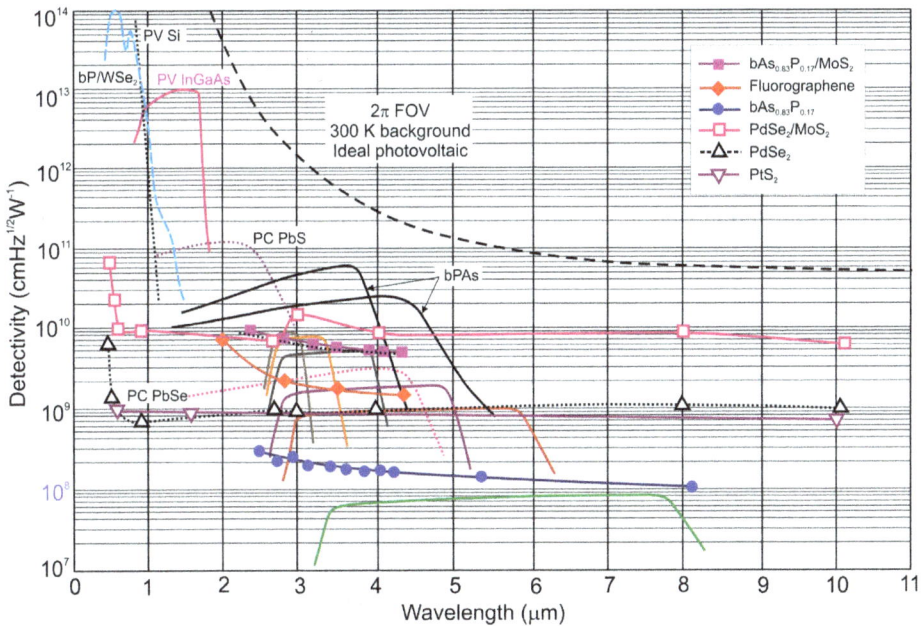

FIGURE 9.17 Room-temperature spectral detectivity curves of the commercially available photodetectors [PV Si and InGaAs, PC PbS and PbSe, HgCdTe photodiodes (solid lines – Reference 35)]. Also, the experimental data for different types of 2D material photodetectors are included. PC – photoconductor, PV – photodiode (after Reference 29).

However, the layered-material photodetectors are characterised by limited linear dynamic range of operation and slow response time.

Figure 7.43 also compares the experimental detectivity values published in literature for different types of single-element 2D material photodetectors operated at room temperature with theoretically predicted curves for P-i-N HOT HgCdTe photodiodes. The potential properties of HOT HgCdTe photodiodes, operated in longer wavelength infrared range (above 3 μm), guarantee achieving more than order of magnitude higher detectivity (above 10^{10} Jones) in comparison with the value predicted by Rule 07.

9.3.2 Thermal Detectors

Thermal detectors are classified according to the operating schemes as thermopiles, bolometers and pyroelectric detectors.

The basic structure of a thermoelectric graphene photodetector design is shown in Figure 9.18 [36]. This device, made of a sheet of graphene with dual split-backgates, develops a photovoltage across electrodes M1–M2 as a function of the voltage applied to the backgates. The device shows photoresponse even at 10.6 μm. Multiple graphene detectors are combined into the thermopile composed of an infrared absorber (made of a $SiO_2/Si_3N_4/SiO_2$ combination) that is suspended from the substrate, a series of thermal arms that connect the absorber and the surroundings, with interleaved p- and n-type graphene channels on top – see Figure 9.18(c). The fabrication of a free-standing absorber membrane was made after undercutting the silicon underneath with an isotropic etching.

Figure 9.19 compares the detectivity and the response time of graphene thermopiles with different types of state-of-the-art thermal-detector technologies, including bolometers (VO_x, etc.), thermopiles (poly-Si, Al, thermoelectric materials, etc.) and pyroelectric devices (PZT and other piezoelectric materials). For more advanced thermal-detector technologies, the detectivity magnitude at room temperature is in the order of $\sim 10^8$–10^9 cmHz$^{1/2}$/W. As is shown, the performance of current graphene thermopile technology is considerably inferior in comparison with the state-of-the-art thermal detectors and is below 10^6 cmHz$^{1/2}$/W. However, the theoretically predicted performance is even better than today's state-of-the-art technologies. For example, a 10-nm thick absorber with good mechanical stability and 50 per cent absorption achieved through nano-photonic structures, would make graphene thermopiles better than any existing bolometers.

The main difficulty in development of high sensitivity graphene bolometers is the weak variation of electrical resistance versus temperature. Recently published papers by El Fatimy *et al.* [37] have shown that graphene quantum dots on SiC exhibit extremely high variation of resistance versus temperature due to quantum confinement, higher than 430 MΩ/K at 2.5 K leading to responsivities 1×10^{10} V/W for THz region. In hot electron bolometers with quantum dots in epitaxial graphene, the bandgap is induced via quantum confinement (without the need of gates) using a simple single layer structure. Figure 9.20(a) presents the *NEP* for 0.15 THz versus temperature from 2.5 K to 80 K calculated for a 30 nm and a 150 nm quantum dots. The *NEP* is approximately one order of magnitude lower than the best commercial cooled bolometer and much faster in response time (a few nanoseconds, compared to milliseconds for commercial bolometers). These quantum dot bolometers operate in very broad spectral range from THz to ultraviolet radiation with responsivity being independent versus wavelength – see Figure 9.20(b). Similar to hybrid photodetectors (see Figure 9.14), drop of reponsivity versus absorber power is also observed for graphene bolometers [see Figure 9.20(b)].

Graphene with the lowest mass per unit area of any material, extreme thermal stability and an unmatched spectral absorbance, generates interest as active bolometer absorbers. However, due to its weak temperature-dependent electrical resistivity, it has failed to challenge the state-of-the-art at room temperature. Both the speed and sensitivity are inversely proportional to the thermal resistance, so a sensitive bolometer is often slow. A common method to modify the speed and sensitivity is to change the thermal resistance between the bolometer and its environment.

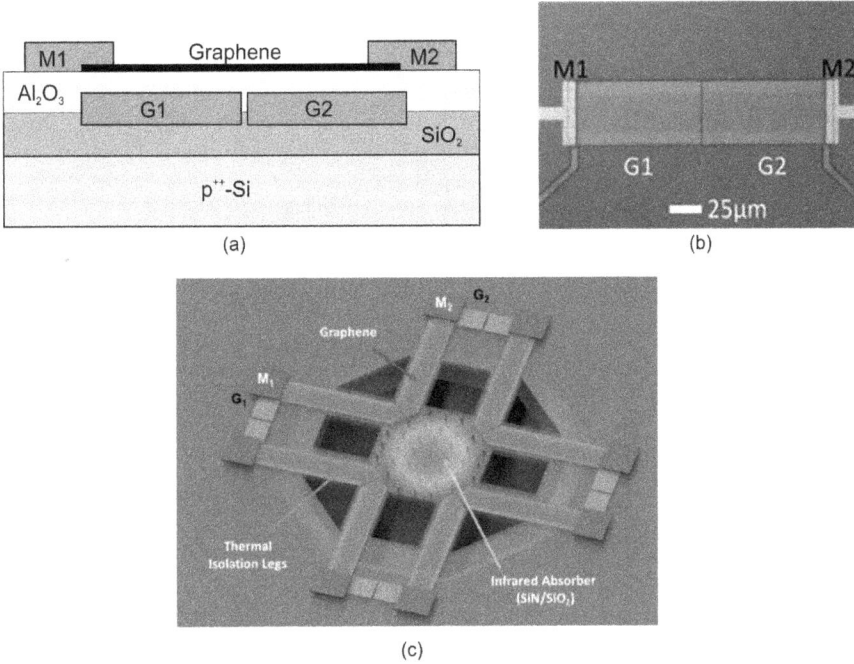

(a)

(b)

(c)

FIGURE 9.18 Thermoelectric graphene photodetector: schematic graphene split-gate thermopile with supported substrate (a) and its microscopic image (b). M1 and M2 are metal contacts to graphene, and G1 and G2 are split gates that electrostatically dope the graphene channel to form a p-n junction. Graphene thermopile with suspended IR absorber (c); the square in the centre is the dielectric absorber. The whole structure is suspended on the substrate to reduce the thermal conductance in the vertical direction (after Reference 36).

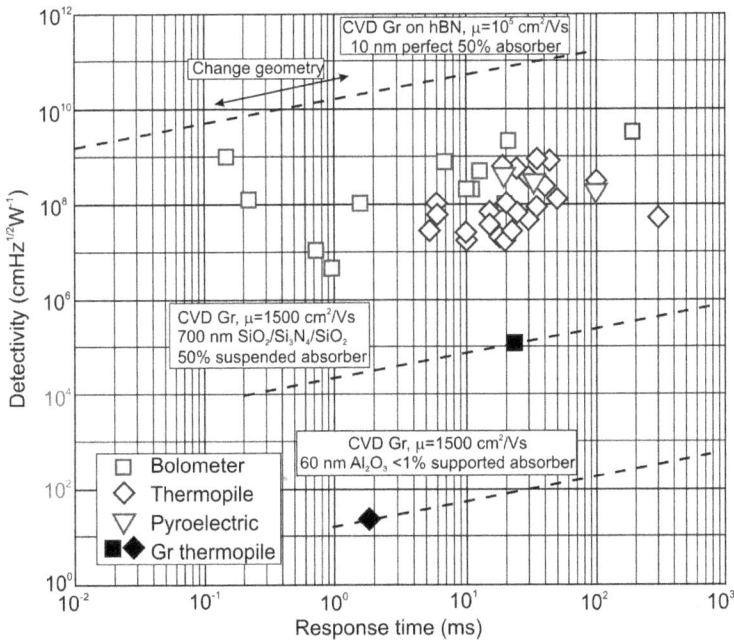

FIGURE 9.19 Detectivity versus response time for different technology nodes of graphene thermopiles in comparison with mainstream uncooled thermal IR detectors (after Reference 36).

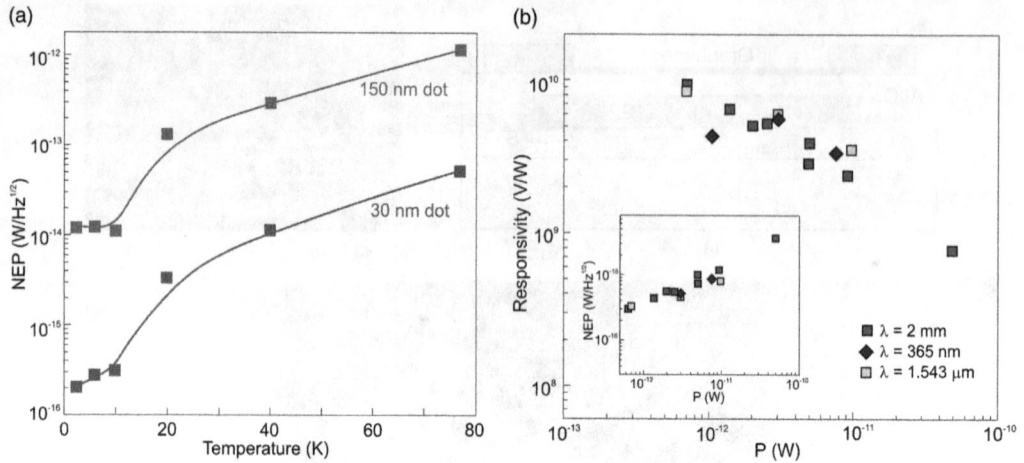

FIGURE 9.20 Quantum dot bolometers: *NEP* versus temperature at 0.15 THz for 30 nm and 150 nm quantum dots (a) (adapted after Reference 37) and responsivity versus absorbed power at different wavelength. Inset: *NEP* versus absorbed power at selected wavelengths (b) (adapted after Reference 38).

REFERENCES

1. *International Roadmap for Devices and Systems. 2018 Update. More Moore.* https://irds.ieee.org/images/files/pdf/2018/ 2018IRDS_MM. pdf.
2. N. Briggs, S. Subramanian, Z. Lin, X. Li, X. Zhang, K. Zhang, K. Xia, D. Geohegan, R. Wallace, L.-Q. Chen, M. Terrones, A. Ebrahimi, S. Das, J. Redwing, C. Hinkle, K. Momeni, A. van Duin, V. Crespi, S. Kar, and J.A. Robinson, "A roadmap for electronic grade 2D materials", *2D Mater.* 6, 022001 (2019).
3. F. Bonaccorso, Z. Sun, T. Hasan, A. C. Ferrari, "Graphene photonics and optoelectronics", *Nature Photon.* 4, 611–622 (2010).
4. K.S. Novoselov, A.K. Geim, S.V. Morozov, D. Jiang, Y. Zhang, S.V. Dubonos, I.V. Grigorieva, and A.A. Firsov, "Electric field effect in atomically thin carbon films", *Science* 306, 666–669 (2004).
5. F. Xia, H. Yan, and P. Avouris, "The interaction of light and graphene: Basic, devices, and applications", *Proc. IEEE* 101(7), 1717–1731 (2013).
6. J.-H. Chen, C. Jang, S. Xiao, M. Ishigami, and M. S. Fuhrer, "Intrinsic and extrinsic performance limits of graphene devices on SiO_2,", *Nat. Nanotechnol.* 3, 206–209 (2008).
7. R.R. Nair, P. Blake, A.N. Grigorenko, K.S. Novoselov, T.J. Booth, T. Stauber, N.M.R. Peres, and A.K. Geim, "Fine structure constant defines visual transparency of graphene", *Science* 320, 1308 (2008).
8. X. Li, L. Tao, Z. Chen, H. Fang, X. Li, X. Wang, J.-B. Xu, and H. Zhu, "Graphene and related two-dimensional materials: Structure-property relationships for electronics and optoelectronics", *Appl. Phys. Rev.* 4, 021306-1–31 (2017).
9. T. Low and P. Avouris, "Graphene plasmonic for terahertz to mid-infrared applications", *ACS Nano* 8(2), 1086–1001 (2014).
10. V. Nicolosi, M. Chhowalla, M.G. Kanatzidis, M.S. Strano, and J.N. Coleman, "Liquid exfoliation of layered materials", *Science* 340:1226419 (2013).
11. J. Wang, H. Fang, X. Wang, X. Chen, W. Lu, and W. Hu, "Recent progress on localized field enhanced two-dimensional material photodetectors from ultraviolet-visible to infrared", *Small* 13, 1700894 (2017).
12. X. Wang, Y. Sun, and K. Liu, "Chemical and structural stability of 2D layered materials", *2 D Mater.* 6, 042001 (2019).
13. M. Buscema, J.O. Island, D.J. Groenendijk, S.I. Blanter, G.A. Steele, H.S.J. van der Zant, and A. Castellanos-Gomez, "Photocurrent generation with two-dimensional van der Waals semiconductor", *Chem. Soc. Rev.* 44, 3691–3718, 2015.

14. M. Long, P. Wang, H. Fang, and W. Hu, "Progress, challenges, and opportunities for 2D material based photodetectors", *Adv. Funct. Mater.* 1803807 (2018).

15. F. Wang, Z. Wang, L. Yin, R. Cheng, J. Wang, Y. Wen, T.A. Shifa, F. Wang, Y. Zhang, X. Zhan, and J. He, "2D library beyond graphene and transition metaldichalcogenides: a focus on photodetection", *Chem. Soc. Rev.* 47(4) 2018, DOI: 10.1039/c8cs00255j

16. J. Cheng, C. Wang, X. Zou, and L. Liao, "Recent advances in optoelectronic devices based on 2D materials and their heterostructures", *Adv. Optical Mater.* 7, 1800441 (2019).

17. K.F. Mark and J. Shan, "Photonics and optoelectronics of 2D semiconductor transition metal dichalcogenides", *Nat. Photonics* 10, 216–226 (2016).

18. S. Manzeli, D. Ovchinnikov, D. Pasquier, O.V. Yazyev, and A. Kis, "2D transition metal dichalcogenides", *Nat. Rev. Mater.* 2(8), 1–15 (2017).

19. L. Pi, L. Li, K. Liu, Q. Zhang, H. Li, and T. Zhai, "Recent progress on 2D noble-transition-metal dichalcogenides", *Adv. Funct. Mater.* 29, 1904932 (2019).

20. Z. Yang, J. Dou and M. Wang, "Graphene, transition metal dichalcogenides, and perovskite photodetectors", http://dx.doi.org/10.5772/intechopen.74021.

21. W. Zhang, Z. Huang, W. Zhang, and Y. Li, "Two-dimensional semiconductors with possible high room temperature mobility", *Nano Res.* 7, 1731–1737 (2014).

22. Y. Zhao, J. Qiao, Z. Yu, P. Yu, K. Xu, S.P. Lau, W. Zhou, Z. Liu, X. Wang, W. Ji, and Y. Chai, "High-electron-mobility and air-stable 2D layered $PtSe_2$ FETs", *Adv. Mater.* 29, 1604230 (2017).

23. M.R. Habib, W. Chen, W.-Y. Yin, H. Su, and M. Xu, "Simulation of transition metal dichalcogenides, in *Two Dimensional Transition Metal Dichalcogenides. Synthesis, Properties, and Applications*, pp. 135–172, edited by N.S. Arul and V.D. Nithya, Springer, Singapore, 2019.

24. X. Yu, P. Yu, D. Wu, B. Singh, Q. Zeng, H. Lin, W. Zhou, J. Lin, K. Suenaga, Z. Liu, and Q.J. Wang, "Atomically thin noble metal dichalcogenide: a broadband mid-infrared semiconductor", *Nat. Commun.* 9, 1545 (2018).

25. L.-H. Zeng, D. Wu, S.-H. Lin, C. Xie, H.-Y. Yuan, W. Lu, S.P. Lau, Y. Chai, L.-B. Luo, Z.-J. Li, and Y.H. Tsang, "Controlled synthesis of 2D palladium diselenide for sensitive photodetector applications", *Adv. Funct. Mater.* 29, 1806878 (2019).

26. P. W. Bridgman, "Two new modifications of phosphorus", *J. Am. Chem. Soc.* 36(7), 1344–1363 (1914).

27. X. Ling, H. Wang, S. Huang, F. Xia, and M.S. Dresselhaus, "The renaissance of black phosphorus", *PNAS* 112(15), 4523–4530 (2015).

28. Y. Akahama, S. Endo, and S. Narita, "Electrical properties of black phosphorus single crystals", *J. Phys. Soc. Jpn.* 52(6), 2148–2155 (1983).

29. A. Rogalski, M. Kopytko, and P. Martyniuk, "2D material infrared and terahertz detectors: status and outlook", *Opto-Electron. Rev.* 28, 107–154 (2020).

30. B. Liu, M. Köpf, A.N. Abbas, X. Wang, Q. Guo, Y. Jia, F. Xia, R. Weihrich, F. Bachhuber, F. Pielnhofer, H. Wang, R. Dhall, S.B. Cronin, M. Ge, X. Fang, T. Nilges, and C. Zhou, "Black arsenic–phosphorus: layered anisotropic infrared semiconductors with highly tunable compositions and properties", *Adv. Mater.* 27, 4423–4429 (2015).

31. G. Konstantatos, M. Badioli, L. Gaudreau, J. Osmond, M. Bernechea, F.P. Garcia de Arquer, F. Gatti, and F.H.L. Koppens "Hybrid graphene-quantum dot phototransistors with ultrahigh gain", *Nat. Nanotechnol.* 7, 363–368 (2012).

32. F.H.L. Koppens, T. Mueller, Ph. Avouris, A.C. Ferrari, M.S. Vitiello and M. Polini, "Photodetectors based on graphene, other two-dimensional materials and hybrid systems", *Nat. Nanotechnol.* 9, 780–793 (2014).

33. M. Dyakonov and M.S. Shur, "Shallow water analogy for a ballistic field effect transistor: new mechanism of plasma wave generation by the dc current", *Phys. Rev. Lett.* 71, 2465–2468 (1993).

34. W. Guo, S. Xu, Z. Wu, N. Wang, M.M.T. Loy, and S. Du, "Oxygen-assisted charge transfer between ZnO quantum dots and graphene", *Small* 9, 3031–3036 (2013).

35. https://vigo.com.pl/wp-content/uploads/2017/06/VIGO-Catalogue.pdf.

36. A. Nourbakhsh, L. Yu, Y. Lin, M. Hempel, R.-J. Shiue, D. Englund, and T. Palacios, "Heterogeneous integration of 2D materials and devices on a Si platform", in *Beyond-CMOS Technologies for Next Generation Computer Design*, pp. 43–84, edited by R.O. Topaloglu and H.-S.P. Wong, Springer, 2019.

37. A. El Fatimy, R.L. Myers-Ward, A.K. Boyd, K.M. Daniels, D.K. Gaskill, and P. Barbara, "Epitaxial graphene quantum dots for high-performance THz bolometers", *Nat. Nanotechnol.* 11, 335–338 (2016).

38. A. El Fatimy, A. Nath, B.D. Kong, A.K. Boyd, R.L. Myers-Ward, K.M. Daniels, M.M. Jadidi, T.E. Murphy, D.K. Gaskill, and P. Barbara, "Ultra-broadband photodetectors based on epitaxial graphene quantum dots", *Nanophotonics* 7(4), 735–740 (2018).

10 Terahertz Detectors

The terahertz (THz) range of electromagnetic spectrum still presents a challenge for both electronic and photonic technologies and is often described as the final unexplored area of spectrum. This radiation is frequently treated as the spectral region within frequency range $v \approx 0.1–10$ THz (see Figure 7.1).

The THz region of the electromagnetic spectrum has proven to be one of the most elusive. Being situated between infrared light and microwave radiation, THz radiation is resistant to the techniques commonly employed in these well-established neighbouring bands. Historically, the major use of THz spectroscopy has been by chemists and astronomers in the spectral characterisation of the rotational and vibrational resonances and thermal-emission lines of simple molecules. Terahertz receivers are also used to study the trace gases in the upper atmosphere, such as ozone and the many gases involved in ozone depletion cycles, such as chloride monoxide. Air efficiently absorbs in a wide spectral THz region (except for narrow windows around $v \approx 35$ GHz, 96 GHz, 140 GHz and 220 GHz, and others, see Figure 10.1 [1]). THz and millimetre waves are efficient at detecting the presence of water and thus are efficient at discriminating different objects on human bodies (water content of human body is about 60%), as the clothes are transparent. In the longer wavelength region (cm wavelength region) even persons hiding behind a wall (not very thick), can be visualised. It should be mentioned that about half of the luminosity of the universe and 98 per cent of all the photons emitted since the Big Bang belong to THz radiation [2]. This relict radiation carries information about the cosmic space, galaxies, stars and planets formation [3].

The past twenty years have seen a revolution in THz systems, as advanced materials research new and higher-power sources, and the potential of THz for advanced physics research and commercial applications has been demonstrated. Numerous recent breakthroughs in the field have pushed THz research to centre stage. As examples of milestone achievements can be included in the development of THz time-domain spectroscopy (TDS), THz imaging, and high-power THz generation by means of nonlinear effects [4–7]. Research involved with THz technologies is now receiving increasing attention, and devices exploiting this wavelength band are set to become increasingly important in a diverse range of human activity applications (e.g., security, biological, drugs and explosion detection, gases fingerprints, imaging, etc.). Nowadays, THz technology is also of much use in fundamentals science, such as nanomaterials science and biochemistry. This is based on the fact that THz frequencies correspond to single and collective excitations in nanoelectronic devices and collective dynamics in biomolecules.

DOI: 10.1201/9781003263098-10

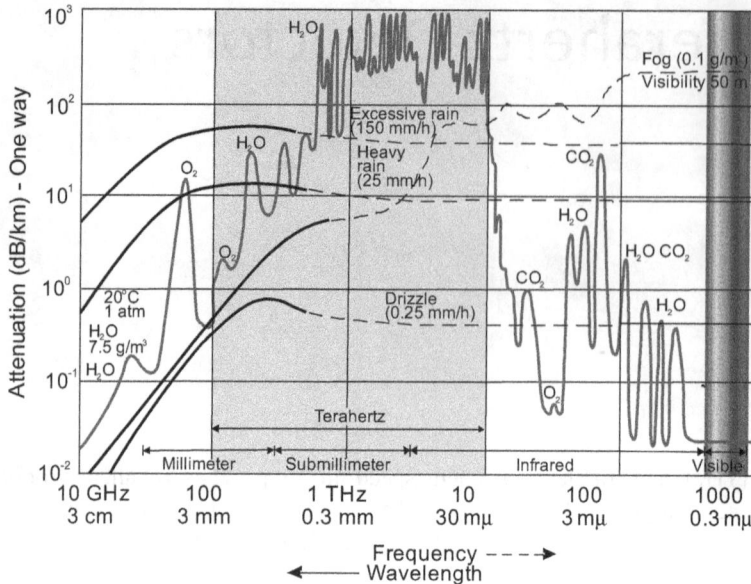

FIGURE 10.1   Attenuation of Earth atmosphere from visible to radiofrequency band region (after Reference 1).

10.1   ROOM TEMPERATURE THZ DETECTORS

In the development of THz imaging systems, particular attention is devoted to the realisation of sensors with a large potential for real-time imaging while maintaining a high dynamic range and room-temperature operation. CMOS technology process is especially attractive due to their low price tag for industrial, surveillance, scientific and medical applications. However, CMOS THz imagers developed thus far have mainly operated single detectors based on lock-in technique to acquire raster-scanned imagers with frame rates on the order of minutes. With this in mind, much recent development is directed towards three types of focal plane arrays (FPAs):

- Schottky barrier diodes (SBDs) compatible with the CMOS process;
- field effect transistors (FETs) relying on plasmonic rectification phenomena; and
- adaptation of infrared bolometers to the THz frequency range.

An important issue for an FPA is pixel uniformity. It appears however, that the production of monolithically integrated detector arrays encounters so many technological problems that the device-to-device performance variations and even the percentage of non-functional detectors per chip tend to be unacceptably high.

The performance of monolithically integrated detector arrays with room temperature THz detectors is summarised in Table 10.1. SBDs respond to the THz electric field and usually generate an output current or voltage through a quadratic term in their current-voltage characteristics. In general, the noise equivalent power (*NEP*) of SBD and FET detectors is better than that of Golay cells and pyroelectric detectors around 300 GHz. Both the pyroelectric and the bolometer FPAs with detector response times in the millisecond time range are not suited for heterodyne operation. FET detectors are clearly capable in heterodyne detection with improving sensitivity. Diffraction aspects predict FPAs for higher frequencies (0.5 THz and above) and in conjunction with large *f*/# optics.

Below, a short description of different kinds of uncooled THz detectors is presented [8]. Further insight on *NEP* values of state-of-the-art of direct detectors at room temperature is provided in Figure 10.2 [9].

TABLE 10.1
Parameter of Some Uncooled THz Detectors

Device type	Electrical responsivity (V/W)	Conditions	NEP (W/Hz$^{1/2}$)
Schottky diodes			
ErAs/InGaAlAs spiral planar antenna	-	Zero bias, 639 GHz	4.0×10^{-12} $NEDT$ = 120 mK
InGaAs log-spiral antenna	~200 for system estimate 10^3 intrinsic for the diode	0.8 THz	5.0×10^{-12}
VDI Model: WR2.8 ZBD	1500	260–400 GHz	2.7×10^{-12}
VDI Model: WR1.5ZBD	750	500–750 GHz	5.1×10^{-12}
VDI Model: WR1.0 ZBD	200	750–1100 GHz	20×10^{-12}
VDI Model: WR0.65 ZBD	100	1100–1700	40×10^{-12}
Bolometers			
$Hg_{0.8}Cd_{0.2}Te$ HEB	0.30 at 17 mV bias, 36 GHz 96 for 0.89 THz, 13 mV bias	Room temperature	2.2×10^{-9} for 17 mV bias, 35 GHz 7.4×10^{-9} for 0.89 THz, 12 mV bias
Si_xGe_y:H	170	0.934 THz, uncooled	0.2×10^{-9}
Vanadium oxide	-	Uncooled	320×10^{-12} at 4.3 THz, 9×10^{-13} @ 7.5–14 μm
Niobum film	21	3.6 mA bias, 1 kHz mod, 300 K	1.10×10^{-10}
Ti, antenna-coupled microbolometer	-	10 kHz chop, 1.04 mA bias, 300K	1.5×10^{-11}
Nb_5N_6	400	0.4 mA bias, > 10 kHz	9.8×10^{-12}
Vanadium oxide array	1.5×10^4	1 V bias, 130 μm, uncooled	2.00×10^{-10}
Nb, polymide, antenna coupled	450	< 1 THz	1.5×10^{-11}
Al/Nb; antenna coupled	85	1 kHz mod, 1.6 mA bias	2.5×10^{-11}
Fee-standing Nb bridge antenna coupled	210 (average over 10 devices)	650 GHz	12.5×10^{-12}
Pyroelectrics			
Philips P5219 deuterated L-alanine TGS	321	10 Hz mod; amplifier with gain of 4.8, 91 GHz	3.1×10^{-8}
QMC instr	18 300 1200	10 Hz mod; 1.89 THz, < 20 Hz mod	4.4×10^{-10}
$LiTaO_3$	-	530 GHz, Melectron Model SPH-45	2.0×10^{-9}
Golay cells			
Tydex Golay Cell GC-1X	100 000	21 Hz chper	1.4×10^{-10}
Microtech Instruments	10000	12.5 Hz chopper	10×10^{-8}
Micro-array, layer by layer, polimer membranes over Si	-	30 Hz mod 105 GHz	300×10^{-9}
Tydex Golay Cell, 6-mm-diameter diamond window		10 Hz mod	7.0×10^{-10}

(continued)

TABLE 10.1 (Continued)
Parameter of Some Uncooled THz Detectors

Device type	Electrical responsivity (V/W)	Conditions	NEP (W/Hz$^{1/2}$)
CMOS-based and plasma detectors			
BiCMOS SiGe, 0.25 μm HBT	Current R_i 1 A/W at 0.7 THz	3×5 array, chopper 125 kHz	50×10^{-12} at 0.7 THz
BiCMOS SiGe, 0.25 μm NMOS	Voltage R_v 80 kV/W at 0.6 THz	3×5 array, chopper 16 kHz	300×10^{-12} at 0.6 THz
CMOS SiGe, 65 nm NMOS	Voltage R_v 140 kV/W at 0.87 THz	32×32 array, chopper 5 kHz	100×10^{-12} at 0.87 THz
CMOS SiGe, 65 nm NMOS	Voltage R_v 0.8 kV/W at 1 THz	3×5 array, chopper 1 kHz	66×10^{-12} at 1 THz
CMOS-SBD, 130 nm	Voltage R_v 0.323 kV/W at 0.28 THz	4×4 array, chopper 1 kHz	29×10^{-12} at 0.28 THz
CMOS-SBD, 65 nm	-	1 element; 1 MHz mod	42×10^{-12} at 0.86 THz
CMOS, 150 nm, NMOS	Voltage R_v at 4.1 THz	1 element	133×10^{-12} at 4.1 THz
InGaAs HEMT	Voltage R_v 23 kV/W at 200 GHz	1 element	0.5×10^{-12} at 200 GHz
Asymmetric dual-grating gate InGaAs HEMT	Voltage R_v 6.4 kV/W at 1.5 THz	1 element	50×10^{-12} at 1.5 THz

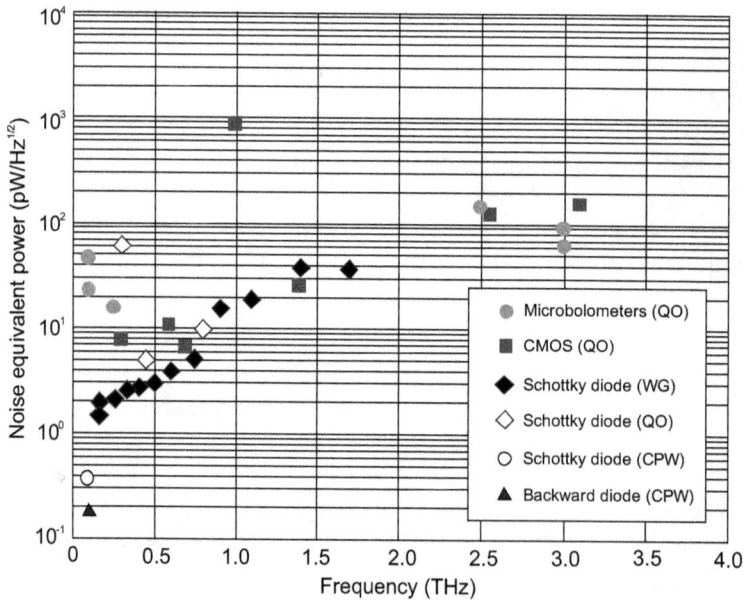

FIGURE 10.2 State-of-the-art direct terahertz detectors at room-temperature. Shown are Schottky diodes mounted in a waveguide (WG), in quasi-optical configuration (QO), in on-wafer measurements (CPW – coplanar waveguide), CMOS FET (QO), microbolometers (QO), and heterostructure backward diodes.

10.1.1 SCHOTTKY BARRIER DIODES

In spite of achievements of other kind of detectors for THz waveband, the Schottky barrier diodes (SBDs) are among the basic elements in THz technologies. They are used either in direct detection or as nonlinear elements in heterodyne receiver mixers operating in a temperature range of 4–300 K. The cryogenically cooled SBDs were preferably used in mixers in the 1980s and early 1990s, later to be widely replaced by superconductor-insulator-superconductor (SIS) or hot electron bolometer (HEB) mixers, in which mixing processes are similar to that observed in SBDs but, for example, in SIS structures the rectification process is based on quantum-mechanical photon-assisted tunnelling of quasiparticles (electrons). The nonlinearity of SBD *I-V* characteristic (the current increases exponentially with the applied voltage) is the prerequisite for mixing to occur.

Historically, first Schottky-barrier structures were pointed contacts of tapered metal wires (e.g., a tungsten needle) with a semiconductor surface (the so-called crystal detectors). Due to limitation of whisker technology, such as constraints on design and repeatability, starting in the 1980s, the efforts were made to produce planar Schottky diodes with air-bridge fingers [see Figure 10.3(a)]. This design has been among the most important steps toward a practical Schottky diode mixer for THz frequency applications, with several thousand diodes on a single chip and where parasitic losses such as the series resistance and the shunt capacitance are minimised. To achieve good performance at high frequencies the diode area should be small. Reducing junction area one reduces junction capacitances to increase operating frequency. But, at the same time, one increases the series resistance.

Using advanced technology, the diodes are integrated with many passive circuit elements (impedance matching, filters and waveguide probes) onto the same substrate. By improving the mechanical arrangement and reducing loss, the planar technology is pushed well beyond 300 GHz up to several THz. For example, Figure 10.3(b) shows photographs of a bridged four-Schottky diodes' chip arrayed in a balanced configuration to increase power handling.

An alternative method of Schottky barrier formation has been elaborated by molecular beam epitaxy (MBE) *in-situ* deposition of a semimetal (ErAs) on semiconductor (InGaAs/InAlAs on InP substrates) to reduce the imperfections that give rise to excess low-frequency noise, particularly $1/f$ noise [10]. Excellent *NEP* performance for this III-V semiconductor SBD has been reported (1.4 pW/Hz$^{1/2}$ at 100 GHz). By using interband tunnelling, a heterojunction backward diode demonstrated 49.7 kV/W responsivity and 0.18 pW/Hz *NEP* at 94 GHz [11]. More recently Han et al. [12] have demonstrated fully functional CMOS imager operating near or in the sub-millimetre-wave frequency range (see Figure 10.4). The 4×4 array increases the imaging speed by 4 to 8 times, due to fewer mechanical scan steps.

The experimental active THz imaging arrangement is shown in Figure 10.5. The most of papers presented characterisations of FPAs using monochromatic THz sources such as quantum cascade

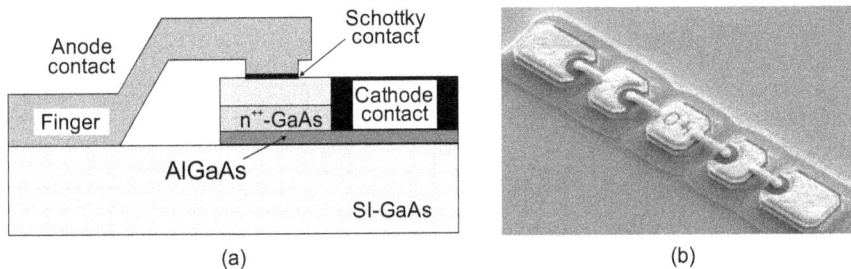

FIGURE 10.3 GaAs Schottky barrier diode: (a) schematic of a planar diode and (b) a four-diode chip array.

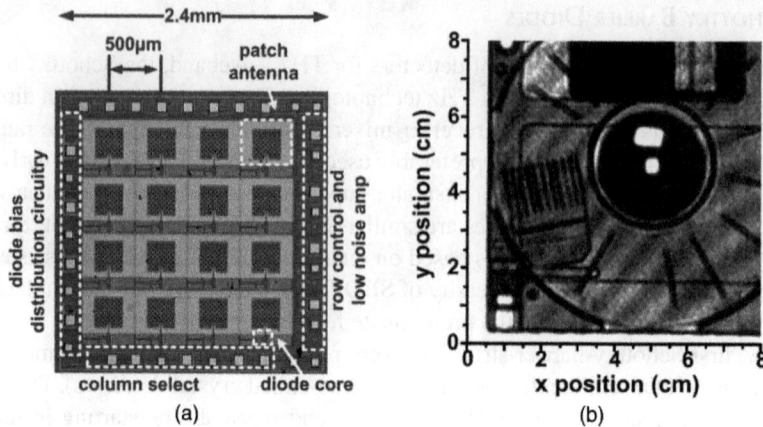

FIGURE 10.4 CMOS SBD 280-GHz imager: die photos of the array (a) and an image of music greeting card obtained (after Reference 12).

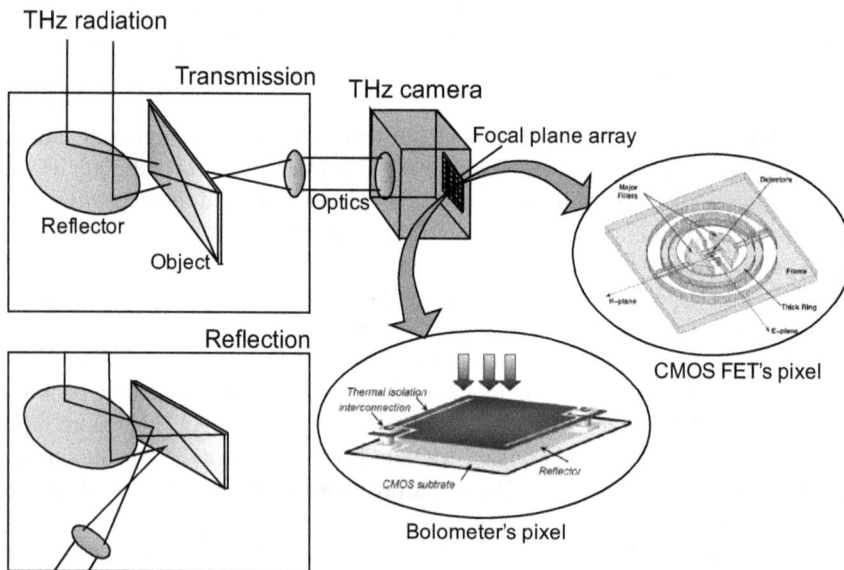

FIGURE 10.5 Experimental setup of THz imaging system. Cutaway depicts alternative reflection mode setup.

lasers (QCLs) or far infrared optically pumped lasers delivering mW-range powers. As Figure 10.5 shows, the reflected beam backlights an object with a maximum area and the transmitted light is collected by a camera lens. The focal plane is positioned behind the camera lens, making the object plane in front of the lens. Also shown is the modified reflection mode setup, where a specular reflection is collected by the repositioned lens and camera.

10.1.2 FIELD EFFECT TRANSISTOR AND CMOS-BASED DETECTORS

The use of field-effect transistors (FETs) as a THz detector is described in section 9.2. The large-scale interest in using FETs started around 2004 after the first experimental demonstration of

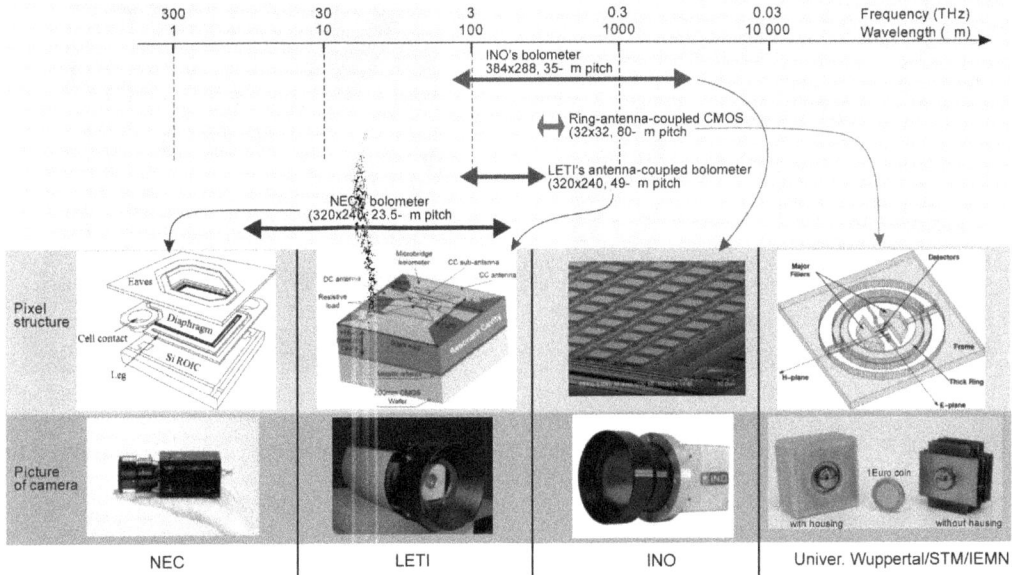

FIGURE 10.6 Development status of uncooled THz focal plane arrays.

sub-THz and THz detection in silicon-CMOS FETs. Two years later it was shown that Si-CMOS FETs can reach a *NEP* value that is competitive with the best conventional room temperature THz detectors. At present the advantages of Si-CMOS FET technology (room temperature operation, very fast response time, easy on-chip integration with read-out electronics and high reproducibility) lead to the straight-forward array fabrication [13, 14].

The first CMOS FPA used to capture transmission-mode THz video streams in real-time without the need for raster scanning and source modulation has been fabricated. A camera with 32×32 pixel array fully integrated in a 65-nm CMOS process technology has been demonstrated [15] (see right side of Figure 10.6). Each 80-μm array pixel consists of a differential on-chip ring antenna coupled to NMOS direct detector operated well-beyond its cut-off frequency. The camera chip has been packed together with a 41.7-dBi silicon lens in a 5×5×3 cm^3 camera module. In continuous-wave illumination the camera achieves a responsivity of 100–200 kV/W and a total *NEP* of 10–20 nW/Hz$^{1/2}$ up to 500 frames per second (fps) at 856 GHz.

Leti has developed complementary THz arrays based on CMOS FETs, either in direct or heterodyne detection [16]. For direct detection an innovative readout architecture is elaborated to take advantage of the large pixel pitch (240×240 μm^2) to enhance the flexibility and the sensitivity. Video sequences up to 100 frames per second have been achieved. Fast scanning of large field of view of opaque scenes has been achieved in a body scanner prototype. Each individual image acquired in real-time corresponds to a 40×60 mm^2 surface at the scene level. In order to cover the size of a chest, one mirror is successively moved in order to compose a 5×5 tiled array of individual images. A human trunk of a typically 20×30 cm^2 surface has been successfully scanned in less than 10 seconds (see Figure 10.7) to identify metallic and ceramic objects concealed under a shirt [17].

Although currently FET-based THz detectors presents poorer sensitivities than bolometer THz detectors, however, FET-based THz detection using standard low-cost CMOS technology appears to be an interesting way to benefit from THz imaging advantages. FET FPAs do not require vacuum packaging.

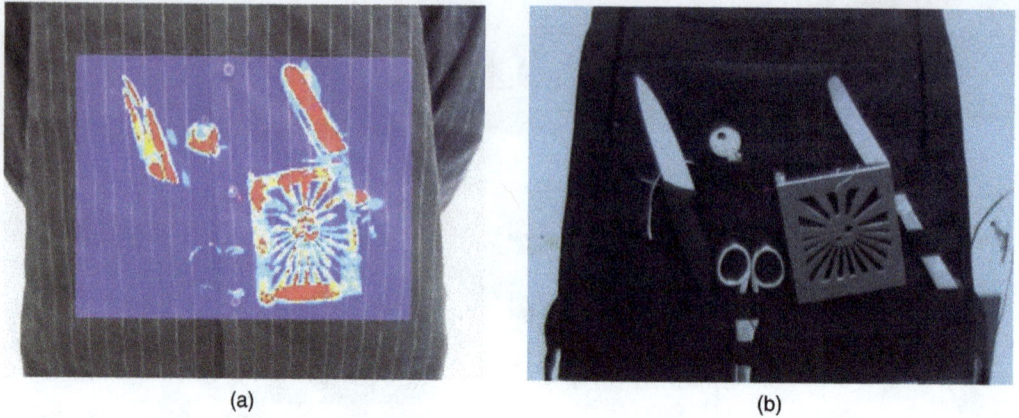

(a)   (b)

FIGURE 10.7 Large field of view fast scanning THz image acquired within less than 10 seconds by the scanner demonstrator (a) and visible photograph (b).

10.1.3 MICROBOLOMETERS

An impressive promising technology is also coming from commercially available microbolometer arrays. Adaptation of infrared microbolometers to the THz frequency range after the successful demonstration of active THz imaging in 2006 [18] entailed that in the period 2010–2011 three different companies/organisations announced cameras optimised for the >1-THz frequency range: NEC (Japan) [19], INO (Canada) [20] and Leti (France) [21]. The number of vendors is expected to increase soon.

Different designs of THz bolometer pixels have been proposed. NEC's pixel is divided into two parts (see left side of Figure 10.6): a silicon readout integrated circuit (ROIC) in the lower part, and a suspended microbridge structure in the upper part. The microbridge has a two-storied structure. The bottom is composed of a diaphragm and two legs, while the top (eaves) structure is formed on the diaphragm to increase the sensitive area and fill factor. The diaphragm and the eaves absorb THz radiation. The diaphragm is composed of VO_x bolometer thin film, SiN_x passivation layers and TiAlV electrodes, while the eaves structure is composed of SiN_x layer and a TiAlV thin film THz absorption layer.

A schematic of one Leti pixel of an amorphous silicon microbolometer array is shown in the top centre of Figure 10.6. The 50-μm pitch is associated with quasi-double-bowtie antennas to a thermometer microbridge structure derived from the standard IR bolometer. The membrane is suspended over the substrate by arms and pillars. In order to enhance the antenna gain, an equivalent quarter-wavelength resonant cavity is realised under antennas with an 11-μm thick SiO_2 layer deposited over the metallic reflector. To ensure electric contact between the bolometer pillars and CMOS metal upper contacts, the vias are etched through an 11-μm cavity and then metalised.

Figure 10.8 summarises the *NEP* values for bolometer FPAs fabricated by three vendors. The FPAs optimised for 2–5 THz exhibit impressive *NEP* values below 100 pW/Hz$^{1/2}$. It can be seen that wavelength dependence of *NEP* is quite flat below 200 μm. Further improvement of performance is possible by increasing the number of pixels and modification of the antenna design while preserving pixel pitch, ROIC and technological stack. Similarly, Figure 10.9 compares *NEP* values of existing THz photon detectors dominating the market. In both figures performance of graphene-based detectors also are included. At the present stage of technology, the most effective graphene THz detectors employ plasma rectification effect in FETs, where plasma wave in the channel are excited by incoming THz wave modulating the potential difference between gate and source/drain and being rectified via non-linear coupling and transfer characteristics in FET. FETs indeed provide

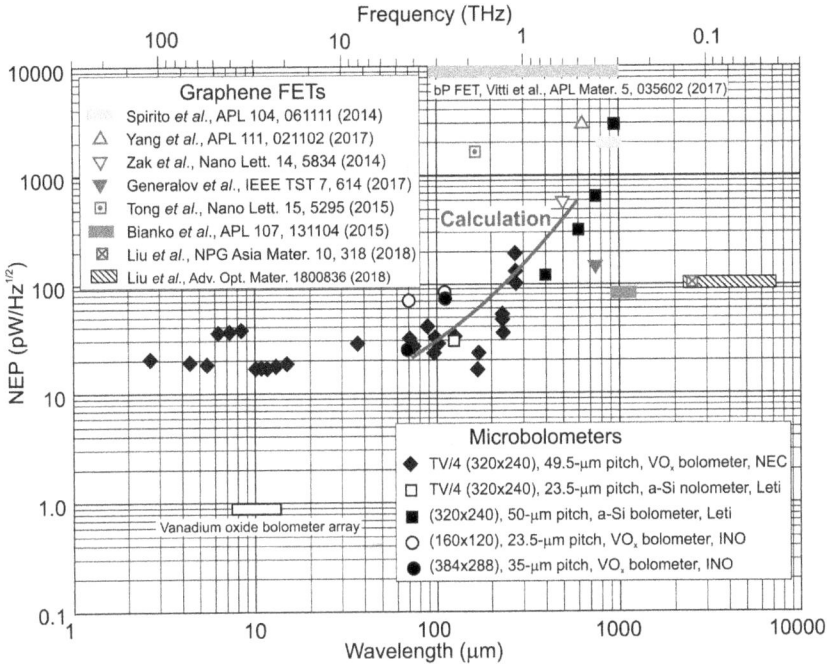

FIGURE 10.8 NEP spectral dependence for microbolometer THz FPAs and graphene FET detectors (after Reference 22).

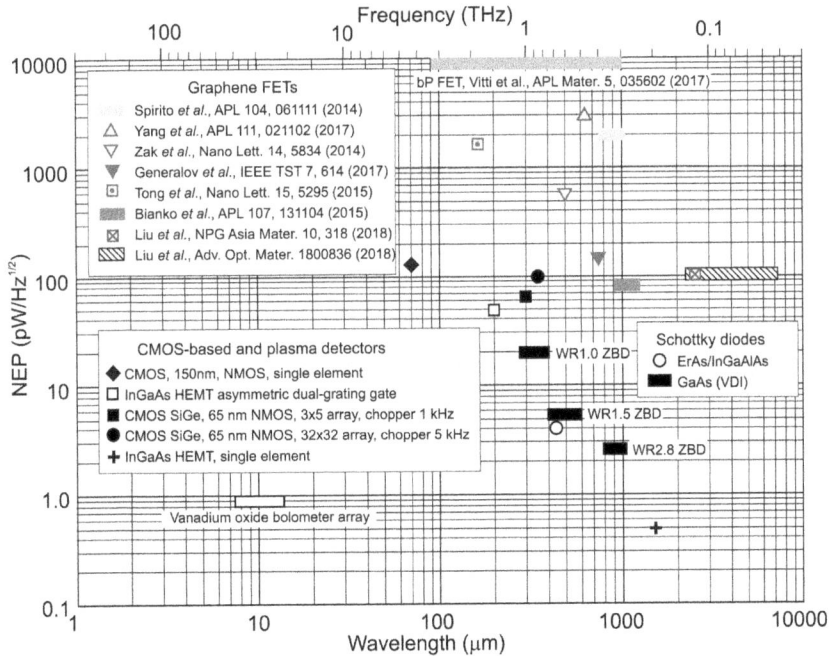

FIGURE 10.9 NEP spectral dependence for different photon THz (CMOS-based, Schottky diodes) and graphene FET detectors (after Reference 22).

some advantages at THz frequencies, namely the inherent scalability and the combination of a fast response and high frequency operation. For comparison, the performances of Schottky diodes are strongly affected by parasitic capacitances and usually show a dramatic cut-off above 1 THz.

10.2 EXTRINSIC SEMICONDUCTOR DETECTORS

Research and development of extrinsic IR photodetectors have been ongoing for more than 50 years. In the 1950s and 1960s, germanium could be made purer than silicon. Today, the problems with producing pure Si have been largely solved. Si has several advantages over Ge.

For wavelengths longer than 40 μm there are no appropriate shallow dopants for silicon; therefore, germanium devices are still of interest for very long wavelengths (see section 7.5.6). At the same time, the operating temperature must be reduced to less than 2 K.

The standard planar hybrid architecture, commonly used to construct near and mid-infrared focal-plane arrays [23], is not suitable for far IR detectors where readout glow, lack of efficient heat dissipation, and thermal mismatch between the detector and the readout could potentially limit their performance. Usually, the far-infrared arrays have a modular design with many modules stacked together to form a 2-dimensional array. The achievement of low *NEP* values in the range of a few parts 10^{-17} WHz$^{-1/2}$ is made possible by advances in crystal growth development and control of the residual minority impurities down to 10^{10} cm^{-3} in a doped crystal. As a result, a high lifetime and mobility value, and thus a higher photoconductive gain, have been obtained.

The Infrared Astronomical Satellite (IRAS), the Infrared Space Observatory (ISO), and for the far-infrared channels the Spitzer-Space Telescope (Spitzer) have all used bulk germanium photoconductors. In the Spitzer mission a 32×32-pixel Ge:Ga unstressed array was used for the 70-μm band, while the 160 μm band had a 2×20 array of stressed detectors [24]. The detectors are configured in the so-called Z-plane to indicate that the array has substantial size in the third dimension.

An innovative integral field spectrometer, called the Field Imaging Far-Infrared Line Spectrometer (FIFI-LS) was developed for the Herschel Space Observatory and SOFIA – see Figure 10.10. To accomplish this, the instrument has two 16×25 Ge:Ga arrays, unstressed for the 45–110 μm range and stressed for the 110 to 210 μm range [25].

The Photodetector Array Camera and Spectrometer (PACS) is one of the three science instruments on ESA's far infrared and sub-millimetre observatory (Herschel Space Laboratory). Apart from two Ge:Ga photoconductor arrays, it employs two filled silicon bolometer arrays with 16×32 and 32×64 pixels, respectively, to perform integral-field spectroscopy and imaging photometry in the 60–210 μm wavelength regime [26]. Median *NEP* values are 8.9×10^{-18} W/Hz$^{1/2}$ for the

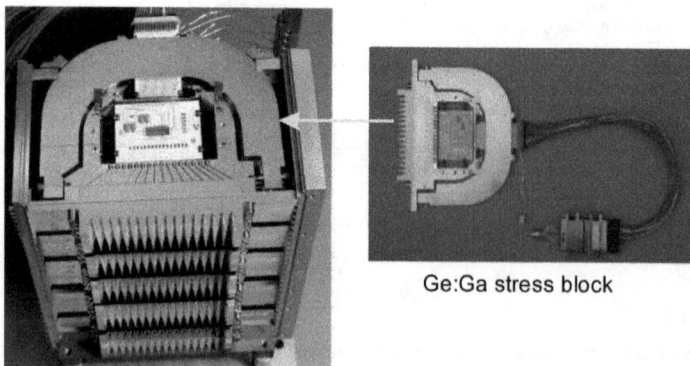

Ge:Ga stress block

FIGURE 10.10   PACS photoconductor focal plane array. The 25 stressed and low-stress modules of PACS instrument (corresponding to 25 spatial pixels) in the red and blue arrays are integrated into their housing.

TABLE 10.2

Performance of Si:As BIB FPAs fabricated in several formats for both ground and space based applications (after Reference 27)

Parameter	Si:As BIB	Phenix	MIRI	Aquarius-1k
Applications/Users	Ground-based telescopes ESO, Univer. of Tokyo	Space telescopes JAXA	Space telescopes JWST, NASA	Ground-based telescopes ESO, Univer. of Arizona
Format	320×240	1024×1024 2048×2048	1024×1024	1024×1024
Pixel size	50 μm	25 μm	25 μm	30 μm
ROIC type	DI	SFD	SFD	SFD
Fill factor	≥ 95%	≥ 95%	≥ 98%	≥ 98%
ROIC input referred noise	$< 1000e_{RMS}$	$6{-}20e_{RMS}$	$< 10{-}30e$	Low gain $< 1000e_{RMS}$ High gain $< 100e_{RMS}$
Integration capacity	7 or $20{\times}10^6$ e-	$3{\times}10^6$ e-	$2{\times}10^5$ e-	1 or $11{\times}10^6$ e-
Max. frame rates	100 to 500 Hz	0.1 Hz	0.1 Hz	120 Hz
Number of outputs	16 or 32	4	4	16 or 64
Packaging	LCC	LCC	Module	Module – 2 side buttable

DI – direct injection, SFD – source follower per detector, e⁻ - electron, RMS - root mean square, LCC - leadless chip carrier.

stressed and $2.1{\times}10^{-17}$ W/Hz$^{1/2}$ for the unstressed detectors, respectively. The detectors are operated at ~1.65 K. The readout electronics is integrated into the detector modules – each linear module of 16 detectors is read out by a cryogenic amplifier/multiplexer circuit in CMOS technology but operates at temperature 3–5K.

The design of BIB detectors offers a number of advantages over conventional extrinsic photoconductors: the high absorption coefficient of the absorbing layer means that detectors with comparatively small active volumes can be made, providing low susceptibility to cosmic rays without compromising quantum efficiency. Also, due to the heavy doping of the active layer, the impurity band increases in width, thereby effectively decreasing the energy gap between the impurity band and the conduction band. BIB arrays are mainly used for ground- and space-based far-infrared astronomy. Both low- and high-flux version of the BIB detector have been elaborated by significant modifications of the detector design. These adjustments included changes in doping profiles and layer thickness and tailoring buried contact resistivity to allow for the larger current densities in the higher photon flux environment. Extrinsic silicon arrays for high-background applications are less developed than that for low-background applications.

Impressive progress has been achieved, especially in Si:As BIB array technology with format as large as 2048×2048 and pixels as small as 18 μm; operated in spectral band up to 30 μm at about 10 K. The characteristics of the most advanced Si:As BIB arrays for astronomy are summarised in Table 10.2. Figure 10.11 shows the evolution of BIB detector arrays at RVS.

10.3   SEMICONDUCTOR BOLOMETERS

Cooled silicon bolometers demonstrate broadband and nearly flat spectral response in the 1–3000 μm wavelength range. They are easier to fabricate with high operability, good uniformity, and lower cost, but they have low operating temperatures (4.2–0.3 K). During fabrication of bolometers, their area, operating temperature, thermal time constant and thermal conductance are adjusted to meet the specific design requirements. Present-day technology exists to produce arrays of hundreds of pixels

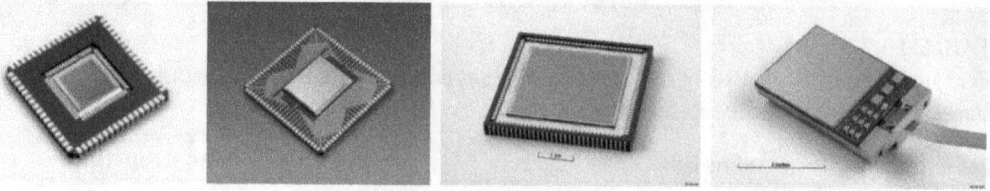

FIGURE 10.11 Evolution of BIB FPAs at RVS. From left to right: SIRTF 256×256, CRC774 320×240, Aquarius-1k 1024×1024, and Phoenix 2048×2048 devices (after Reference 27).

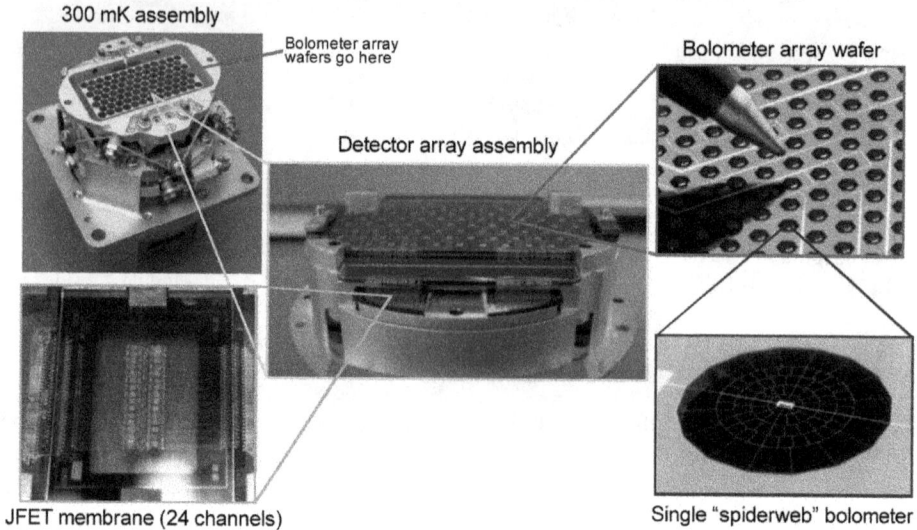

FIGURE 10.12 Bolometer array of the Spectral and Photometric Imaging Receiver (SPIRE).

that are operated in many experiments, including NASA Pathfinder ground-based instruments, and balloon experiments.

The thermistors are typically fabricated by lithography on membranes of Si or SiN. The impedance is selected to a few MΩ to minimise the noise in JFET amplifiers operated at about 100 K. Limitation of this technology is an assertion of thermal mechanical and electrical interface between the bolometers at 100–300 mK and the amplifiers at ≈ 100 K. Usually, JFET amplifiers are sited on membranes that isolate them so effectively that the environment remains at much lower temperatures (about 10 K) – see Figure 10.12. In addition, the equipment at 10 K is itself thermally isolated from nearby components at 0.1–0.3 K.

In bolometer metal films that can be continuous or patterned in a mesh absorb the photons. The patterning is designed to select the spectral band, to provide polarisation sensitivity or to control the throughput. Different bolometer architectures are used. In close-packed arrays and spider web, the pop-up structures or two-layer bump bonded structures are fabricated.

At present, high-performance bolometer arrays for the far IR and sub-mm spectral ranges are available. For example, the Herschel/PACS instrument uses a 2048-pixel array of bolometers and is an alternative to JFET amplifiers [28]. The architecture of this array is vaguely similar to the direct hybrid mid-infrared arrays, where one silicon wafer is patterned with bolometers, each in the form of a silicon mesh.

10.4 PAIR BRAKING PHOTON DETECTORS

One of the methods of photon detection consists in using superconducting materials. If the temperature is far below the transition temperature, T_c, most of electrons in them are banded into Cooper pairs. Photons with energies exceeding the binding Cooper pair energies in the superconductor, 2Δ (each electron must be supplied an energy Δ), can break these pairs, producing quasiparticles (electrons) [see inset of Figure 10.13(a)]. When the bias voltage is increased to the gap voltage, the Cooper pairs on one side of the junction can break up into two quasiparticles, which then tunnel to the other side of the junction before recombining, resulting in a sharp increase in current. This process resembles the interband absorption in semiconductors, with the energy gap equal to 2Δ, when the photons are absorbed and electron-hole pairs are created.

Several structures of pair braking detectors that use different ways to separate quasiparticles from Cooper pairs have been proposed. Among them are superconductor-insulator-superconductor (SIS) and superconductor-insulator-normal metal (SIN) detectors and mixers, radio frequency (RF) kinetic inductance detectors, and superconducting quantum interference device (SQUID) kinetic inductance detectors. Superconducting detectors offer many benefits: outstanding sensitivity, lithographic fabrication, and large array sizes, especially through the development of multiplexing techniques. The basics physics of these devices and progress in their developments are described in Reference [29].

The SIS detector is a sandwich of two superconductors separated by a thin (≈ 20 Å) insulator, which is schematically shown in Figure 10.13(c). Nb and NbTiN are almost exclusively used as superconductors for the electrodes. For a standard junction process, the base electrode is 200-nm sputtered Nb, the tunnel barrier is made using a thin 5-nm sputtered Al layer which is either thermally oxidised (Al_2O_3) or plasma nitridised (AlN). The counterelectrode is 100-nm sputtered Nb or reactively sputtered NbTiN. Typical junction areas are about 1 μm^2.

SIS tunnel junctions are mainly used as mixers in heterodyne type mm and sub-mm receivers, because of their strong non-linear I-V characteristic. They can be also used as direct detection detectors. The operating temperature of SIS junctions is below 1 K: typically $T \leq 300$ mK. However, up to now SIS detectors are difficult to integrate into large arrays.

Progress in development of large-format, high-sensitivity focal plane arrays is especially promising with two detector technologies: transition-edge superconducting (TES) bolometers (see next section) and microwave kinetic inductance detectors (MKIDs) based on different principles of superconductivity. Multiple instruments are currently in development based on arrays up to 10,000 detectors using both time-domain multiplexing (TDM) and frequency-domain

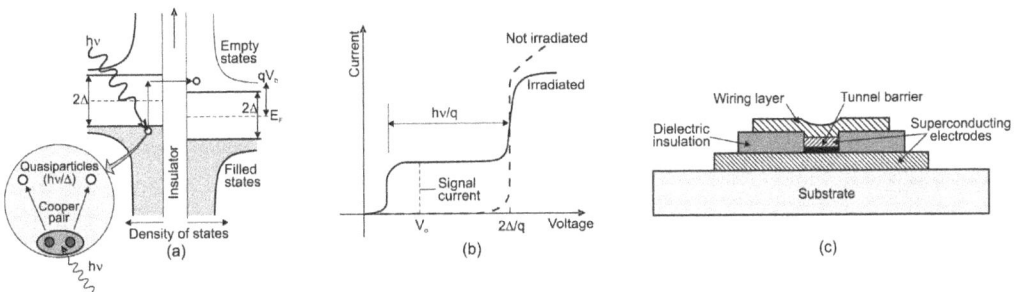

FIGURE 10.13 SIS junction: (a) energy diagram with applied bias voltage and illustration of photon assisted tunnelling, (b) current-voltage characteristic of a non-irradiated and irradiated barrier [the intensity of the incident radiation is measured as an excess of the current at a certain bias voltage V_o – schematic creation of quasiparticle is shown inside (a)], and (c) a cross section of a typical SIS junction.

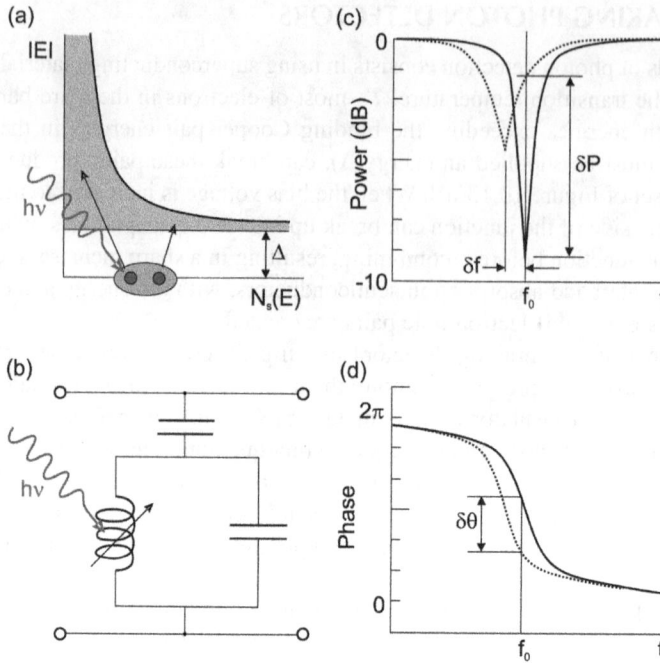

FIGURE 10.14 An illustration of the operational principle behind a MKID.

multiplexing (FDM) with superconducting quantum interference devices (SQUIDs) [30]. Both sensors show the potential to realise the very low ~10^{-20} W/Hz$^{1/2}$ sensitivity needed for space-borne spectroscopy.

A MKID is essentially a high-Q resonant circuit made out of either superconducting microwave transmission lines or a lumped element LC resonator (fabricated from thin aluminium and niobium films). In the first case, a meandered quarter-wavelength strip of superconducting material is coupled by means of a coupling capacitance to a coplanar waveguide through-line used for excitation and readout. Lumped elements are instead created from an LC series resonant circuit inductively coupled to a microstrip feed line placed in a high-frequency resonant circuit (see Figure 10.14). Photons hitting an MKID break Cooper pairs, which changes the surface impedance of the transmission line or inductive element, producing a number of quasiparticles. This causes the resonant frequency and quality factor to shift an amount proportional to the energy deposited by the photon. The amplitude (c) and phase (d) of a microwave excitation signal sent through the resonator. The change in the surface impedance of the film following a photon absorption event pushes the resonance to lower frequency and changes its amplitude. The energy of the absorber photon can be determined from the degree of phase and amplitude shift. The readout is almost entirely at room temperature and can be highly multiplexed; in principle hundreds or even thousands of resonators could be read out on a single feedline [31,32].

10.5 SUPERCONDUCTING HEB AND TES DETECTORS

Among superconducting detectors used for terahertz down-conversions, hot-electron-bolometer (HEB) mixers have attracted attention. Their low local-oscillator (LO) power consumption (less than 1 μW), near-quantum-limited noise performance and ease of fabrication have placed them above competing technologies in the quest for implementation of large-format heterodyne arrays.

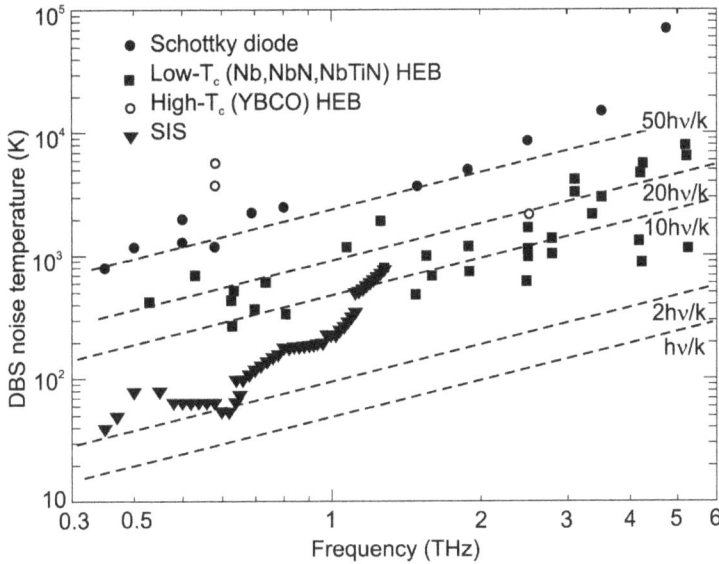

FIGURE 10.15   DSB noise temperature of Schottky diode mixers, SIS mixers, and HEB mixers operated in terahertz spectral band (after Reference 34).

In principle, HEB is quite similar to the transition-edge sensor (TES) bolometer, where small temperature changes caused by the absorption of incident radiation strongly influence resistance of biased sensor near its superconducting transition. The main difference between HEBs and ordinary bolometers is the speed of their response. High speed is achieved by allowing the radiation power to be directly absorbed by the electrons in the superconductor, rather than by using a separate radiation absorber and allowing the energy to flow to the superconducting TES via phonons, as ordinary bolometers do. After photon absorption, a single electron initially receives the energy $h\nu$, which is rapidly shared with other electrons, producing a slight increase in the electron temperature. In the next step, the electron temperature subsequently relaxes to the bath temperature through emission of phonons.

In comparison with TES, the thermal relaxation time of the HEB's electrons can be made fast by choosing a material with a large electron-phonon interaction. The development of superconducting HEB mixers has led to the most sensitive systems at frequencies in the terahertz region, where the overall time constant has to be a few tens of picoseconds. These requirements can be realised with a superconducting microbridge made from NbN, NbTiN, or Nb on a dielectric substrate [33].

Generally, in terahertz receivers, the noise of a mixer is quoted in terms of a single-sideband (SSB), T^{SSB}, or double-sideband (DSB), T^{DSB}, mixer noise temperature. The DSB noise temperatures achieved with Schottky diode mixers, SIS mixers, and HEB mixers operated in terahertz spectral band are presented in Figure 10.15 [34]. The noise temperature of SBD receivers has essentially reached a limit of about 50 $h\nu/k$ in frequency range below 3 THz. Above 3 THz, there occurs a steep increase, mainly due to increasing losses of the antenna and reduced performance of the diode itself.

Figure 10.16(a) presents an example cross-section view of NbN mixer chip. About 150-nm thick Au spiral structure is connected to the contact pads. The superconducting NbN film extends underneath the contact layer/antenna. The central area of a mixer chip shown in Figure 10.16(b) is manufactured from a 3.5-nm thick superconducting NbN film on a high resistive Si substrate [33]. The active NbN film area is determined by the dimensions of the 0.2-μm gap between the gold contact pads. The NbN microstrip is integrated with a planar antenna patterned as log-periodic spiral.

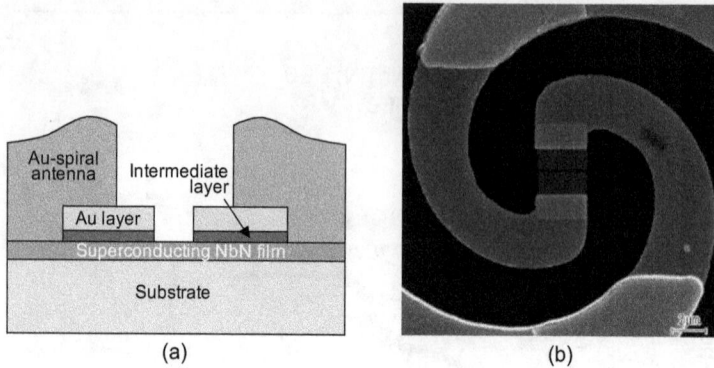

FIGURE 10.16 NbN HEB mixer chip: (a) cross-section view and (b) SEM micrograph of the central area of mixer.

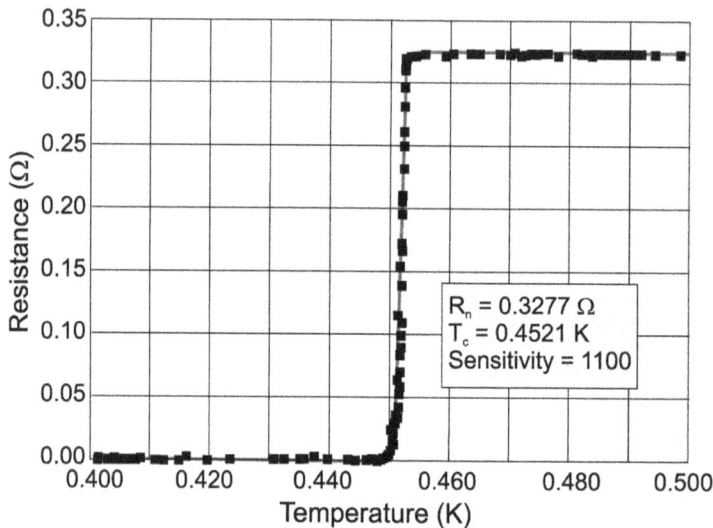

FIGURE 10.17 Resistance versus temperature for a high-sensitivity TES Mo/Au bilayer with superconducting transition at 444 mK.

The name of the TES bolometer is derived from its thermometer, which is based on thin superconducting films held within the transition region, where it changes from the superconducting to the normal state over a temperature range of a few milliKelvin (see Figure 10.17) [35]. Changes in temperature transition can be set by using a bilayer film consisting of a normal material and a layer of superconductor (e.g., thin Mo/Au, Mo/Cu, Ti/Au, etc.). Such a design enables diffusion of the Cooper pairs from the superconductor into the normal metal and makes it weakly superconducting – this process is called the proximity effect. As a result, the transition temperature is lowered relative to that for the pure superconducting film ($T < 200$ mK). Thus, in principle, the TES bolometers are quite similar to the HEBs.

TES bolometers are superior to current-biased particle detectors in terms of linearity, resolution and maximum count rate. At present, these detectors can be applied to THz photons counting because of their high sensitivity and low thermal time constant. Membrane isolated TES bolometers are capable of reaching a phonon $NEP \approx 4 \times 10^{-20}$ W/Hz$^{1/2}$. The current generation of sub-orbital experiments

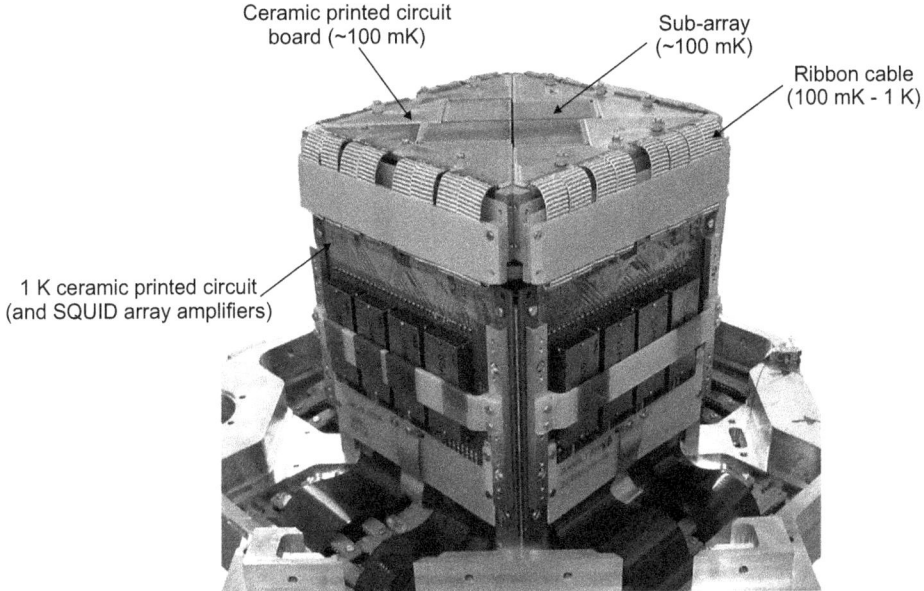

FIGURE 10.18 SCUBA-2 mounted on the James Clerk Maxwell Telescope on Mauna Kea, Hawaii. The instrument weighs 4.5 tonnes and is 3 m high. The massive blue box contains the camera and keeps it cold at about 0.1 K. Submillimetre light from the telescope enters through a small window on the left-hand side (behind the white bars) and is directed onto the two sets of detectors operated at wavelengths of 450 and 850 μm. The top figure shows the photograph of four sub-array modules folded into position in a focal plane unit. Each SCUBA-2 array is made of four side-buttable sub-arrays, each with 1280 (32×40) transition-edge sensors. The principal components are also highlighted.

largely relies on TES bolometers. An important feature of this sensor is that it can operate in a wide spectral band between the radio and gamma rays.

The most ambitious example of TES bolometer array is that used in the Submillimetre Common-User Bolometer Array camera (SCUBA-2), with 10,240 pixels [30]. Operated at wavelengths of 450 and 850 μm, the camera has been mounted on the James Clerk Maxwell Telescope in Hawaii (see Figure 10.18). Each SCUBA-2 array is made of four side-buttable sub-arrays, each with 1280 (32×40) transition-edge sensors.

10.6   FAR-INFRARED INSTRUMENTS FOR ASTRONOMY

Progress in THz detector sensitivity has been impressive over more than half a century, which is shown in Figure 10.19(a) in the case of bolometers used in far-IR and sub-mm-wave astrophysics [36]. The *NEP* value has decreased by a factor of 10^{12} in 80 years, corresponding to improvements by a factor of two every two years. Individual detectors achieved photon noise limited performance for ground-based imaging in the 1990s. The photon noise from astrophysical sources, achievable in space with a cold telescope, $\sim 10^{-18}$ W/$\sqrt{\text{Hz}}$, is now within demonstrated sensitivities. Far-infrared spectroscopy from a cold telescope, however, requires sensitivity $\sim 10^{-20}$ W/$\sqrt{\text{Hz}}$ to reach the astrophysical photon noise limit.

The development of pixel arrays has been comparably revolutionary [36, 37]. Figure 10.19(b) shows an increase in the number of pixels over the last three decades. Detector arrays have doubled in format every 20 months over the past 10 years, producing arrays with pixels now numbering in the thousands. A steady increase in overall observing efficiency is expected in the near future.

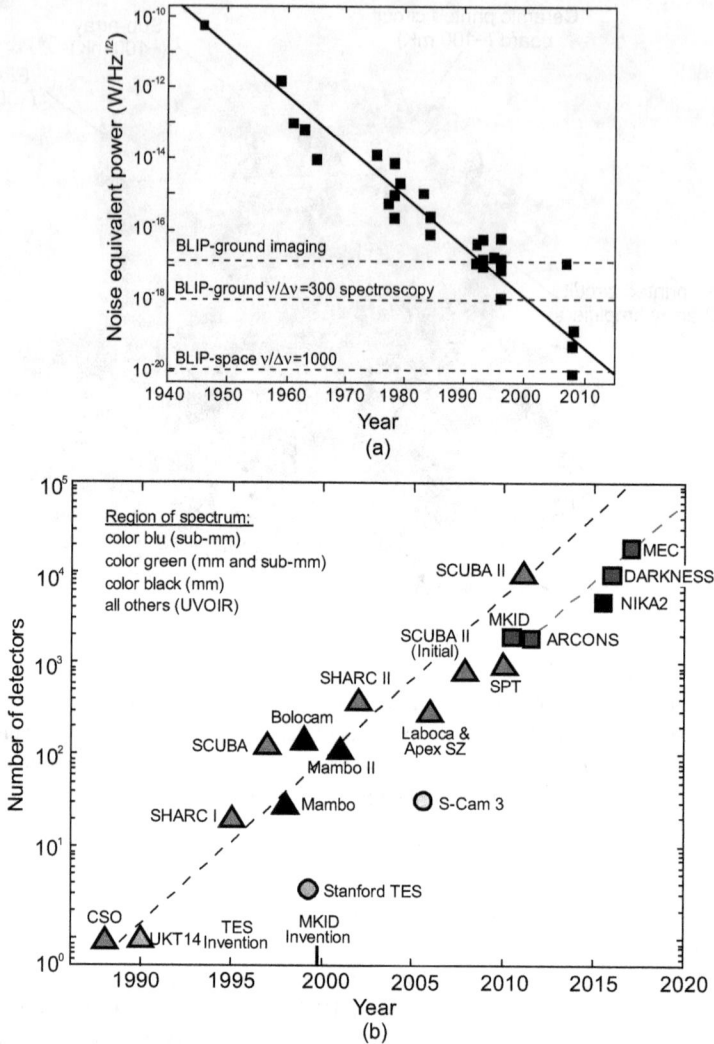

FIGURE 10.19 Trends in development of THz detectors: (a) improvement of the bolometer NEP-value for more than half a century (sensitivity doubled every 2 years over the past 80 years), (b) detector arrays have doubled in format every 20 months over the past 10 years; green symbol indicates current expectation (adapted after Reference 30).

The largest TES arrays currently in operation are the SCUBA 2 arrays, and these array sizes have already been surpassed by MKID instruments in commissioning. The only devices for which large-scale arrays are currently and cost effectively realisable are MKIDs, and array scalability has been demonstrated [37].

All ground-based (ground telescopes) and atmospheric-based observing platforms (planes like SOFIA, balloons) suffer from photon noise from atmospheric emission. The only way to perform competitive far-infrared (FIR) observations are space-based platforms. A rich history of space-based FIR observatories is described in Reference 38. Four examples of satellites that observe at far-infrared wavelengths are shown in Figure 12.20. Table 10.3 gathers selected examples of far-infrared instruments and their characteristics along with some required for future missions.

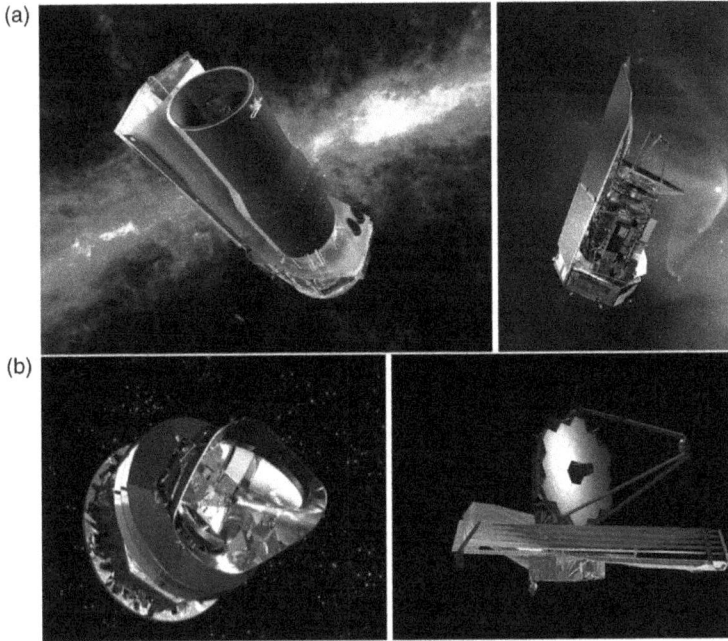

FIGURE 10.20 Four examples of satellites that observe at mid/or far-infrared wavelengths: (a) Spitzer and Herschel and (b) Planck and JWST, which also use V-groove radiators (thermal shields) to achieve passive cooling up to < 40 K.

TABLE 10.3
Selected Examples of Sensitivities Achieved by Far-Infrared to Millimetre-Wave Detector Arrays, along with Some Required for Future Missions (After Reference 38)

Observatory and instrument	Waveband (μm)	Aperture (m)	T_{aper} (K)	T_{det} (K)	NEP (W/$\sqrt{Hz}$)	Detector technology	Detector count	Notes
JCMT-SCUBA	450/850	15	275	0.1	2×10^{-16}	Bolometers	91/36	
JCMT-SCUBA2	450/850	15	275	0.1	2×10^{-16}	TES	5000/5000	
APEX-ArTeMis	200 to 450	12	275	0.3	4.5×10^{-16}	Bolometers	5760	
APEX-A-MIKID	350/850	12	275	0.3	1×10^{-15}	KIDs	25,000	
APEX-ZEUS2	200 to 600	12	275	0.1	4×10^{-17}	TES	555	$R \sim 1000$
CSO-MAKO	350	10.4	275	0.2	7×10^{-16}	KIDs	500	Low-$/pix
CSO-Z-Spec	960 to 1500	10.4	275	0.06	3×10^{-18}	Bolometers	160	
IRAM-NIKA2	1250/2000	30	275	0.1	1.7×10^{-17}	KIDs	4000/1000	
LMT-ToITEC	1100	50	275	0.1	7.4×10^{-17}	KIDs	360	Also at 1.4,2.1 mm
SOFIA-HAWC+	40 to 250	2.5	240	0.1	6.6×10^{-17}	TES	2560	
SOFIA-HIRMES	25 to 122	2.5	240	0.1	2.2×10^{-17}	TES	1024	Low-res channel
BLAST-TNG	200 to 600	2.5	240	0.3	3×10^{-17}	KIDs	2344	
Herschel-SPIRE	200 to 600	3.5	80	0.3	4×10^{-17}	Bolometers	326	
Herschel-PACS bol.	60 to 210	3.5	80	0.3	2×10^{-16}	Bolometers	2560	
Herschel-PACS phot.	50 to 220	3.5	80	1.7	75×10^{-18}	Photoconductors	800	$R \sim 2000$
Planck-HFI	300 to 3600	1.5	40	0.1	1.8×10^{-17}	Bolometers	54	

(*continued*)

TABLE 10.3 (Continued)
Selected examples of sensitivities achieved by far-infrared to millimetre-wave detector arrays, along with some required for future missions (after Reference 38)

Observatory and instrument	Waveband (μm)	Aperture (m)	T_{aper} (K)	T_{det} (K)	NEP (W/$\sqrt{Hz}$)	Detector technology	Detector count	Notes
SuperSpec	850 to 1600	-	N/A	0.1	1.0×10^{-18}	KIDs	~100	$R < 700$
SPACEKIDS	-	-	N/A	0.1	3×10^{-19}	KIDs	1000	
SPICA-SAFARI	34 to 210	3.2	<6	0.05	2×10^{-19}		4000	
SPIRIT	25 to 400	1.4	4	0.05	1×10^{-19}		~100	
OST-imaging	100 to 300	5.9 to 9.1	4	0.05	2×10^{-19}		~10^5	
OST-spectroscopy	100 to 300	5.9 to 9.1	4	0.05	2×10^{-20}		~10^5	$R \sim 500$

REFERENCES

1. A.H. Lettington, I.M. Blankson, M. Attia, and D. Dunn, "Review of imaging architecture", *Proc. SPIE* 4719, 327–340 (2002).
2. A.W. Blain, I. Smail, R.J. Ivison, J.-P. Kneib, and D.T. Frayer, "Submillimetre galaxies", *Phys. Rep.* 369, 111–176 (2002).
3. D. Leisawitz, W.C. Danchi, M.J. DiPirro, L.D. Feinberg, D.Y. Gezari, M. Hagopian, W.D. Langer, J.C. Mather, S.H. Moseley, M. Shao, R.F. Silverberg, J.G. Staguhn, M.R. Swain, H.W. Yorke, and X. Zhang, "Scientific motivation and technology requirements for the SPIRIT and SPECS far-infrared/submillimeter space interferometers", *Proc. SPIE* 4013, 36–46 (2000).
4. P.H. Siegel, "Terahertz technology", *IEEE Trans. Microwave Theory Tech.* 50, 910–928 (2002).
5. E. Bründermann, H.-W. Hübers, and M. F. Kimmitt, *Terahertz Techniques*, Springer-Verlag, Heidelberg, 2012.
6. *Handbook of Terahertz Technology for Imaging, Sensing and Communications*, edited by D. Saeedkia, Woodhead Publishing Limited, Oxford, 2013.
7. F. Sizov and A. Rogalski, "THz detectors", *Prog. Quantum Electron.* 34, 278–347 (2010).
8. E.R. Brown and D. Segovia-Vargas, "Principles of THz direct detection", in *Semiconductor Terahertz Technology: Devices and Systems at Room Temperature Operation*, pp. 212–253, edited by G. Carpintero, L.E. Garcia Muñoz, L. Hartnagel, S. Preu, and A.V. Räisäinem, Wiley, Chichester, 2015.
9. A. Westlund, "Self-switching diodes for zero-bias terahertz detection", *Thesis*, Chalmers University of Technology, Gothenburg, March 2015; http://publications.lib.chalmers.se/records/fulltext/214629/214 629.pdf.
10. E.R. Brown, A.C. Young, J. Zimmerman, H. Kazemi, and A.C. Gossard, "High-sensitivity, quasi-optically-coupled semimetal-semiconductor detectors at 104 GHz", *Proc. SPIE* 6212, 621205 (2006).
11. Z. Zhang, R. Rajavel, P. Deelman, and P. Fay, "Sub-micro area heterojunction backward diode millimeter-wave detectors with 0.18 pW/Hz$^{1/2}$ noise equivalent power", *IEEE Microw. Wireless Compon. Lett.* 21, 267–269 (2011).
12. R. Han, Y. Zhang, Y. Kim, D.Y. Kim, H. Shichijo, E. Afshari, and O. Kenneth, "280 GHz and 860 GHz image sensors using Schottky-barrier diodes in 0.13μm digital CMOS", *IEEE Inter. Solid-State Circuits Confer.* 253–253 (2012).
13. W. Knap and M.I. Dyakonov, "Field effect transistors for terahertz applications", in *Handbook of Terahertz Technology*, edited by D. Saeedkia, pp 121–155, Woodhead Publishing, Cambridge, 2013.
14. W. Knap, D. Coquillat, N. Dyakonova, D. But, T. Otsuji, and F. Teppe, "Terahertz plasma field effect transistors", in *Physics and Applications of Terahertz Radiation*, pp. 77–100, edited by M. Perenzoni and D.J. Paul, Springer, Dordrecht, 2014.

15. R. Al Hadi, H. Sherry, J. Grzyb, Y. Zhao, W. Förster, H.M. Keller, A. Carhelin, A. Kaiser, and U.R. Pfeiffer, "A 1 k-pixel video camera for 0.7–1.1 terahertz imaging applications in 65-nm CMOS", *IEEE J. Solid-State Circuits* 47, 2999–3012 (2012).

16. F. Simoens, J. Meilhan, J.-A. Nicolas, "Terahertz real-time imaging uncooled arrays based on antenna-coupled bolometers or FET developed at CEA-LETI", *J. Infrared Millimeter Terahertz Waves* 36, 961–985, 2015.

17. www.leti-cea.fr/cea-tech/leti/Documents/Rapport%20scientifique/DOPT_annual%20research%20report%202015.pdf.

18. A.W.M. Lee, B.S.Williams, S. Kumar, Q. Hu, and J.L. Reno, "Real-time imaging using a 4.3-THz quantum cascade laser and a 320×240 microbolometer focal-plane array", *IEEE Photonics Technol. Lett.* 18, 1415–1417 (2006).

19. N. Oda, "Uncooled bolometer-type terahertz focal-plane array and camera for real-time imaging", *C. R. Phys* 11, 496–509 (2010).

20. M. Bolduc, M. Terroux, B. Tremblay, L. Marchese, E. Savard, M. Doucet, H. Oulachgar, C. Alain, H. Jerominek, and A. Bergeron, "Noise-equivalent power characterization of an uncooled microbolometer-based THz imaging camera", *Proc. SPIE* 8023, 80230C-1–10 (2011).

21. D.-T. Nguyen, F. Simoens, J.-L. Ouvrier-Buffet, J. Meilhan, and J.-L. Coutaz, "Broadband THz uncooled antenna-coupled microbolometer array—electromagnetic design, simulations and measurements", *IEEE Trans. Terahertz Sci. Technol.* 299–305 (2012).

22. A. Rogalski, M. Kopytko, and P. Martyniuk, "2D material infrared and terahertz detectors: status and outlook", *Opto-Electron. Rev.* 28, 107–154 (2020).

23. A. Rogalski, *Infrared and Terahertz Detectors*, CRC Press, Boca Raton, 2019.

24. E.T. Young, J.T. Davis, C.L. Thompson, G.H. Rieke, G. Rivlis, R. Schnurr, J. Cadien, L. Davidson, G.S. Winters, and K.A. Kormos, "Far-infrared imaging array for SIRTF", *Proc. SPIE* 3354, 57–65 (1998).

25. A. Poglitsch, R.O. Katterloher, R. Hoenle, J.W. Beeman, E.E. Haller, H. Richter, U. Grozinger, N. M. Haegel, and A. Krabbe, "Far-infrared photoconductors for Herschel and SOFIA", *Proc. SPIE* 4855, 115–128 (2003).

26. A. Poglitsch and B. Altieri, "The PACS instrument", in *Astronomy in the Submillimeter and Far Infrared Domains with the Herschel Space Observatory,* edited by L. Pagani and M. Gerin*, EAS Publications Series,* 34, pp. 43–62, 2009.

27. R. Mills, E. Beuville, E. Corrales, A. Hoffman, G. Finger, and D. Ives, "Evolution of large format impurity band conductor focal plane arrays for astronomy applications", *Proc. SPIE* 8154, 81540R-1–10 (2011).

28. N. Billot, P. Agnese, J.L. Augueres, A. Beguin, and A. Bouere, O. Boulade, C. Cara, C. Cloue, E. Doumayrou, L. Duband, B. Horeau, I. Le Mer, J.L. Pennec, J. Martignac, K. Okumura, V. Reveret, M. Sauvage, F. Simoens, and L. Vigroux, "The Herschel/PACS 2560 bolometers imaging camera", *Proc. SPIE* 6265, 62650D (2006).

29. J. Zmuidzinas and P.L. Richards, "Superconducting detectors and mixers for millimeter and submillimeter astrophysics", *Proc. IEEE* 92, 1597–1616 (2004).

30. J.J. Bock, "Superconducting detector arrays for far-infrared to mm-wave astrophysics", http://cmbpol.uchicago.edu/depot/pdf/ white-paper_j-bock.pdf.

31. P. Day, H.G. LeDuc, B.A. Mazin, A. Vayonakis, and J. Zmuidzinas, "A broadband superconducting detector suitable for use in large arrays", *Nature* 425, 817–821 (2003).

32. B.A. Mazin, "Microwave kinetic inductance detectors: The first decade", *The Thirteenth International Workshop on Low Temperature Detectors-LTD13.* AIP Conference Proceedings, Volume 1185, Issue 1, pp. 135–142

33. G.N. Gol'tsman, Yu.B. Vachtomin, S.V. Antipov, M.I. Finkel, S.N. Maslennikiv, K.V. Smirnov, S.L. Poluakov, S.I. Svechnikov, N.S. Kaurova, E.V. Grishina, and B.M. Voronov, "NbN phonon-cooled hot-electron bolometer mixer for terahertz heterodyne receivers", *Proc. SPIE* 5727, 95–106 (2005).

34. H.-W. Hübers, "Terahertz heterodyne receivers", *IEEE J. Sel. Top. Quantum Electron.* 14, 378–391, 2008.

35. D.J. Benford and S.H. Moseley, "Superconducting transition edge sensor bolometer arrays for submillimeter astronomy", *Proceedings of the International Symposium on Space and THz Technology*, www.eecs.umich.edu/ ~jeast/benford_2000_4_1.pdf.

36. M. Harwit, G. Helou, L. Armus, C.M. Bradford, P.F. Goldsmith, M. Hauser, D. Leisawitz, D.F. Lester, G. Rieke, and S.A. Rinehart, "Far-Infrared/Submillimeter astronomy from space tracking an evolving universe and the emergence of life", https://asd.gsfc.nasa.gov/cosmology/spirit/FIR-SIM_Crosscutting_White_Paper.pdf.

37. E.G.P. O'Connora, A. Shearera, and K. O'Brien, "Energy-sensitive detectors for astronomy: Past, present and future", *New Astron. Rev.* 87, 101526 (2019).

38. D. Farrah, K.E Smith, D. Ardila, C.M. Bradford, M. Dipirro, C. Ferkinhoff, J. Glenn, P. Goldsmith, D. Leisawitz, T. Nikola, N. Rangwala, S.A. Rinehart, J. Staguhn, M. Zemcov, J. Zmuidzinas, J. Bartlett. S. Carey, W.J. Fischer, J, Kamenetzky, J. Kartaltepe, M. Lacy, D.C. Lis, L. Locke, E. Lopez-Rodriguez, M. MacGregor, E. Mills, S.H. Moseley, E.J. Murphy, A. Rhodes, M. Richter, D. Rigopoulou, D. Sanders, R. Sankrit, G. Savini, J.-D. Smith, and S. Stierwalt, "Review: far-infrared instrumentation and technological development for the next decade", *J. Astron. Telesc. Instrum. Syst.* 5(2), 020901 (2019).

11 Direct and Advanced Detection Systems

The optical radiation receiver consists of a photodetector and a preamplifier connected to signal-processing circuits. The photodetector converts the optical radiation into an electrical signal, which is amplified before further processing to extract useful information carried by the optical signal. The preamplifier must have a low noise level and a sufficiently wide bandwidth to undistort the shape of the input waveforms. Designing a low-noise photoreceiver is a difficult task. It is required to minimise the noise contribution from various sources such as background noise, photodetector leakage current, thermal noise of biasing resistors and transistor noise. If the photodetector is an element whose equivalent diagram can be treated as a current source, the noise minimisation is achieved by increasing the biasing resistors value, reducing the capacitance, and minimising the leakage current. For bipolar transistors it is very important to choose the collector current optimal value. It often turns out that as a result of minimising noise, the system bandwidth has become so narrowed that it is no longer sufficient to transfer the transmitted signal without its distortion. The way out of this situation can be to introduce appropriate changes to the system and use appropriately selected elements with a low noise, both active and passive.

11.1 SELECTION OF ACTIVE AMPLIFICATION ELEMENTS

The active element in preamplifiers can be a bipolar or a field-effect transistor, or an integrated circuit with an input on a bipolar junction transistors (BJT), field effect transistors (FET) or metal-oxide semiconductor field effect transistors (MOSFET). The main selection criteria are the source impedance value and the transmitted frequencies range [1]. It is difficult to say authoritatively which active component is best suited for a given application. The nomogram presented in Figure 11.1 may provide some facilitation in the selection. For detectors with the lowest resistances, it is convenient to use a transformer or use transistors (preamplifiers) connected in parallel in order to match the source resistance to the optimal resistance, which means the one at which the amplifier makes the least noise contribution to the noise generated in the source resistance.

Bipolar transistors are most useful for low to medium source-resistance values. Additionally, they can be adjusted by an appropriate selection of the collector current [2]. For higher values of the source resistance, field-effect transistors work best due to the extremely low level of the noise current I_n. MOSFETs transistors are used for the highest values of the resistance R_s. Speaking of BJT, FET, or MOSFET transistors, one should also refer to integrated amplifiers in which the input element is the appropriate transistor.

The most important parameter of each receiving device is its sensitivity, understood as the ability to detect low-intensity signals. For small signals reaching the receiver, a very important issue is the noise optimisation, i.e., obtaining the maximum signal-to-noise (S/N) ratio. Since the first stages of complex electronic devices have the most significant impact on the system overall noise level, very

DOI: 10.1201/9781003263098-11

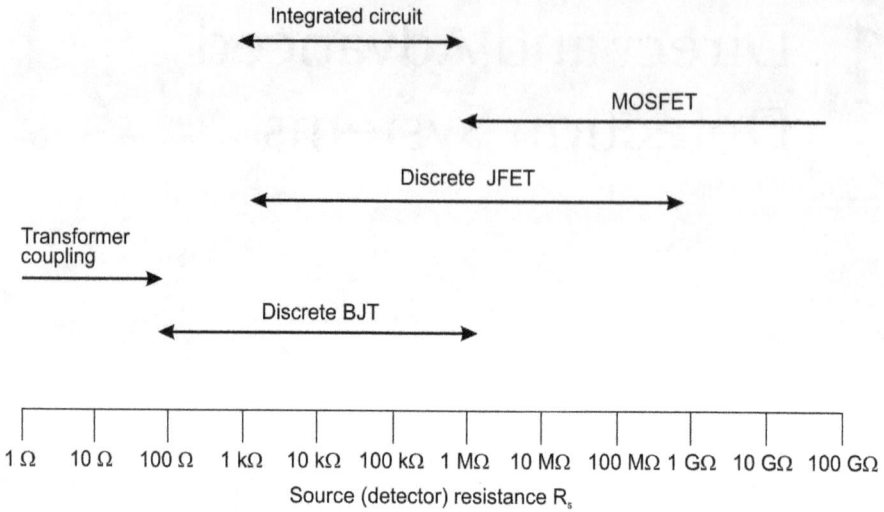

FIGURE 11.1 Nomogram for selecting the amplifier input element (after Reference 1).

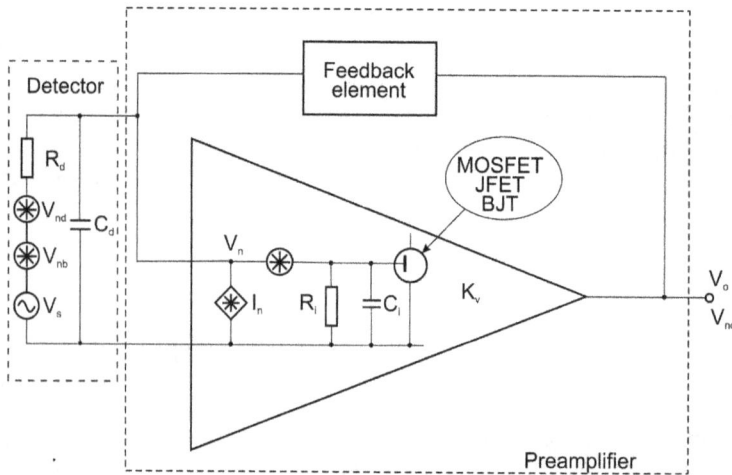

FIGURE 11.2 Noise equivalent diagram of the photodetector-preamplifier circuit: R_i, C_i – the preamplifier input resistance and capacity, respectively (after Reference 2).

strict requirements are placed on preamplifiers. The preamplifier optimal solution is obtained on the basis of an analysis of the individual noise sources contribution to the total equivalent input noise of the detector-preamplifier circuit and calculations of the equivalent input noise. The equivalent diagram is shown in Figure 11.2. The equivalent noise level at the input of the photodetector pre-amplifier (PD-PA) circuit is uniquely determined by the detector noise V_{nd}, the background noise V_{nb}, and the equivalent noise sources V_n and I_n characterising the preamplifier. Preamplifier is treated as noiseless, and the two substitute noise sources placed at its input represent all possible noise inputs from the circuit elements. With uncorrelated noise components, in the low frequency range, the total equivalent noise at the input of the FD-PA circuit is determined by the equation

$$V_{ni}^2 = V_{nd}^2 + V_{nb}^2 + V_n^2 + I_n^2 R_d^2, \tag{11.1}$$

where R_d is the detector resistance. In the higher frequency range, the detector impedance must be taken into account.

The detectors are characterised by an internal (own) noise and a noise generated by the incident radiation stream. The main source of an input noise of signal processing circuits in photoreceivers is the first (input) transistor used in the preamplifier circuit (Figure 11.2). This transistor noise contribution to the total equivalent input noise of the photoreceiver depends on detector impedance. Based on Eq. (11.1), it can be assumed that if the input stage transistor has a high noise current, it cannot work with a high resistance detector. A high value of the input transistor noise current causes a large substitute input noise (high $I_n R_d$ value) on the detector high resistance. A low impedance detector will work well with a low voltage noise preamplifier (negligible $I_n R_d$ value).

The total equivalent input noise $V_{ni\text{-}preamp}$ for a voltage preamplifier is given by the equation

$$V_{ni-preamp} \approx \left\{ \left[\frac{V_n R_i}{R_i + R_d} \right]^2 + \left(I_n \frac{R_i R_d}{R_i + R_d} \right)^2 \right\}^{1/2}, \tag{11.2}$$

where R_i is the input resistance of the preamplifier. If $R_i \gg R_d$, then

$$V_{ni-preamp} \approx \left[V_n^2 + \left(I_n R_d \right)^2 \right]^{1/2}. \tag{11.3}$$

For transimpedance preamplifiers, the total equivalent input noise is in the form of a current source expressed by the equation

$$I_{ni-preamp} \approx \left\{ \left[\frac{I_n R_d}{R_i + R_d} \right]^2 + \left[\frac{V_n \left(R_i + R_d \right)}{R_i R_d} \right]^2 \right\}^{1/2}. \tag{11.4}$$

Assuming that the input resistance R_i of the transimpedance amplifier is very low, Eq. (11.4) takes the form of

$$I_{ni-preamp} = \left[I_n^2 + \left(\frac{V_n}{R_d} \right)^2 \right]^{1/2}. \tag{11.5}$$

The noise voltage transferred to the transimpedance preamplifier output is equal to the product of the total equivalent current noise $I_{ni\text{-}preamp}$ and the transimpedance Z_t of the preamplifier. The current and voltage noise for low-noise transistors operating in a common emitter (source) system is shown in Figure 11.3. The current noise for MOSFET transistors can be neglected.

Characteristics of the noise sources I_n, V_n as a function of frequency for low-noise BJT, unipolar (JFET) field-effect transistors, and integrated circuits are usually provided by manufacturers. Noises of integrated circuits made in a CMOS technology (complementary metal-oxide semiconductor) are usually measured or determined based on the knowledge of the technological process and geometric dimensions. Typically, in the required photoreceiver bandwidth, these characteristics are not flat. The increase in noise is observed both in the low and high frequency range. In the low-frequency range, this increase is due to type $1/f$ noise. Therefore, to calculate the RMS value of the noise

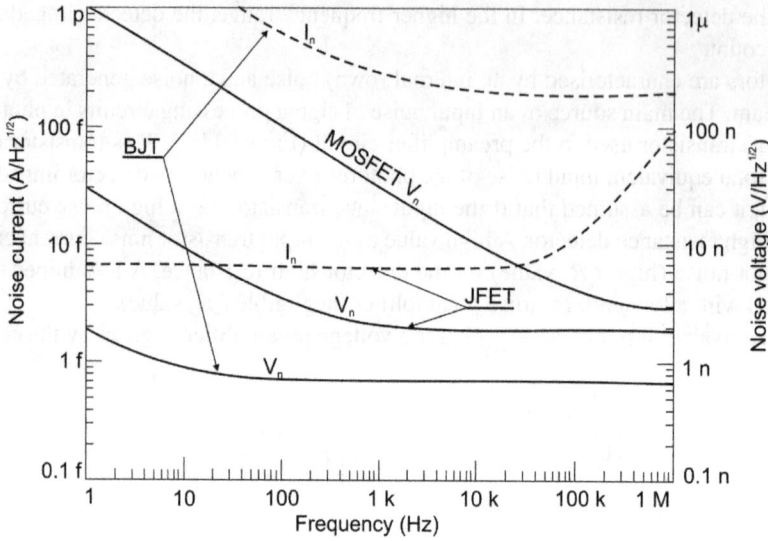

FIGURE 11.3 Current and voltage noise for low-noise BJT, unipolar JFET, and MOSFET transistors as a frequency function (after Reference 3).

voltage at the circuit output, one should know the input noise spectral density distribution and the frequency response $K_v(f)$ of the preamplifier.

For a voltage amplifier, the RMS value of the output noise voltage is given by the equation

$$V_{no}^2 = \int_{f_l}^{f_u} K_v^2(f) V_{ni-preamp}^2(f) df, \tag{11.6}$$

and for a transimpedance amplifier with the transimpedance Z_t

$$V_{no}^2 = \int_{f_l}^{f_u} Z_t^2(f) I_{ni-preamp}^2(f) df. \tag{11.7}$$

Figure 11.4 shows the dependence of the ratio of preamplifier (or input transistor noise) to detector thermal (Johnson's) noise as a function of detector resistance for BJT, JFET, and MOSFET amplifiers, in a common emitter or a common source configuration [3].

It can be noticed that there are some ranges of detector resistance for which the preamplifier noise is lower than the detector thermal noise. Further reduction of a JFET transistor noise below the detector resistance thermal noise even for values greater than 100 MΩ can be achieved by lowering their operating temperature. This is due to a decrease in the transistor gate current value. For any given detector, the values of the thermal noise voltage V_{nt} and the resistance R_d are determined by detector type (they cannot be changed). However, it is possible to change the parameters V_n and I_n of the designed preamplifier. Thus, minimisations of the input noise of the circuit it possible. Changes in the values V_n and I_n are made by choosing adequate elements in the preamplifier circuit. In the case of a photoreceiver using several gain stages, the first stage (when it has a correspondingly high power gain) contributes to the substitute input noise sources V_n and I_n as a rule. This condition is usually met. The V_n and I_n values are primarily determined by the V_{nT} and I_{nT} parameters of the active

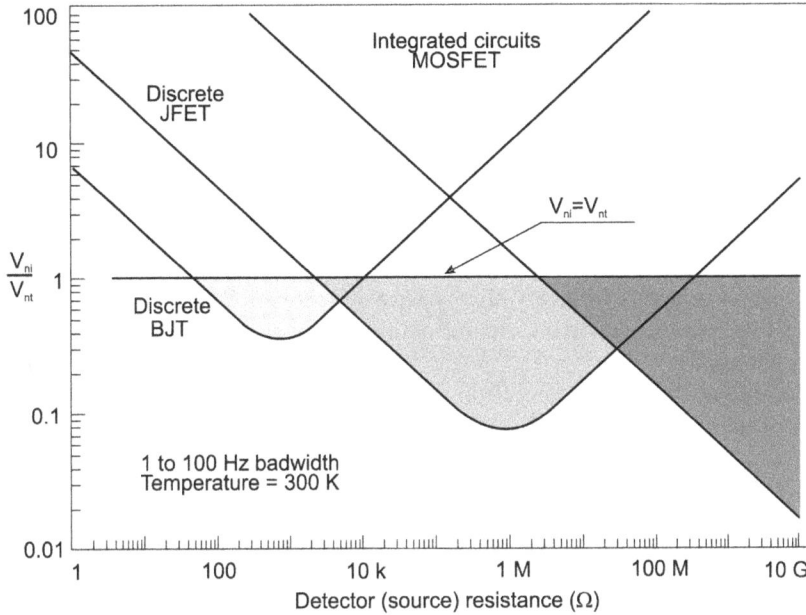

FIGURE 11.4 Dependence of the ratio of the equivalent input noise of BJT, JFET, and MOSFET transistors to the thermal noise of the detector on the detector resistance (after Reference 3).

element used (e.g., transistor). Influence of the noise coming from the transistor biasing circuit (base bias) may be neglected in some cases (with the so-called noiseless biasing). Therefore, the noise figure minimisation will consist in balancing the share of the V_n and I_n sources.

In practice, this means that the selection of the active element used in the input stage is made depending on the value of the detector resistance R_d. The selected element must have such V_{nT} and I_{nT} parameters that they meet the following relation:

$$V_{nT} = I_{nT} R_d. \tag{11.8}$$

Then, the amplifier makes the smallest noise contribution in relation to the noise generated by the detector resistance.

The noise factor is determined by the equation [1]

$$F_{opt} = 1 + \frac{V_n I_n}{2kT\Delta f}, \tag{11.9}$$

and, in this case, it reaches the minimum value. The value of the detector resistance for which the above-mentioned relationships occur is called the optimum resistance (preamplifier noise resistance) and denoted R_o. Noise resistance is not any existing resistance. It is only an abstract concept that helps to quickly find the detector resistance corresponding to the minimum noise factor. Usually, the situation should be reversed, that is, if one has a given value of the detector resistance R_d, then by changing, for example, the transistor collector current value, the condition $V_n = I_n R_s$ can be obtained.

On the basis of the above considerations, it is possible to draw conclusions concerning the division of preamplifiers, which, due to the type of active element used in the input stage, will be applied in practice to individual detector types. For low-resistance detectors (from tens of Ω to 1 kΩ), circuits with bipolar transistors at the input are mainly used because they are characterised by small values of V_n and greater than FETs values of I_n. Sometimes, in order to lower the optimum resistance value R_o, a parallel connection of several active elements or entire amplifiers is used [4]. In the range of average detector resistance, from 1 kΩ to 1 MΩ, the preamplifiers FET input stages can be used. For high resistance, from 1 MΩ to 1 GΩ detectors, low I_n-value transistors are especially recommended. Such requirements fulfil JFET and MOSFET transistors. MOSFET transistors are also suitable for detectors with very high resistances (above 1 GΩ).

Table 11.1 lists the most important features of operational amplifiers made in the BJT, FET, and MOSFET technology.

Figure 11.5 shows the dependence of op amp AD743 type total equivalent input noise on the resistance R_s of the signal source. For detectors with low resistance the amplifier voltage noise V_n dominates, for higher values of R_s the share of the detector thermal noise V_t increases, while for the highest values of R_s, $I_n R_s$ component dominates.

Some of the input stages of photoreceivers use preamplifiers built with discrete elements, that is, low noise transistors. It is caused, among other things, by the fact that the voltage noise V_n of the preamplifiers obtained then is $2^{1/2}$ times lower than the noise of preamplifiers built on operational amplifiers. However, the use of discrete elements requires a more detailed analysis of individual transistor technologies properties.

There are some differences between p-n-p and n-p-n transistors in terms of their use in low-noise detection circuits. The p-n-p transistors have a lower base-spreading resistance resulting from a higher electron mobility in the n-type region and a lower noise voltage compared to n-p-n detectors

---

TABLE 11.1
Properties of Operational Amplifiers Made in the BJT, FET and MOSFET Technology

Detector resistance	Technology	Technology properties
10 Ω – 1 kΩ	BJT	Low input impedance compared with JFET and MOSFET Low noise voltage High noise current Low $1/f$ corner (e.g., for AD 797 ~ 100 Hz) I_n ~ 2 pA/Hz$^{1/2}$, V_n ~ 0.7 nV/Hz$^{1/2}$ Examples of amplifiers: LT 1028, AD 797, AD 4898
1 kΩ – 1 MΩ	JFET	High input impedance (> 10 MΩ) Low noise current Higher noise voltage compared to BJT Higher $1/f$ corner (e.g., for LTC 6268 ~ 100 kHz) I_n ~ 3 fA/Hz$^{1/2}$, V_n ~ 1 nV/Hz$^{1/2}$ Examples of amplifiers: LTC 6268, ADA 4637-1, AD 8620
A few MΩ	JFET and MOSFET	
Above 10 MΩ	MOSFET	Very high input impedance (> 1 GΩ) High $1/f$ corner High noise voltage Low noise current I_n = 0.5 f A/Hz$^{1/2}$, V_n = 4.5 nV/Hz$^{1/2}$ (e.g., for MAX 4475 at f = 1 kHz)

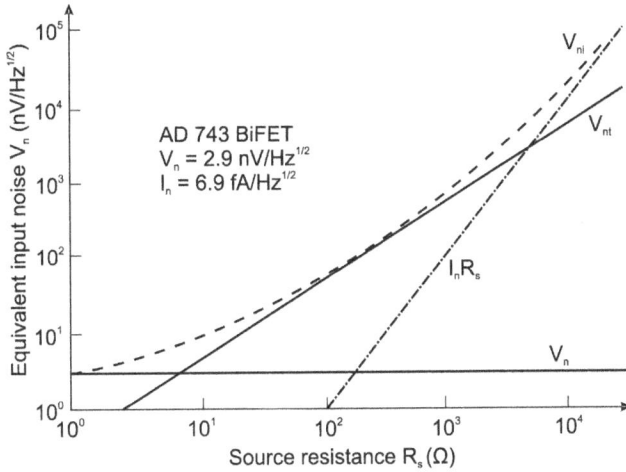

FIGURE 11.5 Dependence of the total equivalent input noise of the op amp AD743 type on the source (detector) resistance (after Reference 1).

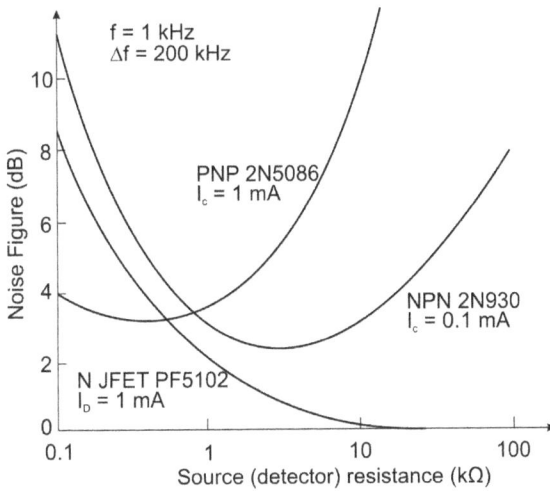

FIGURE 11.6 Dependence of the noise figure on the detector resistance for p-n-p, n-p-n, and JFET transistors (after Reference 7).

and, therefore, should be used for low-resistance detectors. On the other hand, n-p-n transistors have a slightly higher current amplification factor and a higher cut-off frequency, therefore they are recommended for use with detectors with higher resistance (Figure 11.6). In recent years, however, a small group of n-channel JFETs have been developed, for which the noise voltage was below 1 nV/Hz$^{1/2}$ [5–7], and thus a level comparable to, and sometimes lower than, voltage noise in BJT transistors.

In some applications, detection systems with a very high response speed and high signal amplification are required. In this case, HBTs (heterojunction bipolar transistors) and HEMT (high-electron mobility transistors) are recommended [8]. Preamplifiers designed to work with detectors are called front-end electronics [9]. Depending on their configuration, there is voltage, current (transimpedance), and charge preamplifiers.

11.2 VOLTAGE PREAMPLIFIERS

There are many different preamplifiers. The basic systems are voltage mode preamplifiers built on bipolar or FET transistors. Figure 11.7(a) shows a simplified scheme of a preamplifier with a bipolar transistor, while Figure 11.7(b) with a FET transistor. Detector load resistance R_L is a resistance resulting from the parallel connection of the biasing R_1 and R_2 resistors of the base (gate) and the bias resistance R_b of the detector.

Figure 11.8 gives a replacement diagram of the FD-PA circuit which shows that the voltage at its output is determined by the equation

$$V_o = V_i K_v = I_{ph} R_{eq} K_v, \tag{11.10}$$

where V_i is the voltage at the voltage amplifier input, the value of which depends on a photocurrent generated in the detector and the equivalent resistance R_{eq} resulting from the parallel connection of the load resistance R_L and the input resistance R_i of the preamplifier.

Criteria for selecting the optimal load resistance R_L of the detector can be summarised as follows: a high R_L value allows for a large output signal, while a low R_L value provides a wide bandwidth and allows for a greater dynamic input signal.

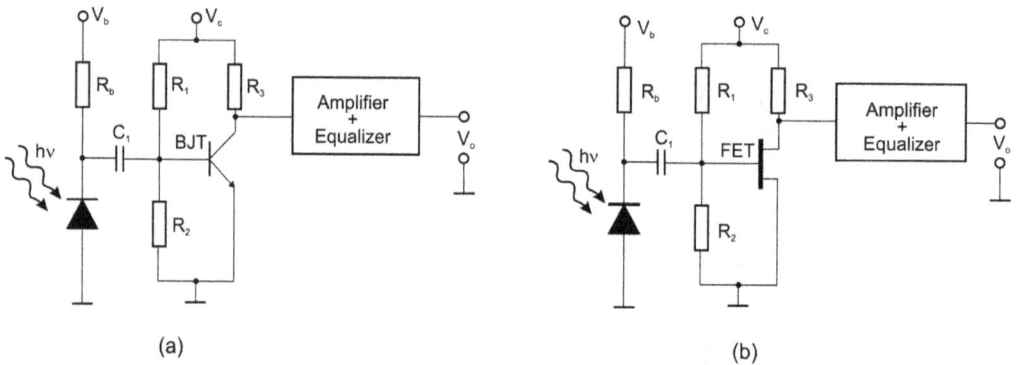

FIGURE 11.7 Simple input circuits of the photoreceiver: (a) preamplifier with a bipolar transistor, (b) preamplifier with a field-effect transistor.

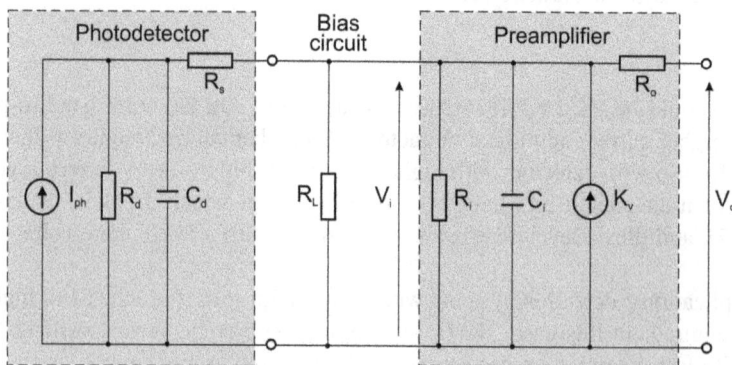

FIGURE 11.8 Equivalent scheme of the photodetector-preamplifier circuit.

The upper limit frequency of the input stage of such a photoreceiver is the following:

$$f_{g3dB} = \frac{1}{2\pi R_{eq} C_{eq}}, \tag{11.11}$$

where C_{eq} is the equivalent capacitance resulting from the parallel connection of the photodiode capacitance and the input capacitance of the transistor.

The input resistance of the FET is significant – usually from 1 to 100 MΩ, so it can be practically neglected when determining R_{eq}. For an amplifier with a FET transistor, it can, therefore, be assumed that $R_{eq} = R_L$. The input resistance of the bipolar transistor takes values in the order of a few kΩ. Therefore, it is not advisable to omit it in the calculation of the equivalent resistance R_{eq}.

Its influence is so significant that it can remarkably change the bandwidth expressed by Eq. (11.11). In contrast to the FET transistor, the input resistance in the BJT can be selected by design, by setting the base current value of

$$R_i = \frac{kT}{qI_B}, \tag{11.12}$$

where I_B is the base current of the transistor.

In preamplifiers with bipolar transistors, the thermal noise is created in the base-spreading resistance and base-biasing resistors. The shot noise, on the other hand, is related to the base current and collector [10]. In voltage preamplifiers with a field-effect transistor, the thermal noise source is the drain-source channel resistance and the gate biasing resistors. The cause of the shot noise is the gate leakage current.

The FET transistor noise power increases with the third power of a bandwidth, while the noise associated with a low base leakage bipolar transistor only increases its power with a bandwidth square. It follows that in the high-frequency range, bipolar transistors introduce less noise than field-effect transistors and are, therefore, more advantageous in this respect in many applications.

In the lower frequency range, FET transistors have better noise properties. In general, the best results are obtained by using FET transistors up to 25–50 MHz, and above this value, the transition to bipolar transistor technology [11].

Voltage preamplifiers can be divided into low and high input impedance preamplifiers. In the input stages of photoreceivers with low input impedance preamplifiers, the signal source is loaded with low impedance (e.g., 50 Ω). Time constant determined by the detector load resistance and the preamplifier input capacitance determines the bandwidth that should be matched to the signal band.

Although preamplifiers with a low input resistance may have a wide bandwidth, they do not provide high sensitivity of the photoreceiver. Photoreceivers with preamplifiers with a low input resistance are of limited use, especially where a wide bandwidth is required.

Figure 11.9(a) shows a low-input impedance preamplifier operating in a common base (CB) configuration. It was used in a CLC 5509 integrated circuit [12]. This circuit provides a wide bandwidth with a very low equivalent input noise voltage of 0.58 nV/Hz$^{1/2}$ at $f = 12$ MHz. It has been designed for signal sources with a resistance of 50–200 Ω.

Figure 11.9(b) shows a preamplifier with very high input impedance and low noise. The preamplifier uses a low noise JFET transistor (IF 9030) working in a common source circuit. In this case, 5.6 nV/Hz$^{1/2}$, 1.4 nV/Hz$^{1/2}$, 0.6 nV/Hz$^{1/2}$, and 0.5 nV/Hz$^{1/2}$ noise voltages were obtained for 0.1 Hz, 1 Hz, 10 Hz and 1 kHz, respectively [13].

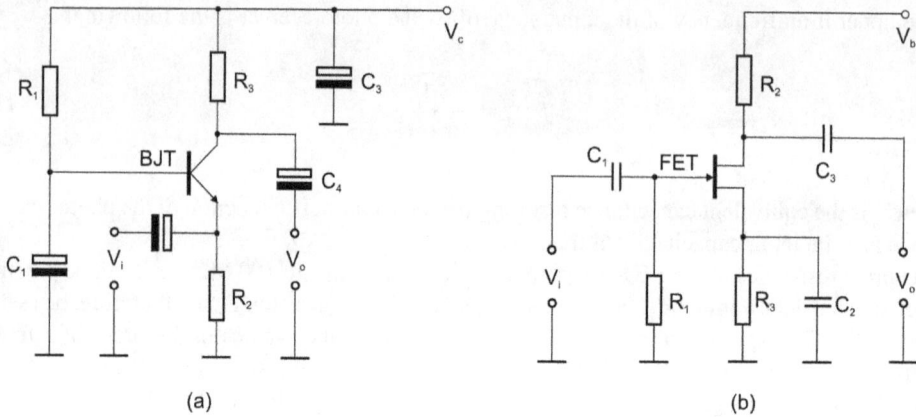

FIGURE 11.9 Voltage preamplifiers: (a) common base circuit, (b) common source circuit.

Equalisers are used in voltage amplifiers to shape frequency characteristics. When designing a pre-amplifier with a high input resistance, all possible noise sources are minimised. This is achieved by

- selection of a resistor biasing the detector due to the minimum level of thermal noise;
- selection of an input active element (due to low noise level, high-upper limit frequency, the highest possible current amplification factor and the lowest possible input capacity); and
- proper selection of the active element operating point.

The primary motivation to increase the preamplifier input impedance is to reduce thermal noise. However, high R_L resistances narrow the photoreceiver input stage bandwidth. It should be emphasised that a preamplifier with high input impedance provides a high load resistance for the detector and, therefore, does not provide a large dynamic range. When a highly sensitive, low dynamic range photoreceiver is needed, the use of a preamplifier with high input impedance is most appropriate.

It is not easy to build a low-noise preamplifier for low-resistance detectors. Note that the thermal noise of a 20 Ω resistance detector is 0.57 nV/Hz$^{1/2}$, so it is less than the voltage noise obtained for the best operating transistors or amplifiers.

The way out of this situation may be to build a preamplifier where input stage transistors (or operational amplifiers) will be connected in parallel [14]. In this case the RMS value of the preamplifier input noise voltage will be expressed by the equation

$$V_{ntotal} = V_n \left(n \right)^{-1/2},$$ (11.13)

where V_n is the RMS noise voltage of a single amplifier, and n is the number of elements used. The above assumption is correct when using transistors or operational amplifiers of the same type.

Figure 11.10 shows a diagram of a preamplifier in which eight-paralleled 2SK 3557–6 type transistors were used in the input stage. As a result of these transistors parallel connection, an input noise voltage of 0.6 nV/Hz$^{1/2}$ for $f = 100$ Hz was obtained [4]. It is equivalent to the RMS value of the resistor thermal noise voltage of about 20 Ω.

11.3 TRANSIMPEDANCE PREAMPLIFIERS

Voltage preamplifiers discussed in the previous section do not provide good linearity and dynamics of signal changes and a wide frequency band. There are known PD-PA circuits operating in the

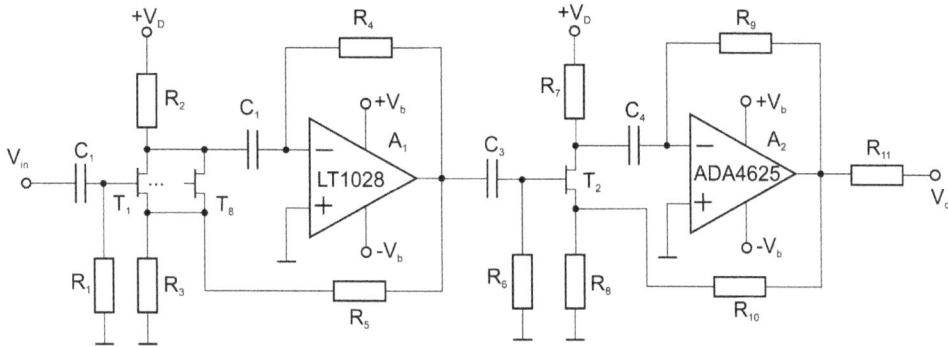

FIGURE 11.10 Diagram of a preamplifier for detectors with a very low resistance (after Reference 4).

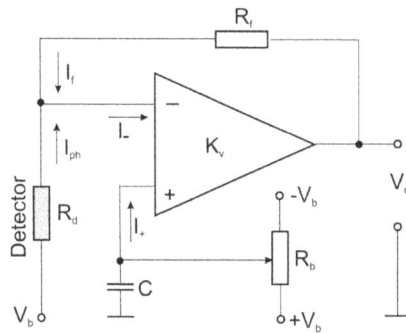

FIGURE 11.11 Schematic diagram of a transimpedance amplifier.

current-voltage converter that are free from disadvantages of previous circuits. The schematic diagram of the transimpedance preamplifier is shown in Figure 11.11. In this circuit, the detector resistance was denoted by R_d. It can be a photodiode, as well as a photoconductive detector. Depending on the type of detector and its specific applications, it can be biased from the source V_b or connected to the circuit ground.

The current produced by the detector flows through an R_f resistor placed in a feedback loop. When designing this type of circuit, one has to take under consideration a certain error caused by the input bias current of the amplifier, which is algebraically added to the input current.

The operational amplifier works in such a way, that the voltage difference between the reversing input and the non-reversing input equals zero. The potentiometer R_b is used to set the output voltage to zero in the absence of detector lighting. It can also be used to compensate for a fixed component at the circuit output caused by background radiation. If we assume that the voltage at the non-reversing input is equal to zero, then the voltage V_d is also equal to zero.

Usually, the input bias current is negligible, thus,

$$I_{ph} \approx -I_f. \tag{11.14}$$

Using Ohm's law we obtain

$$\frac{V_b - V_d}{R_d} = -\frac{V_o - V_d}{R_f}. \tag{11.15}$$

Therefore,

$$V_o = -\frac{R_f}{R_d}V_b = -I_{ph}R_f = -R_I\Phi_e R_f. \tag{11.16}$$

Eq. (11.16) is valid for low frequencies. The output voltage of the transimpedance preamplifier is directly proportional to the photocurrent and resistance in the feedback circuit. In order to obtain high output signal voltages, the feedback resistance can be increased up to hundreds of kilohms without the risk of non-linear processing. The transimpedance amplifier has a wide dynamic range regardless of the photoelectric current value. The photocurrent is proportional to the power Φ_e of the incident radiation, so the preamplifier output voltage will change linearly with the accuracy determined by the feedback loop. Thus, it is possible to process optical signals with powers varying in the range of many orders of magnitude linearly.

Optimal parameters of a photodetector cooperating with a transimpedance amplifier are very often limited by the amplifier parameters, such as input bias current, gain-bandwidth product, input noise voltage and input noise current. Bipolar amplifiers have typical bias currents of 3–100 nA. It is important for detection of a signal with the level of a single nW. This current must then be compensated. Alternative to the bipolar transistor are JFET transistors whose typical bias currents are of the order of a single pA (and even smaller ones, e.g., for LTC6268 ± 3 fA).

The bias currents of FET transistors increase by 2 to 5 times with an increase in temperature from 5°C to 10°C, while the bias currents of bipolar transistors decrease with increasing temperature [15]. Therefore, the use of bipolar transistors should be considered when operating at high temperatures. The upper cut-off frequency of the photodiode-preamplifier circuit is essentially determined by the time constant $R_f C_{eq}$ (where C_{eq} is the equivalent capacity of the photoreceiver input stage).

When forcing with a rectangular light pulse [Figure 11.12(a)] for large values of input capacitances, at a certain frequency, the phenomenon of boosting the photodetector-preamplifier circuit response may occur [Figure 11.12(b)]. The increase in the output voltage in this frequency range results in significant oscillations in response to the input light pulse.

The boost of the system frequency response is a function of the gain-bandwidth product and the ratio of the feedback capacitance C_f to the input capacitance (mainly junction capacitance C_j). The boost size can be reduced by increasing the feedback capacity. The same effect can be obtained by reducing C_j by using the reverse bias. The gain boost reduction can also be obtained by widening the preamplifier bandwidth.

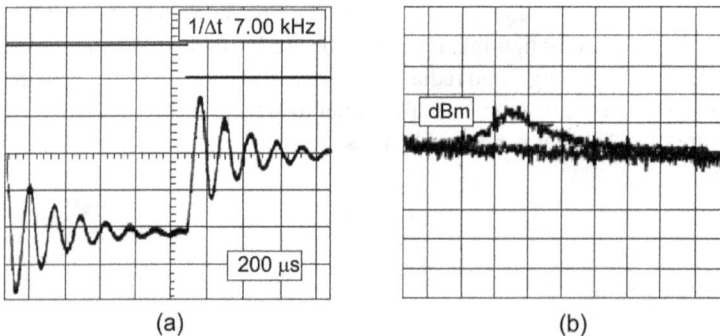

(a)   (b)

FIGURE 11.12 Forcing the photodiode-preamplifier circuit with a rectangular light pulse (a) and its response (b).

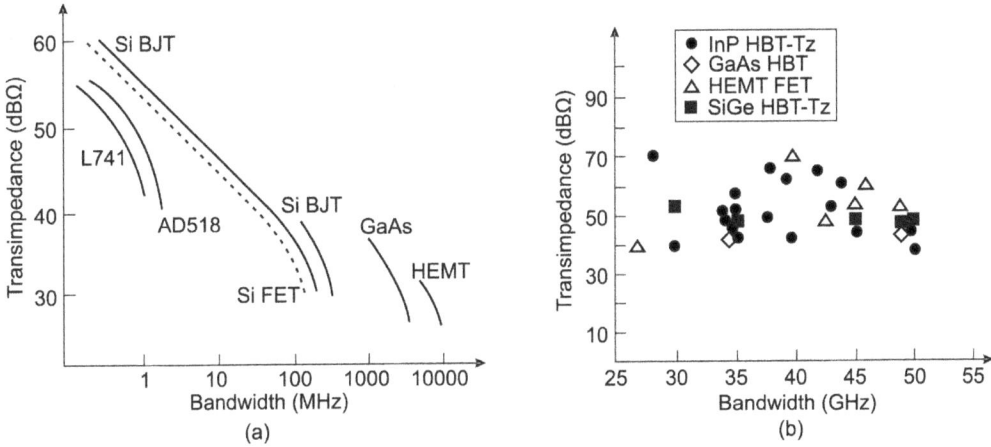

FIGURE 11.13 Relation between: (a) the bandwidth of transimpedance preamplifiers and (b) the transimpedance for transistors and integrated circuits made in various technologies (after Reference 17).

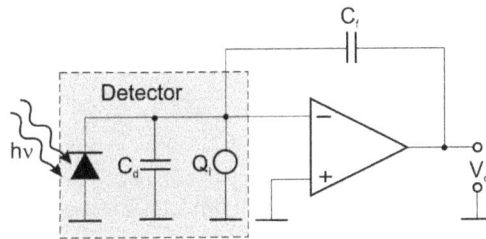

FIGURE 11.14 Diagram of a charge preamplifier.

Figure 11.13 shows the frequency response for transimpedance preamplifiers which use transistors and operational amplifiers made in various technologies. Up to 300 MHz, BJT, and FET transistors, as well as integrated circuits with BJT and FET transistors made of silicon are used in the input stage. Slightly wider bandwidths are obtained for integrated circuits in which bipolar transistors are used [Figure 11.13(a) [16]]. In the frequency range above 1 GHz, active elements made of InP, GaAs, SiGe and HEMT transistors are used [Figure 11.13(b)].

11.4 CHARGE PREAMPLIFIERS

A charge preamplifier, also known as a charge-sensitive preamplifier (CSP), belongs to the category of integrating amplifiers. This preamplifier should have high input resistance, high gain and low self-noise. A simplified diagram of the charge preamplifier is shown in Figure 11.14.

The charge amplifier basic parameter is a conversion factor (charge gain) which is expressed as the ratio of the maximum value of the voltage V_{omax} at the output of this circuit to the charge excitation Q_i:

$$k_q = \frac{V_{omax}}{Q_i}. \tag{11.17}$$

The voltage value at the output of the CSP system depends on the value of the capacitance C_f and the integration time, but does not depend on the capacitance of the detector C_d:

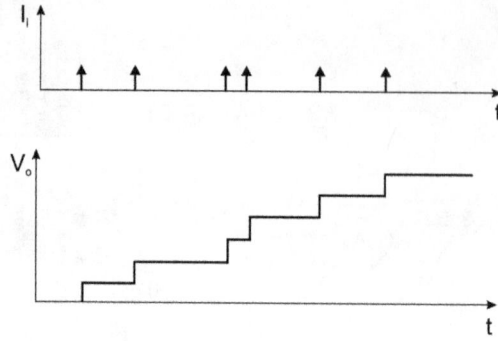

FIGURE 11.15   Illustration of the input signal and the waveform of the output voltage of a charge preamplifier.

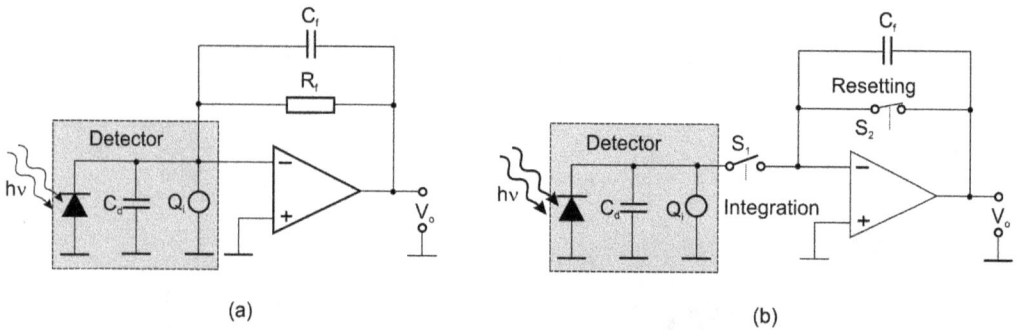

FIGURE 11.16   Schematic diagram of the CSP circuit: (a) with a resistor in the feedback loop, (b) with a "key" in the feedback loop.

$$V_o = -\frac{Q_i}{C_f} = -\frac{1}{C_f}\int_0^t I_{ph}\,dt, \qquad (11.18)$$

where $1/C_f$ is the charge preamplifier sensitivity and t is the integration time. A preamplifier with this structure has become known as a preamplifier with a non-resistive feedback loop.

A detector produces a stochastic sequence of current pulses, the amplitude of which depends on the intensity of the measured radiation. After some time, however, the preamplifier may reach a saturated state (Figure 11.15), similar to a pulse sequence detection. In this situation, the capacitor C_f should be discharged by means of additional circuits. This disadvantage is devoid of the systems shown in Figure 11.16.

The resistor R_f ensures a dynamic discharge of the capacitor C_f. Its value should be as high as possible and the time constant $R_f C_f$ should be greater than the measured pulse duration. It determines the lower limit frequency of the analysed preamplifier [18]:

$$f_{-3dB} = \frac{1}{2\pi R_f C_f} = \frac{1}{2\pi\tau}. \qquad (11.19)$$

Ideally, the voltage rise time at the integrator output should be equal to the charge accumulation time in the detector capacity. In the case of the circuit shown in Figure 11.16(b), discharge of the capacitor C_f takes place using the switch S_2 at the end of the signal measurement period. Thus, the system is ready for the next measurement.

More information about this type of circuit will be provided during the analysis of signal-reading circuits for CMOS arrays. Operational amplifiers used in CSP systems should have a very low input noise current and very low input bias currents. Otherwise, there is a load on the signal source and a voltage drop at the preamplifier output. Careful selection of passive elements, as well as type and design of the PCB also plays an important role, that is, the choice of material for the PCB, the number of layers of the PCB or the way the tracks are arranged.

11.5   FIRST STAGES OF PHOTORECEIVERS

There are two general types of detectors: thermal and photon. These photodetectors are used with many types of preamplifiers. The choice of a circuit's configuration for the preamplifier is largely dependent upon the system application. The concept of the photoreceiver input stage is understood as a system consisting of a detector, detector bias system and a low-noise preamplifier. In this chapter we will discuss preamplifiers designed for various detectors, both thermal and photon.

11.5.1   PHOTORECEIVERS WITH PHOTON DETECTORS

Both voltage and transimpedance preamplifiers can be used to amplify signals received from photo-conductive detectors. Figure 11.17 shows a simplified scheme of the input stage of a photoreceiver with a voltage preamplifier. In this circuit, the detector is connected to the load resistance R_L and biased from a low-noise voltage source. This detector forms a voltage divider with a load resistance and can be connected interchangeably.

The photoconductive detector resistance decreases with the increasing irradiance E_e and is as follows:

$$R_d = R_{dark} - kE_e, \tag{11.20}$$

where R_{dark} is the dark resistance of the detector, k is the constant depending on the detector area and sensitivity.

The value of the current flowing in a voltage divider is given by the equation

$$I = \frac{V_b}{R_{dark} + R_L}, \tag{11.21}$$

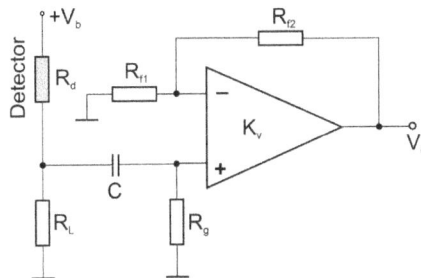

FIGURE 11.17   Simplified schematic diagram of the photoreceiver input stage with a voltage preamplifier.

hence, the voltage variation on the load resistance relative to the variation in the photodetector resistance is as follows:

$$dV_{R_L} = \frac{R_L}{\left(R_{dark} + R_L\right)^2} V_b dR_{dark}.$$ (11.22)

If the condition is met,

$$R_L \ll R_g \gg \left(2\pi fC\right)^{-1},$$ (11.23)

this preamplifier gain is frequency independent, and the output voltage is given by the equation

$$V_o = \left[\frac{R_L}{\left(R_{dark} + R_L\right)^2}\right]\left[\frac{R_{f1} + R_{f2}}{R_{f1}}\right]V_b kE_e.$$ (11.24)

It is directly proportional to the detector irradiation intensity.

Eq. (11.24) shows that the photovoltage increases linearly with an increase in the voltage biasing the photoconductor. However, too high of a voltage (detector bias current) may cause the detector temperature to rise (due to Joule heat). The increase in the detector temperature may, therefore, cause both unstable operation and deterioration of parameters. Figure 11.18 shows a signal–noise relationship and an detectivity of the detector bias voltage.

As the bias voltage increases, both the signal and the noise increase. Exceeding the photoresistor specified bias voltage causes a stronger increase in noise than in signal. For a given type of detector there is, therefore, a well-defined value of the bias voltage at which the signal-to-noise ratio reaches its maximum value. The load resistance determines many parameters of the photoreceiver input stage. The optimal value selection for this resistance, therefore, depends

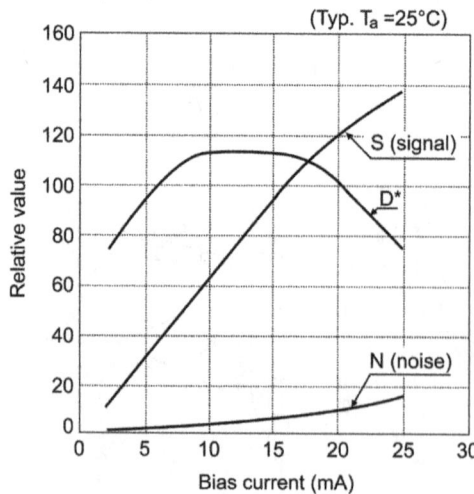

FIGURE 11.18 Dependence of the signal, noise, and detectivity on the bias voltage of the InSb photoconductor (after Reference 19).

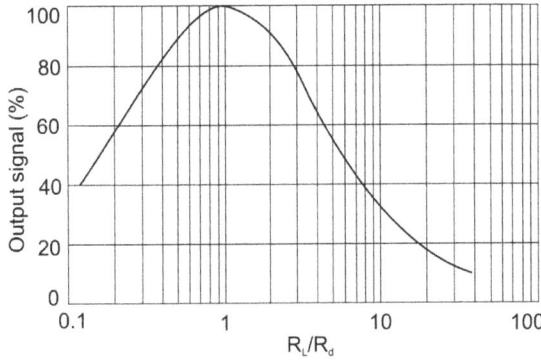

FIGURE 11.19 Dependence of the output signal on the ratio of the load resistance to the PbS detector resistance.

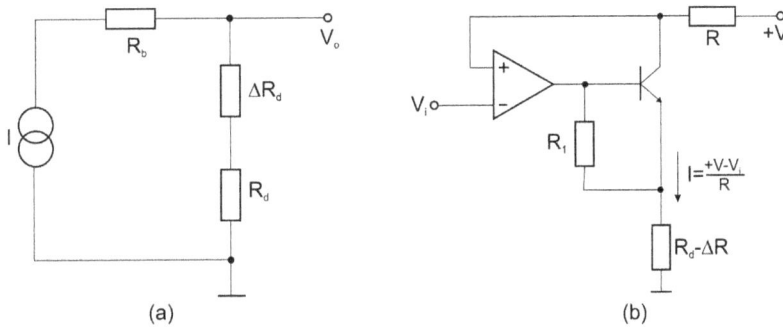

FIGURE 11.20 Photoconductive detector biasing system: (a) from a current source, (b) from a precise current source.

on the specific application. The photoresistor load resistance value together with the shunt capacitance determines the upper limit frequency of the photoreceiver input stage. A high cut-off frequency can be achieved with a low load resistance. However, a low value for this resistance is a source of high thermal noise. This noise value can significantly exceed the detector noise. This will significantly reduce the detectivity value. Thus, in order to obtain low thermal noise, a high load resistance must be used.

Figure 11.19 shows the output signal dependence on the ratio of the load resistance to the photodetector dark resistance. The maximum value of the output signal can be obtained if the load resistance is equal to the detector resistance R_d.

The photoconductive detector can also be biased from a precise current source (Figure 11.20). The current supply to the detector can be very precisely stabilised by means of an operational amplifier operating in a current source configuration. In a system with a current source, the output voltage is equal to

$$V_o = I\left(R_d - \Delta R_d\right). \tag{11.25}$$

Transimpedance amplifiers are also used to amplify signals received from photoconductive detectors. A simplified schematic diagram of the photoreceiver input stage with the transimpedance preamplifier is shown in Figure 11.21. In this case, the detector is galvanically connected to the

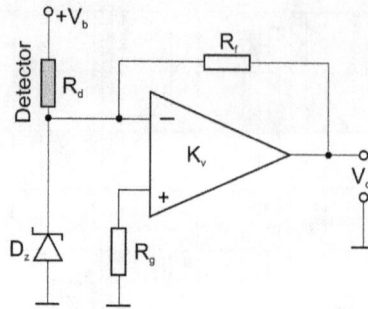

FIGURE 11.21 Simplified schematic diagram of a transimpedance preamplifier for photoconductive detectors.

op amp inverting input. The detector is powered by a DC voltage source. If voltage is applied to the photoconductive detector, the dark current flows even in the absence of lighting. Value of this current strongly depends on a detector temperature. The increase in the detector temperature causes a generation of additional carriers in a semiconductor conduction band. Therefore, the detector temperature should be controlled. It is especially important for detectors made of semiconductors with a narrow bandgap [20]. The Zener diode D_z is used to protect the operational amplifier input against overvoltage. In order to limit a differential input offset voltage of the operational amplifier, a non-inverting input was connected via the resistor R_g to the circuit ground.

Assuming that the voltage at the amplifier inverting input equals zero, the current flowing through the detector is given by the equation

$$I_c = \frac{V_b}{R_d}.$$

(11.26)

This current also flows through the feedback resistor and creates a voltage at the preamplifier output:

$$V_o = \frac{R_f V_b}{R_d}.$$

(11.27)

The dark current flowing through the detector is given by the equation

$$I_{dark} = \frac{V_b}{R_{dark}}.$$

(11.28)

So, the total current is equal to

$$I_c = I_{ph} + I_{dark}.$$

(11.29)

If the dark current is subtracted from the total current, then we get a photocurrent. The radiation modulation is commonly used to separate the useful signal current from the total current that is received at the output of the preamplifier. It is provided by a chopper which is placed in a beam of radiation incident on the detector surface. In some applications, the radiation source may be internally modulated.

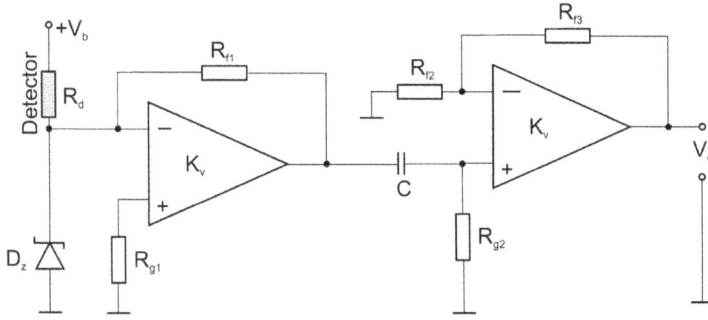

FIGURE 11.22 Two stage AC coupled transimpedance preamplifier for photoconductive detectors.

To isolate the AC component from the total current signal, AC coupling must be used. As the transimpedance preamplifier is galvanically connected to the signal detector, a coupling capacitor should be placed at its output. This type of solution makes it possible to remove a slow-changing component and a constant component from the background and dark current.

Figure 11.22 shows a two-stage preamplifier with a capacitive coupling. The first stage of the amplification path uses a transimpedance preamplifier and the second stage uses a non-inverting voltage amplifier.

The voltage signal received at the output of the first stage of the preamplifier is given by the equation

$$V_{o1} = -\left(\frac{R_{f_1}}{R_{dark}} V_b \right)\left(1 + \frac{kE_e}{R_{dark}} \right). \tag{11.30}$$

Transforming Eq. (11.30), we obtain

$$V_{o1} = -\left(\frac{R_{f1}}{R_{dark}} V_b + \frac{R_{f1}}{R_{dark}^2} kE_e V_b \right). \tag{11.31}$$

The first component represents the DC component, while the second component represents the AC component of the signal. This voltage value is directly proportional to the supply voltage and resistance in the feedback circuit and inversely proportional to the detector dark resistance.

If the condition is met,

$$R_{g2} \gg (2\pi f C)^{-1}, \tag{11.32}$$

then, the voltage at the output of the preamplifier is the following:

$$V_o = \frac{R_{f_1}}{R_{dark}^2} \frac{R_{f_2} + R_{f_3}}{R_{f_2}} kE_e V_b. \tag{11.33}$$

It is directly proportional to the intensity of irradiation.

The analysis of the above-mentioned circuits operation shows that the detector DC power supply and the photocurrent voltage reading are characterised by a high non-linearity of operation and an easy saturation of the detection circuit. Moreover, such a circuit is sensitive to temperature fluctuation, which causes changes in a photoconductive detector resistance. Much better is the detector constant voltage supply and the current reading by a transimpedance preamplifier. It maintains a constant voltage value on the detector and, thus, provides a constant photoelectric amplification, as well as a constant sensitivity over a wide range of lighting and operating temperature changes.

Detection circuits with high dynamics of input signal changes use Wheatstone bridge circuits (Figure 11.23). The Wheatstone bridge is a precise circuit used to measure small changes in resistance. It is characterised by a high output impedance and, therefore, it is necessary to use operational amplifiers in a configuration of an instrumentation amplifier (with identical, high impedances of both inputs) to amplify their output voltage.

The resistor R_b is used to ensure the optimum value of the detector bias current, the resistor R_{adjust} – to balance the bridge in the absence of detector lighting – and the resistor R_{lin} – to extend a linear range of the circuit operation. Teledyne company recommends this type of detection circuits for low-resistance HgCdTe photoresistors [21].

Let us now consider preamplifiers for photodiodes. Photodiode can operate in a photovoltaic [Figure 11.24(a)] or photoconductive mode (Figure 11.24(b)). In the first case, there is no voltage source supplying the photodiode, while in the second case, the photodiode is supplied from a DC voltage source and is loaded with the resistance R_L. Different preamplifiers are used depending on the mode of operation of a photodiode.

Figure 11.25 shows load lines for a photodiode operation in a photovoltaic and photoconductive mode. The photodiode operating point results from the intersection of the load line with the I-V characteristics. If the photodiode works in a photovoltaic circuit, the load line passes through the origin of the coordinate system and intersects the photodiode characteristics in the fourth quadrant of the coordinate system. When $R_L = \infty$, the load line coincides with the abscissa axis. It is possible

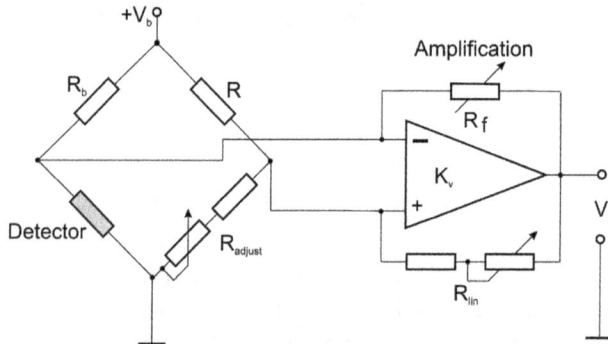

FIGURE 11.23 Preamplifier with a photoresistor located in a Wheatstone bridge.

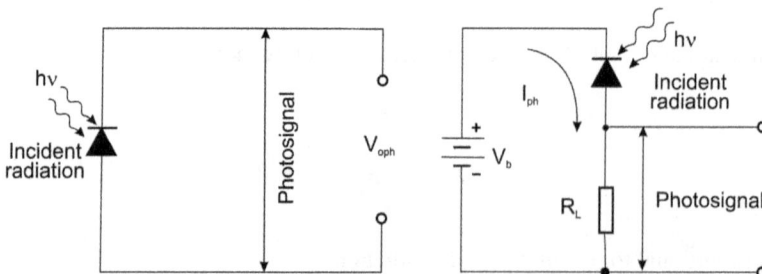

FIGURE 11.24 Photodiode circuit: (a) a photodiode is open, (b) a photodiode is reverse biased.

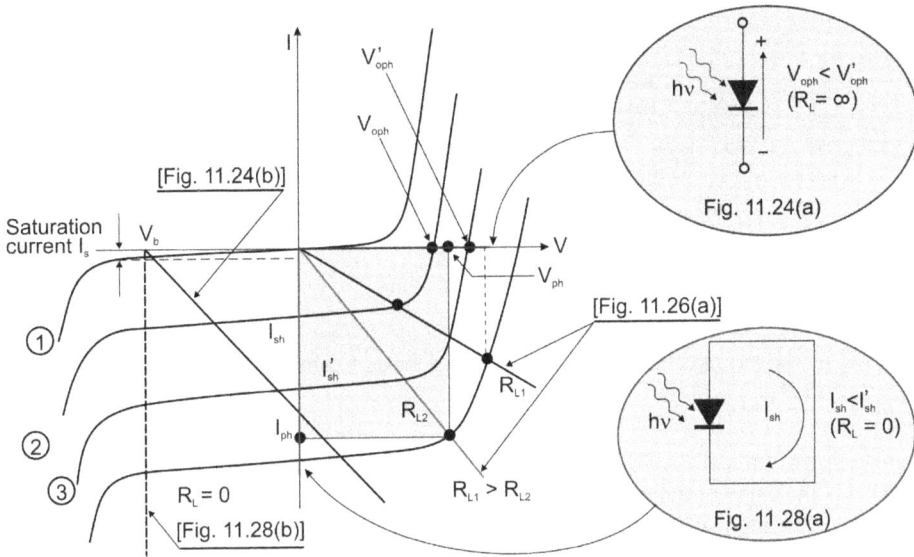

FIGURE 11.25 Current-voltage characteristics of photodiodes with load lines.

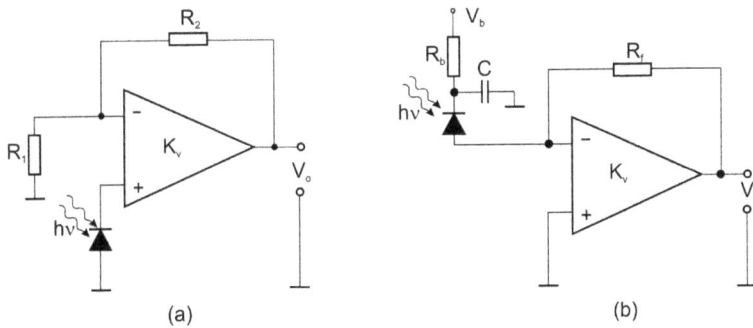

FIGURE 11.26 Schematic diagram of the preamplifier allowing the photodiode to work: (a) in the fourth quarter of the characteristics I-V, (b) in the third quarter of the characteristics I-V.

to read the voltage V_{oph}. The voltage at which the I-V characteristic crosses the abscissa is called the open-circuit voltage V_{oph}. It changes logarithmically with a change of the incident radiation power. For lower load-resistance values, the photodiode working point is determined by the voltage V_{ph} and the photocurrent I_{ph}. In this case, it is possible to measure both the voltage V_{ph} and the current I_{ph}. The value of the resistance R_L, for which the product $V_{ph}I_{ph}$ takes the maximum value, should be treated as the optimal resistance R_{Lopt}.

Figure 11.26(a) shows a simplified preamplifier schematic diagram that allows the photodiode to work in the fourth quarter of the I-V characteristics. If the input impedance of the operational amplifier is greater than the shunt resistance of the photodiode, the operating condition in the so-called "open circuit" will be met. The voltage at the preamplifier output is determined by the equation

$$V_o = \frac{R_1 + R_2}{R_1} \frac{kT}{q} ln\left[\frac{I_{ph} + I_s}{I_s}\right], \tag{11.34}$$

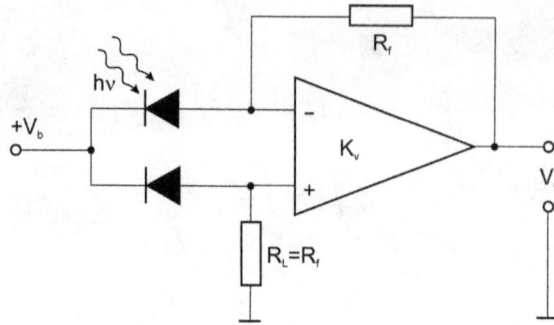

FIGURE 11.27 The way of compensation of the photodiode dark current.

and changes logarithmically as a function of the incident radiation intensity. The disadvantage of this solution is the exponential dependence of the saturation current I_s on the detector temperature. Therefore, in many applications the detector temperature must be precisely stabilised. The photovoltaic range of work is mainly used in solar cells.

When the photodiode operates in a photoconductive mode [Figure 11.26(b)], the load line is determined by the photodiode bias voltage V_b and the current value $I = V_b/R_L$. The load line slope depends on the load resistance value. If the photodiode is reverse biased with the voltage V_b, then, even in the absence of illumination some dark current flows – I_{dark}, which is the shot noise source. Increase in illuminance causes an increase in the I_{ph} current. For high load resistance values, a non-linear dependence of the photocurrent on the incident radiation power is obtained. In this case, the total current is equal to the sum of the short circuit current and the dark current:

$$I_c = R_I A E_e + I_{dark}. \tag{11.35}$$

The voltage at the preamplifier output is directly proportional to the detector current and is the following:

$$V_o = R_I A E_e R_f + I_{dark} R_f. \tag{11.36}$$

If the V_b voltage biasing the photodiode equals zero, the second component in this expression can be omitted.

Dark current compensation can also be achieved by using an additional photodiode with identical parameters that should be connected to the second input of the operating amplifier (Figure 11.27) [22].

If the photodiode works with zero load resistance [Figure 11.28(a)] and no supply voltage (it corresponds to the load line coinciding with the ordinate axis), then, the output current is directly proportional to the irradiance. This current is called the photodiode short-circuit current and is described by the equation

$$I_{sh} = R_I A E_e. \tag{11.37}$$

A load resistance close to zero is provided by the transimpedance preamplifier. The short-circuit current is characterised by a very good linearity in relation to changes in the irradiance. Linearity is determined by the type of photodiode and the type of circuit in which it operates. It is possible

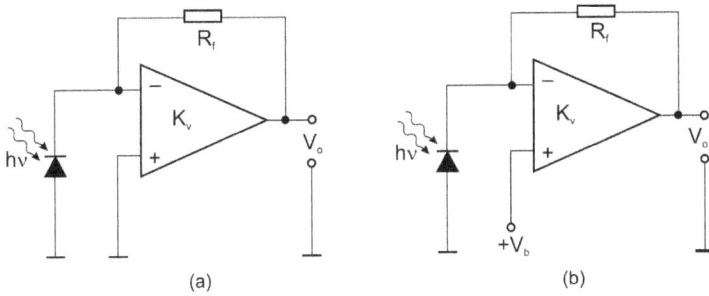

FIGURE 11.28 Photodiode operation with a *I-V* converter: (a) without biasing, (b) with reverse biasing.

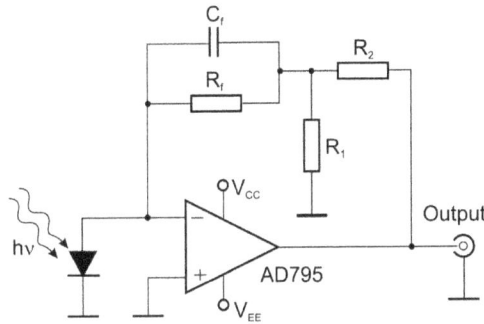

FIGURE 11.29 Photodiode preamp employing a T network for added gain.

to obtain a satisfactory linearity in terms of changes in the incident radiation power from a few pW to mW.

Linearity is limited from the bottom by the *NEP* value and from the top by the load resistance and supply voltage. The circuit shown in Figure 11.28(b) has the advantages of that shown in Figure 11.28(a), and, at the same time, ensures a constant value of the photodiode bias voltage. For an ideal amplifier, the voltage drop across the photodiode is equal to the bias voltage V_b. The use of reverse bias reduces the photodiode junction capacitance, and, thus, increases the upper frequency of the photoreceiver input stage. Another advantage of this circuit is a slight increase in the input signal dynamic range. In order to obtain a high gain of the *I-V* converter, it is necessary to use the high value resistor R_f. It should be taken into account that the existing parasitic capacities increase the time constant and reduce the bandwidth. This disadvantage is absent in a T-bridge feedback network preamplifier in a feedback loop (Figure 11.29). In this circuit, by using not very large resistor values, it is possible to obtain high gain values and improve its stability [23].

Now let us look at the preamplifiers used for photomultiplier tubes (PMTs). During measurements with photomultiplier tubes, it is often the case that the output signals are too small in amplitude to be correctly recorded with an oscilloscope. The most natural action in this case is to increase the photomultiplier gain by increasing the voltage at its divider supplying individual electrodes (Figure 6.7). However, this method of obtaining a higher amplitude signal that can be correctly recorded with an oscilloscope is only effective for recordings below the cut-off gain. When this is exceeded, the photomultiplier can be easily removed from the linear operation mode and switched to the digital mode of operation PMT. Moreover, as the PMT supply voltage increases, the number of dark counts increase, and the signal-to-noise ratio deteriorates. Therefore, the most effective way to increase the amplitude of output signals from such an instrument is to use a low-noise broadband preamplifier.

The current value obtained from the PMT anode for a single electron emitted from the photocathode is

$$I(t) = \frac{-qG}{\tau} \exp\left(\frac{-t}{\tau}\right),$$

(11.38)

where G is the photomultiplier gain, q is the electron charge and τ is the decay time constant.

Current signal conversion into voltage can be obtained by applying the load resistance at the photomultiplier output (Figure 11.30). Figure 11.30(a) shows a circuit with a DC connection between PMT and a voltage preamplifier, while the circuit shown in Figure 11.30(b) uses an AC coupling. The voltage value obtained on R_L is equal to the product of the photocurrent obtained from the anode I_{pha} and the load resistance R_L (Figure 11.31).

For higher values of load resistance, higher voltage amplitude is obtained, however, the time of signal decay increases, and undesirable effects appear (voltage reduction between the last dynode and anode and deterioration of PMT linearity [24]). Therefore, in most cases, the resistor R_L should be used so that the voltage drop does not exceed 1V [25].

The value of the resistor R_L together with the equivalent capacitance C_{eq} resulting from the parallel connection of the output capacitance PMT, the stray capacitance and the input capacitance of the preamplifier determine the high-range cut-off frequency f_c of this circuit:

$$f_c = \frac{1}{2C_{eq}R_L}.$$

(11.39)

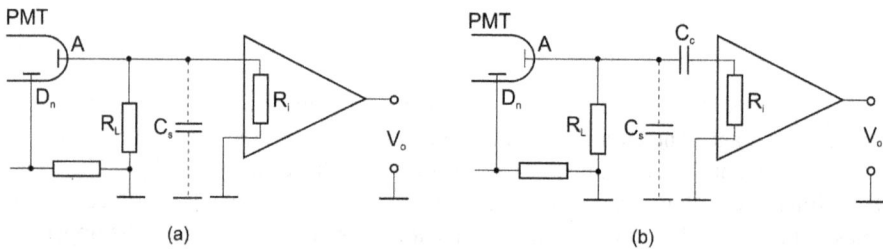

(a)   (b)

FIGURE 11.30 Preamplifier internal input resistance: (a) DC connection of PMT with the preamplifier, (b) AC connection of PMT with the preamplifier; where A – anode, D_n – last dynode (after Reference 24).

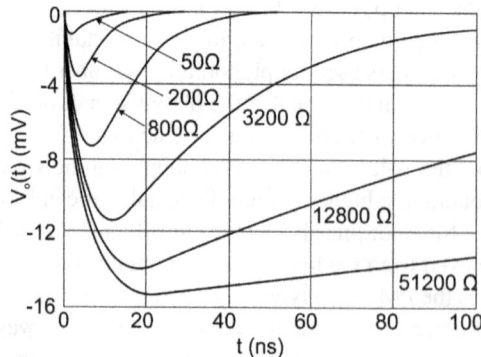

FIGURE 11.31 The shape of a signal obtained on the PMT load resistance (after Reference 25).

The above expression is valid if the load resistance R_L is much less than the input resistance of the preamplifier. If this condition is not met, then the value of the effective load resistance results from the parallel connection of the resistance R_L and the input resistance R_i of the preamplifier.

The following conclusions can be drawn from the above analyses:

- to detect optical signals of a short duration and a high repetition frequency, use a low-value load resistance (e.g., 50 Ω) and try to minimise the stray capacity,
- to obtain a linear relationship between the voltage on the R_L resistance and the power of incident radiation, the value of this resistance must be selected so that the voltage drop caused by the photocurrent maximum value does not exceed a few per cent (e.g., 1 V) of the voltage between the last dynode and anode;
- to obtain a greater responsivity of the detection circuit, the resistor R_L of a higher value should be used. However, it should not exceed the value of the preamplifier input resistance.

The photomultiplier tube can be treated as a current source with high resistance, therefore the use of a voltage preamplifier will not provide a sufficiently wide bandwidth and a desired gain. A better solution is to use a transimpedance preamplifier, a stray capacitance preamplifier, or a charge preamplifier. The choice of a specific type of preamplifier depends on intensity, duration and frequency of the received pulses of optical radiation.

A simplified diagram of the transimpedance preamplifier to the photomultiplier is shown in Figure 11.32.

Advantages of using a transimpedance amplifier are discussed in section 11.4. In order to minimise the influence of external interference, a photomultiplier with a power supply system should be placed in a common shielded housing. In addition, the following points should be noted: connection between the PMT and the preamplifier should not be made using trace on the printed circuit board, but a low-noise coaxial cable terminated with a teflon plug; low-noise FET transistors should be used in the input stage of the preamplifier; a low-noise metal resistor with a minimum temperature coefficient of resistance should be used in the feedback loop; PCB board should be made on a glass-epoxy laminate.

The most effective preamplifier for these detectors is the parasitic-capacitance preamplifier shown in Figure 11.33 [2]. It has high input impedance (above 1 MΩ). The parasitic capacitance is presented by the detector and preamplifier input (typically 10–50 pF).

The resulting signal is a voltage pulse having amplitude proportional to the total charge in detector pulse. This type of preamplifiers is sensitive to small changes in the parasitic capacitance. The rise time is equal to the duration of the detector current pulse. A resistor connected in parallel with the input capacitance causes an exponential decay of the pulse. A preamplifier follower is included as a buffer to drive the low impedance of a coaxial cable at the output. These preamplifiers are highly recommended for photomultiplier tubes, microchannel plates (MPTs), and scintillation detectors.

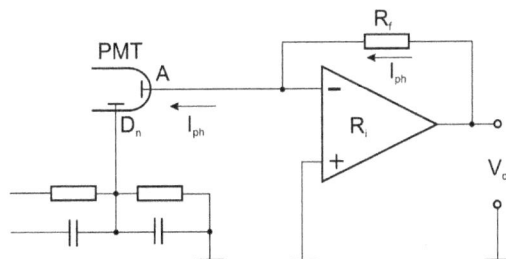

FIGURE 11.32 Current-to-voltage conversion circuit using operational amplifier (after Reference 24).

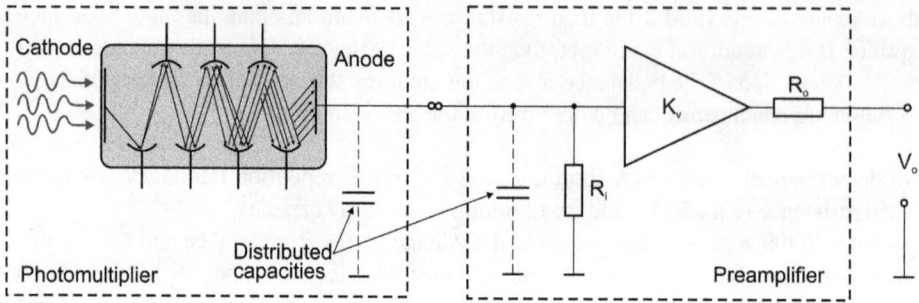

FIGURE 11.33 A simplified diagram of the parasitic-capacitance preamplifier (after Reference 2).

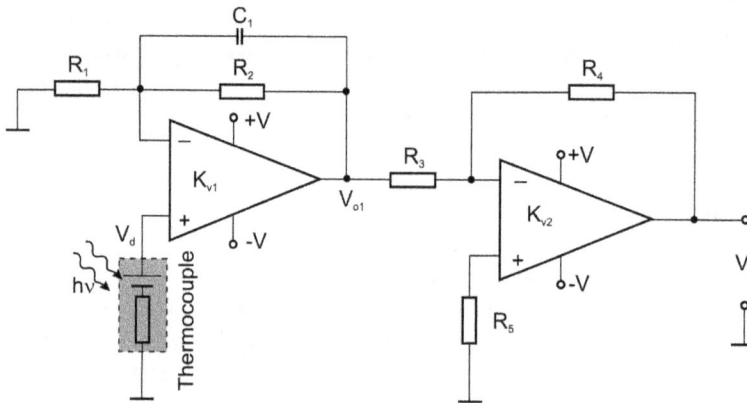

FIGURE 11.34 Simplified schematic diagram of a voltage DC coupled preamplifier for thermopile detectors.

For most of the energy spectroscopy application, charge-sensitive preamplifiers are preferred. These are discussed in Section 11.4.

11.5.2 PHOTORECEIVERS WITH THERMAL DETECTORS

This subsection discusses preamplifiers for thermocouples, bolometers and pyroelectric detectors.

Low-noise preamplifiers are used to amplify the signal from thermopiles and are optimised for a noise voltage. Examples of circuit solutions are shown in Figures 11.34 and 11.35. The output signal from the first stage of the preamplifiers is determined by the equation

$$V_{o1} = \left[\frac{R_1 + R_2}{R_1} \right] R_v A \Phi_e, \tag{11.39}$$

where R_v is the voltage responsivity of the thermopile.

The voltage signal at the second stage output equals

$$V_o = \left[\frac{R_1 + R_2}{R_1} \right] \frac{R_4}{R_3} R_v A \Phi_e. \tag{11.40}$$

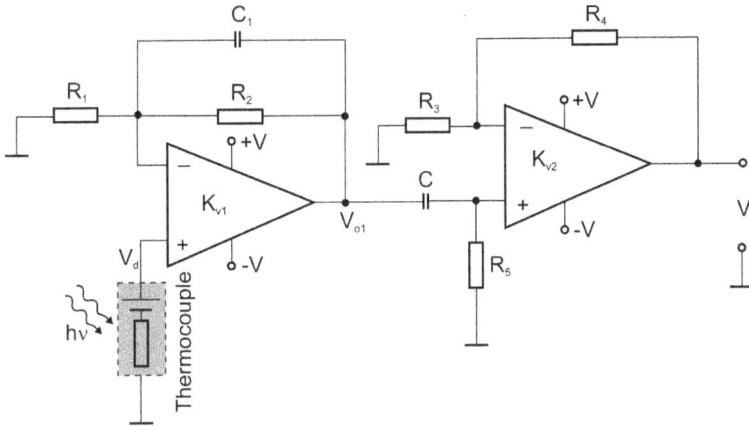

FIGURE 11.35   Capacitive coupled two stage preamplifier designed to amplify the signal from a thermopile.

The output signal voltage RMS value is directly proportional to the voltage responsivity of thermopile, photosensitive surface, and irradiance.

The cut-off frequency for this circuit depends on the value of the components in the C_1R_2 feedback loop:

$$f_{gr} = \frac{1}{2\pi C_1 R_2}. \tag{11.40}$$

Figure 11.35 shows a simplified schematic diagram of the AC coupled preamplifier. For this solution, the output voltage for low frequencies is given by the following equation:

$$V_o = \left[\frac{R_1 + R_2}{R_1}\right]\left[\frac{R_3 + R_4}{R_3}\right] R_v A E_e. \tag{11.41}$$

Radiation reaching the photoreceiver with the AC circuit should be modulated with a frequency of a single Hz.

Figure 11.36 shows a diagram of a preamplifier circuit designed to amplify the signal from a thermopile proposed by Dexter company [26]. The input stage uses a differential pair of low-noise bipolar transistors MAT-01 type. These transistors have a very low noise voltage and are, therefore, suitable for use with thermopiles.

Thermopiles are often used to measure temperature of a source-emitting infrared radiation. The voltage signal received from a thermopile depends not only on the source temperature but also on the ambient temperature. These phenomena must also be taken into account when designing an input stage of a photoreceiver in which this type of detector is used.

Additional electronic circuits should remove the output signal, which depends on the ambient temperature and provides a signal proportional to the source temperature [27]. The above disadvantage is devoid of the signal processing system, the diagram of which is shown in Figure 11.37. This circuit uses a thermistor to measure the ambient temperature. A thermopile voltage signal is fed to a non-inverting input of the op-amp, while voltage from the voltage divider $(R_{th} - R_d)$ is fed to the inverting input of this amplifier. As a result, the voltage signal from the ambient temperature is compensated [28].

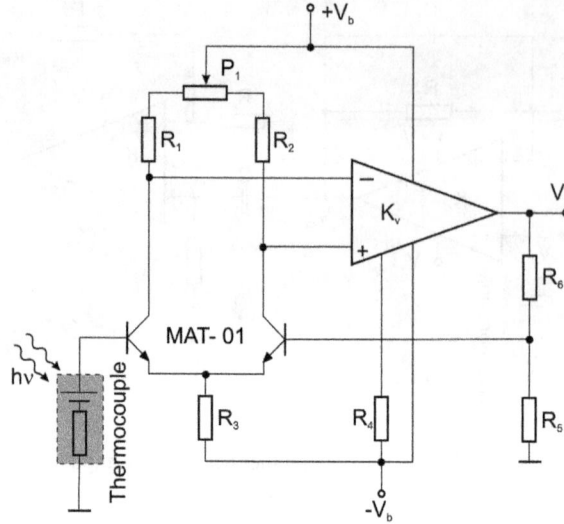

FIGURE 11.36   Diagram of a thermopile preamplifier.

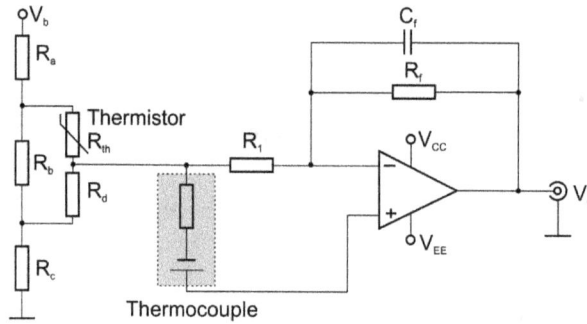

FIGURE 11.37   Schematic diagram of a thermopile preamplifier with the ambient temperature signal compensation.

In order to ensure greater accuracy in measuring the temperature of the infrared source under test, microprocessor-based systems shall be used.

Bolometers occupy a very important place among thermal detectors. As mentioned in Section 4.3.3, infrared light radiated from an object is absorbed by the bolometer absorber layer, causing the bolometer resistance to decrease. The incident light level can be read out as a voltage signal by low noise preamplifier. Currently, microbolometer arrays and CMOS readout integrated circuit are mainly used.

Figure 11.38 shows a typical preamplifier from one pixel of microbolometer arrays. This circuit has a reference resistance that is equivalent to the bolometer resistance, and both are connected in series. Changes in current equivalent to changes in the bolometer resistance are converted to voltage signals by a charge preamplifier [28].

The last group of circuits discussed here are preamplifiers for pyroelectric detectors. The electric charge formation on the pyroelectric detector electrodes as a result of the incident radiation can be recorded by a voltage or a current amplifier. Due to the fact that the electric charge generated in the pyroelectric detector is neutralised over time, the measurement of incident radiation is only possible using a modulated beam. The modulation frequency can range from 0.01 Hz to 1000 Hz.

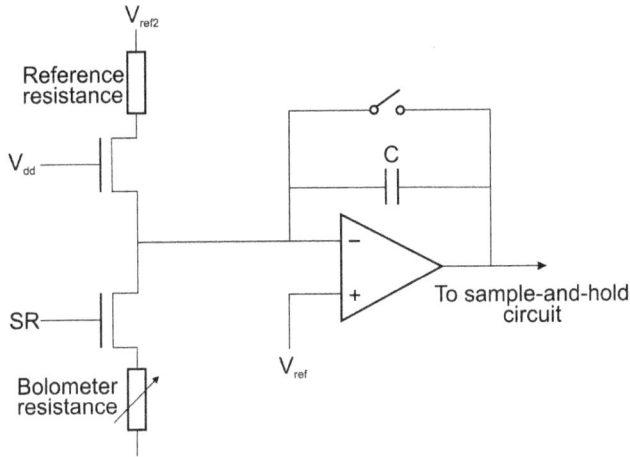

FIGURE 11.38   Diagram of a bolometer preamplifier – one pixel.

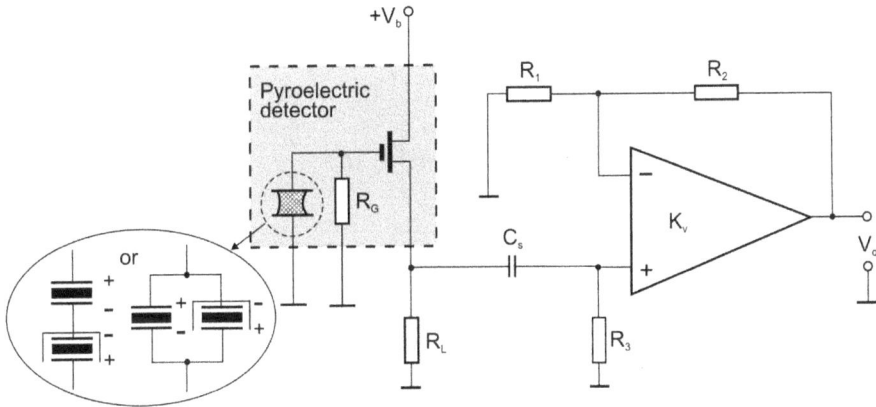

FIGURE 11.39   Diagram of a preamplifier with a pyroelectric detector, which is integrated with the FET transistor and the gate resistor R_G.

Very often this type of detector is mounted together with a transistor in standard TO 5 and TO 39 transistor housings. Inside the housing a resistor biasing the transistor gate is also mounted. The value of this resistor, depending on the application, can range from 50 to 10^{12} Ω. Most often, a FET or MOSFET transistor mounted near the detector is used for signal amplification. Usually, their input resistance is much higher than the detector parallel resistance. Accidental resistance and the capacity of the replacement scheme determine the detector electrical time constant, which defines the upper-limit frequency of the photodetector preamplifier system. This frequency is called the cut-off frequency.

The amplifier with the FET transistor can operate in a source follower or a current converter in which feedback is used instead of the gate biasing resistor. This achieves a system bandwidth widening without compromising the detector detectivity.

A diagram of electrical connections of the pyroelectric detector operating as a voltage source is shown in Figure 11.39. In this type of operation, the pyroelectric detector is connected to a signal preamplifier with high input impedance. Voltage generated on the detector electrodes is applied to the source follower gate. Increase in voltage at the gate of this transistor causes the flow of a drain-source current, and, at the same time, the increase in voltage on the resistance R_L. Voltage changes on the R_L resistor, caused by changes in the incident radiation power, are transmitted by the coupling capacitor to the voltage amplifier input. The pyroelectric detector is placed in a common housing with a FET transistor and R_G resistor. The resistor R_L is outside the housing.

If the condition is met,

$$R_L \ll R_3 \gg \left[2\pi f C_S \right]^{-1},$$ (11.42)

then, the voltage at the output of the preamplifier is the following:

$$V_o = \left[\frac{R_1 + R_2}{R_1} \right] R_v A E_e.$$ (11.43)

If the pyroelectric detector is not integrated with the source follower, then a voltage preamplifier with high input impedance should be used (Figure 11.40). In order to obtain high sensitivity, the preamplifier input resistance should be greater than the detector parallel resistance.

Voltage at the output of the first stage of the preamplifier V_{o1} is determined by the equation

$$V_{o1} = \left[\frac{R_1 + R_2}{R_1} \right] R_v A E_e.$$ (11.44)

It may fluctuate with changes in the ambient temperature. This problem can be solved by keeping the detector at a constant temperature (which is not always possible), connecting a compensating element to an active element and using alternating current feedback to the second amplification stage. If

$$R_5 \gg \left[2\pi f C_1 \right]^{-1},$$ (11.45)

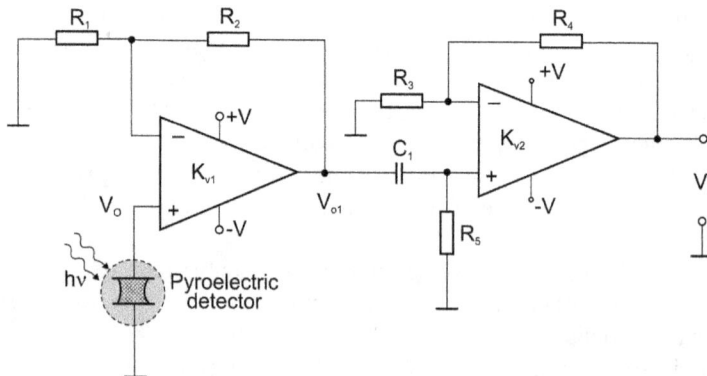

FIGURE 11.40   Preamplifier with a pyroelectric detector scheme.

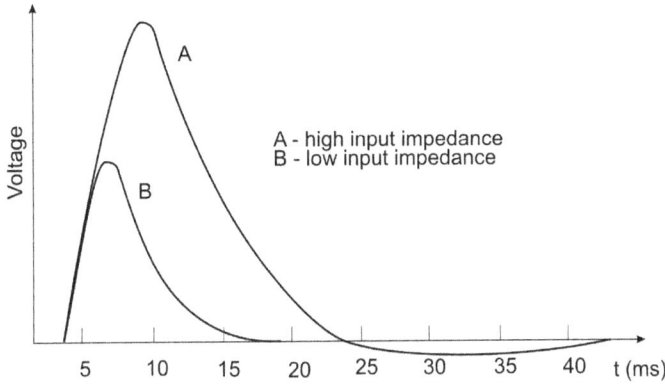

FIGURE 11.41 Voltage changes at the preamplifier output for two input impedance values.

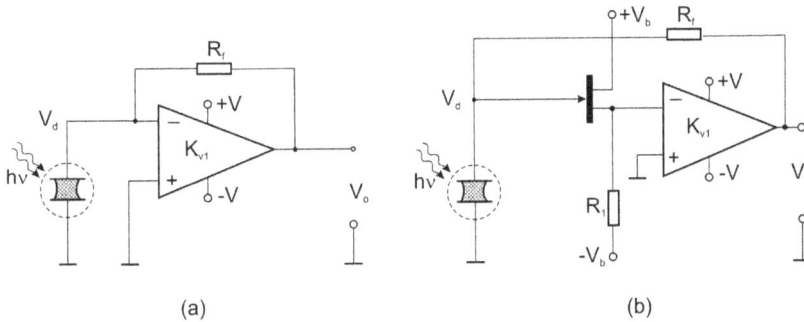

FIGURE 11.42 Diagrams of the pyroelectric detectors operating as a current source.

where f is the modulation frequency, then

$$V_o = \left[\frac{R_1 + R_2}{R_1} \right]\left[\frac{R_3 + R_4}{R_3} \right] R_v AE_e. \qquad (11.46)$$

In practical measuring systems, there is a need to switch the input resistance. Lowering the input resistance is used when a signal with a higher repetition frequency needs to be measured (Figure 11.41, wave B). In this case, the response time is shortened and, therefore, pulses appearing in succession do not overlap. However, using a lower input resistance will reduce the photoreceiver input stage sensitivity. Such circuits reduce the electrical time constant in proportion to the gain of the open-loop amplifier. Due to short response times and high permissible detector power densities, they have found application in high-power laser radiation detection systems.

The connection schemes of the pyroelectric detector operating as a current source are shown in Figure 11.42.

11.6 NOISE MODELS OF FIRST STAGES OF OPTICAL DETECTION SYSTEMS

Many factors determine the sensitivity of a photoreceiver. One of them is the ubiquitous noise. Signal amplification is always accompanied by at least the same noise amplification; moreover, each amplifier adds its own noise to the signal. Thus, increased amplification of a signal cannot be accompanied by improvement of its power-to-noise ratio. On the other hand, as this ratio worsens, the signal becomes increasingly difficult to distinguish. In this chapter is a noise analysis of photodetectors using so-called direct detection.

Creation of a photoreceiver input stage noise model usually begins with considering the equivalent electrical circuit of a given signal source, detector power supply circuit and preamplifier. Such an equivalent circuit for alternating current should consider all impedances of the circuit and the signal source. Each resistance and current source should be assigned a corresponding noise generator in the form of equivalent sources. Resistances introduce a thermal and excess noise. Current sources are characterised by shot noise, $1/f$ type noise, and other excess type noise. The purpose of studying the equivalent noise scheme is to calculate the equivalent input noise. It is advantageous to consider the photodetector-preamplifier circuit as a whole. During the analysis, it is necessary to consider the detector-preamplifier coupling circuits and the preamplifier itself. Finding the noise equivalent diagram of the coupling circuit usually does not present any major difficulties, and as for the amplifier, we have the input noise voltage V_n and the noise current I_n. Taking into account the noise of the detector, the coupling circuit, and the preamplifier, it will be possible to determine the total equivalent input noise of the photoreceiver.

Determination of the equivalent noise at the photoreceiver input takes place in three stages:

- determination of the total noise at the output;
- calculation of the total power amplification; and
- determination of the equivalent input noise as a quotient of output noise and power amplification.

This chapter is devoted to the noise models of photoreceivers' input stages, therefore, a noise in a photoreceiver with voltage and transimpedance amplifiers was determined. The noise models of receivers with p-n, p-i-n, and avalanche photodiodes are also discussed, paying special attention to the possibility of obtaining a high ratio of signal power to the noise power.

Simplified schematic diagrams of the first stages of photoreceivers with voltage preamplifiers based on bipolar and field-effect transistors are shown in Figure 11.7. Based on the schematic of a voltage preamplifier built on bipolar transistors, a noise equivalent circuit of the first stage of a photoreceiver is proposed in Figure 11.43. The signal current generator I_{ph} represents the detected signal. Noises in a detector (photodiode) are represented by three noise generators: I_{nph} is the shot noise originating from the photocurrent, I_{nd} is the shot noise from a dark current, and I_{nb} is the shot

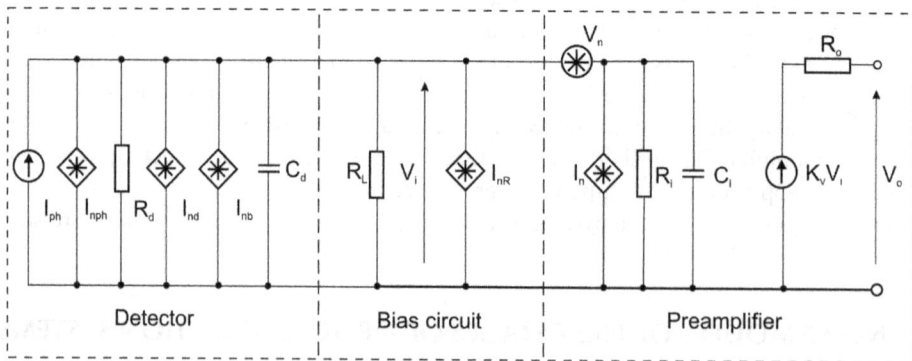

FIGURE 11.43 Equivalent scheme of the photodetector-voltage-type preamplifier circuit (C_d is the detector capacity, and R_i and C_i are the input resistance and capacitance of the preamplifier, respectively).

noise from background current $I_b = R_v A E_e$. The load (bias) resistor R_L affects both the level of the detector signal and its noise. The noise current generator I_{nR} is the thermal noise current and excess noise of the load resistance R_L. Since the thermal noise of I_{nR} is inversely related to the square root of the resistance, R_L must be large. For the lowest-noise system, at very low frequency, the detector will be the dominant noise source, but at higher frequencies amplifier noise becomes increasingly important.

A preamplifier is shown as a controlled voltage source with the gain K_v and two noise equivalent sources V_n and $I_{n'}$. In the photoreceiver first stage, the detector current produces the input voltage V_i across the resistance R_L and the capacitance C_d connected in parallel with it. If R_d and $R_i \gg R_L$, the transmittance function of this circuit is described by the equation

$$\frac{V_o}{I_{ph}} = \frac{K_v R_L}{\left((\omega R_L C_{eq})^2 + 1 \right)^{1/2}}, \tag{11.47}$$

where $C_{eq} = C_d + C_i$.

In the low frequency range, the output voltage is the following:

$$V_o = I_{ph} R_L K_v. \tag{11.48}$$

Voltage at the circuit output is proportional to the photocurrent, the detector load resistance and the preamplifier voltage gain. Unfortunately, due to the fact that capacitances C_d and C_i exist in the photoreceiver input stage, the gain depends on the frequency. The system 3-dB cut-off frequency is given by the following equation:

$$f_{-3dB} = \frac{1}{2\pi R_L C_{eq}}. \tag{11.49}$$

The voltage rise time is as follows:

$$t_r = 2.2 R_L C_{eq} = \frac{2.2}{2\pi f_{-3dB}} = \frac{0.35}{f_{-3dB}}. \tag{11.50}$$

Figure 11.43 shows the signal-to-noise ratio in the first stage of the photoreceiver with a voltage amplifier is

$$\frac{S}{N} = \frac{I_{ph}^2}{I_{nph}^2 + I_{nd}^2 + I_{nb}^2 + I_n^2 + \dfrac{4kT\Delta f}{R_L} + \left(\dfrac{V_n}{R_L}\right)^2}. \tag{11.51}$$

In the numerator there is a photocurrent, while in the denominator there is a total equivalent input noise of the photodetector-preamplifier circuit. The first three components define respectively the shot noise coming from photocurrent, detector dark current, and background, respectively; the fourth component is the preamplifier current noise, the fifth is the thermal noise of the resistance R_L and the last one is the preamplifier voltage noise. Achieving a large signal-to-noise ratio in the

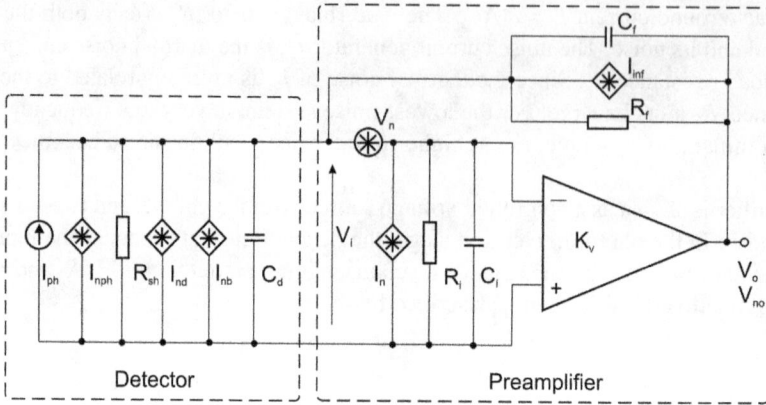

FIGURE 11.44 Equivalent scheme of the first stage of the photoreceiver with a transimpedance preamplifier.

input stage of the photoreceiver with a voltage preamplifier is possible for high resistances R_L and low current noise I_n of the preamplifier. Of course, obtaining a low contribution of the fifth and sixth component in the total equivalent input noise, respectively, comes at the expense of narrowing the photoreceiver bandwidth.

Figure 11.44 shows the equivalent noise scheme of the photoreceiver first stage with a transimpedance preamplifier. In this circuit, the detector noise sources are identical to the case in Figure 11.43, except that R_{sh} is the detector parallel resistance.

Preamplifier noise is represented by the voltage source V_n and the current I_n. Thermal noise from the feedback resistor is presented as a current source:

$$I_{nf} = \left(\frac{4kT\Delta f}{R_f} \right)^{1/2}.$$

(11.52)

It is desirable that the thermal noise of the resistor R_f is less than the detector thermal noise. Thus, the following relation should be fulfilled:

$$R_f > R_{sho} \frac{T_{R_f}}{T_{det}},$$

(11.53)

where R_{sho} is the detector resistance at zero bias voltage, T_{Rf} is the temperature of the resistor R_f, T_{det} is the detector temperature.

If the resistor R_f has the same temperature as the detector, considering the thermal noise, its value should be higher than the detector resistance. A high value of the resistor R_f provides a high transimpedance which can also lead to a saturation of the preamplifier.

If a photon noise from the photocurrent is greater than a thermal noise of the resistor R_f, then the condition is satisfied:

$$\frac{4kT\Delta f}{R_f} < 2qI_{ph}\Delta f.$$

(11.54)

Therefore,

$$R_f > \frac{2kT_{R_f}}{qI_{ph}}. \tag{11.55}$$

Eqs. (11.53) and (11.55) should be used to determine the initial transimpedance value of the preamplifier. Feedback resistor should be carefully selected, taking into account a drift and a $1/f$ noise. Large area resistors have a low $1/f$ noise, however large dimensions may not be acceptable in some applications. Before the designer decides on a given type of resistor, he should carefully measure it, both in terms of $1/f$ noise and temperature stability. This is very important because variations in transimpedance as a function of temperature can be perceived as a noise. The value of the feedback resistor should therefore be as high as possible but providing a bandwidth for a signal. After selecting the feedback resistor, a low-noise differential amplifier should be selected.

The voltage V_i at the preamplifier input is proportional to the photocurrent:

$$V_i = I_{ph}Z_d, \tag{11.56}$$

where Z_d is the detector impedance.

The voltage at the output of this circuit depends on the ratio of the impedance in the feedback circuit to the impedance of the detector and amounts to

$$V_o = -V_i \frac{Z_f}{Z_d}, \tag{11.57}$$

where

$$Z_f = \frac{R_f}{1 + j\omega R_f C_f}. \tag{11.58}$$

The voltage at the transimpedance amplifier output is equal to the product of the photocurrent and the impedance Z_f, thus,

$$V_o = -I_{ph}Z_f = -\frac{I_{ph}R_f}{1 + j\omega\tau_f} = -\frac{I_{ph}R_f}{1 + \omega^2\tau_f^2} + j\frac{I_{ph}R_f\omega\tau_f}{1 + \omega^2\tau_f^2}, \tag{11.59}$$

where $\tau_f = R_f C_f$. The imaginary part of Eq. (11.59) shows a phase of the output voltage. In order to simplify the analysis, this component will be omitted in the following considerations.

The voltage amplitude at the circuit output is equal to the modulus of Eq. (11.59) and is as follows:

$$|V_o| = (V_o V_o^*)^{1/2} = \frac{|I_{ph}|R_f}{(1 + \omega^2\tau_f^2)^{1/2}}. \tag{11.60}$$

The 3-dB cut-off frequency of the circuit under consideration is given by the equation

$$f_{-3dB} = \frac{1}{2\pi\tau_f}. \tag{11.61}$$

Note that the voltage at the preamplifier output is independent of the detector resistance and capacitance.

If the condition is met,

$$\tau_d = R_{sh}C_d \gg R_fC_f, \tag{11.62}$$

then the frequency characteristics of a photodetector-preamplifier circuit is determined by the time constant R_fC_f.

We will try to assess the contribution of individual noise sources to the total noise of the considered system. Photocurrent noise I_{nph}, dark current noise I_{nd}, background current noise I_{nb}, and preamp noise current I_{nph} are transferred to the preamplifier output in the same way as a photocurrent. Thus, the following equations determine the voltage of the noise output from these sources:

$$\left\langle V_{nph}^2 \right\rangle^{1/2} = \frac{\left\langle I_{nph}^2 \right\rangle^{1/2} R_f}{\left(1+\omega^2\tau_f^2\right)^{1/2}}, \tag{11.63}$$

$$\left\langle V_{nd}^2 \right\rangle^{1/2} = \frac{\left\langle I_{nd}^2 + I_{nb}^2 \right\rangle^{1/2} R_f}{\left(1+\omega^2\tau_f^2\right)^{1/2}}, \tag{11.64}$$

$$\left\langle V_{In}^2 \right\rangle^{1/2} = \frac{\left\langle I_n^2 \right\rangle^{1/2} R_f}{\left(1+\omega^2\tau_f^2\right)^{1/2}}. \tag{11.65}$$

The contribution of the preamplifier noise voltage to the total circuit output noise can be calculated using Eq. (11.60):

$$\left\langle (V_{no})^2 \right\rangle^{1/2} = \left\langle \left[V_n\left(f\right)\right]^2 \right\rangle^{1/2} \frac{R_f}{R_{sh}} \left(\frac{1+\omega^2\tau_d^2}{1+\omega^2\tau_f^2}\right)^{1/2}. \tag{11.66}$$

The thermal noise I_{nf} of the feedback resistor when transferred to the preamplifier output gives the following voltage:

$$\left\langle U_{nf}^2 \right\rangle^{1/2} = \frac{\left\langle I_{nf}^2 \right\rangle^{1/2} R_f}{\left(1+\omega^2\tau_f^2\right)^{1/2}} = \left(\frac{4kTR_f df}{1+\omega^2\tau_f^2}\right)^{1/2}. \tag{11.67}$$

RMS value of the output noise voltage is equal to the root of the sum of squares of the individual noise sources:

$$\left\langle \left(V_{no}^{calk} \right)^2 \right\rangle^{1/2} = \left[(V_{nph})^2 + (V_{nd})^2 + (V_{In})^2 + (V_{no})^2 + V_{nf})^2 \right]^{1/2}. \tag{11.68}$$

After dividing the total output noise determined by Eq. (11.68) by the system transimpedance, we obtain the expression for the total input equivalent noise current:

$$I_{ni}^{calk} = \left(I_{nph}^2 + I_{nd}^2 + I_{nb}^2 + I_n^2 + \frac{4kT\Delta f}{R_f} + \left(\frac{V_n}{R_f} \right)^2 \right)^{1/2}. \tag{11.69}$$

The total equivalent input noise is the sum of the noise mean squares from: photocurrent $- I_{ph}$, detector dark current $- I_d$, background current $- I_b$, thermal noise of the resistor $- R_f$, and current and voltage noise of the preamplifier. Thus, the signal-to-noise ratio will take the form of

$$\frac{S}{N} = \frac{I_{ph}^2}{I_{nph}^2 + I_{nd}^2 + I_{nb}^2 + I_n^2 + \dfrac{4kT\Delta f}{R_f} + \left(\dfrac{V_n}{R_f} \right)^2}. \tag{11.70}$$

As already mentioned, in a photoreceiver with a transimpedance amplifier, an identical frequency response can be obtained with the resistance R_f higher than the resistance R_L that occurs in a photoreceiver with a voltage amplifier. Thus, after comparing Eqs. (11.51) and (11.70), it can be seen that for the same frequency response, the signal-to-noise ratio is higher for the transimpedance amplifier than for the voltage amplifier. In practice, this means that transimpedance amplifiers can have a wider bandwidth with a noise performance comparable to high input impedance amplifiers.

Figure 11.45 presents noise equivalent circuit of the first stage of a photoreceiver with a charge-sensitive amplifier (CSA). In the preamplifier, a low-noise JFET or CMOS transistor or an operational amplifier with input on these transistors should be used. In the equivalent circuit, one can distinguish the detector shot noise from photocurrent I_{ph}, detector dark current I_d, background radiation I_b, shot noise from leakage current of gate I_g of the transistor, voltage noise V_n of the transistor and thermal noise V_{nRf} of the feedback resistance R_f. The current source I_{ng} represents the current noise of the transistor. A root mean square value of the current derived from shot noise of the detector currents and the transistor gate leakage current is as follows:

$$I_n^2 = 2q \left(I_{ph} + I_d + I_b + I_g \right) \Delta f. \tag{11.71}$$

Noise of the transistor is described by

$$V_n = \frac{8}{3} kT \frac{1}{g_m} + \frac{k_f}{C_{ox}^2 WLf}, \tag{11.72}$$

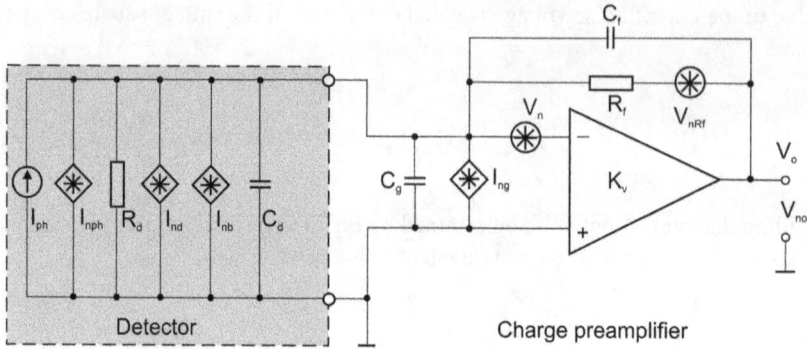

FIGURE 11.45 Noise equivalent circuit of the first stage of a photoreceiver with the CSA.

where g_m is transistor transconductance, k_f is the $1/f$ noise coefficient, W and L are the width and length of the transistor gate, respectively, C_{ox} is gate oxide capacitance. The first component in Eq. (11.72) determines the channel resistance thermal noise, while the second component determines the $1/f$ noise [29]. From Figure 11.45, the total noise output voltage can be determined as

$$V_{no}^2 = V_n^2 \left(1 + \frac{C_{in}}{C_f}\right)^2 + \left[I_n^2 + \left(\frac{V_{nR_f}}{R_f}\right)^2\right] \frac{1}{\left(sC_f\right)^2}, \qquad (11.73)$$

where $C_{in} = C_d + C_f + C_g$ is the input capacitance of the CSA.

The first term (transistor voltage source) is constant over entire range of frequency. It is amplified by the noise gain, which is given by $(1+C_{in}/C_f)^2$. The second noise component decreases with increasing frequency and is not dependent on the input capacitance. In the detector read-out electronics, a shaper stage is also integrated. This stage is inserted to filter the CSA output signal to improve SNR value, to add more gain, to shorten the pulse duration and to reduce the possibility of pile-up pulses. Detailed information about the noise models of the CSA circuit can be found in Reference 30 and Reference 31.

11.7 MAXIMISATION OF SIGNAL TO NOISE RATIO IN PHOTORECEIVERS

Figure 11.46 shows a block diagram of an optical radiation receiver designed for a direct detection including various noise sources. Most of the noise sources shown are found in both p-n, p-i-n, and avalanche photodiodes.

The background radiation noise is of great importance for the propagation of infrared radiation in the atmosphere. In the case of fiber-optic communication, they are very low and often overlooked. In the avalanche photodiode, an additional noise appears due to the random nature of the internal amplification mechanism. Therefore, at the beginning, we will discuss the noise occurring in receivers built with the use of p-n and p-i-n photodiodes. In p-n and p-i-n photodiodes, the shot noise of the photocurrent I_{ph} and the dark current I_d is the basic noise source. If it is necessary to consider the photocurent I_b from the background, then the mean square value of the total shot noise is given by the equation

$$I_{ntotal}^2 = 2q\left(I_{ph} + I_d + I_b\right)\Delta f. \qquad (11.74)$$

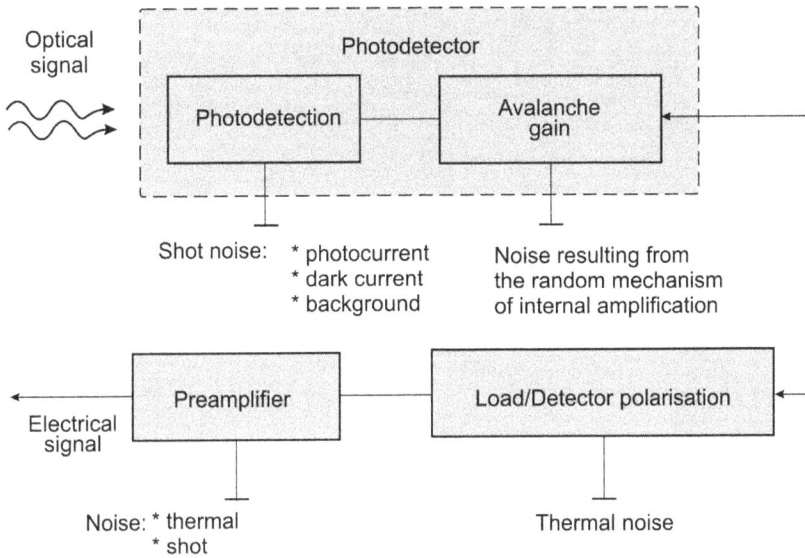

FIGURE 11.46 Optical radiation receiver model including noise sources.

Background current is equal to the current responsivity multiplied by the radiation power of the background ($I_b = R_I\Phi_b$), while the RMS value of the noise current is given by the equation $I_{nb} = (2q\Delta f I_b)^{1/2}$. Thermal noise of the detector load resistance and the noise of the preamplifier active elements may also play an important role in these photoreceivers.

The preamplifier noises V_n and I_n can be replaced by a single current source:

$$I_{na}^2 = \frac{1}{\Delta f}\int_0^{\Delta f}\left(I_n^2 + V_n^2\left|Y\right|^2\right)df, \qquad (11.75)$$

where Y is the input admittance of the amplifier.

As shown earlier, photodiodes can work with both voltage and transimpedance preamplifiers. For the equivalent schemes shown in Figures 11.43 and 11.44, the expression for the signal-to-noise ratio takes the form of

$$\frac{S}{N} = \frac{I_{ph}^2}{2q\left(I_{ph}+I_d+I_b\right)\Delta f + \dfrac{4kT\Delta f}{R_L} + I_{na}^2}. \qquad (11.76)$$

The first component determines the shot noise from a photocurrent, dark current and background, the second one – the thermal noise of the detector load resistance, and the third one – the preamplifier noise. For the circuit shown in Figure 11.44, the resistance $R_L = R_f$.

Let us now consider a few specific cases. Suppose the average signal current is greater than the dark current, so we can remove I_d from Eq. (11.76). Such a situation occurs when the dark current is insignificant and the received optical power is high. Let us also assume that the shot noise current greatly exceeds the thermal noise current, which occurs especially at high optical power levels.

This means that we can omit the component $4kT\Delta f/R_L$. If, in addition $I_{na}^2 << 2q\Delta f\left(I_{ph}+I_d\right)$, then the expression for the signal-to-noise ratio will be simplified to the form of

$$\frac{S}{N} = \frac{I_{ph}}{2q\Delta f}.$$
(11.77)

If we use the equation determining the photocurrent dependence on the incident radiation power, then Eq. (11.77) will take the form of

$$\frac{S}{N} = \frac{\eta \Phi_e \lambda}{2hc\Delta f} = \frac{\eta A E_e \lambda}{2hc\Delta f}.$$
(11.78)

A photoreceiver whose the signal-to-noise ratio of which is described by Eq. (11.78), is limited only by a shot noise or simply – we say that the photoreceiver is quantum limited. Unfortunately, a high optical power does not always reach the photoreceiver. If the optical signal power is low, then the shot noise is negligible in relation to the thermal noise, and Eq. (11.78) takes the form of

$$\frac{S}{N} = \frac{R_L(\eta q \Phi_e / h\nu)^2}{4kT\Delta f}.$$
(11.79)

This is the case where the photoreceiver is limited by a thermal noise or, simply, it is thermally conditioned.

After analysing Eq. (11.79), it can be seen that the signal-to-noise ratio increases in direct proportion with the square of the optical power received, that is, if the optical power increases by $\Delta \Phi_e$ [dB], the signal-to-noise ratio will increase by $2\Delta \Phi_e$ [dB]. It follows that, in this case, relatively small changes, for example in path-transmission efficiency, result in significant differences in the amplitude level of the received signal.

In quantum limited systems, an increase in optical power by $\Delta \Phi_e$ [dB] results in an improvement in the signal-to-noise ratio only by the amount of $\Delta \Phi_e$ [dB], because the dependence of the signal-to-noise ratio on the incident radiation is linear [Eq. (11.78)].

Let us now look at the effect of load resistance on the signal-to-noise ratio. Figure (11.43) highlights the resistance R_d shunting the current source of the detector, the load resistance R_L, and the preamplifier input resistance R_i. The lowest of these resistances has the greatest impact on loading the detector current source. Reducing the load resistance deteriorates the signal-to-noise ratio [Eq. (11.76)]. However, it should be remembered that increasing the load resistance, although it improves the signal-to-noise ratio, narrows the receiver bandwidth and lowers the permissible signal dynamics. Its influence is especially important at low levels of the radiation received [Eq. (11.79)].

When the source resistance is equal to the load resistance, the signal power to noise power ratio is reduced by 50 per cent compared to that obtained with a high load resistance. In some applications, it is possible to replace the resistance R_L with an inductance that does not introduce thermal noise. Obviously, the above analysis does not apply to a transimpedance preamplifier, the input resistance of which is obtained by feedback.

Linking the preamplifier noise I_{na}^2 with the load resistance R_L enables the introduction of the noise factor F_n [dB] expressed in this equation:

$$F_n = 1 + \frac{I_{na}^2}{I_{nt}^2}.$$
(11.80)

After summing up the thermal noise of the load resistance I_{nt}^2 and the amplifier noise I_{na}^2, the following equation is obtained:

$$I_{nt}^2 + I_{na}^2 = \frac{4kT\Delta f F_n}{R_L}.$$

(11.81)

Substituting the above relationship into Eq. (11.76), we obtain

$$\frac{S}{N} = \frac{I_{ph}^2}{2q\left(I_{ph} + I_d + I_b\right)\Delta f + \dfrac{4kT\Delta f F_n}{R_L}}.$$

(11.82)

An increase in the value of this ratio is obtained for lower values of the preamplifier noise factor F_n and a higher value of the load resistance.

Let us now consider effect of shunt capacitances on the signal-to-noise ratio. Although capacitance is virtually noise-free, it can cause an increase in the equivalent input noise. A shunt capacitance does not affect the detector signal-to-noise ratio because it decreases the detector signal and noise equally, but not the following preamplifier noise.

Consider the noise equivalent circuit, including shunt capacitance, shown in Figure 11.47. In this circuit, the signal source with the resistance R_d is represented by the generator V_s, and the noise voltage source V_{nd}. Preamplifier noise was described by means of the current source I_n connected in parallel to the detector and the voltage source V_n connected in series with the resistance R_d of the detector. Capacitance C is connected in parallel with the detector. It is equal to the sum of the detector junction capacitance and the preamplifier input capacitance.

The total output noise level for the circuit shown in Figure 11.47 is as follows:

$$V_{no}^2 = V_{nd}^2\left(\frac{1}{1+\omega^2 R_d^2 C^2}\right) + V_n^2 + I_n^2\left(\frac{R_d^2}{1+\omega^2 R_d^2 C^2}\right).$$

(11.83)

The power gain is determined by equation

$$K_v^2 = \frac{1}{1+\omega^2 R_d^2 C^2}.$$

(11.84)

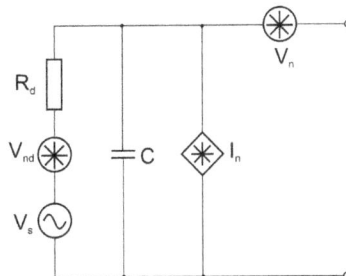

FIGURE 11.47 Shunt capacitance along with preamplifier and detector models.

We calculate the total input noise by dividing V_{no}^2 by K_v^2, hence,

$$V_{n\,input}^2 = V_{nd}^2 + \left(1 + \omega^2 R_d^2 C^2\right)V_n^2 + I_n^2 R_d^2. \tag{11.85}$$

As can be seen from Eq. (11.85), although the capacitor does not add noise, the preamplifier noise voltage V_n is increased by the shunt capacitance. The total input noise floor increases by a term of $\omega^2 R_d^2 C^2 V_n^2$.

Finally, let us analyse the signal-to-noise ratio in the first stage of photoreceivers with avalanche photodiodes. The high sensitivities of avalanche photodiodes can be obtained due to the phenomenon of avalanche multiplication. An internal amplification mechanism greatly increases a signal current generated in the output of the detector and improves the signal-to-noise ratio. However, it does not affect the noise from the load resistance, as well as from amplifier noises. Avalanche amplification increases the noise coming from dark current and quantum noise to such an extent that they can become decisive factors for a correct operation of the photoreceiver [32]. This is because the random carrier multiplication mechanism introduces an additional noise in the form of increased shot noise, exceeding the level resulting only from the original generation of non-equilibrium carriers.

The dominant noise source in the avalanche photodiode is a shot noise that is multiplied similarly to the signal. However, as the signal power increases in proportion to M^2, the noise power increases in proportion to M^{2+x}. The factor x takes values in the range of 0.03–0.5 for a silicon avalanche photodiode and within the range of 0.7–1.0 for an avalanche photodiode made of germanium or elements of III-V groups.

One of the parameters characterising the avalanche photodiode is an excess noise factor or multiplication factor:

$$F(M) = M^x. \tag{11.86}$$

It depends on the type of material the photodiode is made of, design features of the photodiode, and type of carriers (electrons or holes) playing a dominant role in the multiplication process.

There are many equations that describe the multiplication factor of the excess APD photodiode. Smith et al. gives the following relation [33]:

$$F(M) = M\left[1 - (1-k)\left(\frac{M-1}{M}\right)^2\right], \tag{11.87}$$

where k is the ratio of the hole ionisation factor to the electron ionisation factor.

If the ionisation is caused by holes, then,

$$F(M) = M\left[1 + \left(\frac{1-k}{k}\right)\left(\frac{M-1}{M}\right)^2\right]. \tag{11.88}$$

For silicon photodiodes $k \cong (0.02\text{–}0.1)$, and for germanium photodiodes, the coefficient k is in the range of (0.3–1.0).

An important characteristic of avalanche photodiodes is dependence of the avalanche multiplication factor M on the reverse bias voltage and temperature. Such characteristics are usually provided by photodiode manufacturers.

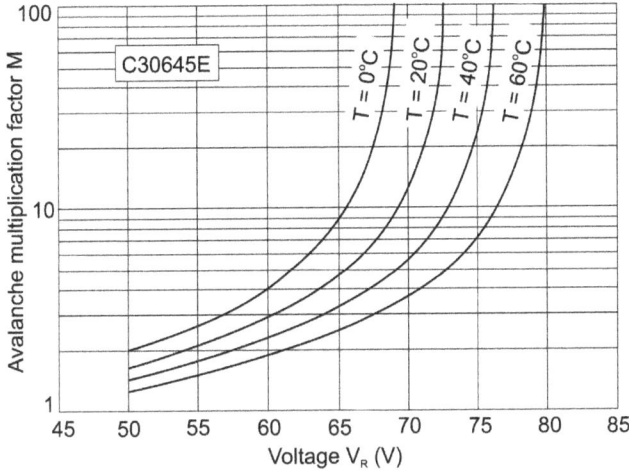

FIGURE 11.48 Avalanche multiplication factor of the InGaAs/InP type C30645E photodiode as a function of reverse bias voltage for different temperatures (after Reference 35).

Figure 11.48 shows an example of a dependence of the InGaAs/InP photodiode avalanche multiplication factor as a function of the reverse bias voltage for different temperatures [34]. The figure shows that in order to maintain a constant value of the avalanche photodiode sensitivity with changing temperature, the bias voltage should be regulated. For this purpose, specialised avalanche photodiode power supply systems are manufactured.

The average square value of the total shot noise is given by the relation

$$I^2_{n\,shot} = 2q\Delta f \left[\left(I_{ph} + I_{db} + I_{b} \right) M^2 F \left(M \right) + I_{s} \right],$$
(11.89)

where I_{db} is the bulk component of the primary dark current, and I_{s} is the surface leakage current component of the dark current.

Eq. (11.89) shows that the surface component of the dark current I_{s} is not multiplied. Instead, the photocurrent I_{ph}, the background current I_{b}, and the volume component of the primary dark current I_{db} are multiplied.

If the load resistance thermal noise and the preamplifier noise are added to the shot noise of the avalanche photodiode, we obtain the total noise level of the avalanche photodiode input stage. Knowing the total noise, we can determine the signal-to-noise ratio:

$$\frac{S}{N} = \frac{M^2 I^2_{ph}}{2q\Delta f \left(I_{ph} M^2 F \left(M \right) + I_{s} + \left(I_{db} + I_{b} \right) M^2 F \left(M \right) \right) + \frac{4kT\Delta f}{R_L} F_{n}}.$$
(11.90)

If we assume that $F(M) = M^x$, thus,

$$\frac{S}{N} = \frac{M^2 I^2_{ph}}{2q\Delta f \left(I_{ph} M^{2+x} + I_{s} + \left(I_{b} + I_{db} \right) M^{2+x} \right) + \frac{4kT\Delta f}{R_L} F_{n}}.$$
(11.91)

The numerator of this equation is photocurrent, and the denominator is noise. The first component of the denominator is the shot noise and the second one is the load resistance thermal noise along with the preamplifier noise. Rearranging Eqs. (11.91), we obtain

$$\frac{S}{N}(M) = \frac{I_{ph}^2}{2q\Delta f\left(I_{ph} + I_b + I_{db}\right)M^x + 2q\Delta f I_s M^{-2} + \dfrac{4kT\Delta f F_n}{R_L}M^{-2}}.$$ (11.92)

This equation shows that the first component of the denominator increases with an increase in the avalanche multiplication factor, while the second component decreases. Thus, there exists an optimum value of the avalanche multiplication factor M_{op} at which the signal-to-noise ratio takes the maximum value.

From calculations of the extreme of the function (11.92), it follows that

$$M_{op}^{2+x} = \frac{4kTF_n}{xqR_L\left(I_{ph} + I_d\right)}.$$ (11.93)

Figure 11.49 presents exemplary characteristics, showing the dependence of signal current, thermal noise, shot noise and total noise on the avalanche multiplication factor M. For low values of the avalanche multiplication factor, a signal from the radiation incident on the detector is lower than the resultant noise. Thermal noise dominates in this range, which means that the resultant noise current practically does not change with this coefficient increase. For high values of the avalanche multiplication factor, the thermal noise significance decreases remarkably, while a shot noise share increases.

There is a well-defined value of the avalanche multiplication factor, and, therefore, the supply voltage, at which the signal-to-noise ratio is the highest. This corresponds to the case where the

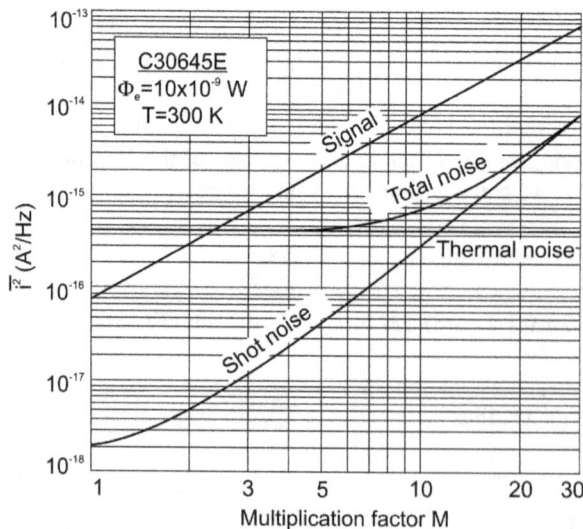

FIGURE 11.49 Dependence of signal current, thermal noise, shot noise, and total noise on the avalanche multiplication factor M for the InGaAs/InP photodiode C30645E type for $P = 10$ nW (after Reference 2).

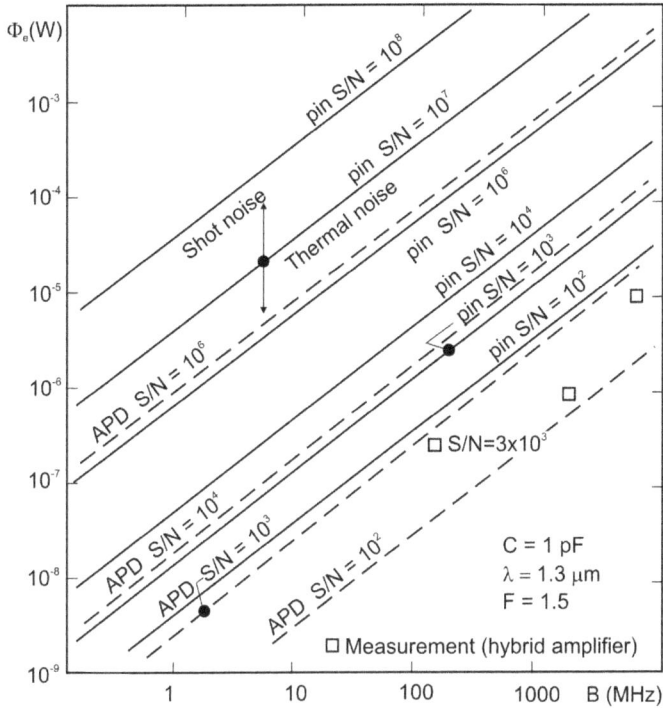

FIGURE 11.50 Sensitivity of receivers with the p-i-n photodiode (solid lines) and the avalanche photodiode with optimal gain (dashed lines) (after Reference 34).

distance between the "signal" line and the "total noise" curve is the largest. Of course, these parameters will change with temperature changes due to the fact that the photodiode dark current and the avalanche multiplication factor show a strong dependence on temperature.

In order to maintain a constant value of the avalanche multiplication factor as a function of temperature changes, the photodiode supply voltage should be changed and the temperature coefficient of changes in this voltage depends on the type of material the photodiode is made of. Therefore, specialised power supplies are used to power the avalanche photodiodes. A detailed analysis concerning the selection of the optimal working point of the avalanche photodiode and the systems used to stabilise the photoreceiver input stage sensitivity can be found in the literature [35, 36]. Figure 11.50 shows the receiver sensitivity with an avalanche photodiode and a p-i-n photodiode.

There is an improvement in the sensitivity for small signals and low signal-to-noise ratios. In the range of strong signals, the avalanche photodiodes sensitivity may even be lower than that of p-i-n photodiodes due to a faster noise increase.

11.8 MONOLITHIC AND HYBRID PHOTORECEIVERS

Integrated photoreceivers can be divided into two main groups: monolithic photoreceivers and hybrid photoreceivers (Figure 11.51). Monolithic photoreceivers consist of a detector, a high input impedance preamplifier or a transimpedance preamplifier, and one or more amplification and matching stages. Such a circuit is very convenient to use, because it is a ready-made, carefully designed, proven and made a complete optical receiver input circuit.

The use of an integrated photoreceiver significantly reduces the possibility of introducing external interference through the leads connecting the detector to the amplifier. In the integrated

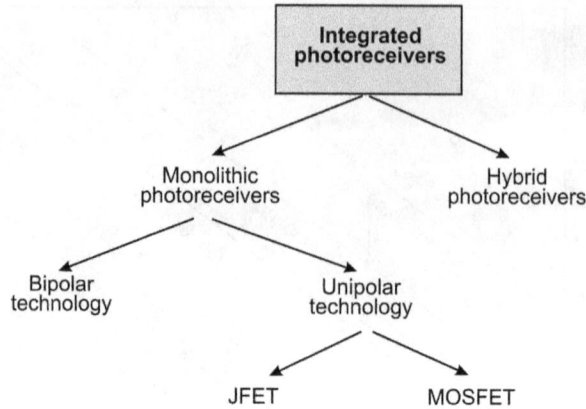

FIGURE 11.51 Division of integrated photoreceivers.

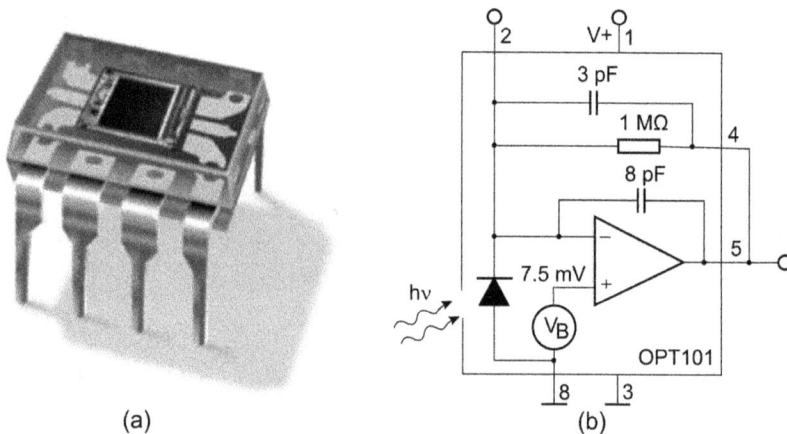

FIGURE 11.52 Monolithic photoreceiver: (a) photo, (b) scheme.

photoreceiver, these connections are very short and well shielded. Figure 11.52 shows an example of the photoreceiver input stage which was made in the monolithic technology [37, 38].

Hybrid photoreceivers consist of separately manufactured photodiode and amplifier circuits, which are then assembled and connected in a common, compact housing. This can be, for example, a combination of a p-i-n photodiode with a high input impedance amplifier or a transimpedance amplifier on a ceramic substrate. The housings used are, for example, popular and convenient double-row sockets for mounting on printed circuit boards. Figure 11.53 shows an example of a photoreceiver that was made using hybrid technology [39, 40].

11.9 PHOTON COUNTERS

Photomultipliers and avalanche photodiodes have found application not only in detection systems for measuring very low photon fluxes, but also in photon counters. The photon flux that reaches these detectors produces a pulse signal at their output. Amplitude and shape of this pulse depend on the optical radiation intensity (Figure 11.54). If the radiation intensity is high, then at the output of the photomultiplier there is a phenomenon of summation of a large number of independent pulses generated by photons falling on a photocathode surface [41]. As a result of superimposing these

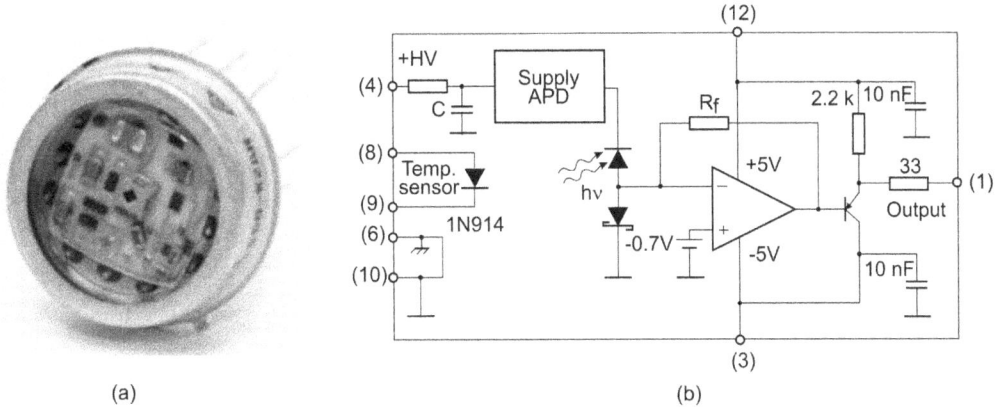

(a)   (b)

FIGURE 11.53 Hybrid photoreceiver: (a) photo, (b) scheme.

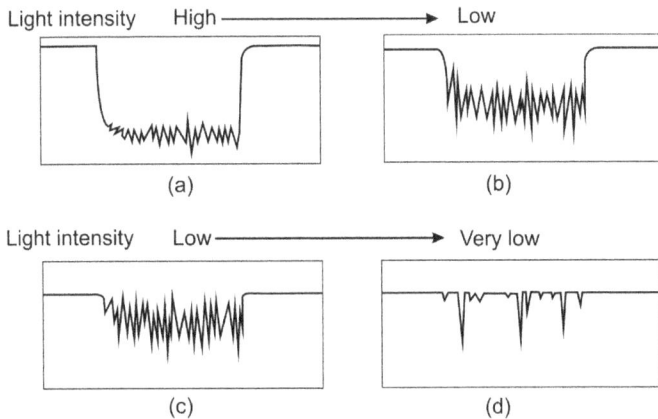

FIGURE 11.54 Photomultiplier response to an optical radiation pulse of different intensity: (a–c) analogue mode, (d) digital mode.

pulses, we will obtain a voltage waveform which is shown in Figure 11.54(a). In this case, a high signal-to-noise ratio was obtained. As the radiation intensity decreases, the signal-to-noise ratio decreases [Figure 11.54(b) and 11.54(c)]. This type of photomultiplier work is called the analogue mode. If the radiation intensity continues to decrease, the photomultiplier output will receive discrete pulses [Figure 11.54(d)]. This type of a PMT work is called the digital count mode or a photon counting region.

Typical detection systems with photomultiplier tubes are shown in Figure 11.55 [41]. The signal processing system shown in Figure 11.55(a) consists of a DC preamplifier, a low-pass filter, an A/D converter and a computer. In systems with an optical radiation modulation, in particular in optical communication, systems with pulse amplifiers and fast A/C converters are used [Figure 11.55(b)]. At very low radiation intensity, individual pulses from detected photons are amplified. For this purpose, detection systems are used, a diagram of which is shown in Figure 11.55(c). The number of pulses counted is directly proportional to the number of incident photons.

In practical systems, there is noise in addition to the useful signal. Its presence causes the so-called "dark pulses" to appear at the photomultiplier output. In simple detection systems, they will interfere with the useful signals.

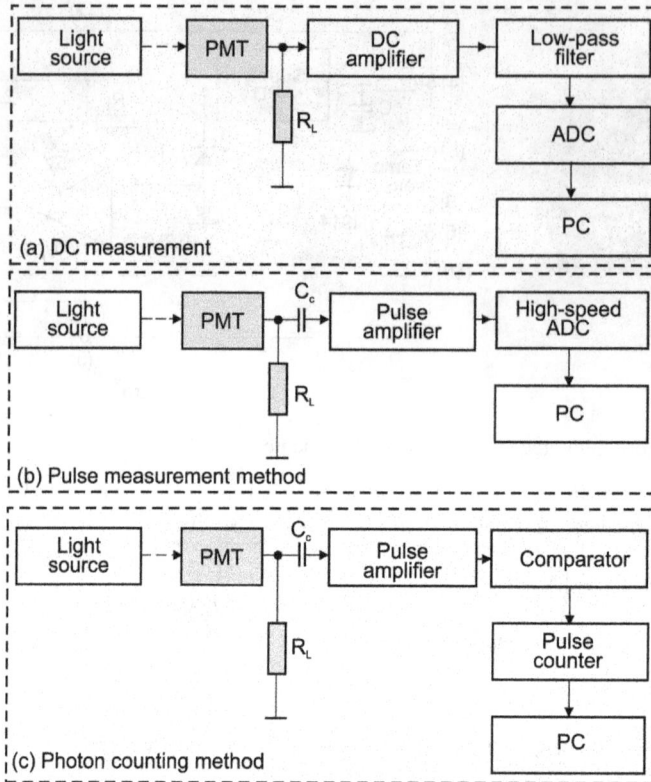

FIGURE 11.55 Typical optical radiation detection systems used for photomultipliers: (a) with a direct current path, (b) with a pulse amplifier, and (c) with a photon counter (after Reference 41).

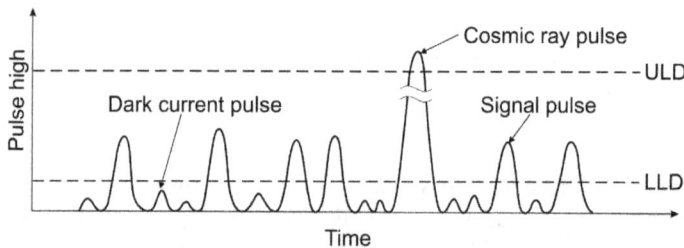

FIGURE 11.56 Voltage waveform at the output of the pulse amplifier in the circuit shown in Figure 11.55(c), where LLD means lower-level discrimination, ULD means upper-level discrimination (after Reference 42).

Discriminators are used to limit dark pulse counts. Then, their output will show only those pulses whose amplitude exceeds the set threshold. They are then counted in the pulse counter (Figure 11.56) [42]. Sometimes there are interference pulses of very high amplitude. They may come from cosmic radiation. In order to limit their influence, the upper level discrimination (ULD) comparisons was introduced. The system, in which two levels of discrimination are used, is called the pulse height distribution (PHD).

In the PHD method, it is very important to select the lower-level discrimination (LLD) value and the upper ULD discrimination level. The lower level of discrimination should be higher than the amplitude of a vast majority of noise pulses. In such a designed circuit, pulses will be counted, the amplitude of which is between the LLD and the ULD.

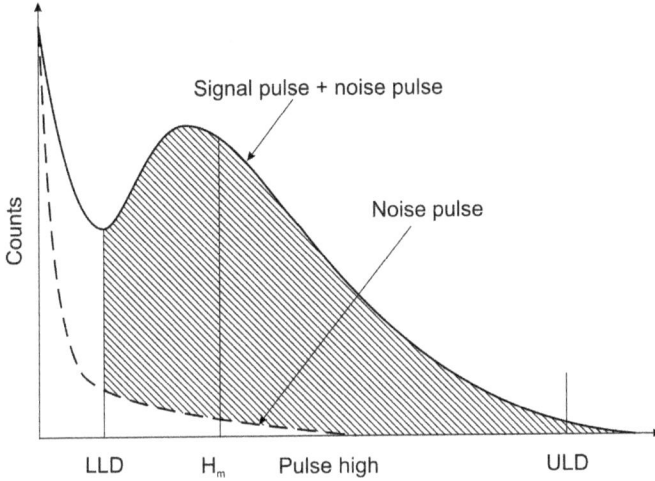

FIGURE 11.57 Typical distribution of the number of pulses of given amplitude at the photomultiplier output (after Reference 42).

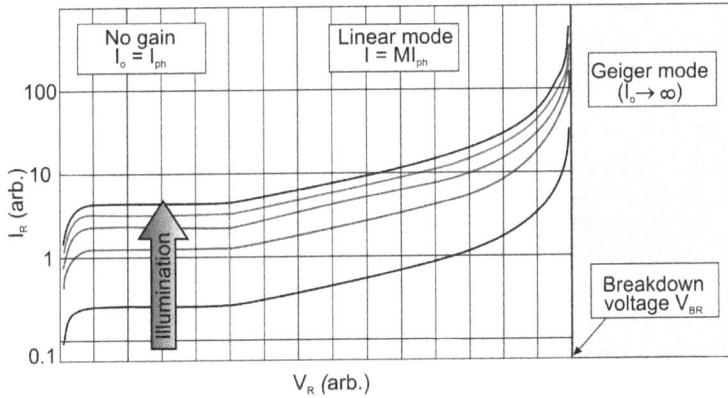

FIGURE 11.58 Current-voltage characteristics of an avalanche photodiode with a marked area of linear mode and Geiger mode (after Reference 44).

Figure 11.57 shows a typical distribution of the number of pulses at the photomultiplier output depending on their amplitude. Analysis of the literature shows that the LLD should be 1/3 of the average amplitude of the detected H_m pulses, while the ULD – three times the H_m value [42].

Avalanche photodiodes are also used to detect a very low intensity optical radiation (power less than pW). They can work in a linear mode and as photon counters in "Geiger" mode (Figure 11.58). In the linear mode the supply voltage of the APDs photodiodes is lower than the breakthrough voltage, that is, $V_R < V_{BR}$, and the output current is proportional to the primary current (I_{ph}) and to the avalanche multiplication factor M:

$$I_o = I_{ph}M. \tag{11.94}$$

Avalanche photodiodes operating in the linear mode, which is a standard area of the APD work, are characterised by a very high sensitivity and a short response time. They are used, among others, in laser rangefinders, lidars, spectroscopy, and fast and highly sensitive optical radiation receivers.

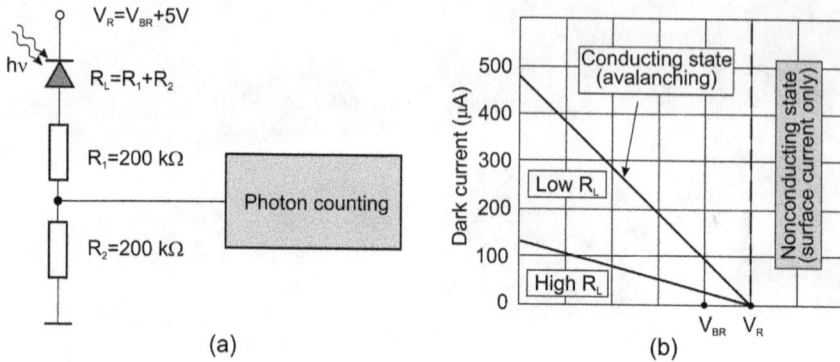

FIGURE 11.59 APD power supply scheme: (a) passive photodiode pulse quenching circuit, (b) simple APD loads.

In the Geiger mode, the APD operating point is selected so that the value of the reverse bias voltage V_R is greater than the breakdown voltage $V_R > V_{BR}$ [43]. Then, a very large current will flow through the 'illuminated' avalanche photodiode, which may cause it permanent damage (Figure 11.58 [44]). To prevent this phenomenon, special passive and active pulse-quenching circuits are used. We will call them passive or active pulse-quenching circuits (PPQC or APQC for short).

Before we go on to discuss these systems, let us assume that the photodiode has a current with an acceptable value, not exceeding the latching current. The value of this current can be limited by resistors in the PPQC system. This system should be designed in such a way that, in the absence of APD lighting and small dark currents, the photodiode is in the off state. If the photodiode is illuminated, the current will flow rapidly and generate a pulse at its output. The photodiode can also be "turned on" due to the existence of volume carriers generating dark pulses. Therefore, avalanche photodiodes intended for use in photon counters should be particularly selected in terms of a low volume value of dark currents. If the number of dark pulses is very small, then a Geiger mode photodiode can be used for a single photon counting.

Figure 11.59 shows a scheme of a passive avalanche photodiode pulse suppression circuit (a) and simple loads of this circuit (b). In the absence of "lighting" of the photodiode, there is the voltage V_R on its cathode. There is no current flowing in the pulse suppression circuit. If there is a stream of photons on the APD surface, then the current flowing through R_1 and R_2 resistors will cause appropriate voltage drops and 'switching off' the photodiode. Photodiode voltage drops to $V_R - I_d R_L$. The APD current decay rate is conditioned by the time constant resulting from the values of resistance R_1 and R_2 and capacity of the circuit. Photodiode readiness to count successive photons is also conditioned by this time constant and $V_R - V_{BR}$ voltage difference. Typical value of the photodiode off time is in the order of several hundred ns, while the return time of the system for counting subsequent photons (time resolution) is of about 400 ps. The jitter is of the same order of magnitude as the voltage rise time of the photodiode.

For the currents $(V_R - V_{BR})/R_L$ much higher than the lock current I_{latch}, the photodiode remains in the avalanche (conduction) region. If the current $(V_R - V_{BR})/R_L$ is much smaller than I_{latch}, the photodiode immediately goes to a non-conductive area. For large R_L values, the photodiode operating point is in a non-conductive area and only a surface component of the noise current flows through the photodiode.

In order to shorten the photodiode dead time, active circuits are used to quench the photodiode pulses. In this case, transistors are used instead of the load resistance. When counting photons, the transistor is off, while when the APD returns to the active state the transistor is on [45, 46]. Response times of the system are mainly determined by the transistor switching on and off times. The resolution of active extinguishing circuits is of about 20 ps.

11.10   ADVANCED METHODS OF SIGNAL DETECTION

The first stages of the photoreceivers discussed in section 11.6 are called direct detection circuits. In order to design a photoreceiver that can detect very low intensity optical signals, it is necessary to analyse the equivalent scheme of its first stage and perform optimisation in order to obtain the minimum value of the equivalent input noise and the maximum value of the signal-to-noise ratio (Section 11.7).

If the photoreceiver input stage so designed makes it impossible to detect optical signals, then other methods of detection should be used. Thus, this chapter is devoted to detection methods that allow the detection of optical signals below the noise level. We called them advanced detection methods.

11.10.1   Signal Averaging

When measuring a small repetitive or steady-state signal in the presence of noise, we can often improve the results by making a number of measurements and taking their average. Figure 11.60 presents a scheme of signal detection system for steady-state signals with an analogue integrator.

If radiation from both a signal source and the background is incident on a detector surface, the desired signal will appear with noise at the detector output. It is amplified in a preamplifier and next reaches the integrator input. Let us assume that before beginning the measurement cycle, the voltages at inputs of both the differential amplifier and the integrator and the integrator output are all equal to zero. If a voltage V_i appears at the integrator input, a current I_1 will flow through the resistor R. This current causes changes the capacitor C, to give a voltage $V_o(T)$ at the circuit output, where

$$V_o(T) = -\frac{1}{RC}\int_0^T V_i dt + V_o(0),$$ (11.95)

where $V_o(0)$ is the initial voltage at the capacitor at $t = 0$ and $RC = \tau$ is the time constant of the integrator.

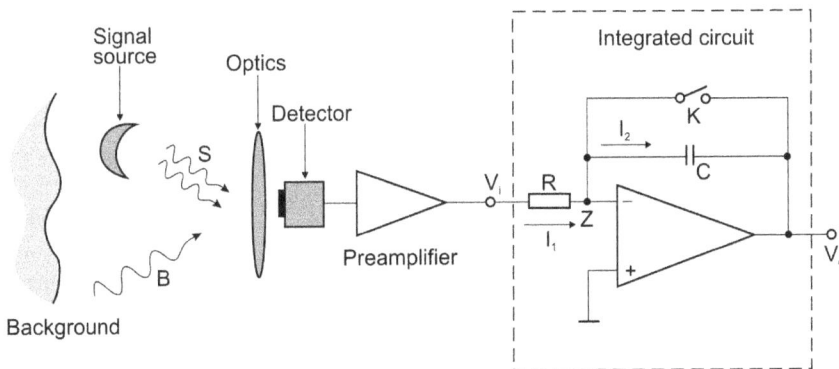

FIGURE 11.60   Analogue integrator used to collect detected signal level.

The voltage at the system output is inversely proportional to the time constant. In practice, the capacitor C is short-circuited at the beginning of a measuring cycle by means of the switch K. So, the second constant term of equation (11.95) can be omitted. Opening the switch K initiates the measuring cycle, during which the signal integration occurs. If the assumption is made that there is a constant voltage of the value v at the system input, then, after a time t, the output voltage will be directly proportional to the product vt. Thus, the signal-to-noise ratio at the integrator output takes a form

$$\frac{S}{N} = v\left(\frac{2t}{S_n}\right)^{1/2},$$

(11.96)

where S_n is the input white noise power density. This equation tells that the signal-to-noise ratio can increase linearly with the square root of the integration time t (for $t \ll RC$).

The integrating process in mathematical form corresponds to taking a series of measurements and summing each of the received values. If we make N measurements, each integrated over the period t, and then the received results are added, the signal-to-noise ratio is described as

$$\frac{S}{N} = v\left(\frac{2Nt}{S_n}\right)^{1/2}.$$

(11.97)

In this case, signal-to-noise ratio increases proportionally to square root of a number of the performed measurements (or the total measurement time Nt). Similarly as in equation (11.97), the time constant of an integrator does not affect the value of a signal-to-noise ratio. In real conditions, the value of the time constant should be chosen to ensure the desired level of the output signal after an appropriate integration time t [47].

One disadvantage of the simple integrator is that $1/f$ noise, electronic offsets, and background light-level charges can all degrade the performance. We shall now describe another signal recovery method that avoids these problems.

11.10.2 Phase Sensitive Detection

Phase sensitive detection (PSD) is a commonly used measurement method that allows the reception of optical signals of very low intensity in the presence of undesirable background or noise (especially $1/f$ noise) [48]. It is used even in conditions where the signal amplitude is lower than the noise level (for periodic signals).

To understand the purposefulness of using phase-sensitive detection, let us consider the following example. For this, let us assume that we have a sinusoidal signal with an amplitude of 10 nV and a frequency of 10 kHz. This signal is fed to a preamplifier with a 100 kHz frequency response, a voltage gain of 1000 V/V and an input noise voltage of 5 nV/Hz$^{1/2}$. For the analysed system, the signal amplitude at the preamplifier output is 10 μV (10 nV×1000 V/V). On the other hand, the noise amplitude is 1.6 mV (5 nV/Hz$^{1/2}$×(100 kHz)$^{1/2}$×1000 V/V). Thus, this circuit makes it impossible to detect a signal with such small amplitude. In the next step, connect a filter with a centre frequency of 10 kHz and a quality factor (Q factor) of 100 to the output of the preamplifier. The frequency response of this filter is 100 Hz (10 kHz/100). The amplitude of the signal at the output of the filter will be 10 μV, while the noise voltage will decrease to 50 μV (5 nV/Hz$^{1/2}$(100 Hz)$^{1/2}$×1000). In this case, we will not detect a signal with such a small amplitude either.

Now let us connect a phase-sensitive amplifier to the output of the preamplifier, which contains a low-pass filter with a bandwidth of 0.01 Hz. In this case, the noise amplitude is 0.5 μV (5 nV/Hz$^{1/2}$× (0.01Hz)$^{1/2}$×1000), while the signal amplitude remains at the same level. We have obtained a signal to noise ratio of 20, so it is possible to detect a signal with such small amplitude. We will discuss how this system works later in this chapter.

A diagram of a typical phase-sensitive detection system is shown in Figure 11.61. The measuring system consists of a radiation source, a chopper with a controller, a detector, a low-noise preamplifier and a lock-in amplifier (LIA).

The idea of operation of the phase-sensitive detection system is shown in Figure 11.62. There are five main stages: optical chopper, detection, signal amplification, phase-sensitive demodulation and reconstruction of the examined signal. Phase-sensitive amplifiers play a very important role in PSD detection systems. They are available commercially in single-phase and dual-phase (LIA) variants, as well as in analogue and digital technology [49–56]. First, let us get acquainted with the construction and working principle of the analogue LIA amplifier.

Figure 11.63 shows a simplified diagram of a typical phase-sensitive amplifier. It consists of two paths: signal and reference, a phase-sensitive detector and an output amplifier. This circuit is called single-phase LIA amplifier. The signal path is designed to amplify the tested signal and limit its

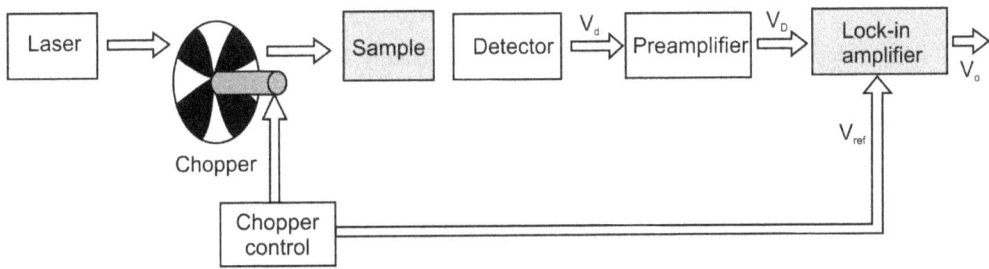

FIGURE 11.61 Diagram of the phase-sensitive detection system.

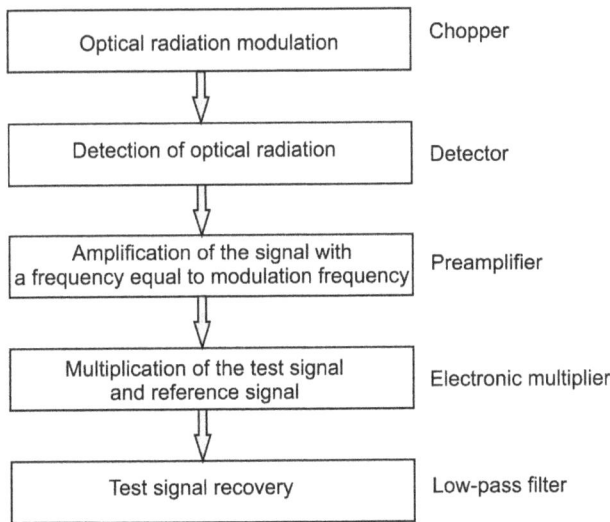

FIGURE 11.62 Idea of PSD operation.

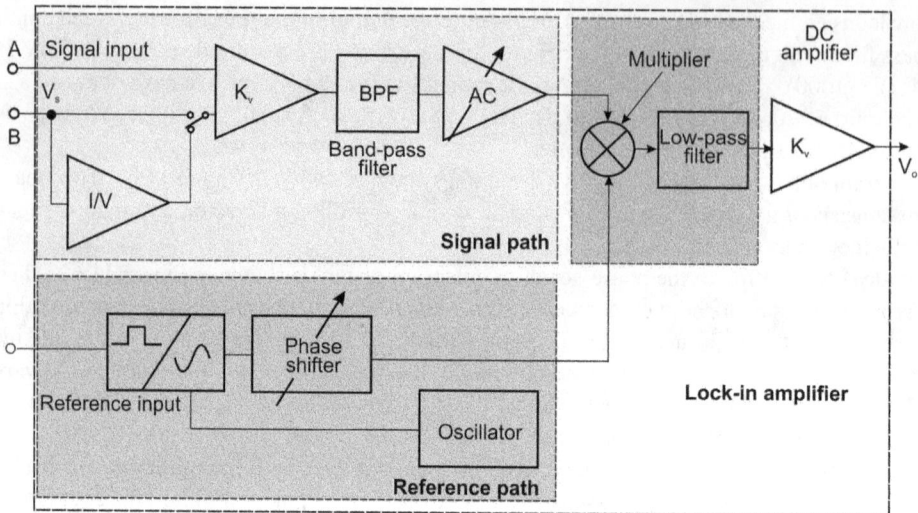

FIGURE 11.63   A simplified diagram of a phase-sensitive amplifier.

bandwidth in order to improve the signal-to-noise ratio. Usually, it is built of a current and/or voltage preamplifier, a band-pass filter (BPF) and an AC amplifier with adjustable gain [52].

A particularly important role is played by the phase-sensitive detector (PSD), that is, a sub-assembly consisting of a mixer and a low-pass filter. There are three technical solutions of PSD detectors, in which the multiplication circuit is made in the following technology: analogue, with a digital switch and digital [48]. Analogue technology multipliers are rarely used due to their non-linear nature of operation, high noise, and therefore lower ability to detect low-level signals.

The idea behind the operation of these detectors is to rectify the input signal synchronously with the reference signal; hence, the name synchronous rectifier. Their main advantage is that they are easy to manufacture and can operate over a very wide dynamic range of the measured signal [53]. The purpose of the low-pass filter is to remove unwanted harmonics and noise in order to faithfully reproduce the measured DC signal. The reference path includes a sine former, a phase shifter and a local sinusoidal generator. The reference channel is used to shape a sinusoidal signal when receiving a sawtooth or square wave signal from the outside, remove higher harmonics and provide a phase shift so as to be phase-compatible with the signal under test. As a rule, a phase shifter allows a phase shift of more than 360 degrees. This is usually done by smooth phase adjustment: from 0 to 95 degrees and 3 step-phase shifts of 90 degrees. The reference signal can also be produced by a sinusoidal generator inside a phase-sensitive amplifier.

Let us now examine the working principle of the LIA amplifier. We assume that the measured signal has the form of sinusoidal wave described by the formula

$$V_{sig} = V_s K_v cos\left(2\pi f_s t + \varphi\right), \tag{11.98}$$

and the reference signal

$$V_{ref} = V_R cos\left(2\pi f_R t\right). \tag{11.99}$$

After multiplying these signals, we will get at the mixer output

$$V_{MX} = \frac{1}{2}V_s K_v V_R \left[\cos\left(2\pi\left(f_s - f_R\right) + \varphi\right) + \cos\left(2\pi\left(f_s + f_R\right) + \varphi\right)\right].$$ (11.100)

If the condition $f_s = f_R$ is satisfied, then

$$V_{MX} = \frac{1}{2}V_s K_v V_R \left[\cos\left(\varphi\right) + \cos\left(2\pi 2 f t + \varphi\right)\right].$$ (11.101)

At the output of the low-pass filter we get a constant component which is directly proportional to the amplitude of the measured voltage and the reference voltage

$$V_{MX} = \frac{1}{2}V_s K_v V_R \cos\varphi.$$ (11.102)

The output signal depends on the phase difference between the measured signal and the reference signal – hence, the name of the phase-sensitive detection.

By using a phase shifter it is possible to make the phase difference between the measured signal and the reference signal equal to zero, then

$$V_{MX} = \frac{1}{2}V_s K_v V_R.$$ (11.103)

Let us now turn to the principle of operation of the LIA two-phase amplifier. In this case, it contains a second PSD detector, a 90° phase shifter and two functional blocks that enable the voltage of the tested signal and the phase value between the measured signal and the reference signal to be determined. A simplified diagram of this amplifier is shown in Figure 11.64.

Let us assume that the measured signal has the form of a sine wave described by the formula (11.98), and the reference signal has the form of the formula (11.99). After the multiplication of these signals, at the output of the demodulator X, we will get a signal described by the formula (11.100). In turn, at the output of the demodulator Y we get

$$V_{MY} = V_s K_v \cos\left(2\pi f_s t + \varphi\right)\left(-V_R \sin\left(2\pi f_R t\right)\right)$$ (11.104)
$$= \frac{1}{2}V_s K_v V_R \left[\sin\left(2\pi\left(f_s - f_R\right) + \varphi\right) - \sin\left(2\pi\left(f_s + f_R\right) + \varphi\right)\right].$$

If $f_s = f_R$, then

$$V_{MX} = \frac{1}{2}V_s K_v V_R \left[\cos\left(\varphi\right) + \cos\left(2\pi 2 f t + \varphi\right)\right].$$ (11.105)

$$V_{MY} = \frac{1}{2}V_s K_v V_R \left[\sin\left(\varphi\right) - \sin\left(2\pi 2 f t + \varphi\right)\right].$$ (11.106)

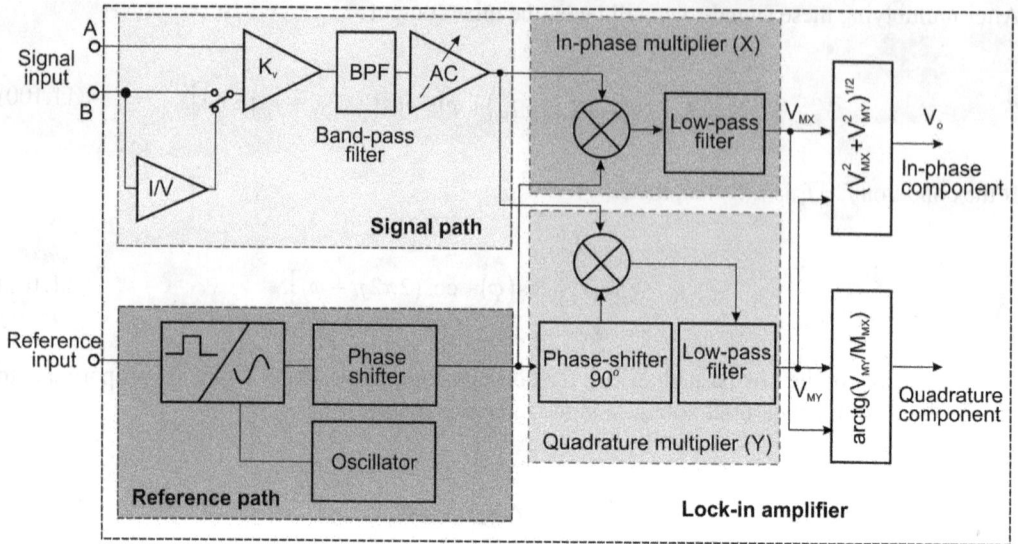

FIGURE 11.64 Simplified scheme of a two-phase-sensitive amplifier.

At the output of low-pass filters we get two constant components (X and Y), which are directly proportional to the amplitude of the measured voltage and the amplitude of the reference voltage:

$$V_{MX} = \frac{1}{2} V_s K_v V_R \cos\varphi, \qquad (11.107)$$

$$V_{MY} = \frac{1}{2} V_s K_v V_R \sin\varphi. \qquad (11.108)$$

For this configuration, the phase difference between the test signal and the reference signal need not be constant and given with high accuracy. However, in a single-phase system, its changes caused by various factors are a source of voltage-measurement error. The LIA two-phase amplifier does not have this drawback, because the amplitude of the output signal and the phase are calculated from the formulas

$$V_o = \left(V_{MX}^2 + V_{MY}^2 \right)^{1/2} = \frac{1}{2} V_s V_R K_v, \qquad (11.109)$$

$$\varphi = arctan \left(\frac{V_{MY}}{V_{MX}} \right). \qquad (11.110)$$

A large selection of LIA amplifiers is offered by Stanford Research Systems. More recent developments have used digital signal processing techniques. These instruments are referred to as digital instruments or DSP (Digital Signal Processing instruments). The general scheme of digital PSD amplifiers is similar to the layout shown in Figure 11.64. In these amplifiers, analogue filters, analogue current preamplifiers (I/V converters) and voltage preamplifiers are used in the

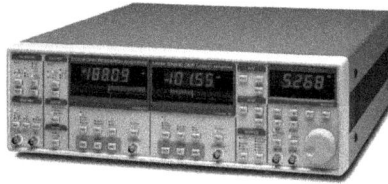

FIGURE 11.65 Photograph of digital LIA amplifier type SR 830 from Stanford Research System.

measurement channel [52]. The amplified analogue signal is sampled with a 16-bit A/D converter. The signal processed in this way is sent to the in-phase mixer and to the quadrature mixer digital PSD detector. The generator is made in the form of tables with the values of the sine and cosine functions. All signal processing takes place inside the DSP.

The photograph of the digital amplifier LIA type SR 830 from Stanford Research System is shown in Figure 11.65 [54]. This instrument enables measurements in the range from 1 mHz to 102.4 kHz. The input signal dynamic range is over 100 dB. The output filter enables to obtain time constants from 10 µs to 30,000 s (24 dB/octave).

The advantages of these digital amplifiers include

- high stability, both temperature and time, of the internal generator frequency;
- low distortion introduced by the synphase and quadrature PSD detectors; and
- high stability, both in terms of temperature and time, of the output voltage.

Phase-sensitive detection systems have found numerous applications in scientific research and in various extremely low-intensity signal detection systems [55–58]. Consider an example where the LIA amplifier is used in a system capable of detecting trace concentrations of gases. In direct absorption spectroscopy (DAS) systems, there is very little absorption of laser radiation at low gas concentrations. Therefore, small changes in irradiance are also observed at the output of the test sample [Figure 11.66(a)]. They are so small that it may be difficult to measure them. Therefore, it is necessary to use ultra-sensitive absorption detection techniques [57,58]. One of these is multi-pass spectroscopy, in which high sensitivity is achieved by extending the optical radiation path in the measurement cell.

A further improvement in the sensitivity of the detection system can be achieved with the use of wavelength modulation absorption spectroscopy (WMAS) circuits using the LIA in the "$2f$" mode of operation. This mode is based on the fact that the LIA system does not analyse the f_{mod} component, but $2 \times f_{mod}$. The WMS system uses wavelength modulation of the laser radiation.

At the beginning, the spectral range of the radiation source is adjusted to the wavelength range in which the absorption line of the tested gas is present [Figure 11.66(b)]. Next, the wavelength modulation procedure is carried out with a linear signal with the sinusoidal component of the f_{mod} frequency plotted. When the tested gas is placed between the laser and the detector, then the modulation of radiation amplitude occurs with a function determined by the shape of its absorption characteristics in the tested wavelength range. It is caused by the dependence of the gas absorption cross-section on the wavelength. At the point where the absorption line of the tested gas is located, not only the f_{mod} modulating signal-frequency component will appear at the photodetector output, but also the $2 \times f_{mod}$ signal. The radiation modulated in this way is supplied to the input of LIA amplifier, in which the so-called "$2 \times f_{mod}$" detection occurs (Figure 11.67).

The signal value indicated by the LIA amplifier reaches the maximum value for the absorption line of the measured gas [Figure 11.66(d)]. However, the f_{mod} component at this point will have a value of zero. Therefore, this method enables the detection of a very small change in radiation power

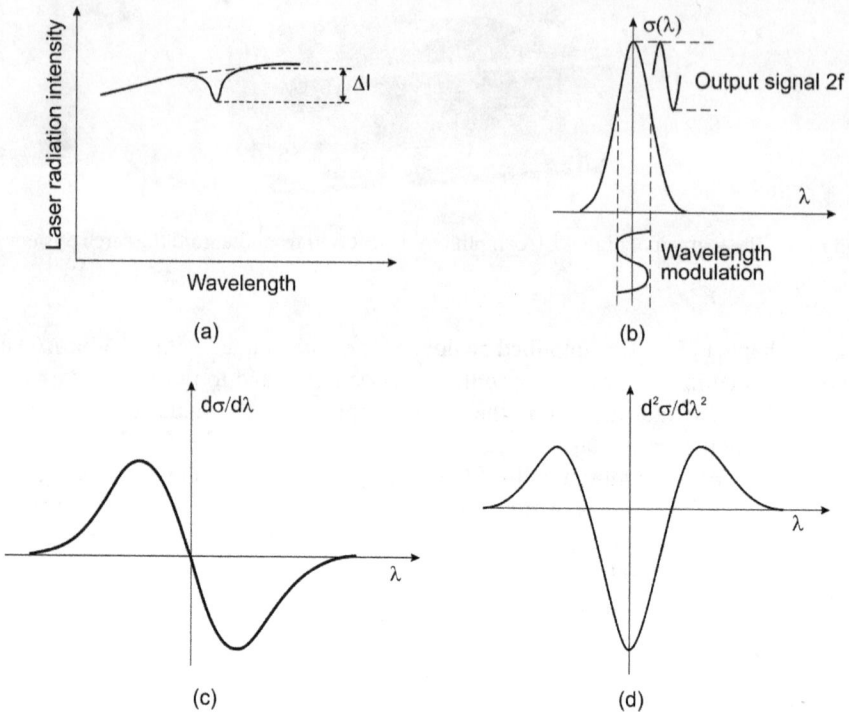

FIGURE 11.66 Measurement of gas concentration: (a) with the DAS method, (b) absorption band of the tested gas (c) first derivative of the absorption band, (d) second derivative of the absorption band.

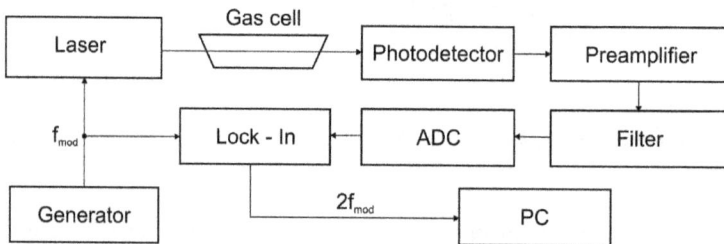

FIGURE 11.67 WMAS circuit diagram.

(caused by the weak absorption line of the tested gas), while maintaining high dynamics of signal changes, limiting the influence of possible interferents and noise. This method achieves detection limits of about 10^{-7} cm^{-1} [58]. The amplitude of the second derivative signal is much greater than the amplitude of the signal obtained in the DAS method, and therefore its measurement allows for increasing the signal-to-noise ratio.

11.10.3 BOXCAR DETECTION SYSTEMS

Phase-sensitive detection systems are used to measure constant intensity and slow-changing signals. In many situations, there is a need to measure the amplitude shape of periodic pulsed signals. In these cases, other measuring methods should be used. One of these methods is the so-called synchronous signal integration (boxcar detection systems, boxcar integrator, boxcar averager or gated integrator [59]). This method enables the measurement of periodic signals, even of complex shapes,

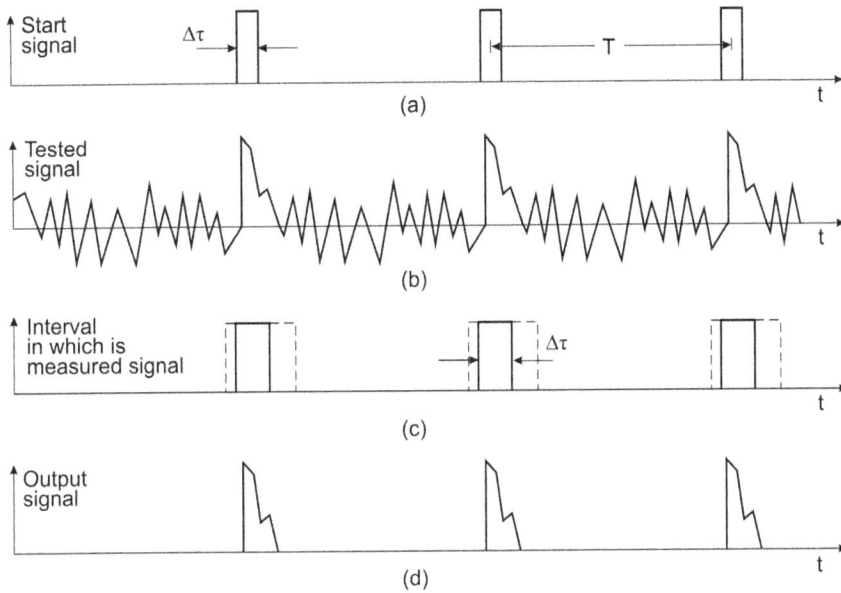

FIGURE 11.68 Time courses in the method with synchronous signal integration: (a) starting signal, (b) measured signal, (c) time interval during which the signal is measured, (d) signal at the output of the detection circuit.

the amplitude of which is lower than the noise level of the input stage of the photoreceiver. In order to apply this method, two basic conditions must be met:

- the tested signal should be periodic; and
- the start signal, which would determine the moment of time when the signal measurement cycle starts, should be provided [Figure 11.68(a)].

The periodicity of the signal in the described method is not absolutely necessary if the information about the moment of appearance of the start signal is known. It can be obtained from a clock generator triggering the signal source, or directly from that source. Figure 11.68 shows the concept of the detection system with synchronous signal integration. A periodic signal is given to the input of the detection system together with a noise of large amplitude [60].

In order to improve the signal-to-noise ratio, first limit the time interval in which the signal will be measured [Figure 11.68(c)], and then repeat the measurements for n periods. This function is implemented by a gated integrator. This integrator consists of a sampling gate (a key) and a RC low-pass filter [Figure 11.69(a)]. Note that if we limit the time of signal measurement to the duration of the sampling gate, then no noise from other time intervals appears at the output of the measurement system [Figure 11.68(d)]. The gated integrator performs two functions: first, it averages the voltage over the gate time, and second, it remembers this voltage value until the next sample is measured. If the key is closed, it starts the process of charging the capacitance C at a rate resulting from the RC time constant [Figure 11.69(b)], called the gate time constant [61].

The integrator should be designed so that the following relation is fulfilled:

$$t_{obs} = t_g \frac{T}{t_m},$$

11.111)

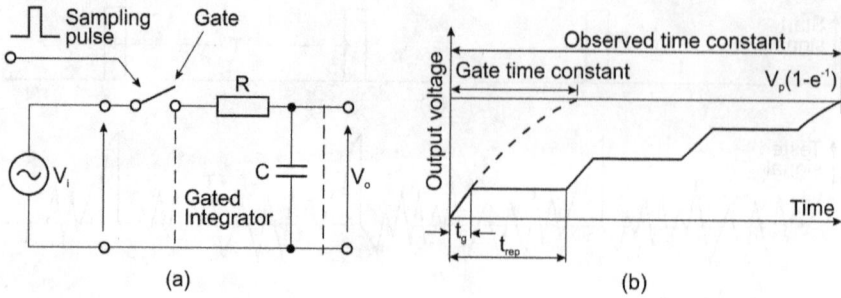

FIGURE 11.69 Gated integrator: (a) schematic diagram, (b) voltage waveform at the output of this circuit.

where t_{obs} is the total measurement time of the signal, t_m is the key-on time, and T is the period of the timing signal. Thus, for a properly designed integrator, the voltage amplitude at its output, during a single measurement cycle, should reach only a few percent of the input voltage amplitude [60].

The integration process removes the high-frequency components of the input signal, thus improving the signal-to-noise ratio. The equivalent noise bandwidth for an *RC* circuit is given by the known relationship

$$\Delta f = \frac{1}{4\tau} = \frac{1}{4RC}. \tag{11.112}$$

After the averaging is completed, the system is set to zero and prepared to measure the next samples.

We can distinguish two types of detection systems with synchronous signal integration:

- static gate work; and
- systems with a dynamic gate (waveform recovery boxcar averager).

The idea of static gate work is shown in Figure 11.70. This circuit is characterised by a constant delay of the gate switching time in relation to the edge of the trigger pulse [59]. Thus, the integration of the signal takes place in well-defined time intervals.

Let us now examine the schematic of a static gate detection system. The diagram of this system is shown in Figure 11.71. This circuit consists of a signal source, a detector-preamplifier circuit, a key, a signal integrator and a control circuit. The control system includes: generator, delay system and multivibrator. The pulses from the control generator are simultaneously applied to the optical signal source and the delay circuit. The signal from the delay circuit triggers the multivibrator, which turns on the key. The key on time depends on the duration of the multivibrator pulse. The source of the signal is usually a laser diode (LD) or a light-emitting diode (LED).

Let us assume that the control generator works with the frequency $f = 1/T$. The delay time of the clock pulse controlling the triggering of the multivibrator is t_d, and the switch-on time of the key is t_m. This time can be programmed with the monostable multivibrator. The front of each clock pulse starts the generation of a light pulse. Figure 11.72 shows the voltage waveforms at the various points of the detection system with synchronous signal integration.

The signal from the detector output after amplification is sent to the electronic key and then to the integrator. The signal $V_k(t)$, that is applied to the integrator is described by the formula

$$V_k(t) \equiv V_D(t) \quad \text{when} \quad t_d \leq t \leq t_d + t_m, \quad V_k(t) \equiv 0 \quad \text{for the others } t. \tag{11.113}$$

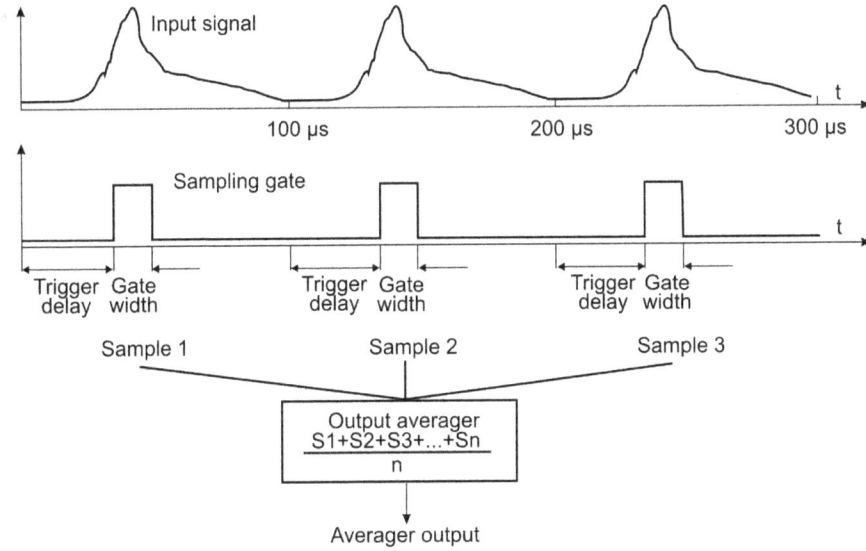

FIGURE 11.70 Idea of static gate circuit operation.

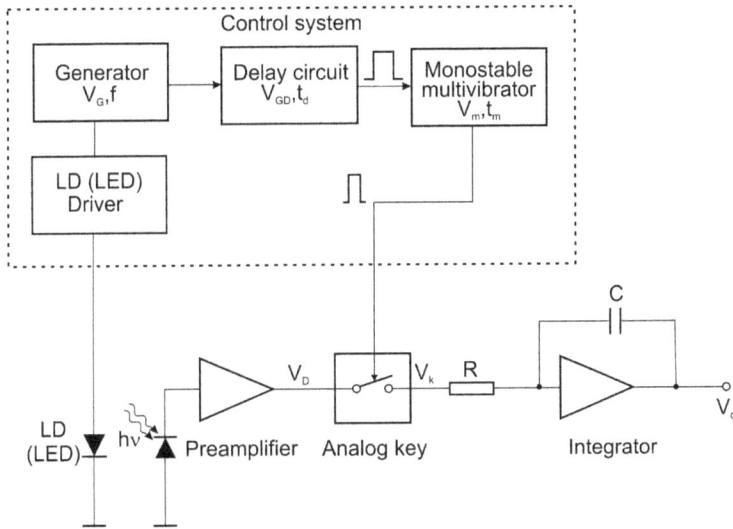

FIGURE 11.71 Analogue synchronous integration system.

Let us try to calculate the voltage at the output of the integrator. Let us assume that the voltage at the output of the integrator is zero at the initial moment and let us carry out measurements for n periods. In order to simplify the initial analysis, let us assume that the system is noiseless. With this assumption, the voltage at the output of the system is

$$V_o\left(t_d\right) = -\frac{1}{RC} n \int_0^T V_k\left(t\right) dt = -\frac{1}{RC} n \int_{t_d}^{t_d+t_m} V_D\left(t\right) dt, \qquad (11.114)$$

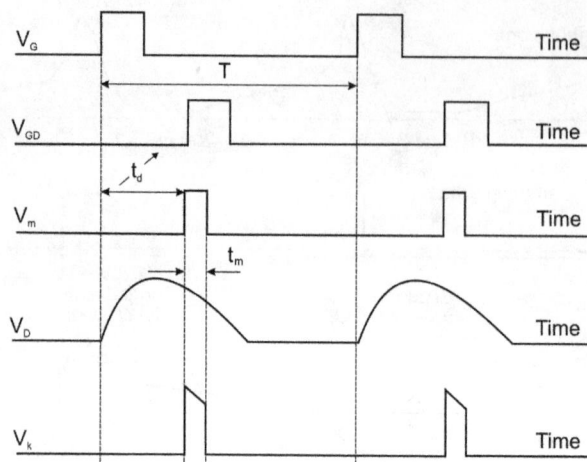

FIGURE 11.72   Waveforms of the signal in individual points in "boxcar" integrator.

where R and C represent the value of the resistance and capacitance of the integrating circuit, respectively. The 'minus' sign is due to the fact that the voltage signal from the output of the analogue key is usually applied to the inverting input of the integrator. If the time interval t_m is sufficiently small, the value of the amplitude of the output signal will not change significantly during the time interval from t_d to $t_d + t_m$. Thus equation (11.114) will take the form

$$V_o\left(t_d\right) = -\frac{n}{RC}V_D\left(t\right)t_m.$$ (11.115)

From this formula it follows that the value of the voltage at the output of the integrating system $V_o(t_d)$ is directly proportional to the instantaneous value of the voltage at the output of the preamplifier $V_D(t)$, the number of measurement periods n, and the duration of the pulse t_m, while inversely proportional to the time constant of the integrator. Thus, the detection system with synchronous signal integration makes it possible to increase the amplitude of the output signal by increasing the number of measurement cycles n.

In practice, the voltage signal will always occur in the presence of unwanted noise $V_{ni}(t)$. The noise is a random process and therefore takes on different values in successive measurement cycles. The noise voltage at the output of a system with synchronous integration is described by the formula

$$V_{no} = k\sum_{i=1}^{m} \int_{t_d}^{t_d+t_m} V_n(iT+t)dt,$$ (11.116)

where $k = -1/RC$, $V_n(iT+t)$ is the noise voltage during the i-th pulse at a time, t, from its start.

Due to its random nature, an average value can be predicted. Using Eq. (11.96), for white noise of power spectral density S_n, the mean value of the noise power for a single measurement cycle is given by

$$P_{no} = \frac{k^2}{2}S_n t_m.$$ (11.117)

Thus, the rms value of the noise voltage at the output of the circuit for a single integration cycle is

$$V_{no} = \left(P_{no}\right)^{1/2} = k\left(\frac{S_n t_m}{2}\right)^{1/2}. \qquad (11.118)$$

The input total noise power will be

$$P_{ni} = S_n \Delta f, \qquad (11.119)$$

where Δf is noise equivalent bandwidth. Therefore, the rms input noise voltage is given by the formula

$$V_{ni} = \left(S_n \Delta f\right)^{1/2}. \qquad (11.120)$$

Transforming equations (11.118) and (11.120) we obtain

$$V_{no} = kV_{ni}\left(\frac{t_m}{2\Delta f}\right)^{1/2}. \qquad (11.121)$$

This expression is only valid if the noise spectrum has a uniform density in the frequency range from f_{min} do f_{max}. Whereby, the condition $f_{min} \ll 1/t_m$, and $f_{max} \gg 1/t_m$ should be satisfied.

After taking the noise into account, the value of the voltage signal at the output of the system with synchronous signal integration after n measurement cycles will be

$$V_0' = nkV_D\left(t_d\right)t_m \pm V_{no}\left(n\right)^{1/2}. \qquad (11.122)$$

Using Equations (11.117) and (11.119), the signal power and noise power, at the output of the system, for a single integration cycle is

$$P_{so} = V_D^2\left(t_d\right)t_m^2 k^2, \quad P_{no} = \frac{k^2}{2}\frac{P_{ni}}{\Delta f}t_m. \qquad (11.123)$$

Therefore, the expression for the signal to noise power ratio becomes

$$\frac{S}{N} = 2\frac{V_D^2\left(t_d\right)}{V_{ni}^2}t_m \Delta f, \qquad (11.124)$$

instead, the ratio of the signal voltage to the noise voltage is

$$\left(\frac{S}{N}\right)_{volt} = \frac{V_D\left(t_d\right)}{V_{ni}}\left(2t_m \Delta f\right)^{1/2}. \qquad (11.125)$$

After n measurement cycles, the signal voltage increases n times, and the RMS value of the noise voltage – $\sqrt{n}$ times. In this case, the ratio of the signal voltage to the noise voltage is

$$\left(\frac{S}{N}\right)_{volt} = \frac{nV_D\left(t_d\right)}{n^{1/2}V_{ni}}\left(2t_m\Delta f\right)^{1/2} = \frac{V_D\left(t_d\right)}{V_{ni}}\left(2nt_m\Delta f\right)^{1/2}, \qquad (11.126)$$

and has risen $\sqrt{n}$ times.

This measurement system is called a synchronous integration system, because the samples are summed synchronously with the measurement cycles of the signal. Systems with synchronous integration are very efficient in recovering information carried by a sequence of periodic pulses whose amplitude is smaller than the noise level of the photodetector-preamplifier system.

The improvement in signal-to-noise ratio S/N obtained by measuring the signal for n cycles comes at the expense of measurement time. This time, for a given delay t_d, will be equal to nT. The disadvantage of the considered method is that most of the time the integrator is not connected to the input. The measurement of the voltage at the output of the photodetector-preamplifier system takes place only in the time interval t_m/T (i.e., when the key is on).

In measuring systems, there is often a need to determine the shape of the tested signal. So let us follow the system with a dynamic gate. The idea behind the operation of this system is presented in Figure 11.73. To do this, follow the algorithm below:

- set a delay time t_d;
- reset the integrator;
- perform signal integration for n pulses of the control generator;
- note the voltage value obtained at the output of the integrator;
- increase time t_d by the value of t_m;
- reset the voltage at the integrator output again;
- perform the measurement for n generator pulses; and
- note the result.

These activities should be repeated until a set of values, $V_0'(t_d)$, is obtained, which will enable the reconstruction of the shape of the measured signal. Thus, in order to measure the pulse shape,

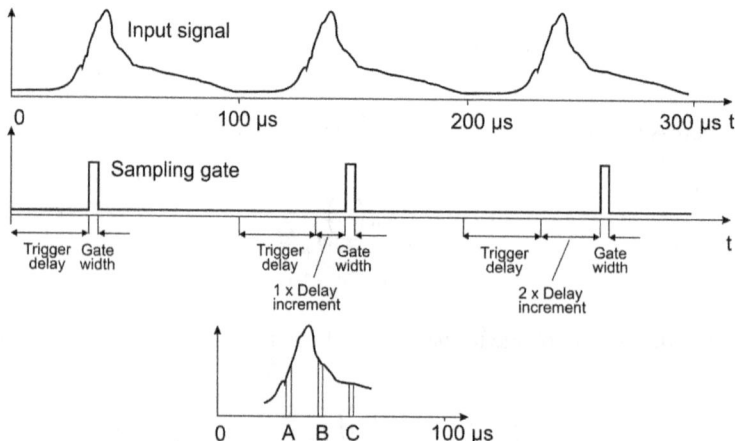

FIGURE 11.73   The idea of operation system with dynamic gate.

the measurement of T/t_m needs to be repeated many times, for each value of t_d. Hence, the time required to measure the pulse shape will be nT^2/t_m. The total measurement time can be reduced by increasing the single sampling time t_m. However, this will reduce the ability to observe the details of the pulse [59].

The signal theory shows that the optimal sampling time should meet the condition

$$t_m \leq \frac{1}{2f_{max}}. \tag{11.127}$$

A smaller value of the time t_m increases the required measurement time, while a higher value limits the possibilities of observing the pulse details. This detection system is not efficient because most of the signal power is lost when the key is open. The multiplexed analogue synchronous integration system does not have this disadvantage [61].

The use of the multiplex method makes the measurement faster and more efficient. However, fully analogue systems are rarely used today. This is because it is difficult to design a circuit with many identical switches and analogue integrators. Moreover, such systems are too expensive. Therefore, digital signal processing methods have developed rapidly in the last few decades. They are cheaper than analogue circuits, and their level of technical utility is difficult to achieve with analogue methods.

Currently there are commercially available cards that perform the functions of detection circuits with synchronous signal integration. A photograph of the four-channel M4i4451-x8 card, which is characterised by high resolution, high sensitivity and a wide dynamic range, is shown in Figure 11.74 [63]. Detailed data on this card can be found in publication [62].

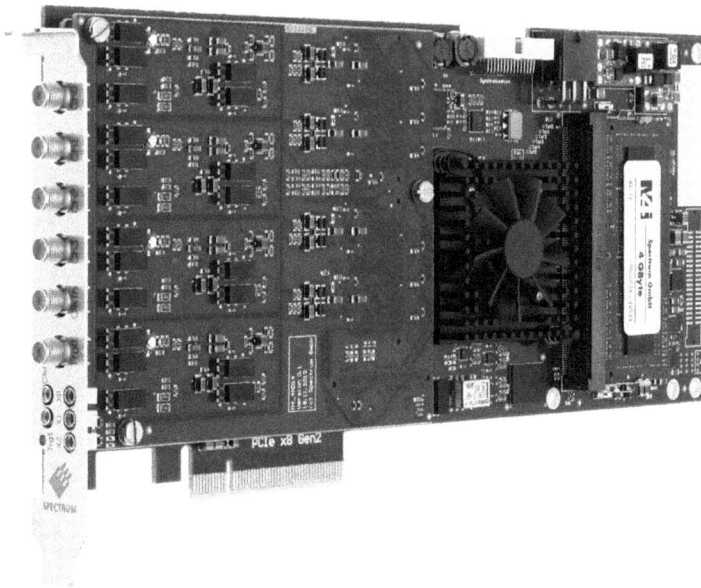

FIGURE 11.74 A photo of a card that performs the functions of detection circuits with synchronous signal integration.

11.10.4 COHERENT DETECTION

So far, we have considered systems that were based on the modulation of the light intensity in a transmitter and direct detection of this in a photoreceiver. It was not essential for the modulated light wave to be a coherent wave and its spectrum could be wide. These systems are simple and cheap, but they have constraints on their transmission possibilities. The photoreceivers decoded only the information connected with the intensity or with the square of the electromagnetic field amplitude, whereas information also can be carried by its phase and frequency. The possible photoreceiver sensitivity results from the basic noise limits, as the noise of the photodetector, preamplifier and background.

To improve the signal-to-noise ratio, it would be an advantage to increase the photocurrent at the detector output. We have already noted that using photoreceivers with APDs had constraints resulting from additional multiplication noises. To avoid problems with direct detection, coherent detection, a method of receiving based on interference of two beams of coherent laser radiation, can be used. Figure 11.75 illustrates the differences between coherent detection and direct detection.

Figure 11.75(a) presents a direct detection system. To narrow the received optical bandwidth, we have applied a filter to limit the spectral range of radiation reaching the detector – Figure 11.75(b). For example, optical filters based on the Bragg effect can have 5-nm bandwidth for 1.56 μm wavelengths, corresponding to a detection band, Δf, equal to 600 GHz [65]. This wide bandwidth of what is a reasonably narrow optical filter illustrates that application of an optical filter cannot easily ensure narrow wavelength selection of a photoreceiver. A widely spaced Fabry-Perot filter can achieve bandwidth of several hundred MHz but is costly and difficult to stabilise, so impractical

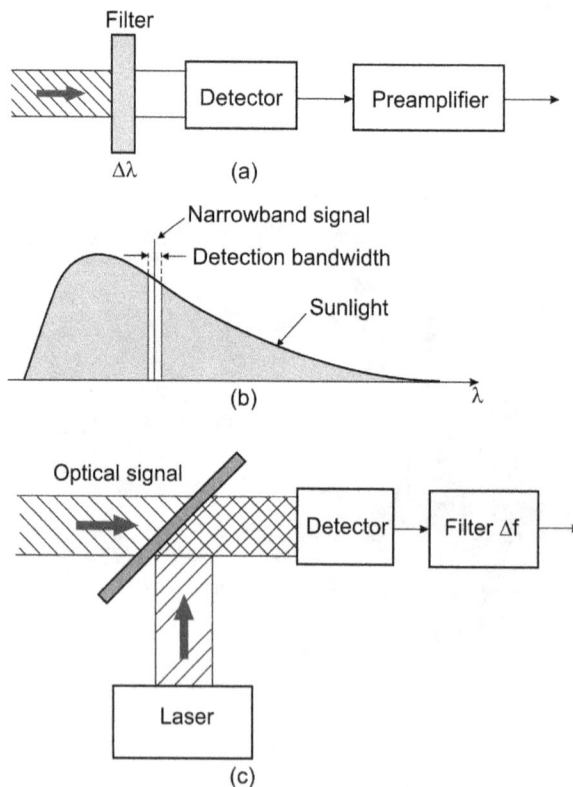

FIGURE 11.75   Comparison of coherent versus incoherent optical detection (after Reference 64).

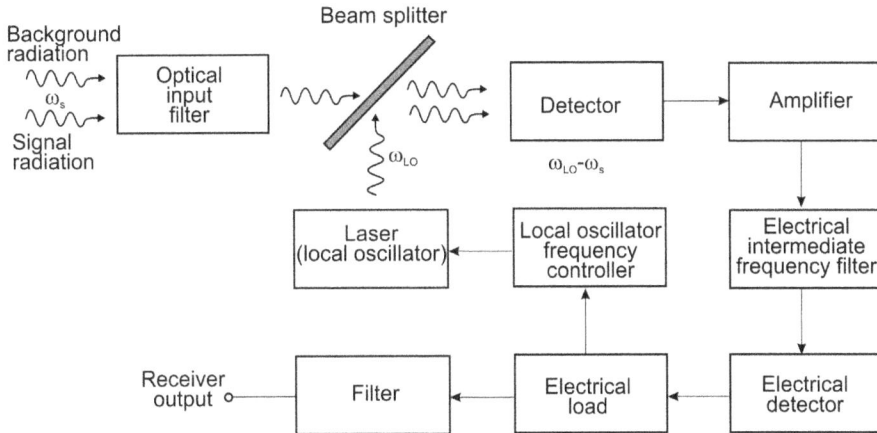

FIGURE 11.76   Block diagram of heterodyne detection optical receiver.

for most systems. However, the simple addition of a beam-splitter and an additional coherent light source, a so-called local oscillator, provides a coherent detection scheme that can use either heterodyne or homodyne detection systems [see Figure 11.75(c)].

Heterodyne detection technique has been commonly used for many years in commercial and domestic radio receivers and also for the microwave range of an electromagnetic spectrum. The main virtues of this method detection are higher sensitivity, higher and more easily obtained selectivity, plus the possibility of detection of all types of modulation and easier tuning over wide ranges [66]. Coherent optical detection has been developed since 1962, but compact and stable production of this system is more difficult, and the system is more expensive and troublesome than its radio-technique equivalent. The basic block diagram of heterodyne optical receiver is shown in Figure 11.76.

Laser radiation containing information is, after being passed through an input optical filter and beam splitter, arranged to coherently combine or 'mix' with a light beam of a local oscillator at the detector surface. A beam-splitter can be made in many ways, the simplest being a glass plate with adequate refraction coefficient. In a general case, a device fulfilling such a role is called a direction coupler, as an analogy to microwave or radio devices. A detector used for signal mixing has to have a square-law characteristic to detecting electronic field of the light, but this is conveniently typical of most optical detectors (photodiode, photoconductor, photomultiplier, APD, etc.). This signal is next amplified. An electrical filter of intermediate frequency (IF) extracts the desired difference component of the signal, which next undergoes a demodulation process. The design and operation principle of the subsequent electrical detector depends on the nature of the modulation of a signal. The signal from a load resistance passes through an output filter to a receiver output and, by means of a local oscillator frequency controller, it controls a laser. A frequency control loop is used for the local oscillator laser to maintain a constant frequency difference $\omega_L - \omega_s = \omega_p$ with the input signal. An indispensable condition for efficient coherent detection is to match the polarisation, and to shape both waveforms of both beams to match the profile of the detector surface.

Expression for the signal-to-noise ratio at the heterodyne detection system with APD for $P_L \gg P_s$ is given by

$$\frac{S}{N} = \frac{2R_i M \sqrt{P_s P_L}}{\left(2q\Delta f M^{2+x} R_i P_L + \dfrac{4kT\Delta fF}{R_L}\right)^{1/2}} \approx \left(\frac{R_i P_s}{q\Delta f M^x}\right)^{1/2}. \qquad (11.128)$$

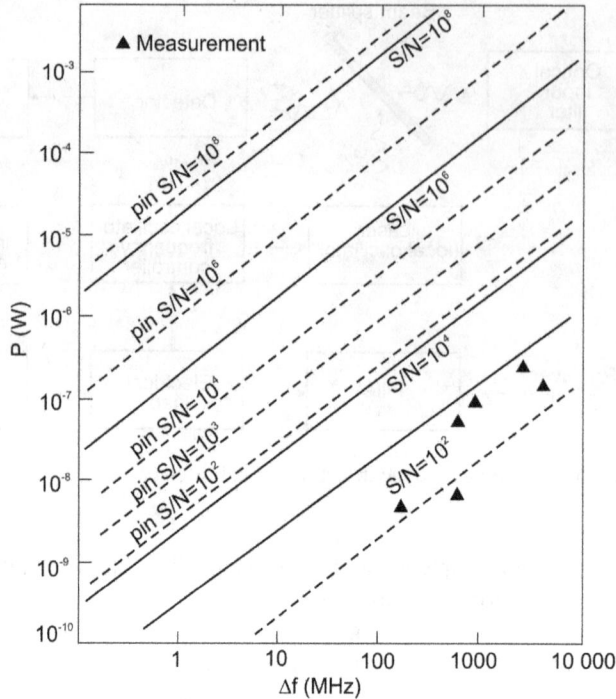

FIGURE 11.77   Sensitivity of the coherent photoreceiver (dashed line) and p-i-n photodiode (solid line) [34].

Assuming a photodiode responsivity $R_i = \eta q / h\nu$, usually in A/W, we have

$$\frac{S}{N} = \frac{\eta P_s}{h\nu\Delta f M^x} = 2\left(\frac{S}{N}\right)_{quanta}. \tag{11.129}$$

Figure 11.77 shows a comparison of coherent detection sensitivity (solid lines) with the sensitivity of direct p-i-n photodiode detection ($M = 1$) for the same values of signal-to-noise ratio. Significant improvement in sensitivity can be observed for weak signals. Higher sensitivity of a detector ensures qualitatively better detection as increased information bit rate or can permit longer communications links to be used between each regenerator circuit. In long-distance fibre telecommunications, however, the use of optical fibre amplifier has taken much of the impetus from development of the coherent receiver, although the latter still have the unique advantage of highly selective narrowband detection.

In heterodyne detection, the spectrum of laser modulation was shifted into an IF range, so selectivity of a photoreceiver depends on the bandwidth of the IF amplifier. This is arranged electronically, so it can easily be sufficiently narrow. Having a narrow IF circuit bandwidth is especially important for detection of multichannel signals.

In practice, the technique of heterodyne detection is used for construction of Doppler velocimeters and laser rangefinders as well as in spectroscopy (particular LIDAR systems). It may yet find application in more telecommunications systems.

If a signal frequency is equal to the frequency of a local oscillator, the IF frequency equals zero. It is a special case of coherent detection, so-called homodyne detection. In a homodyne detection optical receiver (Figure 11.78), the incoming laser carrier is again combined with a reference wave from a local laser on a photodiode surface, but in this case both frequencies are the same.

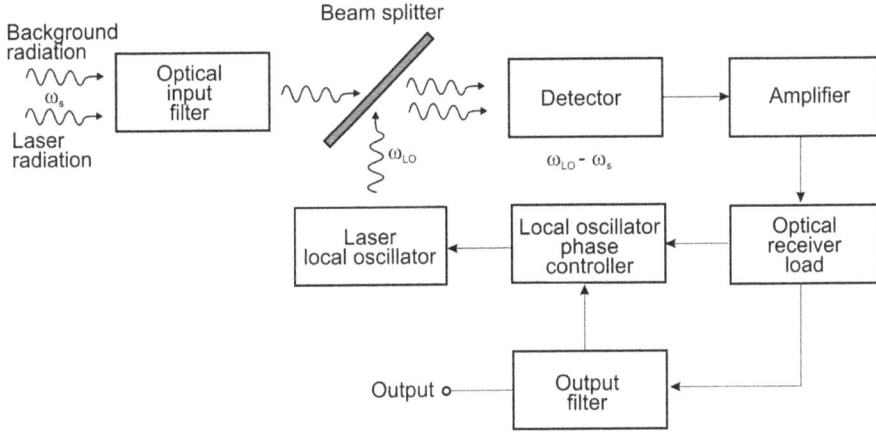

FIGURE 11.78 Block diagram of homodyne detection optical receiver (after 34).

The photodetector current in a homodyne receiver is given by

$$I_{hom} = R_i M \left(P_s + P_L \right) + 2 R_i M \left(P_s P_L \right)^{1/2} \cos \varphi_p \left(t \right).$$ (11.130)

The first component is a direct-current component, but the second one contains the useful information regarding the optical signal. The current at the detector output increases with increase in local oscillator power and with the optical receiver responsivity.

If the local oscillator power is high, the shot noise originating from a signal current, thermal noise and dark-current noise can be omitted. For amplitude modulation we have

$$\frac{S}{N} = \frac{\left(2 R_i M (P_s P_L)^{1/2} \right)^2 R_L}{\left(2 q \Delta f M^{2+x} R_i P_L + 4 k T \Delta f F / R_L \right) R_L} \approx \frac{2 R_i P_s}{q \Delta f M^x} = \frac{2 \eta P_s}{q \Delta f M^x}.$$ (11.131)

As can be seen, the signal-to-noise ratio for homodyne detection is twice as high as heterodyne detection. This is basically because the homodyne detector allows direct addition or subtraction of the electrical fields, depending on whether the signal and local oscillator are in phase or 180° out of phase. With heterodyne detection, the relative phases change linearity with time, and mixing of signals is not effective when signals have 90° or 270° phase differences.

As it results from Eq. (11.130), homodyne detection derives the baseband modulation signal carrying the information directly. Thus, further electronic demodulation is not required.

Homodyne receivers are used in the most sensitive coherent systems. In practice, construction of such receivers is difficult because

- the local oscillator must be locked to keep a constant zero phase difference to the incoming optical signal, and this requires excellent spectral purity; and
- power fluctuation of the local laser must be eliminated.

Constant difference of both laser phases can be achieved using an optical phase-locked loop.

The requirements for spectrum purity are less critical in the diversity systems [65, 67] in which the cosine component current expressed by Eq. (11.130) and also the quadrature current component

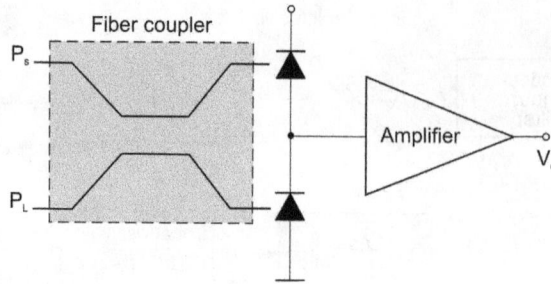

FIGURE 11.79 Balanced mixing receiver with fibre coupler and series connection of the photodiodes.

proportional to $sin\phi_p t$ are produced. A sum of vectors of these currents makes it possible to avoid influence of ϕ_p phase change, but as with the heterodyne system, the SNR suffers when phases are not identical. It has been assumed that the local laser has no amplitude noise. In practice, this type of noise, is often the limiting factor, because the local laser power is strong compared with signal component $2(P_s P_L)^{1/2}$. If detecting these output waves by means of photodiodes, give the corresponding currents

$$I_1 \propto a^2 P_s + b^2 P_L + 2ab\left(P_s P_L\right)^{1/2} \cos\left[2\pi f_s t - \omega_L t + \varphi_s(t) - \varphi_L(t) + \pi/2\right], \quad (11.132)$$

$$I_2 \propto b^2 P_s + a^2 P_L - 2ab\left(P_s P_L\right)^{1/2} \cos\left[2\pi f_s t - \omega_L t + \varphi_s(t) - \varphi_L(t) + \pi/2\right]. \quad (11.133)$$

This noise is contained in the terms $b^2 P_L$ and $a^2 P_L$ respectively. If we assume a symmetrical beam combiner ($a = b$), and the currents I_1 and I_2 are subtracted, then the terms containing P_s and P_L cancel out, and so do their amplitude fluctuations. Due the opposite sign of the third term in equations (11.132) and (11.133), the output signal from the subtractor is doubled. Using the two outputs in this way produces a balanced mixing receiver, using a beam splitter or fibre coupler (Figure 11.79).

In order to make the interference of the signal wave and the local oscillator wave that is received more efficient, their polarisation states must coincide. Due to random vibration in the fibre and temperature changes, mechanical strain in the fibre introduces birefringence, which changes with time. As a consequence, the polarisation state of the signal received changes randomly.

The problems caused by a polarisation mismatch can be overcome in the following ways by

- using a polarisation state controller;
- polarisation scrambling (the polarisation state is deliberately changed at the transmitting end);
- use of polarisation-maintaining fibres (this solution is more expensive); and
- using polarisation diversity (both the local optical wave and signal wave received are split into two orthogonal polarisation states).

PROBLEMS

Example 11.1

An InGaAs photodiode p-i-n has the following parameters: responsivity $R_i = 0.85$ A/W, dark current $I_d = 0.3$ nA, and a bandwidth of 30 MHz. Radiation with a power of 200 nW falls on the detector surface. Find the various noise terms of the photoreceiver and signal-to-noise ratio if $R_L = 10$ kΩ.

Example 11.2

Photoreceiver with p-i-n photodiode has responsivity $R_i = 0.6$ A/W, photocurrent $I_{ph} = 10$ nA and dark current $I_d = 1$ nA. Calculate the *NEP* if the load resistor R_L is 10 kΩ.

Example 11.3

Consider p-i-n photodiode with $I_{ph} = 50$ nA and dark current $I_d = 0.5$ nA. Find the resistance R_L at which the thermal noise will be less than the shot noise.

Example 11.4

A photoreceiver has *NEP* of 2×10^{-13} W/Hz$^{1/2}$. Calculate the optical signal power assuming a signal-to-noise ratio of 1 and the operation bandwidth of 500 MHz.

Example 11.5

Consider the InGaAs p-i-n photodiode used in a photoreceiver as in Figure 11.17 with a load resistance of 10 kΩ. The photodiode dark current is 1 nA. The bandwidth of the photodiode-preamplifier circuit is 1 MHz. Assuming that the preamplifier is noiseless, calculate the SNR when the incident radiant flux is 2 nW and the current responsivity $R_i = 1.1$ A/W at a peak wavelength of 1550 nm.

Example 11.6

For data from Example 11.5 and the preamplifier noise voltage $V_n = 4$ nV/Hz$^{1/2}$, calculate the signal-to-noise ratio.

Example 11.7

Now let us use a transimpedance preamplifier with $R_f = 10$ kΩ and $I_n = 5$ fA/Hz$^{1/2}$. For the data from Example 11.5, calculate the signal-to-noise ratio.

Example 11.8

An InGaAs APD photodiode has the following parameters: unmultiplied dark current $I_d = 0.1$ nA, multiplication $M = 30$, index $x = 0.7$, quantum efficiency $\eta = 0.8$, wavelength $\lambda = 1.55$ μm, and a bandwidth of 1 MHz. Radiation with a power of 1 nW falls on the detector surface. Find signal-to-noise ratio of the photodiode.

Example 11.9

For data from Example 11.5, calculate the signal-to-noise ratio if $R_L = 10$ kΩ.

Example 11.10

Let us consider the influence of the transimpedance preamplifier noise on the signal-to-noise ratio of the APD-preamplifier system, assuming a transimpedance preamplifier with $R_f = 10$ kΩ, $V_n = 1$ nV/Hz$^{1/2}$, and $I_n = 5$ fA/Hz$^{1/2}$. Data as in Example 11.9.

REFERENCES

1. C.D. Motchenbacher and J.A. Connelly, *Low-Noise Electronic System Design*, John Wiley, New York, 1995.
2. A. Rogalski, Z. Bielecki and J. Mikołajczyk, "Detection of optical radiation", in: *Handbook of Optoelectronics*, Vol. 1, pp. 65–123, 2nd edition, edited by J.P. Dakin and R.G.W. Brown, CRC Press, Boca Raton, 2018.
3. J.L. Vampola, "Readout electronics for infrared sensors", in: *The Infrared and Electro-Optical Systems Handbook*, Vol. 3, pp. 285–342, edited by W.D. Rogatto, SPIE Press, Bellingham, 1993.
4. K. Achtenberg, J. Mikolajczyk, Z. Bielecki, "FET input voltage amplifier for low frequency noise measurement", *Metrol. Meas. Syst.* 27(3), 541–557 (2020).
5. "TOSHIBA field effect transistor silicon n channel junction type", www.mouser.com/ds/2/408/6909-57550.pdf.
6. "BF862 N-channel junction FET", www.nxp.com/docs/en/data-sheet/BF862.pdf.
7. "AN-6602 Low Noise JFET – the noise problem solver", Fairchild Semiconductor, www.onsemi.com/pub/Collateral/AN-6602.pdf.
8. S. Prassad, H. Schumacher, and A. Gopinath, *High-Speed Electronics and Optoelectronics*, Cambridge University Press, Cambridge, 2009.
9. L. Rossi, P. Fischer, T. Rohe, and N. Wermes, *Pixel Detectors. From Fundamentals to Applications*, Springer, Heidelberg, 2006.
10. A. Van Der Ziel, *Noise in Measurements*. John Wiley, New York, 1976.
11. H. Kressel, *Semiconductor Devices for Optical Communication*. Topics in Applied Physics, Vol. 39, Springer, Berlin, 1980.
12. "CLC5509 ultra low noise preamplifier", www.elenota.pl/datasheet-pdf/28269/National Semiconductor/CLC5509.
13. F.A. Levinzon, "Ultra-low-noise high-input impedance amplifier for low-frequency measurement applications", *IEEE Trans. Circuits Syst.* 55(7), 1815–1822 (2008).
14. A. Kay, *Operational Amplifier Noise. Techniques and Tips for Analyzing and Reducing Noise*, Elsevier, Oxford, 2012.
15. G. Keiser, *Optical Fiber Communications*, McGraw Hill, Boston, 2000.
16. S. Donati, *Photodetectors: Devices, Circuits and Applications*, Prentice Hall, New York, 2000.
17. P. Kalinowski, J. Mikolajczyk, A. Piotrowski, and J. Piotrowski, "Recent advances in manufacturing of miniaturized uncooled IR detection modules", *Semicond. Sci. Technol.* 34, 033002, 1–49 (2019).
18. B.C. Baker, "Improved noise performance of the ACF2101 switched integrator", Burn-Brown, Application Bulletin, 1993.

19. *InSb Photoconductive Detectors P6606 Series*. Hamamatsu. Cat. No KIRD 1026E11, 2012.

20. A. Rogalski, *Infrared Detectors*, 2nd edition, CRC Press, Boca Raton, 2011.

21. *PB-300 Preamplifiers. Operating instruction*. Teledyne Judson Technologies, 2002.

22. *Analog Devices Circuit Note CN-0272*, AD8065.

23. *Low Power, Low Noise Precision FET Op Amp*, AD795. Analog Devices. Data Sheet, 2019.

24. *Photomultiplier Tubes. Basics and Application*, 3rd edition, Photon is Our Business. Hamamatsu, 2007. www.hamamatsu.com/resources/pdf/etd/PMT_handbook_v3aE.pdf.

25. A.G. Wright, "Why photomultipliers need amplifiers", *Photonics Spectra*, November 2002.

26. *Example Amplifier Circuits*, Dexter Research Center, 2004.

27. *Preamplifiers For Electro-Optic Detectors*. Everett Infrared, 2009.

28. "Thermal detectors", Chapter 07, Hamamatsu Handbook. www.hamamatsu.com/resources/pdf/ssd/e07_handbook_Thermal_detectors.pdf.

29. F.U. Amin, "On the design of an analog front-end for an X-ray detector", Lamberd Academic Publishing, Linkoping, 2009.

30. M. Dahoumane, D. Dauvergne, J. Krimmer, J.L. Ley, E. Testa, and Y. Zoccarato, "A low noise and high dynamic range CMOS integrated electronics associated with double sided silicon strip detectors for a Compton camera gamma-ray detecting system", *IEEE Nuclear Science Symposium and Medical Imaging Conference* (NSS/MIC), 1–6, Seattle, 2014.

31. W.T. Evariste, M.I. Adolphe, T. Daniel, and D.Y. Arnaud, "Noise optimisation of readout front ends in MOS technology with PS circuit", *Asian J. Appl. Sci.* 02, 752–761 (2014).

32. K. Holejko, R. Nowak, "Continuous wave laser celiometer with code modulation for measurements of cloud base height", *Opto-Electron. Rev.* 8, 195–199 (2000).

33. R.G. Smith, C.A. Brackett, and T.A. Reinbold, "Optical detector package", *Bell Syst. Tech. J.* 57(6) 1809–1822 (1978).

34. A. Rogalski, Z. Bielecki, *Detekcja sygnałów optycznych*, wydanie II, PWN (in Polish).

35. Z. Bielecki, "Analysis of operations conditions of avalanche photodiode on signal to noise ratio", *Opto-Electron. Rev.* 5, 249–256 (1997).

36. G.H. Rieke, *Detection of Light: From Ultraviolet to the Submillimeter*, Cambridge University Press, Cambridge, 1994.

37. www.elfadistrelec.pl/Web/WebShopImages/landscape_large/1-/01/texas-instruments-opt-101p.jpg.

38. OPT101 *Monolithic Photodiode and Single Supply Transimpedance Amplifier*, Texas Instruments Product Folder, 2015. www.ti.com/lit/ds/symlink/opt101.pdf.

39. www.excelitas.com/sites/default/files/2019-.05/ProductPhoto_RxModule_C30659-series_AP.jpg

40. C30659 Series_Rev. 1.7-2017.07, Excelitas Technologies, www.excelitas.com/

41. K. Kume, "Optical detectors and receivers", in *Handbook of Optoelectronics*, 2nd edition, Vol. 1, pp. 395–430, edited by J.P. Dakin and R.G.W. Brown, CRC Press, Boca Raton, 2018.

42. *Photomultiplier Tubes, Photonics KK*, Catalog Hamamatsu, 2016.

43. B.F. Aull, A.H. Loomis, D.J. Young, R.M. Heinrichs, B.J. Felton, P.J. Daniels, and D.J. Landers, "Geiger-mode avalanche photodiodes for three dimensional imaging", *Linc. Lab. J.* 13(2), 335–350 (2002).

44. G.M. Williams and A.S. Huntington, "Probabilistic analysis of linear mode vs Geiger mode APD FPAs for advanced LIDAR enabled interceptors", *Proc. SPIE* 6220, 622008 (2006).

45. S. Vasile, R.L. Wilson, S. Shera, D. Shamo, and M.R. Squillante, "High gain avalanche photodiode arrays for DIRC applications", *IEEE Trans. Nuclear Science* 46(4), 849–853 (1999).

46. D. Phelan, J.C. Jackson, R.M. Redfern, A.P. Morrison, and A. Mathewson, "Geiger mode avalanche photodiodes for microarray systems", *Proc. SPIE* 4626, 89–97 (2002).

47. J.C.G. Lesurf, *Information and Measurement*, The Institute of Physics, London, 1995.

48. *Signal Recovery. What is a Lock-in Amplifier*. Technical note TN 1000, 2019. www.ameteksi.com/-/media/ameteksi/download_links/documentations/7210/tn1000_what_is_a_lock-in_amplifier.pdf.

49. *About Lock-in Amplifier. Application Note #3*, Stanford Research Systems, www.thinksrs.com/downloads/pdfs/applicationnotes/AboutLIAs.pdf

50. *Signal Recovery. The Analog Lock-in Amplifier*. Technical note TN 1002, 2008. www.ameteksi.com/-/media/ameteksi/download_links/documentations/5210/tn1002_the_analog_lock-in_amplifier.pdf.

51. *Signal Recovery. Specifying Lock-in Amplifiers*. Technical note TN 1001, 2008. www.ameteksi.com/-/media/ameteksi/download_links/documentations/7210/tn1001_specifying_lock-in_amplifiers.pdf.

52. *Signal Recovery. The Digital Lock-in Amplifier.* Technical note TN 1003. www.ameteksi.com/-/media/ameteksi/download_links/documentations/7270/tn1003_the_digital_lock-in_amplifier.pdf.

53. *Low Lewel Optical Detection Using Lock-in Amplifier Techniques.* Application note AN 1003, Perkin Elmer, www.chem.ucla.edu/~craigim/pdfmanuals/appnotes/an1003 (access 25.11.2019).

54. *Digital lock-in amplifiers.* SR 810 and SR 830 DSP lock-in amplifiers, Stanford Research Systems. https://catalog.orixrentec.jp/pdf/21008900.pdf?id=21008900&ex=pdf&k=0a992f996bdc91f289d858 76a8203e0895cca668

55. *The Lock-In Amplifier: Noise Reduction and Phase Sensitive Detection,* http://old.phys.huji.ac.il/~greenwald/el_lab/labC/LockI.pdf

56. G. Kloos, *Application Lock-in Amplifierin Optics,* SPIE Press, Bellingham, 2018.

57. J. Wojtas, Z. Bielecki, T. Stacewicz, J. Mikołajczyk, and M. Nowakowski, "Ultrasensitive laser spectroscopy for breath analysis", *Opto-Electron. Rev.* 20(1), 77–90 (2012).

58. Z. Bielecki, T. Stacewicz, J. Wojtas, and J. Mikołajczyk, "Application of quantum cascade lasers to trace gas detection", *Bull. Pol. Acad. Sci.: Tech. Sci.* 63(2), 515–525 (2015).

59. Signal Recovery. *What is a boxcar averager.* Technical note TN 1005, 2004. http://123.physics.ucdavis.edu/week_1_files/Boxcar_Averager.pdf.

60. https://studylib.net/doc/18327873/box-car-integrator-%E2%80%A2-the-box-car-integrator-is-used-for.

61. J.D.W. Abernethy, "The boxcar detector", *Wireless World,* 576–579, December 1970, www.keithsnook.info/wireless-world-magazine/Wireless-World-1970/The%20Boxcar%20Detector%20-%20J%20D%20W%20Abernethy.pdf.

62. https://spectrum-instrumentation.com/sites/default/files/download/m4i44_manual_english.pdf

63. https://spectrum-instrumentation.com/sites/default/files/m4i4451-x8.png.

64. A. Rogalski and Z. Bielecki, "Detection of optical radiation", *Bulletin of the Polish Academy of Science. Technical Science* 52(1), 43–66 (2004).

65. J.R. Bary and E.A. Lee, "Performance of coherent optical receivers", *Proc. IEEE* 78(8), 1369–1394 (1990).

66. G.P. Agrawal, *Fiber-Optic Communications Systems,* 3rd edition, John Wiley, New York, 2002.

67. S.F. Jackobs, "Optical heterodyne (coherent) detection", *Amer. J. Phys.* 56, 235 (1988).

68. "Compound semiconductor photosensors", Chapter 06. KIRDB0137EA, Hamamatsu.

12 Focal Plane Arrays

The basic concept of a modern imager system is to form a real image of the scene, detect the variation in the imaged radiation and, by suitable electronic processing, create a visible representation of this variation analogous to conventional television cameras. The charge-coupled device (CCD) and complementary metal-oxide-semiconductor (CMOS) image sensor technologies were invented during the late 1960s and early 1970s. Typical camera construction is similar to a digital video camera. Detectors are only a part of usable sensor systems. Instead of a CCD/CMOS image arrays that video and digital still cameras use, the infrared (IR) camera detector (see Figure 12.1) is a focal plane array (FPA) of micrometer-size pixels made of various material sensitive to infrared (IR) wavelengths. Once a detector is selected, optics (lens) material and filters can be selected to somewhat alter the overall response characteristics of an IR camera system.

12.1 INTRODUCTION

The term "focal plane array" (FPA) refers to an assemblage of individual thousands/millions detector picture elements ("pixels") located at the focal plane of an imaging system. Although the definition could include 1D ("linear") arrays as well as 2D arrays, it is frequently applied to the latter. Usually, the optics part of an optoelectronic images device is limited only to focusing of the image onto the detector's array. These so-called "staring arrays" are scanned electronically, usually using circuits integrated with the arrays. The architecture of detector-readout assemblies has assumed a number of forms, which are described in detail, for example, in References 1–4. The types of readout integrated circuits (ROICs) include the function of pixel deselecting, antiblooming on each pixel, subframe imaging, output preamplifiers and may include yet other functions.

In 1970, Boyle and Smith [5] presented the principle of CCD on a transfer of charge packets in the metal–insulator–semiconductor (MIS) structure. Soon after, Amelio *et al.* [6] developed the first working device. In the 1980s, many CCD instrument solutions were developed for use in video cameras [7,8]. At present, the largest CMOS sensors available commercially for photography are "medium format" with a size of about 44 mm×33 mm. CCDs exist in slightly larger sizes up to 54 mm×40 mm with over 60 million pixels (e.g., 8956×6708, pixel size of 6 μm [9]). Larger sensors for scientific applications may have been produced. CCDs above 3 gigapixels offer the largest formats [10]. The resolution the Legacy Survey of Space and Time (LSST) camera [see Figure 12.2(a)] is high enough that a golf ball can be seen from around 15 miles (24 km) away. The largest-format CMOS arrays contain about 4×10^8 pixels.

Invention of CCD devices had a great impact not only on the development of detection systems for imaging in the visible light range, but also on the development of FPAs working in the IR range. Whereas in the early 1980s the technology of IR detector arrays was developed with dimensions

DOI: 10.1201/9781003263098-12

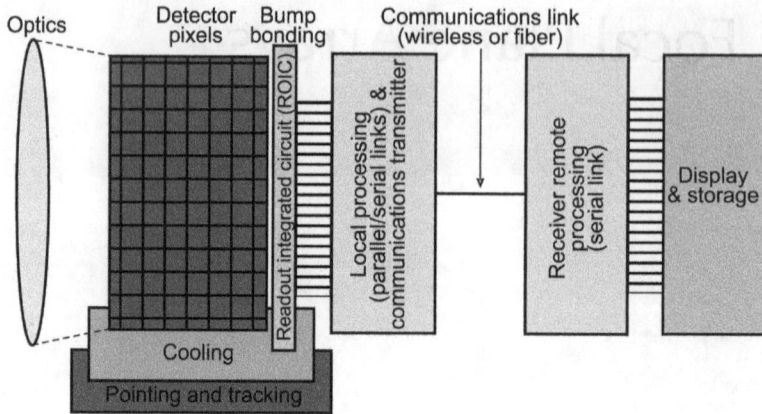

FIGURE 12.1 Schematic representation of an imaging system showing important sub-systems.

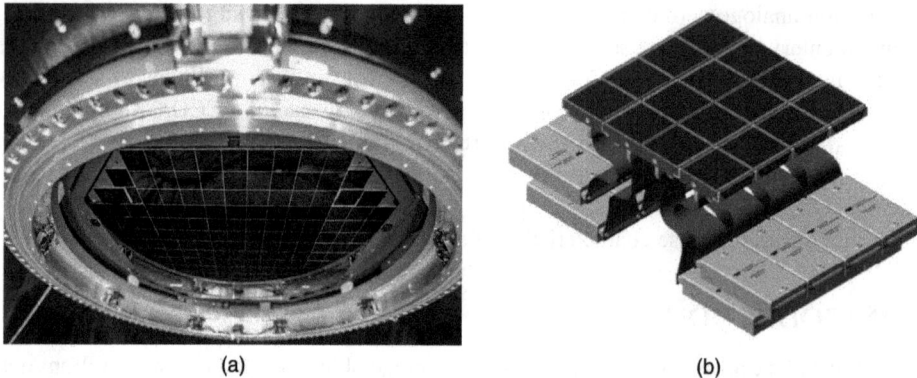

(a)   (b)

FIGURE 12.2 Large format visible and infrared image arrays: (a) the complete focal plane of the future LSST Camera is more than 2 feet wide and contains 189 individual sensors that will produce 3,200-megapixel images. The camera will be installed in Rubin Laboratory (Chile) in 2022; (b) the Euclid HgCdTe focal plane assembly with 16 H2RG arrays and 16 SIDECAR ASIC modules fabricated by Teledyne Imaging Sensors.

of 64×64 pixels, arrays containing about 10^8 pixels are now obtained. The Euclid Near-Infrared Spectrometer and Photometer (NISP) array, which consists of 16 H2RG devices (each with 2k×2k 18-μm pixel size) will be the largest IR array operating in space (67 million pixels): it will be launched soon [11]. These sensor chip assembles (SCAs) were made with a substrate-removed MBE HgCdTe material system with 2.3-μm cut-off wavelength. The SCAs are mounted on a buttable molybdenum package that enables close packing of the 16 flight SCAs in the NISP focal plane [see Figure 12.2(b)].

FPA technology has revolutionised many kinds of imaging, from γ rays to the terahertz and even radio waves, and the rate at which images can be acquired has increased by more than a factor of a billion in many cases. Figure 12.3 illustrates the trend in array size over the past 50 years [12]. Imaging FPAs have been developing in-line with the ability of silicon-integrated circuit (ICs) technology to read and process the array signals, and also to display the resulting image. The progress in arrays has also been steady mirroring the development of dense electronic structures such as dynamic random access memories (DRAMs). Infrared arrays have had nominally the same development rate

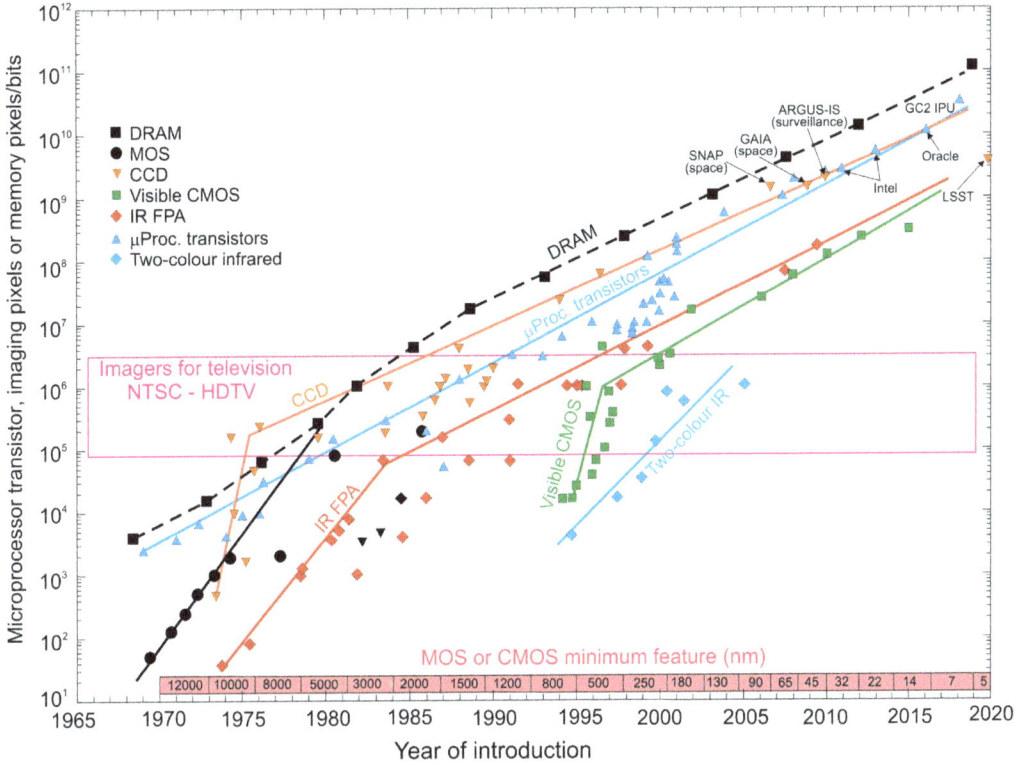

FIGURE 12.3 Imaging array formats compared with the complexity of silicon microprocessor technology and dynamic access memory (DRAM) as indicated by transistor count and memory bit capacity (adapted after Reference 12 with completions). The timeline design rule of MOS/CMOS features is shown at the bottom. Note the rapid rise of CMOS imagers which are challenging CCDs in the visible spectrum. Infrared arrays with size above 100 mega pixels are now available for astronomy applications. Imaging formats of many detector types have gone beyond that required for high-definition TV.

as DRAM ICs, which have followed Moore's Law with a doubling-rate period of approximately 18 months – however, with FPAs lagging DRAMs by about 5–10 years. The 18-month doubling time is evident from the slope of the graph presented in the Figure 12.4, which shows the log of the number of pixels per array as a function of the first year of commercial availability. Array size will continue to increase but perhaps at a rate that falls below the Moore's Law curve. An increase in array size is already technically feasible. However, the market forces that have demanded larger arrays are not as strong now that the megapixel barrier has been broken.

The trend of increasing the pixel's number is likely to continue in the area of large format arrays, constrained only by budgets but not technology. This increase will be continued using a close-butted mosaic of several SCAs. Butting refers to tiling closely together separate pieces of semiconductor to come to one large sensitive array operated as a single image sensor. In most cases butting is used to make imagers that are larger than the largest imager a single wafer can hold.

There are considerable efforts to decrease imaging system size, weight, and power consumption (SWaP) – consequently reducing system cost. The SWaP criterion influences the shrinking of arrays' pixels. Pixel reduction is also mandatory to improve system resolution and reliability. Reduction of the focal plane proportionally to the detector size has not changed the detector's field of view, so in the optics-limited region, smaller detectors have no effect on the system's spatial resolution.

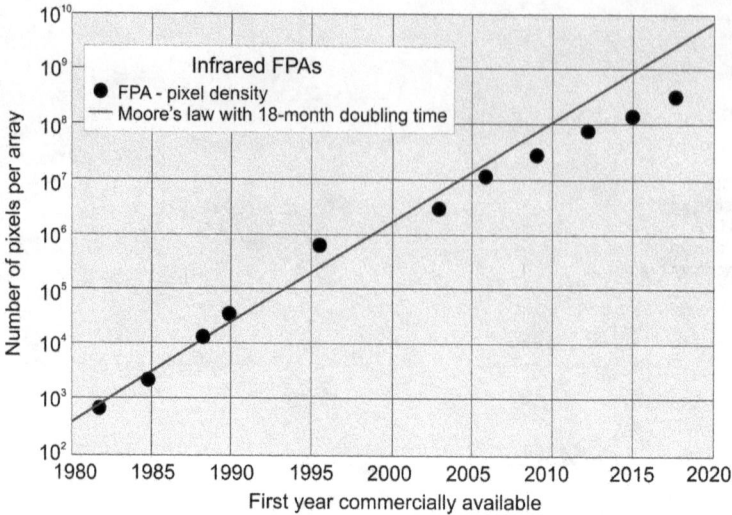

FIGURE 12.4 The number of pixels on an infrared array has been growing exponentially, in accordance with Moore's Law, for 40 years with a doubling time of approximately 18 months. The pixel density of infrared arrays will keep increasing with time but perhaps below Moore's curve.

Currently, various technologies of array detectors with signal processing in the image plane are being developed. In IR devices both scanning systems and staring systems are used. The simplest scanning linear array used in thermal imaging systems consists of a row of detectors [Figure 12.5(a)]. An image is generated by scanning the scene across the strip using, as a rule, a mechanical scanner. At standard video frame rates, at each pixel (detector) a short integration time has been applied, and the total charge is accommodated. In order to achieve a better performance from imaging systems, two-dimensional (2D) detector arrays with signal processing in the image plane of the optical system are used. The staring arrays [Figure 12.5(b)] are scanned electronically.

The scanning system, which does not include multiplexing functions in the focal plane, belongs to the first-generation systems. A typical example of this kind of detector is a linear photoconductive array (PbS, PbSe, HgCdTe) in which an electrical contact for each element of a multielement array is brought off the cryogenically cooled focal plane to the outside, where one electronic channel is used at ambient temperature for each detector element.

The second-generation systems (full-framing systems) being developed at present have at least three orders of magnitude more elements ($> 10^6$) on the focal plane than first-generation systems, and the detector elements are configured in a 2D array. These staring arrays are scanned electronically by circuits integrated with the arrays.

Intermediary systems are also fabricated with multiplexed scanned photodetector linear arrays in use and with, as a rule, time delay and integration (TDI) functions.

In this chapter, we will discuss the principles of operation of linear arrays, CCD and CMOS devices that belong to monolithic arrays, hybrid arrays usually used in infrared systems, and the architecture of FPAs reading systems.

12.2 SMALL ARRAYS

As is marked in the previous section, today's sensors are used in two general configurations: FPAs and arrays of few/tens elements. It is obvious, that small detector assembles are much cheaper than FPA and have a significant dollar-share of the market due to the larger number sold. Table 12.1 compares both sensor configurations.

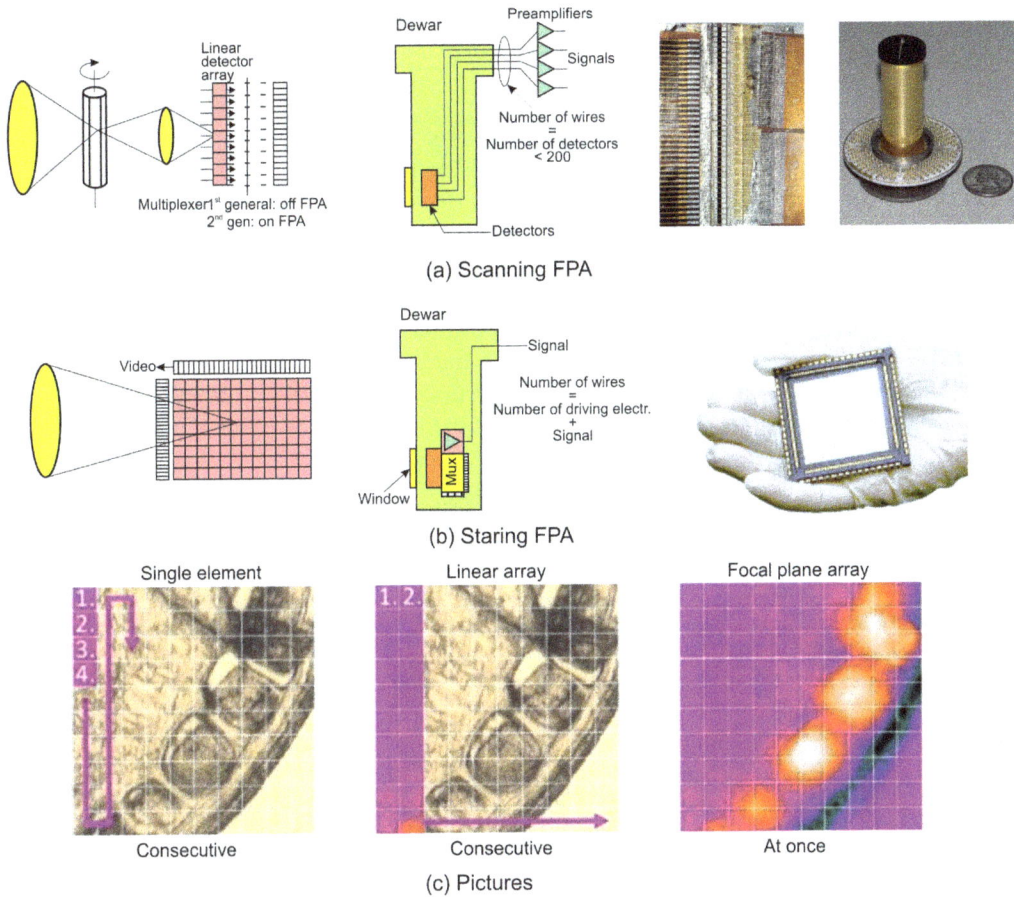

(a) Scanning FPA

(b) Staring FPA

(c) Pictures

FIGURE 12.5 Scanning and staring focal plane arrays. The pictures at the bottom show the working principle of single element, linear array, and focal plane array. As is shown, single-element and line-array approaches are consecutive methods that step by step collect the imaging data.

TABLE 12.1
Comparison of Two General Detector Configurations

Feature	Small detector assembles	FPAs
Detectors (pixels)	A few/tens: 1, 2, 4, 16, 64, 128	Thousand, millions
Relative cost	Low	Expensive
Quantity per year	Many	Few
Electronics	Discrete or small ASICs	ROIC
Primary applications	Various nonimaging and imaging	Imaging

A scanning system [13] is an indispensable component of a device in which the linear arrays are used. A schematic diagram of a conventional serial scan system is shown in Figure 12.5(a). In such a system, the image is mechanically scanned over the surface of discrete detectors. To obtain a TV standard picture, the scanning speed must be high enough. Observation time for a single image pixel is equal to the detector size divided by the scanning speed:

$$\tau_{piksel} = \frac{w}{v_{skan}},$$

(12.1)

where w is the detector size and v_{skan} is the scanning speed.

The signal from each elementary detector is amplified and then multiplexed. In first-generation systems, electrical leads from each elementary array detector are outside the focal plane. In order to increase sensitivity and reduce noise, detectors operating in the IR spectral range are usually cooled. In particularly sensitive systems, important preamplifier components (input FET transistor, feedback resistor) are cooled as well [4].

Preamplifiers for each array detector are made in the form of hybrid circuits composed of discrete elements. A preamplifier is located a few to several millimetres from the detector. It has quite large dimensions, and in the case of cooperation with detectors of high impedance, it is sensitive to electromagnetic disturbances. Such solutions reduce the number of detection channels and arrays surfaces. Typical examples of this type of detection systems are line arrays with PbS, PbSe and HgCdTe photoconductors, containing 64, 128 or 256 detectors [14]. Linear photodiode arrays with Si or InGaAs detectors with a different number of elements are also produced [15].

Intermediate devices between the linear array and the 2D array of detectors are time-delay integration (TDI) systems.

Simple scanning circuits include a single row of detectors that convert scenery lines to an output signal that is then multiplexed to the final video amplifiers. The detector field of view is scanned to image the entire scene. To reduce image flickering, the scene is generally scanned at a rate of 30 to 100 times per second.

Among other things, thermographic devices use detection systems with a serial image analysis, that is, one image line is searched by one n-element linear mosaic. Such a mosaic operating in series is equivalent to a single "super-detector" with a better performance compared to a single detector. To derive the image information, a special TDI signal processing method is used. It consists of a synchronised delaying of signals from successive detectors and then accumulating them.

The signal obtained at the output of the linear array is the sum of signals from the elementary detectors S_e:

$$S_o = \sum_{i=1}^{n} S(i) = nS_e,$$

(12.2)

where n is the number of detectors in the array. The noise, on the other hand, is uncorrelated; hence, the root mean square (RMS) value of the output noise voltage is the root of the sum of the mean square noise voltages of individual detectors:

$$V_{no} = \sqrt{\sum_{i}^{n} V_i^2(i)} = \sqrt{n} V_i^2(i),$$

(12.3)

and $\sqrt{n}$ is greater than the noise of a single detector.

From the above considerations comes the result that the TDI method provides an increase in the signal-to-noise ratio (SNR) compared to the discrete detector. The SNR will be corrected according to the relation

$$SNR \cong \sqrt{n}.$$

(12.4)

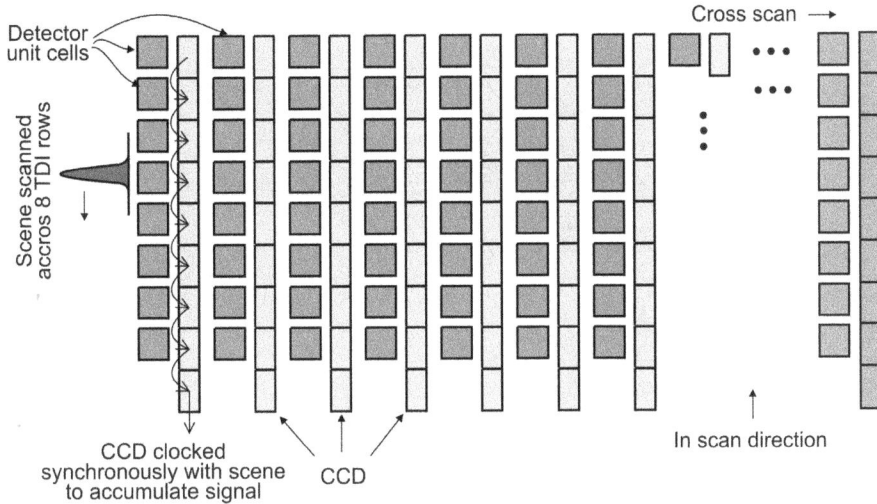

FIGURE 12.6 Diagram of the two-dimensional TDI structure. CCD provides delay between TDI detectors before summing (after Reference 4).

The TDI circuit may be located outside the image plane or as part of the signal processing circuit in the image plane. Figure 12.6 shows a two-dimensional TDI signal-processing array. A typical example of such a system is an HgCdTe detector array consisting of four-line arrays with 288 detectors each. It was optimised for the spectral range of 3–5 μm and 8–10.5 μm [16].

12.3   ARRAYS OF DETECTORS WITH SIGNAL PROCESSING IN THE FOCAL PLANE

FPA architecture is shown in Figure 12.7 [4]. Such a system, apart from radiation detection, also performs various functions related to signal processing from individual detection elements. Electronic circuits performing functions of amplifying, signal integration, background subtraction, component non-uniformity compensation, multiplexing and so on, are called readout integrated circuits (ROIC). Arrays of detectors with signal processing in the image plane are developed in the form of monolithic and hybrid arrays [2,16–19].

12.3.1   MONOLITHIC ARRAYS

In the monolithic approach, both detection of light and signal readout (multiplexing) is done in the detector material rather than in an external readout circuit. The integration of detector and readout onto a single monolithic piece reduces the number of processing steps, increases yields and reduces costs. Common examples of these FPAs in the visible and near infrared (0.7–1.0 μm) are found in camcorders and digital cameras. Two generic types of silicon technology provide the bulk of devices in these markets: charge coupled devices (CCDs) and complementary metal-oxide-semiconductor (CMOS) imagers. CCD technology has achieved the highest pixel counts or largest formats with numbers above 10^9 (see Figure 12.3). CMOS imagers are also rapidly moving to large formats and at present are competed with CCDs. Figure 12.8 shows different architectures of monolithic FPAs.

Currently, low-cost CCD arrays are widely used in cameras, camcorders, scanners, automatic monitoring and control systems, robotics and so forth. Also, for scientific purposes, the range of applications is wide; from imaging the smallest living cells to observing distant stars and

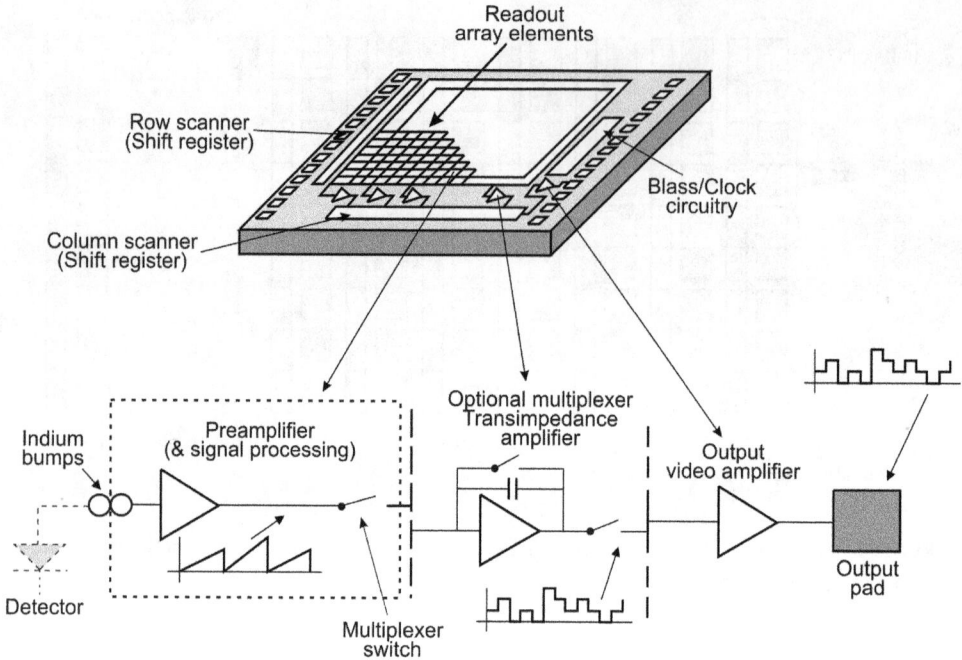

FIGURE 12.7 Diagram of a 2D array of detectors integrated with signal-processing system (signal amplification, data multiplexing, and video output buffering of the signal into a single chip) (after Reference 4).

galaxies (in the latter case, the arrays are placed at the focal points of ground-based and space-based telescopes). Medical applications are also important in mammography, surgery, dentistry and so forth.

A competing technology that has developed over the past twenty years is the CMOS technology. It was developed to produce integrated circuits. However, in the 1990s the work began to adapt this technology to image recording. Its advantage is a relatively simple and cheap production method and the possibility of densely packing transistors as a progress in reducing the design rule. At present, CMOS-based image sensing devices are more preferred owing to their reduced system size and lower power consumption. Sony Corporation has announced its intention to discontinue the delivery/shipment of its CCD image sensors. ·

Figure 12.9 shows the evolution of the CCD and CMOS arrays production growth and their share in the global market [20]. The global image sensors market is estimated to be valued at almost $16 million in 2017 and is forecast to witness a CAGR of 6.2 per cent during 2018–2023. It is expected to move the major market players toward the CMOS technology. Moreover, during the forecast period, the image sensors market will witness robust growth of cameras working in the invisible spectrum application in areas such as surveillance and security, firefighting, medical imaging, and industrial diagnostics.

In the infrared spectral range, the development of monolithic arrays made of semiconductors with a narrow band gap (e.g., HgCdTe, InSb) was undertaken at the end of 1970s. However, their fabrication failed at the end of the 1980s. The main problems were signal handling of the MIS cells, especially in conditions of high background operation; high dark-current density, and difficulties in achieving high charge-transfer efficiency. Especially, the defect-related tunnelling current of the nonequilibrium operated MIS devices is orders of magnitude larger than the fundamental dark current. The MIS capacitor required much higher quality material than the photodiode.

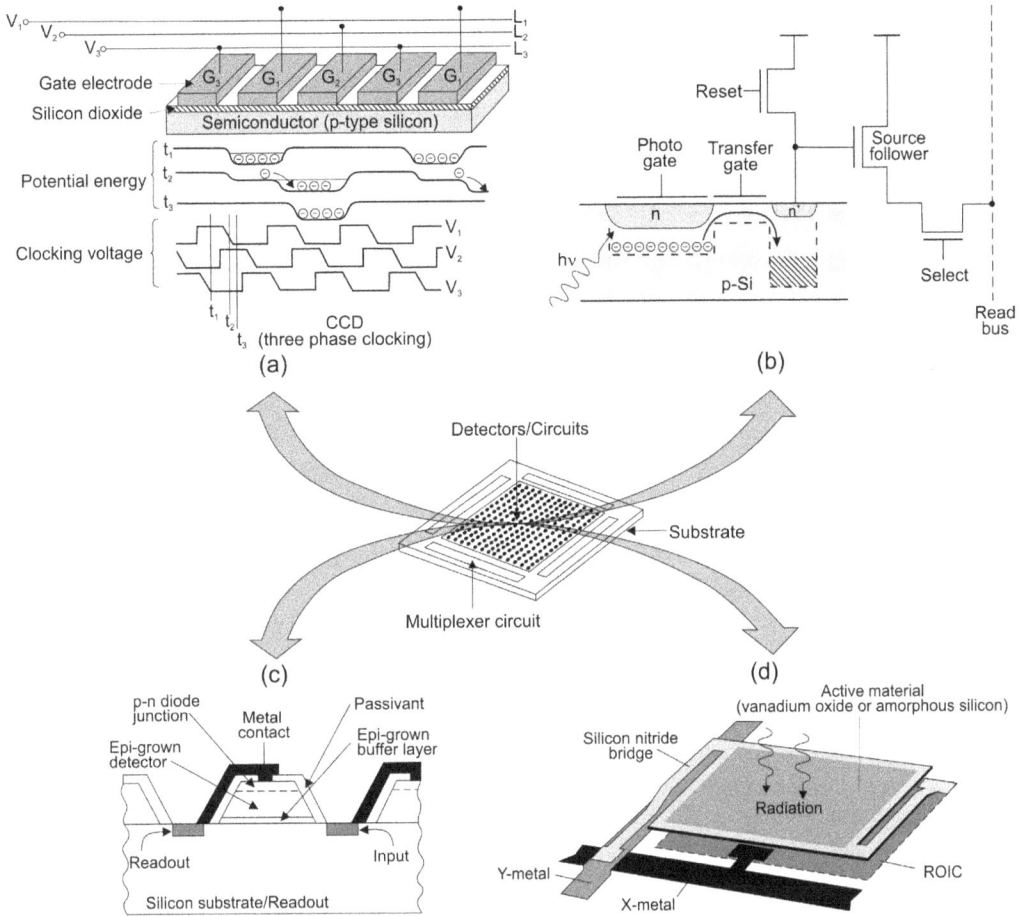

FIGURE 12.8 Monolithic focal plane arrays: (a) CCD, (b) CMOS, (c) heteroepitaxy-on-silicon, and (d) microbolometer.

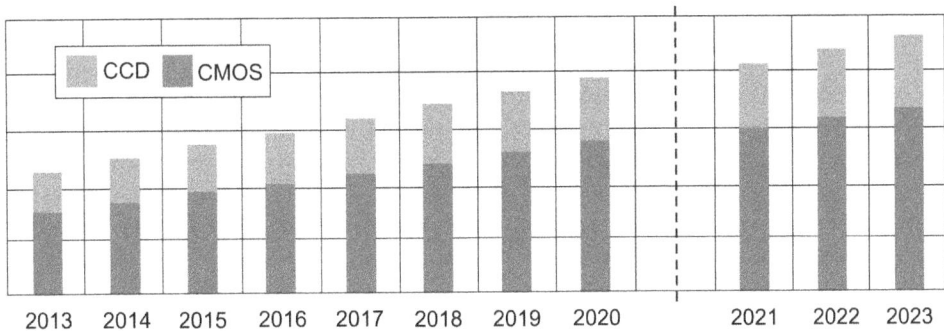

FIGURE 12.9 Evolution of CCD and CMOS global image sensors market (after Reference 20).

The best results in monolithic technology were achieved for silicon FPAs with a Schottky barrier completely compatible with the VLSI silicon technology and in the microbolometer array technology [Figure 12.8(d)]. Development of PtSi Schottky barrier FPAs was stopped in late 2010s [21]. Both dark-current and quantum efficiency have reached their theoretical limits, and no further improvement was expected by refining the material and/or process technologies. Their cost is less attractive when compared with uncooled microbolometer FPAs. Microbolometer arrays fabricated on an industrial scale and used for thermal imaging have covered a significant portion of the global market.

12.3.2 Hybrid Arrays

In the case of hybrid technology, we can optimise the detector material and multiplexer independently. Other advantages of hybrid-packaged FPAs are near-100 per cent fill factors, and increased signal-processing area on the multiplexer chip.

Development of hybrid packaging technology began in the late 1970s [22] and took the next decade to reach volume production. In the early 1990s, fully 2D imaging arrays provided a means for staring sensor systems to enter the production stage. In the hybrid architecture, indium bump bonding with readout electronics provides for multiplexing the signals from thousands or millions of pixels onto a few output lines, greatly simplifying the interface between the vacuum-enclosed cryogenic sensor and the system electronics.

Although focal plane array imagers are very common in our lives, they are quite complex to fabricate. Depending on the array architecture, the process can include over 150 individual fabrication steps. The hybridisation process involves flip-chip indium bonding between the "top" surfaces of the ROIC and detector array. The indium bond must be uniform between each sensing pixel and its corresponding read-out element in order to insure high-quality imaging. After hybridisation, a backside thinning process is usually performed to reduce the amount of substrate absorption. The edges off the gap between the ROIC and FPA can be sealed with low viscosity epoxy before substrate is mechanically thinned down to several microns. Some advanced FPA fabrication processes involve complete removal of the substrate material.

Innovations and progress in FPA fabrication are dependent on adjustments to the material growth parameters. Usually, in-house growth has enabled manufacturers to maintain the highest material quality and to customise the layer structures for multiple applications. For example, since HgCdTe material is critical to many principal product lines, and comparable material is not available externally, most global manufacturers continue to supply their own wafers. Figure 12.10 shows process flow for integrated infrared FPA manufacturing. As is shown, boule growth starts with the raw materials, polycrystalline components. In the case of HgCdTe FPA process, polycrystalline ultrapure CdTe and ZnTe binary compounds are loaded into a carbon-coated quartz crucible. The crucible is mounted into an evacuated quartz ampoule, which is placed in a cylindrical furnace. Large-crystal CdZnTe boules are produced by mixing and melting the ingredients, followed by recrystallising with the vertical gradient freeze method. Their standard diameters reach 125 millimetres. The boule substrate material is then sawn into slices, diced into squares, and polished to prepare the surface for epitaxial growth. Typical substrate sizes up to 8 cm×8 cm have been produced. The HgCdTe layers are usually grown on top of the substrate by MBE or MOCVD. In the case of MOCVD epitaxial technology also large-size GaAs substrates are used. The selection of substrate depends on the specific application. The entire growth procedure is automated, with each step being programmed in advance.

After growing the detector epitaxial structures, the wafers are non-destructively evaluated against multiple quality specifications. They are then conveyed to the array processing line, where the sensing elements (pixels) are formed by photolithographic steps, including mesa etching, surface passivation, metal contact deposition and indium bump formation. After wafer dicing, the FPAs are ready for mating to the ROICs. The ROIC branch of the process is shown in the lower right of Figure 12.10. For each pixel on the detector array, there is a corresponding unit cell on the ROIC to collect the photocurrent and process the signal. Each design is delivered to a silicon

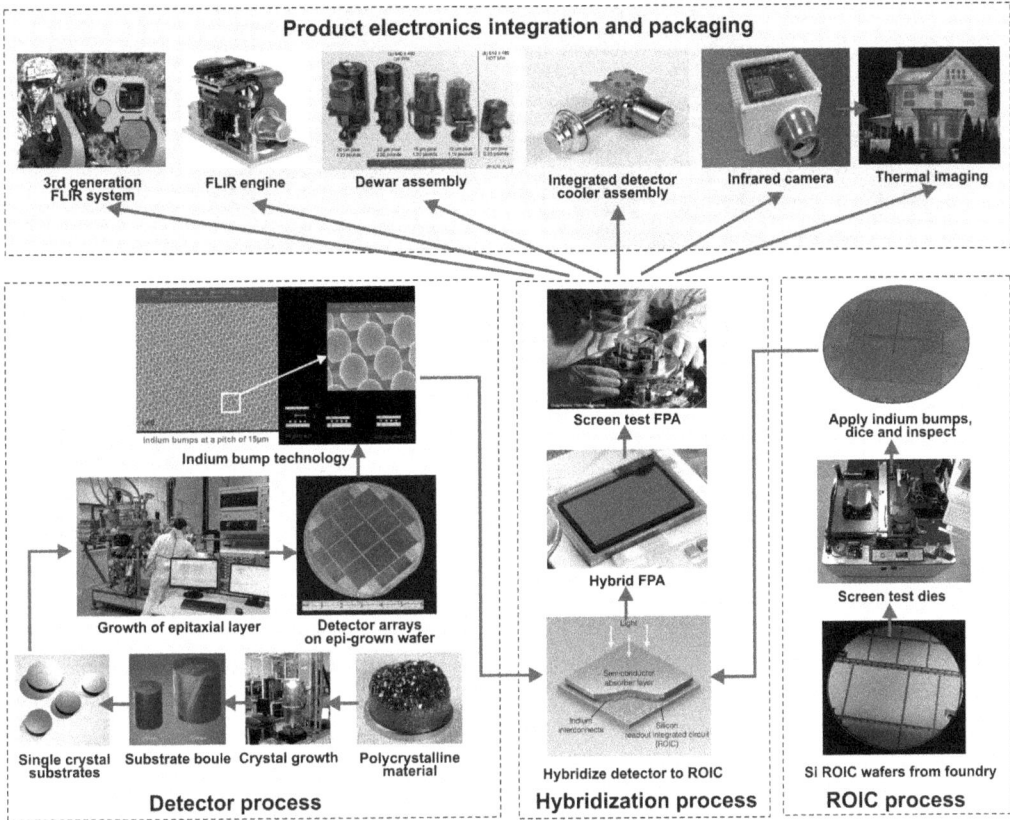

FIGURE 12.10 Process flow for integrated infrared FPA manufacturing.

foundry for fabrication. Next, the ROIC wafers are diced and are ready for mating with the FPA. The most advanced flip-chip bonders, utilising laser alignment and submicron-scale motion control, bring the two chips together (see the centre of Figure 12.10). At present FPAs with a pixel pitch size below 10 μm are aligned and hybridised with high yield. Each FPA with attached ROIC is tested according to a defined protocol and is installed in a sensor module. Finally, associated packaging and electronics are designed and assembled to complete the integrated manufacturing process.

Detector FPA has revolutionised many kinds of imaging from gamma rays to infrared and even radio waves. More general information about background, history, the present stage of technology and trends can be found, for example, in References 2 and 19. Information about the assemblies and applications can be found at various vendor websites.

Different hybridisation approaches are in use today. The most popular is flip-chip interconnect using bump bond [see Figure 12.11(a,c)]. In this approach, indium bumps are formed on both the detector array and the ROIC chip. The array and the ROIC are aligned and force is applied to cause the indium bumps to cold-weld together. In the other approach, indium bumps are formed only on the ROIC; the detector array is brought into alignment and proximity with the ROIC, the temperature is raised to cause the indium to melt, and contact is made by reflow.

Large focal plane arrays with fine-pitched bumps may require substantial force to achieve reliable interconnects, which creates the potential for damaging delicate semiconductor detector layers. Also, there is always a risk of misalignment associated with the joining process and "hybrid slip".

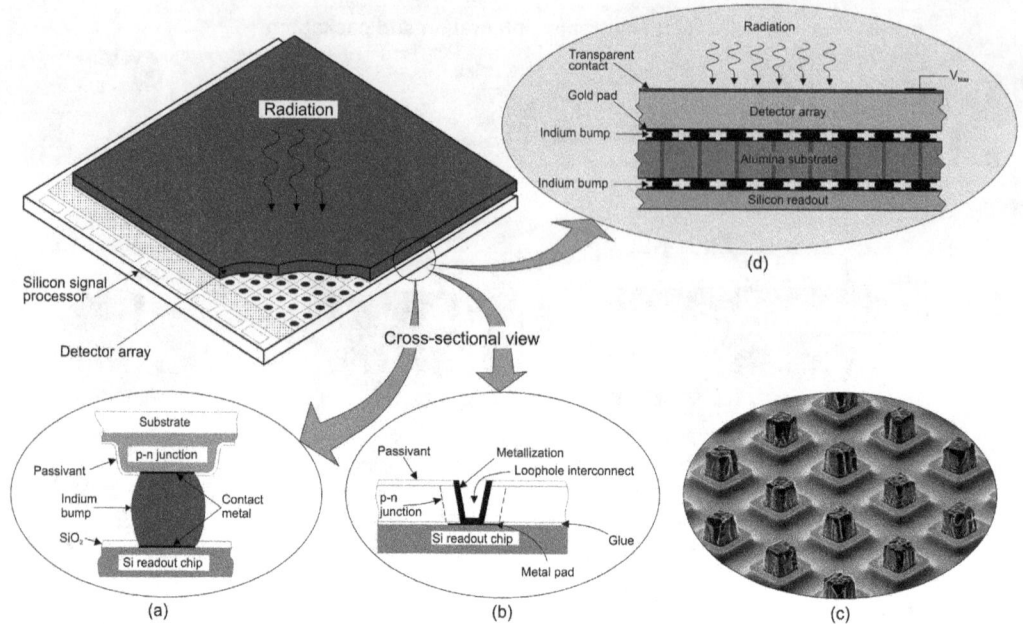

FIGURE 12.11   Hybrid IR FPA interconnect techniques between a detector array and silicon multiplexer: (a) indium bump technique, (b) loophole technique, (c) SEM photo shows mesa photodiode array with indium bumps, and (d) layered-hybrid design suitable for large format far IR and sub-mm arrays.

Some of these issues can be resolved by using a fusion bonding (or direct bond) process, which usually involves a room temperature alignment of wafers via Van der Waals interactions followed by annealing that creates permanent covalent interfacial bonds between upper and lower wafers. The direct bond process requires less than 10 pounds of force (in comparison with > 1000 pounds for indium-based process) to mate the detector and ROIC. This eliminates misalignment errors and many potential problems associated with compression bonder (hybrid slip, layer damage, bump separation, etc.). Fusion bonding is especially used in production of very large arrays up to 10k×12k format and thin active layers (<10 μm). This approach is beneficial for devices with enhanced blue and UV performance and modulation transfer function (*MTF*). The drawback of this method is its extreme sensitivity to surface flatness, roughness and particles.

Recently, an alternative technology based upon adhesive bonding between the active detector layer and support wafer has been introduced. This provides low-temperature bonding and alignment accuracies in the 1–2 μm range. However, the adhesive has to be carefully selected and tested for mechanical rigidity, temperature stability and outgassing, and inter-via connections must be made after bonding and thinning.

Infrared hybrid FPA detectors and multiplexers are also fabricated using loophole interconnection – see Figure 12.11(b) [23, 24]. In this case, the detector and the multiplexer chips are glued together to form a single chip before detector fabrication. The photovoltaic detector is formed by ion implantation, and loopholes are drilled by ion-milling and electrical interconnection between each detector and its corresponding input circuit is made through a small hole formed in each detector. The junctions are connected down to the silicon circuit by cutting the fine, few μm in diameter holes through the junctions by ion milling, and then backfilling the holes with metallisation. A similar type of hybrid technology called VIP (vertically integrated photodiode) was reported by DRS Infrared Technologies (formerly Texas Instruments) [25, 26].

It is difficult to make small pixel pitches (below 10 μm) using bump-bonding interconnect technique, especially when high yield and 100 per cent pixel operability are required. A new facility gives 3D integration process using wafer bonding, where such materials as Si and InP have been monolithically integrated with pixel size down to 6 μm [27].

The detector array can be illuminated from either the front side (with the photons passing through the transparent silicon multiplexer) or backside (with photons passing through the transparent detector array substrate). In general, the latter approach is most advantageous, as the multiplexer will typically have areas of metallisation and other opaque regions that can reduce the effective optical area of the structure. The epoxy is flowed into the space between the readout and the detectors to increase the bonding strength. In the case of backside detector illumination, the transparent substrates are required. When using opaque materials, substrates must be thinned to below 10 μm to obtain sufficient quantum efficiencies and reduce crosstalk. In some cases, the substrates are completely removed. In the "direct" backside illuminated configuration, both the detector array and the silicon ROIC chip are bump-mounted side-by-side onto a common circuit board. The "indirect" configuration allows the unit cell area in the silicon ROIC to be larger than the detector area and is usually used for small-scanning FPAs, where stray capacitance is not an issue.

Readout circuit wafers are processed in standard commercial foundries and can be constrained in size by the die-size limits of the photolithography step and repeat printers. Because of field-size limitations in those photography systems, CMOS imager chip sizes must currently be limited to standard lithographic field sizes of less than 32×26 mm for submicron lithography. To build larger sensor arrays, a new photolithographic technique called *stitching* can be used to fabricate detector arrays larger than the reticle field of photolithographic steppers. The large array is divided into smaller subblocks. Later, the complete sensor chips are stitched together from the building blocks in the reticle. Each block can be photocomposed on the wafer by multiple exposures at appropriate locations. Single blocks of the detector array are exposed at one time, as the optical system allows shuttering, or selectively exposing only a desired section of the reticle.

12.4   BASIC PARAMETERS OF DETECTOR ARRAYS

The configuration of the imaging system is shown in Figure 12.12. On the graph in this figure, A_s and A_d are, respectively, the surfaces of the object and the detector, r is the distance of the object to the lens (system optics), $A_{ap} = \pi D^2/4$ and D are the surface and the diameter of the lens (aperture, entrance-pupil). The detector is placed in the focal plane of the system in the distance $\approx f$ to the entrance pupil. The optic's system is characterised by so-called F-number – that is, $f/\# = f/D$.

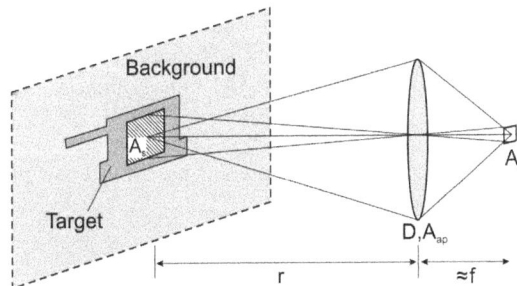

FIGURE 12.12   Imaging system configuration.

Sensitivity is one of the photoreceiver basic parameters that should be given special attention. Depending on the photoreceiver type and purpose, its sensitivity can be defined by the signal-to-noise ratio (SNR) or other related parameters, such as

- D^*–detectivity;
- NEC–noise equivalent charge;
- NEI–noise equivalent irradiance;
- FF–fill factor;
- DR–dynamic range;
- NEDT–noise equivalent difference temperature;
- NEP–noise equivalent power;
- MRTD–minimum resolvable temperature difference; and
- MTF–modulation transfer function.

Definitions of detectivity and NEP are given in chapter 2, so let us define the remaining parameters of FPAs.

12.4.1 Noise Equivalent Charge

NEC is a universal parameter that determines the ROIC input circuit sensitivity. NEC is the equivalent noise related to the input of a photoreceiver derived from the accumulated charge in the storage capacitor during a single frame [4] and NEC is specific to a given bandwidth or frame rate.

If the shot noise of the detector I_{nd} is characterised by a uniform spectral density distribution, then the NEC accumulated during the integration time t_{int} is as follows:

$$NEC_{det} = \frac{I_{nd}t_{int}}{q}. \tag{12.5}$$

NEC can be used to describe not only the detector but also other components of FPAs (e.g., the preamplifier and the downstream signal processing path). For the preamplifier, this parameter is expressed by the equation

$$NEC_{preamp} = \left[I_n^2 + \left(\frac{V_n\left(R_d + R_i\right)}{R_d R_i} \right)^2 \right]^{1/2} \frac{t_{int}}{q}, \tag{12.6}$$

where I_n, V_n, R_d and R_i are the equivalent circuit elements (see Figure 11.2).

A commonly used parameter for determining FPAs sensitivity is the noise equivalent irradiance, NEI, or the equivalent input irradiance providing the unity signal-to-noise ratio at the output of FPAs. The output signal is equal to the RMS value of the output noise for a given frequency and bandwidth of the measuring instrument [4].

NEI is associated with NEC dependency:

$$NEI = \frac{NEC}{\eta A_o t_{int}}. \tag{12.7}$$

Photon/(cm^{2}s) is the unit of NEI.

Other FPAs components can also be described using *NEI*. Similar to the noise analysis of the photoreceiver input stage, it can be written that

$$NEI_{FPAs} = \left(NEI_{sys}^2 - NEI_{ph}^2\right)^{1/2} = \left(NEI_{sys}^2 - \frac{\phi_B}{\eta A_o t_{int}}\right)^{1/2}. \tag{12.8}$$

The first component of Eq. (12.8) describes *NEI* of the entire detection system, while the second component of *NEI* comes from the photon flux incident on a detector surface. This parameter is used to evaluate radiometers and photon counters.

12.4.2 NOISE EQUIVALENT DIFFERENCE TEMPERATURE

For infrared arrays the relevant figure of merit for determining the ultimate performance is not the detectivity, D^*, but the noise equivalent difference temperature (*NEDT*) and the modulation transfer function (*MTF*). We will consider the primary performance metrics of thermal imaging systems: thermal sensitivity and spatial resolution. Thermal sensitivity is concerned with the minimum temperature difference that can be discerned above the noise level. The *MTF* concerns the spatial resolution and answers one question: How small an object can be imaged by the system? The general approach of system performance is given by Lloyd in his fundamental monograph [28].

NEDT is a temperature resolution defined as a difference between the test temperature (circular or rectangular) and a homogeneous background at which the unit ratio of the maximum signal to the effective noise voltage value, at a specific point in the electronic signal processing system, is equal to the unity. *NEDT* is defined as

$$NEDT = \frac{V_n}{\Delta V / \Delta T}, \tag{12.9}$$

where V_n is the RMS noise, ΔV represents the signal measured for the temperature difference ΔT. *NEDT* characterises the detection system sensitivity for low spatial frequencies.

NEDT can be also determined theoretically if the spectral characteristics of the detector detectivity are known [18,29] (see also Example 12.5):

$$NEDT = \frac{4F^2 \Delta f^{1/2}}{A^{1/2} t_{op}} \left[\int_{\lambda_a}^{\lambda_b} \frac{dM}{dT} D^*(\lambda) d\lambda\right]^{-1}, \tag{12.10}$$

where $F = f/D$ is the *f/#*, A is the detector area, t_{op} represents the transmission coefficient of the optical system in the spectral range from λ_a to λ_b, M is the radiant exitance.

In the above considerations it is assumed that the temporal detector's noise is the main source of noise. However, this stipulation is not true for FPAs, where the nonuniformity, u, of the pixels' responses is a significant source of noise. This nonuniformity is a source of fixed-pattern noise (FPN, spatial noise). The main sources of FPN result from a technological dispersion of the parameters of the individual pixels, the parameters of the optics used and the parameters of the ROIC systems. Figure 12.13 shows the dependence of the total *NEDT* on detectivity for different residual nonuniformity, u, assuming 300 K scene temperature and the set of parameters inserted in the figure. The nonuniformity has stronger influence on *NEDT* value than detectivity. It is shown

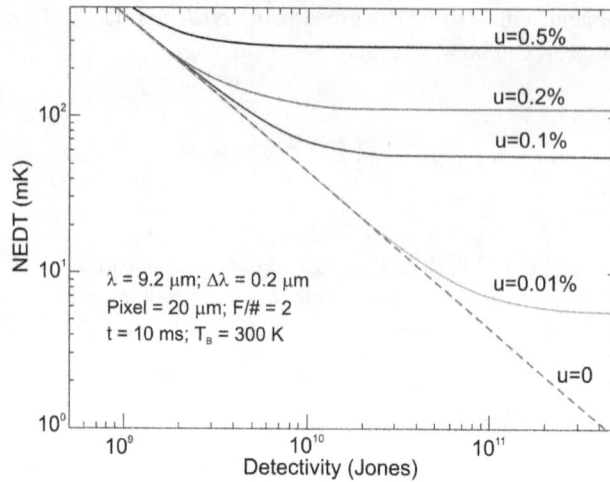

FIGURE 12.13 *NEDT* as a function of detectivity for different levels of nonuniformity $u = 0.01\%$, 0.1%, 0.2%, and 0.5%. Note that for $D^* > 10^{10}$ cmHz$^{1/2}$/W, detectivity is not the relevant figure of merit.

that when the detectivity approaches a value above 10^{10} cmHz$^{1/2}$/W (which is easily obtained at present stage of detector technology), the FPA performance is uniformity limited without correction, and thus essentially independent of the detectivity. Various correction methods are used to reduce the impact of the pixel nonuniformities on the image quality. An improvement in nonuniformity from 0.1 per cent to 0.01 per cent after correction could lower the *NEDT* from 63 to 6.3 mK.

12.4.3 MODULATION TRANSFER FUNCTION

To evaluate the quality of amplifiers, frequency response is used. In acoustic systems it means fidelity of the reproduced sound in relation to the sound generated by the source. By treating an optical system, operating in the visible or infrared range, similar to a system transmitting electrical signals, one can assess how accurately optical signals are transmitted. So, we are interested in measuring the frequency response of the optical system. In this case, the equivalent frequency is the spatial frequency. On the other hand, resolution means the ability of a sensing system consisting of an optical system and a detector to represent a point of an object. It can be a discrete detector, CCD array, CMOS array or hybrid array. It is evaluated by photographing a card containing groups of black and white stripes, dimensions of which gradually decrease. Various tests are used to determine the resolution expressed in pairs of lines per millimetre (lp/mm). Figure 12.14 shows the USAF 1951 test (the name from the designers and the design year: "United States Air Force 1951") [35].

Let us consider what the image of a low-dimensional test looks like. For an ideal system, the signal amplitude at the detection system output should have the shape as shown at the top of Figure 12.15 – the output signal should faithfully reflect the input signal. The white bar corresponds to a signal with the highest amplitude, while the black bar corresponds to a signal with the minimum amplitude. In addition, there is a sharp border of transition between the signals corresponding to white and black for both low and high spatial frequency called Nyquist frequency.

In real detection systems, even for wide stripes, there is no sharp border for the transition between stripes – see middle of Figure 12.15. The less sharp the image, the smoother the transition [30]. The difference between areas with different brightness levels is called the contrast (modulation degree).

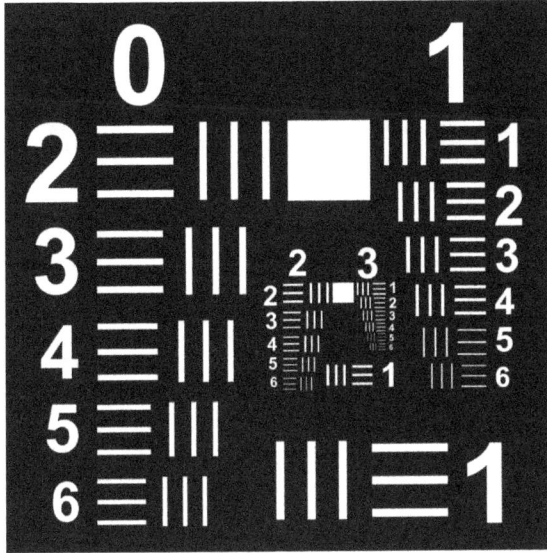

FIGURE 12.14 Example of USAF 1951 resolution test chart.

It depends on the maximum and minimum values of light intensity for a given spatial frequency and is defined as

$$M = \frac{E_{max} - E_{min}}{E_{max} + E_{min}}.$$

(12.11)

When the difference in the reproduction of white and black is clear, then we speak of a high contrast, and when the difference is not clear, of a low contrast (middle of Figure 12.15). In contrast, "narrow bars" will not be visualised as black and white, but as light grey/dark grey. Thus, at more line/mm pairs, the higher the spatial frequency, the smaller the difference in signal intensity between light grey and dark grey. That is, as the spatial frequency increases, the contrast of the image formed by the detection system decreases.

At a certain spatial frequency, we can notice a lack of contrast and the image will become grey. Knowing the object contrast M_{object} and the image contrast M_{image}, the *MTF* function can be determined by

$$MTF = \frac{M_{image}}{M_{object}}.$$

(12.12)

The *MTF* estimates the resolution of an imaging system. In other words, this function characterises the ability of the detection system to transmit the object spatial frequencies, that is, it determines the ability to distinguish details in the analysed image. If the system carries large spatial frequencies, then it means that it is able to recognise a large number of details. It should be stated that the *MTF* function is the best tool to evaluate a given detection system taking into account its resolution and contrast. Its limit value for an ideal optics is determined by a diffraction.

The imaging system *MTF* depends on several components and is dominated by the optics, detector, and display *MTFs* and can be cascaded by simply multiplying the *MTFs* components

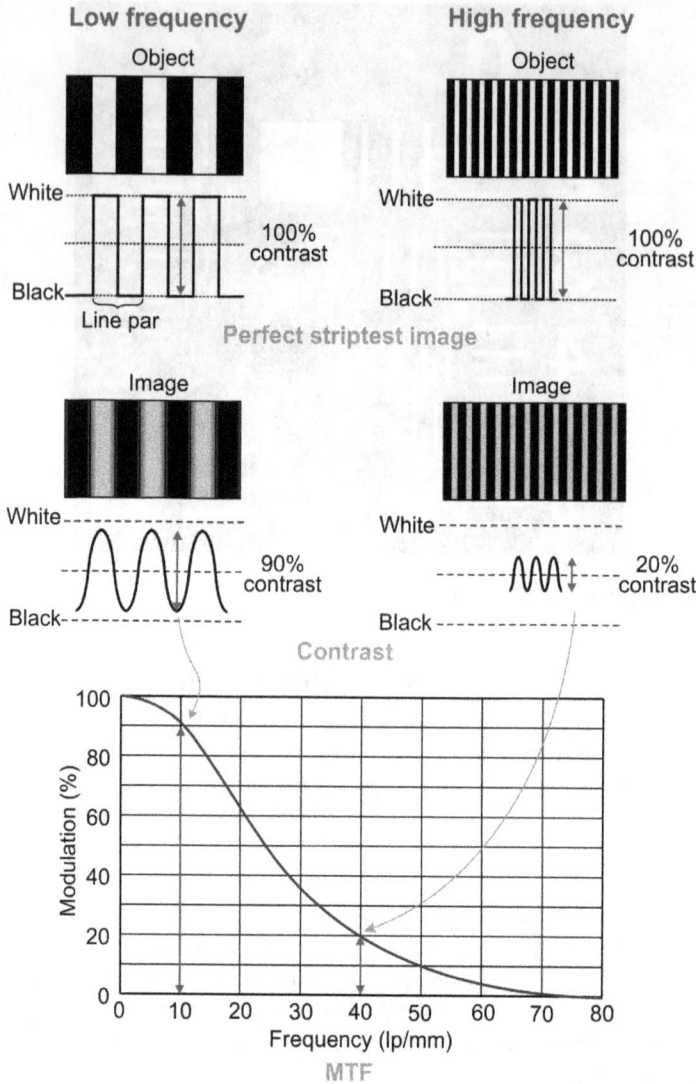

FIGURE 12.15   Idea of the *MTF* measurement.

$$MTF = MTF_{optics} \times MTF_{detector} \times MTF_{display}. \qquad (12.13)$$

Thus, the resultant of the *MTF* function is determined by a component with the lowest resolution.

The *MTF* is usually limited by the size of the detector and the aperture of the optic in spatial frequency terms. The resultant modulation transfer function *MTF* of the total detection system depends mainly on the optics, MTF_{optics}, and the detector $MTF_{detector}$ (Figure 12.16).

12.4.4   MINIMUM RESOLVABLE TEMPERATURE DIFFERENCE

Another parameter, a minimum resolvable temperature difference (*MRDT*) is defined as a temperature difference between the temperature of the four-strip test [with a 7:1 ratio of the height to the

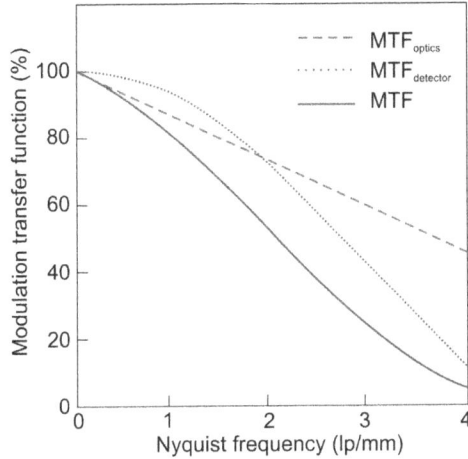

FIGURE 12.16   Example of the modulation transfer function.

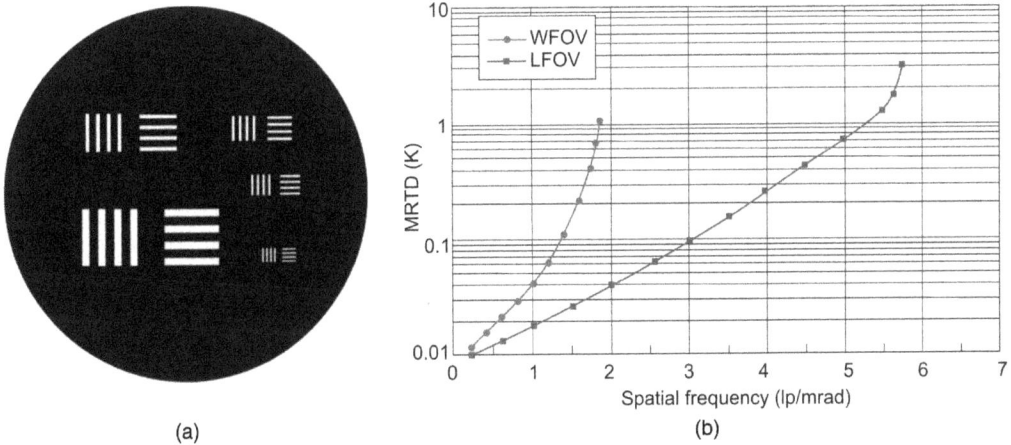

(a)   (b)

FIGURE 12.17   The minimum resolvable temperature difference: (a) sample set of tests, (b) exemplary characteristics of cooled staring thermal imager with two FOV (WFOV and LFOV).

width of a rectangular strip – see Figure 12.17(a)] and the homogeneous background temperature at which the experienced observer distinguishes four test strips using the test observation detection system [31]. *MRDT* is often the preferred figure of merit for imaging sensor in spite of fact that it is a subjective parameter that describes the ability of the imager-human system for detection of low contrast details of the tested object.

The thermal image of a test strip is characterised by the so-called spatial frequency which is expressed in cycles/mrad (the number of temperature changes in an image over a given area). Figure 12.17(b) shows an example test set and the *MRDT* characteristics determined for typical military thermal imagers for airborne surveillance for wide (W) and low (L) field of view (FOV). A camera that has a low *MRDT* value has high thermal resolution and high spatial resolution. Detailed information on testing infrared devices is included in references [32, 33].

The *MRDT* figure of merit comprises both resolution and sensitivity of the thermal imager. Knowing *MRDT* characteristics, the ranges of detection (D), recognition (R), and identification

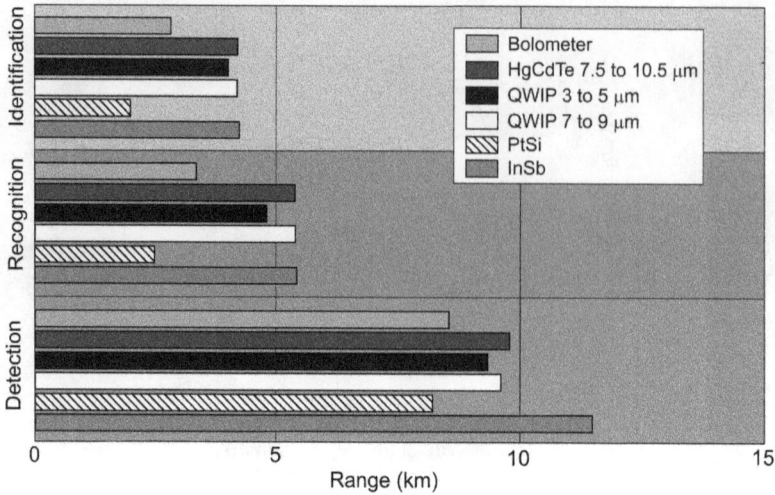

FIGURE 12.18 Comparison DRI ranges for man-sized target assuming atmospheric parameters of a MidLat summer and rural 23 km visibility (adapted after Reference 36).

(I) of a thermal imaging camera can be determined. Thermal imaging systems are used first to detect an object and then to identify it. According to Johnson's criteria [34]

- detection is defined as ability to distinguish an object from the background;
- recognition as ability to classify the object class (animal, human, vehicle, boat ...); and
- identification as ability to describe the object in details (a man with a hat, a deer, a Jeep ...).

The nominal range performance of an infrared camera is calculated for a defined task, standardised target and environmental conditions. The only standardisation available to date is STANAG 4347 [35].

Figure 12.18 is a comparison of various FPAs in detecting, recognising and identifying a man-size target for a canonical tactical sensor ($f/3$, 454 mm focal length, 152 mm aperture operating at 60 Hz). These ranges were calculated using the NVTherm model.

Typically, identification ranges are between two and three times shorter than detection ranges. To increase ranges, better resolution and sensitivity of the infrared systems (and hence the detectors) are required. Further increase of identification ranges can be achieved by using multispectral detection to correlate the images at different wavelengths. For that reason third generation imagers are being developed to extend the range of target detection and identification and to ensure that defence forces maintain a technological advantage in night operations over any opposing force [37].

12.4.5 OTHER PARAMETERS

12.4.5.1 Fill Factor (FF)

The fill factor of an image sensor array can be defined as the ratio of a pixel's light-sensitive area to its total area. CCDs have a 100 per cent fill factor, but CMOS cameras have much less. The lower the fill factor, the less sensitive the sensor is, and the longer exposure/integration times must be. To improve fill-factor, micro-lenses can be added to each pixel to gather light from the insensitive portions of the sensor and focus it down to the active region of pixels, or through backside illumination of the readout where there is no circuitry. The microlens structure may also provide some spectral filtering. In the case of infrared hybrid arrays, independent optimisation of the detector material and multiplexer makes it possible to achieve near-100 per cent fill factors.

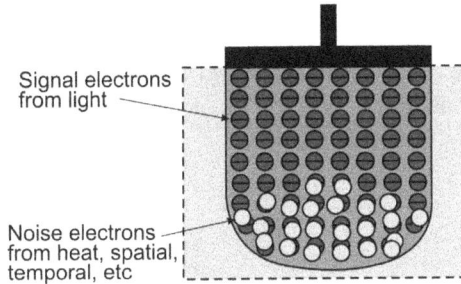

FIGURE 12.19 Illustration of the potential well capacity.

The full well capacity (FWC) determines the amount of photo charge that can be accumulated in a MOS capacitor (Figure 12.19). Its typical value is between 10,000 and 500,000 electrons [38]. This depends mainly on the size of capacitor and determines the maximum value of the signal that can be detected by the CCD detector. On the other hand, a lower limit of the measured signal is determined by the noise of the detector reading system. Knowing both quantities, one can determine the dynamic range of the CCD array. For infrared hybrid arrays, the well capacity is typically in the range of 1×10^6 to 1×10^7 electrons for a 15-μm-pixel design with available node capacities for current CMOS readout designs.

12.4.5.2 Dynamic Range (DR)

The range of signal levels for which the detector is useful provides the dynamic range. The dynamic range of the array quantifies the pixel ability to reproduce both light and dark elements of the recorded scenery. It is defined as the ratio of the maximum value of the signal (which, in most cases, is identical with the maximum number of charges accumulated in the potential well) to the total readout noise in a complete darkness [39]:

$$DR = \frac{well\ capacity\left[e^-\right]}{readout\ noise\left[e^-\right]}. \tag{12.14}$$

Dynamic range can also be expressed in decibels as:

$$DR = 20\log\left(\frac{well\ capacity\left[e^-\right]}{readout\ noise\left[e^-\right]}\right)[\text{dB}], \tag{12.15}$$

then, its value is of the order of 60–100 dB.

To maintain or increase the unit cell's dynamic range will require employing increasingly deeply scaled, higher-density CMOS processes. Higher-density CMOS fabrication processes can also be used to increase in-unit cell processing capacity.

If we assume that the well capacity is 250,000 e-, and the reading noise is 5 e-, then, the dynamic range of the camera is 250 000/5 = 50 000. Table 12.2 shows examples of the potential well capacity, noise, and dynamic range for several CCD sensors.

Detector outputs increase linearly with the input signal over some range of irradiances (Figure 12.20). The highest useful signal might be defined as the point at which a given linearity is exceeded. At large irradiance the output signal saturates. A major source of deviation from linearity is saturation of the detector or electronic circuit.

TABLE 12.2
Examples of the Potential Well Capacity, Noise, and
Dynamic Range Values for Three CCD arrays

Parameter	Sony ICX285AL	Kodak KAI-1020	Kodak KAI-11000
Well capacity [e⁻]	18 000	40 000	60 000
Reading noise [e⁻]	5	9	11
Dynamic range	3600:1	4444:1	5454:1
Dynamic range [dB]	71.1	72.9	74.7

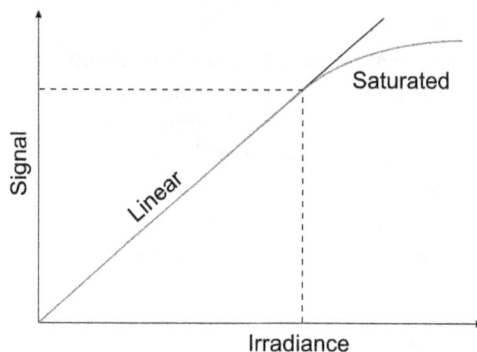

FIGURE 12.20 Signal versus irradiance plot showing linear and saturated regions.

12.4.5.3 Crosstalk

In practice, an array containing small pixels, some signals fall on spots of several pixels. This process is called crosstalk and is generally measured as a percentage of the input or driving signal. A requirement that crosstalk be less than 0.1 per cent would be hard to meet. Figure 12.21 presents an example of the crosstalk due to optical reflection and the electrical coupling.

12.5 CCD IMAGE SENSORS

Since their invention in 1969, CCDs have become the detector of choice for high-quality imaging in a wide range of fields. They have the advantages of excellent resolution, 100 per cent fill factor, greater than 90 per cent peak quantum efficiency, excellent charge-transfer efficiency and very low dark current with sufficient cooling. The importance of the CCD to mankind was recognised by the awarding of a Nobel Prize in Physics in 2009.

The basic element of a monolithic CCD array is a metal-insulator-semiconductor (MIS) structure: Figure 12.22. Used as part of a charge transfer device, an MIS capacitor detects and integrates the generated photocurrent. It is made of three layers:

- conductor (metal);
- insulator (silicon dioxide SiO_2 – oxide); and
- semiconductor (silicon monocrystal).

Here, only n-channel MIS with a p-type substrate is considered, although all of the arguments can be extended to p-channel MIS with appropriate changes. When a bias voltage is applied across a p-type MOS structure, majority charge carriers (holes) are pushed away from the Si-SiO$_2$ interface

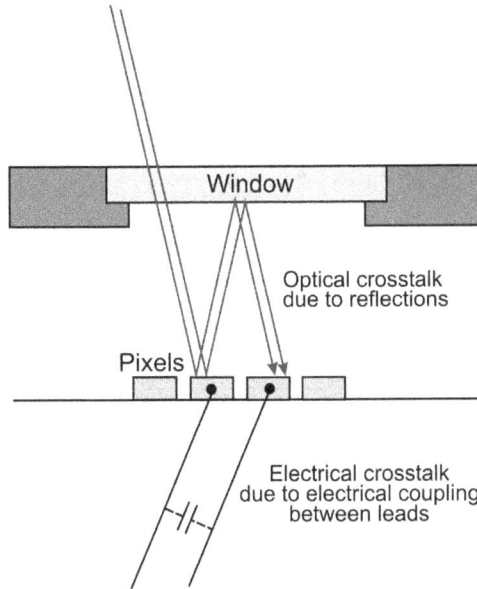

FIGURE 12.21 Crosstalk due to optical and electrical coupling.

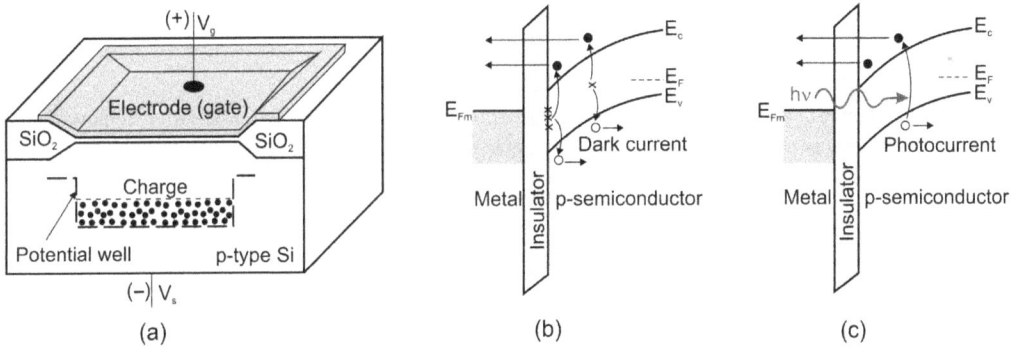

FIGURE 12.22 MIS structure: (a) geometry; a positive bias (inversion bias) is applied for the metal/insulator/ p-type semiconductor example. The current mechanisms of an MIS photodiode (b) without light illumination and (c) with light illumination.

directly below the gate, leaving a region depleted of positive charge and available as a potential energy well for any mobile minority charge carriers (electrons) [Figure 12.22(a)]. The area of the potential well slightly exceeds the gate outline. The surface potential can be controlled by the proper choice of gate voltage, doping density and insulator thickness. The dark current mechanisms for MIS structure represent the currents due to thermal generation in the neutral bulk, the depletion region and via interface states [Figure 12.22(b)]. Also, contribution of the tunnelling current can be appreciable at higher reverse bias.

Under light exposure at the inversion bias, the excess electron-hole pairs are generated in the semi-conductor and contribute to the photocurrent [Figure 12.23(c)]. The electron-hole pairs generated by light are immediately separated, directing the electrons toward the gate and the hole toward the negatively biased substrate bottom. Electrons reside under the oxide layer, and their number is directly proportional to irradiance, time of accumulation of this charge, quantum efficiency and

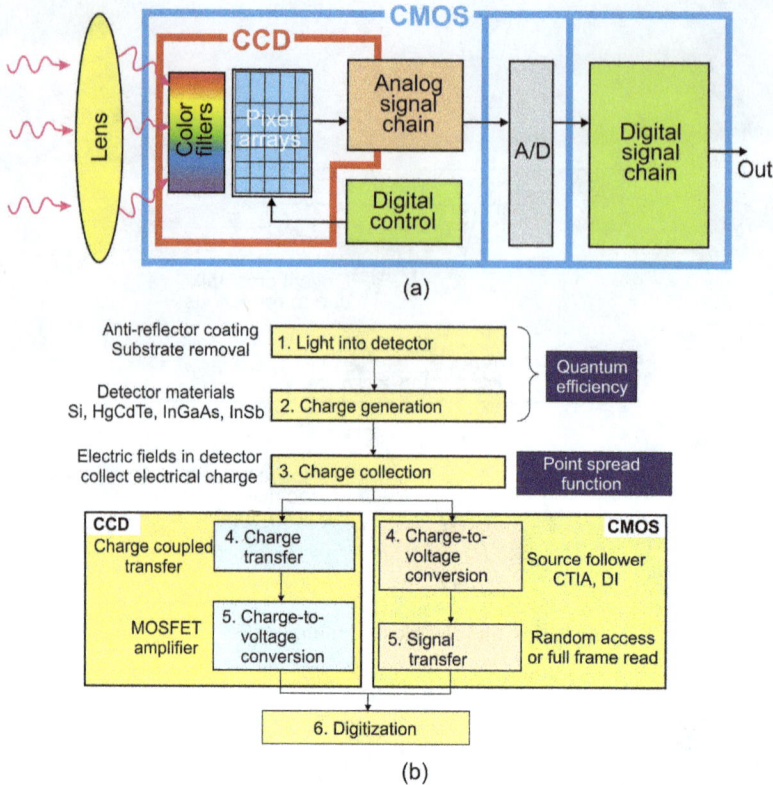

FIGURE 12.23 CCD and CMOS imaging systems: (a) schematic representation showing important subsystems with more functionality on chip for CMOS device, (b) operations of CCD and CMOS devices.

the capacity of the potential well. If the optical radiation intensity is too high, then a potential well overflow and blooming may occur. To prevent this phenomenon, cameras containing a so-called anti-blooming gate have been developed [40].

In order to increase the responsivity of MIS detector, the transparent gates [conducting oxides such as indium tin oxide (ITO) or zinc oxide (ZnO)] for the incident light are incorporated. The other solutions are the metal films with thicknesses of ~10 nm or backside illumination. The gate can also be made of polycrystalline silicon or a highly doped semiconductor. This type of design ensures a better transmission of ultraviolet and visible radiation.

12.5.1 CCD ARRAY OPERATION

CCD technology is very mature with respect to fabrication yield and attainment of near-theoretical sensitivity. CCD technique relies on the optoelectronic properties of a well-established semiconductor architecture: the MOS capacitor. The idea of CCD and CMOS arrays operation is shown in Figure 12.23 and is described in more detail in Figure 12.24.

The first three processes, that is, array illumination, charge generation and charge accumulation are common to both instruments [Figure 12.23(b)]. Both detector technologies use a photosensor to generate and separate the charges in the pixel. The charge is collected in a photodiode or in a MOS capacitor [see Figure 12.8(a,b)]. Beyond that, however, the two sensor schemes differ significantly. During CCD readout, the collected charge is shifted from pixel to pixel all the way to the perimeter. Finally, all charges are sequentially pushed to one common location (floating diffusion), and a single amplifier generates the corresponding output voltages. On the other hand, CMOS detectors

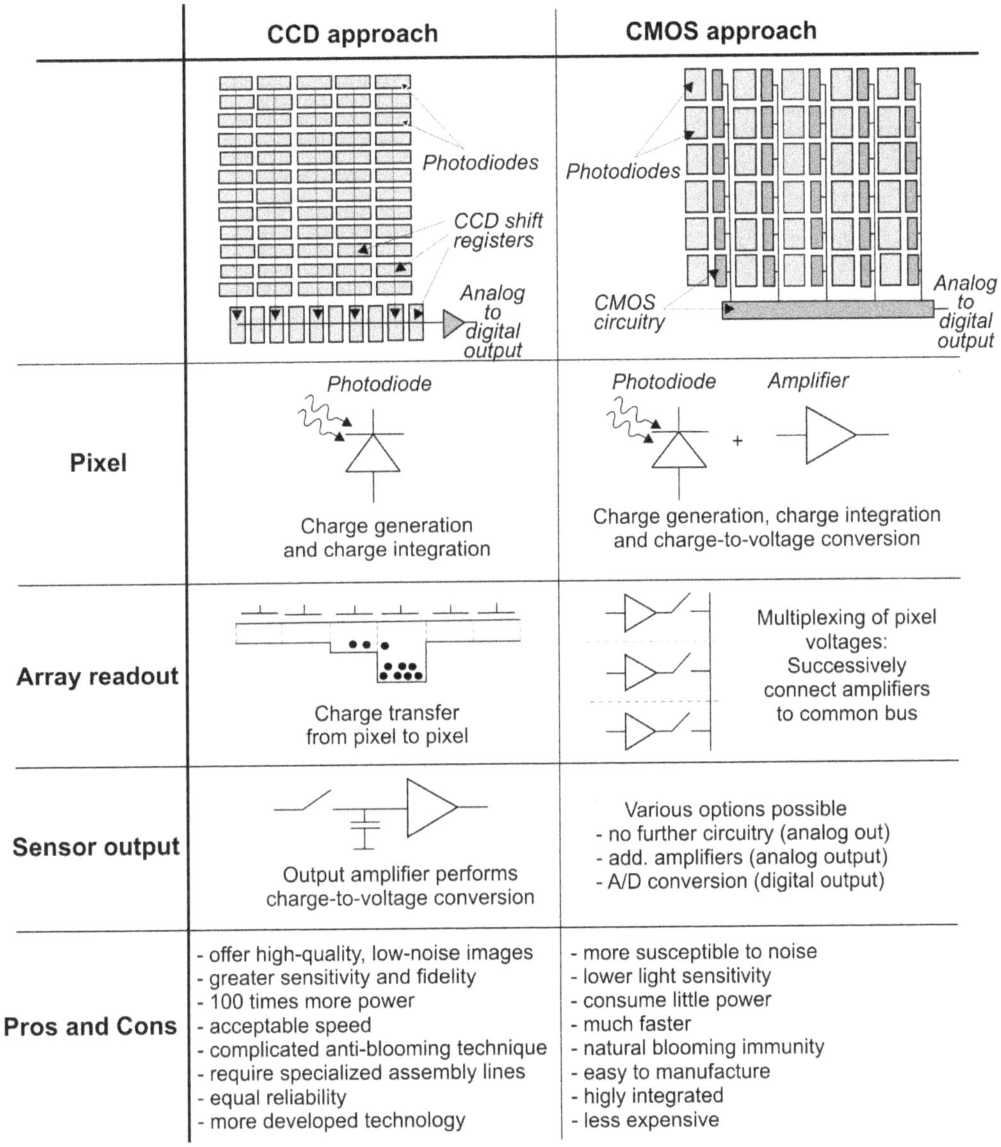

FIGURE 12.24 Comparison between the CCD-based and CMOS-based image sensor approaches.

have an independent amplifier in each pixel [active pixel sensor (APS)]. The amplifier converts the integrated charge into a voltage and thus eliminates the need to transfer charge from pixel to pixel. The voltages are multiplexed onto a common bus line using integrated CMOS switches. Analogue and digital sensor outputs are possible by implementing either a video output amplifier or an analogue-to-digital (A/D) converter on the chip.

The block diagram of a CCD device is shown at the top of Figure 12.24. Electrons generated in the silicon through absorption (charge generation) are collected in the potential energy well under the gate (charge collection). Linear or two-dimensional arrays of these MOS capacitors can therefore store images in the form of trapped charge carriers beneath the gates. The accumulated charges are transferred from potential well to the next well by using sequentially shifted voltage on each gate (charge transfer).

One of the most successful voltage-shifting schemes is called three-phase clocking – see Figure 12.8(a). This register is formed by a cascade of mutually isolated MOS capacitors acting as elementary memory cells. In the considered register, each three consecutive MOS capacitors form an elementary register cell (one image pixel). The capacitors' conductive electrodes connect to the corresponding buses that distribute the phases of the clock waveform: L_1, L_2, L_3. At time t_1, the first electrode, G_1 is biased with the full control voltage, V_1. This means that an inversion area is formed under the electrode. The potential well that it causes can accumulate current carriers. At time t_2, the second electrode L_2 is biased. The potential well induced by it can accumulate current carriers. The size of this layer is so large that it connects to the inversion area under the L_1 electrode. This means that the charges accumulated so far under L_1 will move under L_2 (in the analogy of gravity, balls fall to the lowest place). Their movement occurs through a thin n-type channel produced along the insulator–semiconductor interface. At time t_3, the stored charge in the register is under electrode G_2. There is a zero potential at electrode G_1. Thus, a charge shift to the next register cell has occurred. At the end of the array is a charge-to-voltage converter that faithfully reproduces the image formed by the light incident on the array.

When the shutter is closed (e.g., in a camera), the detection process is finished, and the image is stored in the form of volumetric charges under the electrodes. Now, in a short time, the stored charge is transferred to the memory cell located in the shift register. Charge transfer can occur in several ways: in a two-phase, three-phase, or four-phase cycle [41]. These methods differ in the number of simultaneously applied potentials and in the number of gates making up a single pixel.

The amount of charge carried along CCD can change due to dark current and noise. As a result, the signal level at the CCD device output may be reduced. The crosstalk may also occur because the lost portion of charge may appear in subsequent packets.

The charge transfer efficiency η, understood as the ratio of the amount of charge shifted between neighbouring electrodes to the amount of charge originally accumulated under one of them, is determined by the equation

$$\eta = 1 - \varepsilon, \tag{12.16}$$

where ε is the coefficient of transfer loss or charge transfer inefficiency. It should be noted that the greater the difference between high and low levels of the control signal, the "deeper" the potential well and, thus, the better the electrical charge transport efficiency.

In modern CCD shift registers, the values of η are so close to unity that it is more convenient to use the so-called transfer inefficiency:

$$\varepsilon = 1 - \eta. \tag{12.17}$$

The non-zero value ε implies a charge loss during the transfer, that is, signal attenuation between the initial gathering point and the register output.

The elementary transfer efficiency of CCD shifting registers depends on a number of mainly technological factors (e.g., the distance between the electrodes and the design of the area in which this transfer is performed).

12.5.2   TYPES OF CCD DEVICES

Requirements of reduction pixel size and simplification of the readout circuit have led to more complex architectures of MOS capacitor designs such as pseudo-dual-phase, dual-phase and single-phase control.

In the case of a two-phase circuit, successive gates are made on an oxide layer of varying thickness. This creates a potential gradient along the surface under the two connected gates and allows the charge to be transferred from one gate to another. A valuable advantage of the two-phase CCD shift register is that it allows for a single-level execution of the leads to the cell electrodes. The reader will find other types of CCD instrument control methods in Reference [41].

CCD systems described above are called surface-channel CCD (SCCD) devices because the accumulation and transport of charge take place in the near-surface region. In this type of device, the surface states affect the deterioration of charge-transport efficiency. One reason is the local potential wells (e.g., due to defects in the material, mainly surface states), deeper than those generated by control signals that can trap packages of charge. The second reason results from the application of too-high a frequency of changes of signals, L_1 and L_2.

The defects in the semiconductor material reduce the electron movement speed, and the charge does not keep up with falling into the potential well. As a consequence, the phenomenon of separation of electron packets may occur, which results in distortion of image information. A practical limitation is also the presence of harmful capacitances in CCD structures.

Insufficient efficiency and speed of the charge shift in SCCD devices prevent the production of large-scale integration arrays. The above disadvantages are eliminated by CCD systems with the channel placed deep in the substrate. This type of device is called a buried-channel CCD (BCCD). Increased carrier velocity is then possible due to the fact that the number of defects in the semiconductor depth is much smaller compared to the subsurface layer.

Figure 12.25 shows the cross-section of an elementary register cell of a BCCD device with an n-channel. This channel is made of a depleted n-type semiconductor on a p-type silicon substrate. A large distance between the channel and the gate allows a strong electric field to occur and, thus, to obtain a high charge transfer speed. Thus, BCCD instruments are characterised by high travel efficiency and high speed of operation.

CCD imaging sensors can also be divided according their illumination. These sensors use three basic architectures (see Figure 12.26):

- frontside-illuminated (FSI);
- backside-illuminated (BSI); and
- deep-depletion device.

In FSI CCD light passes through the polysilicon gates that define each pixel and generates an electric charge in the collecting well when pixels are electrically biased. However, due to reflection

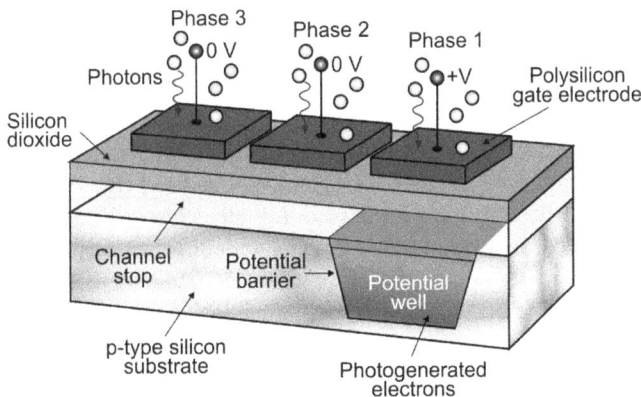

FIGURE 12.25   Cross-section of an elementary cell of a CCD device with a buried channel.

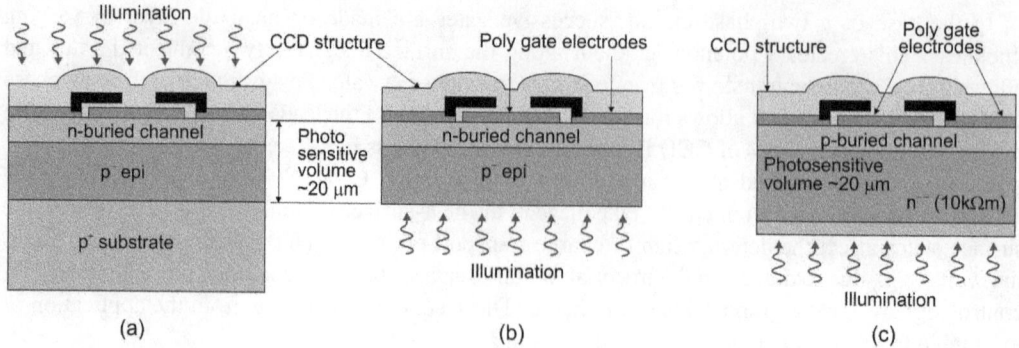

FIGURE 12.26 CCDs technologies: (a) frontside-illuminated CCDs, n-channel on p-type, low resistivity silicon; (b) thinned backside-illuminated CCDs n-channel on p-type, low resistivity silicon; and (c) backside-illuminated deep-depletion CCDs, p-channel on n-type, high resistivity silicon (after Reference 42).

and absorption losses in the poly-gate structure, the quantum efficiency of FSI devices is only 50 per cent (see Figure 7.24). To improve quantum efficiency, the silicon substrate material is uniformly removed to attain approximately 10–15 μm thickness. In this way, an image is focused directly onto the photosensitive area of the CCD without absorption losses in the gate structure [Figure 12.26(b)].

Compared to FSI CCDs, the thinned BSI devices have a higher quantum efficiency with peak > 90 per cent. Further improvement of quantum efficiency can be achieved by using high resistivity silicon with a thickness ranging from 50 to 300 μm [Figure 12.26(c)] in order to produce a larger active photosensitive volume "deeper" in depletion region. This architecture allows fabrication of devices with longer cut-off wavelength.

The noise of CCD instruments manifests as fluctuations in the number of carriers in the charge portion. The main noise mechanisms in CCD elements are the following:

- $1/f$ noise mainly determined by fluctuations of surface states interacting with the charge;
- noise caused by a thermal generation of carriers in a semiconductor;
- photon noise (generated due to photons absorption); and
- noise of a signal readout system and an A/D converter.

Noise caused by a thermal generation of carriers in a semiconductor can be reduced by lowering its operating temperature. For this reason, a thermoelectric cooler (TEC) and a cryogenic cooling – for example, liquid nitrogen in scientific devices – are used. Using TEC and cryogenic coolers, the noise rates of a few electrons/pixel/s and about 1 electron/pixel/h can be achieved, respectively [43]. However, the main sources of noise of CCD arrays come from their signal readout circuitry and A/D converters.

CCD detects light intensity, but not colours. To obtain a colour image, mosaic filters are used in the form of three primary colours: blue (B), green (G) and red (R). As technology developed, various visible (VIS) array designs were developed. Initially, classical Bayer arrays were used, see Figure 12.27(a) and [44, 45], then photosensitive cells with different surfaces were introduced, see Figure 12.27(b), thus improving the quality of the obtained image in different lighting conditions and an additional emerald-coloured filter to increase the image colours tonal range [46]. Light-sensitive elements with a large surface are used to detect low intensity radiation, while elements with a small surface are used in conditions with a bright sunlight. Signals' further processing is performed in the processor in order to obtain an image with the best parameters. These circuits provide better signal dynamics.

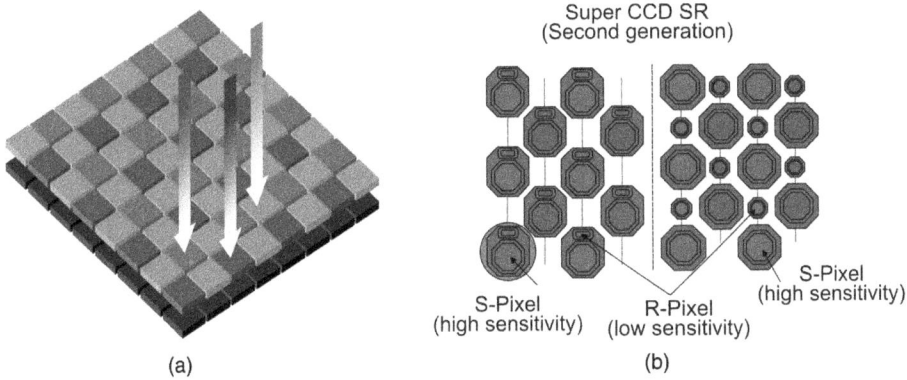

FIGURE 12.27 Types of VIS colour arrays: (a) classic Bayer array and (b) Fuji Super CCD SR array.

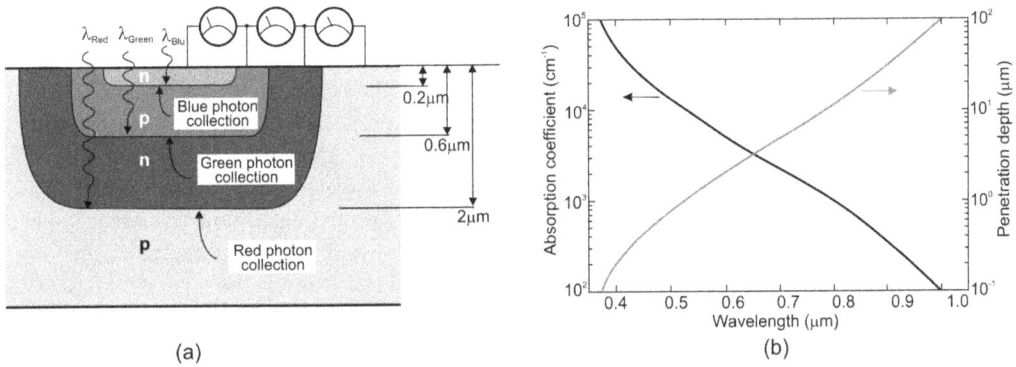

FIGURE 12.28 Schematic illustration of Foveon's sensor stack: (a) cross section of the sensor, and (b) absorption coefficient and penetration depth in silicon.

A new design of visible sensor has been proposed by Foveon and used by the Sigma company. It combines the best of what both film and digital have to offer [47]. This is accomplished by the innovative design of Foveon's X3 direct-image sensors, which have three layers of pixels, just like film has three layers of chemical emulsion; see Figure 12.28 [48]. This silicon sensor is fabricated on a standard CMOS processing line. Foveon's layers are embedded in silicon to take advantage of the fact that red, green and blue light penetrate silicon to different depths (the photodetectors sensitive to blue light are on top, the green sensitive detectors are in the middle, and the red on the bottom), forming the image sensor that captures full colour at every point in the captured image. This is 100 per cent full colour with no interpolation. Figure 12.28(b) plots the absorption coefficient as a function of depth, which is an exponential function of depth for any wavelength. Since the higher energy photons interact more strongly, they have a smaller space constant, and thus the exponential falloff with depth is more rapid.

Foveon's arrays have three times more photosensitive elements compared to the classic array of the same resolution and size. However, a big challenge for technologists is the problem of separating the currents generated by each of the colours. Two other solutions for obtaining colour images are also known. In the first one, the image is obtained by three CCD arrays, each of them containing one R, G, or B filter. This solution is characterised by high resolution, but it is the most technically complicated and expensive. In the second solution, a rotating set of filters is moved over the sensor.

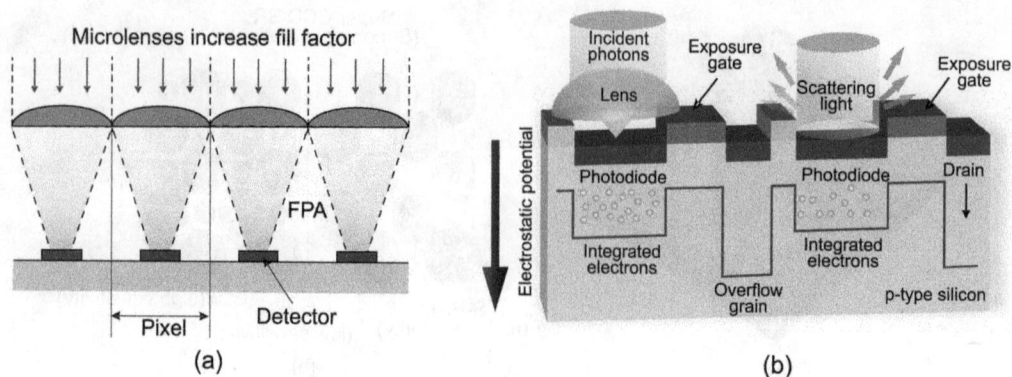

FIGURE 12.29 Cross-sectional drawing of microlensed arrays: (a) general view and (b) design of pixel. Application of microlenses increases the array active area.

This technique is mainly used to register static or slowly changing images due to the low effective processing frequency.

In order to increase the optical fill factor (FF), which is defined as the ratio of the pixel photosensitive area to its total area, microlenses are used (Figure 12.29). They are located above the pixels and focus the incident radiation on the photodetector's surface. In arrays without microlenses and arrays with a low optical FF, only part of radiation falls on the detector active area. Some of this radiation is reflected from the array inactive areas. It is lost, and, in some cases, may be a source of additional noise [49]. In the case of the per-pixel electronics, the area available in the pixel for the detector is reduced, so FF is often limited to 30 to 60 per cent. When the FF is low and microlenses are not used, the light falling elsewhere is either lost or, in some cases, creates artifacts in the imagery by generating electrical currents in the active circuitry. Unfortunately, micro-lenses are less effective when used in low $f/\#$ imaging systems and may not be appropriate for all applications.

Although a microlens improves the pixel sensitivity there are many design challenges associated with the application of micron-scale lens arrays. One key issue is crosstalk, which degrades spatial resolution, colour separation and overall sensitivity. Reducing crosstalk in small pixels has become one of the most difficult and time-consuming tasks in sensor design. At pixel dimensions below 1.45 µm it becomes more difficult in the frontside metallisation of a CMOS sensor and advanced light guiding structures need to be used to reduce crosstalk.

12.5.3 SIGNAL READOUT TECHNIQUES USED IN CCDS

The charge-carrying information about the received signal is converted into voltage at the end of the CCD register. The thus-obtained signal is then sent to an analogue-to-digital (A/D) converter and stored in memory. The first experimental CCD device built by Amelio *et al.* [6] used the technique of injecting a charge into the substrate by biasing one of the gates in such a way as to achieve accumulation. This type of charge detection, however, had limitations in achieving a desired read frequency, noise and processing efficiency. Currently, CCD devices use more advanced signal reading techniques, such as

- floating diffusion amplifier in each pixel;
- system with correlated double sampling (CDS); and
- floating gate amplifier.

12.5.3.1   Floating Diffusion Circuit

One of the simplest and most common output circuits that convert charge to voltage is the floating diffusion equivalent circuit shown in Figure 12.30. It is implemented in each unit cell as shown in the dotted box of the figure. The elementary sensing cell of this circuit consists of detector, capacitor C_{int} of small capacitance, three MOSFET transistors, that is, reset transistor T1, source follower T2 and readout transistor T3. The capacitance C_{int} consists of a follower gate capacitance, mounting capacitances, and detector capacitance. The photocurrent is integrated onto the stray capacitance. Applying Φ_R pulse during the inter-frame time causes transistor T1 to turn on. The capacitance C_{int} is charged to the voltage V_R. The current generated by the detector discharges the capacitor and, therefore, lowers the source follower gate potential. This follower is in the active state only when the pulse ΦE_j is applied to the reading transistor gate. The drain current of the source follower T2 flows through the enable transistor T3 and load resistor outside the array. Currently, very large-scale systems of integration are manufactured, containing floating diffusion amplifiers with a conversion factor exceeding 10 µV/electron.

The amplitude of the voltage at the output of this circuit is given by the equation

$$\Delta V_o = K_W \frac{Q_S}{C_{FD}},$$

(12.18)

where K_W is the source follower gain, Q_S is the amount of charge coming from the signal and C_{FD} is the capacity of the floating diffusion node. C_{FD} capacity is equal to the sum of the follower gate capacity, mounting capacity and detector capacity. An increase in the efficiency of converting charge to voltage can be achieved by reducing the value of this capacitance.

The main source of noise in this circuit is a thermal noise of the reset transistor channel. This noise can be eliminated in a system with double-correlated sampling [50, 51].

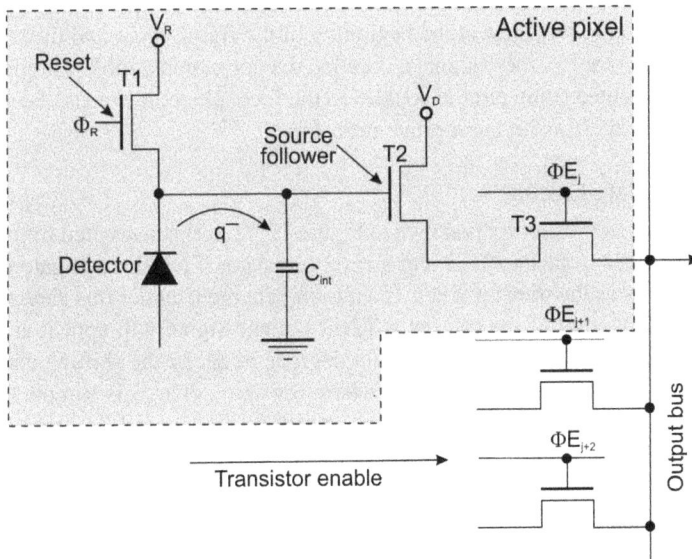

FIGURE 12.30   Diagram of the CCD output circuit from the so-called floating diffusion.

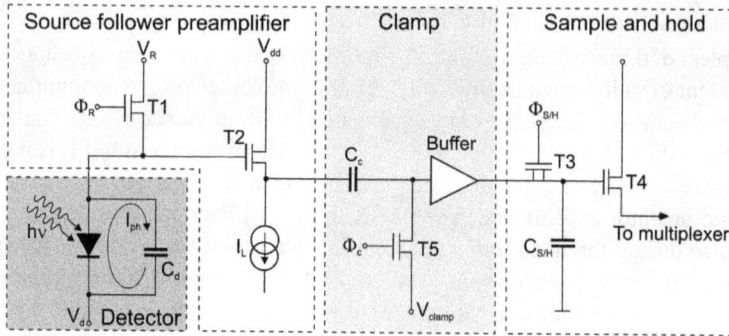

FIGURE 12.31 Correlated double sampling circuit.

12.5.3.2 Correlated Double Sampling Circuit

The dominant source of noise in reading circuits is drift and $1/f$ noise. In order to reduce the noise and increase the signal processing accuracy, a frequent periodic calibration or amplification system resetting is required. Typically, this is done in integrators with a zero reset at the beginning of each integration period.

Figure 12.31 shows a correlated double sampling (CDS) circuit [4]. It consists of a source follower, clamp circuit, sample and hold circuit. In this circuit, the processing is done in two steps. In the first step, at the beginning of the integration period when the T5 key is turned on, a charge proportional to the offset voltage, drift, and low-frequency noise is accumulated in the capacitance C_c. In the second step, at the end of the sampling period, the sample and hold circuit (transistor T3 and capacitance $C_{S/H}$) store the useful signal, taking into account the value of the voltage stored in the capacitance C_c.

From the operating principle of the discussed circuit, the value of voltage stored in the $C_{S/H}$ capacitor is equal to a difference of voltages for the second and first samples, respectively. Since the samples are a short time interval apart, so the offset voltage, drift, and low-frequency noise change slightly, so these factors are eliminated in the subtraction process. The process of double-sampling a signal from a given pixel twice, once at the beginning of the frame cycle and the second time at the end, and using the difference in these signals, is called the correlated double-sampling process. This process can be implemented using circuits located in the focal plane. It can also be realised digitally, outside the detector array using an appropriate processor.

12.5.3.3 Floating Gate Circuit

A diagram of a floating gate amplifier is shown in Figure 12.32. It is constructed from two MOSFETs, that is, a source follower (transistor T2) and a reset transistor T1. The read gate (floating gate) is located in the same row as the transfer gates. If a moving charge is under this gate, then it will cause a change in the gate potential of the transistor T2. A voltage signal will appear at the preamplifier output. The described method of reading does not degrade or decay the shifting charge, so a charge can be detected in many places. An amplifier where the same charge is sampled through several floating gates is called a distributed floating gate amplifier; it was used by Amelio to improve the signal-to-noise ratio [52].

12.5.4 READ-OUT CIRCUITS ARCHITECTURE

The first CCD image sensors were released in 1972–1974 in the United States. As a result of work on these devices, three main varieties of these CCD transducers were developed:

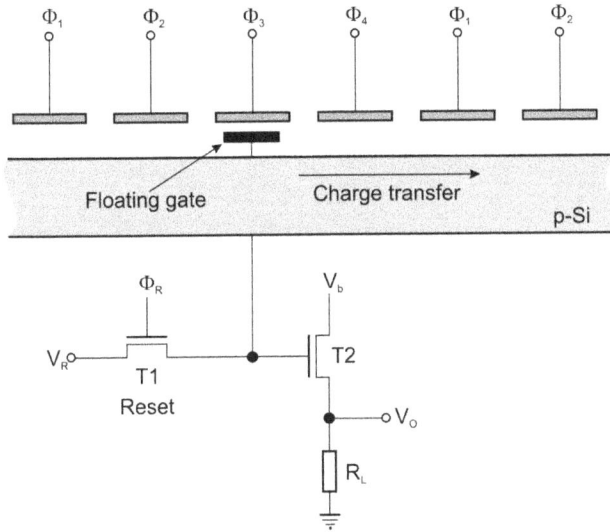

FIGURE 12.32   Floating gate amplifier circuit

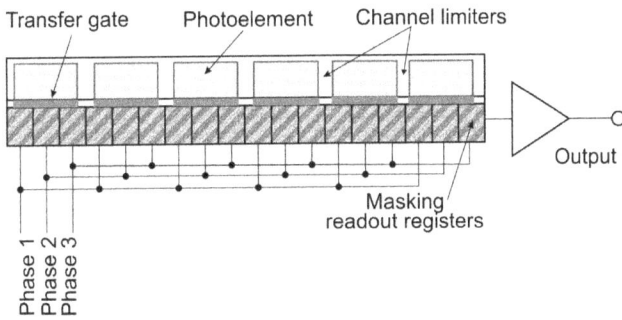

FIGURE 12.33   Linear CCD image sensor.

- full frame (FF);
- frame transfer (FT);
- interline transfer (IL); and
- frame interline transfer (FIT).

Before we discuss the above-mentioned converters, let us first consider a linear array with a three-phase control. This array consists of a photosensitive area, CCD shift register, transfer gates and signal read-out system (Figure 12.33). The register is placed parallel to the photosensitive elements in such a way that one photoelement is coupled by transfer gates with each of the three register items. During image recording, the photosensitive area is isolated from the register.

In order to transfer the charge from the photodetectors to the register, transfer gates are switched on, and the appropriate potential is applied to one of three cells of the register elementary cell. During this time, the voltage is removed from the MOS capacitor gate, which is a photosensitive element. Then, the voltage is removed from the transfer gates, allowing the re-accumulation of charges in the photodetectors. Simultaneously, via a serial register, portions of the charge arrive one by one at the signal readout circuit. In this way, the image from the linear CCD is converted into a time-varying voltage.

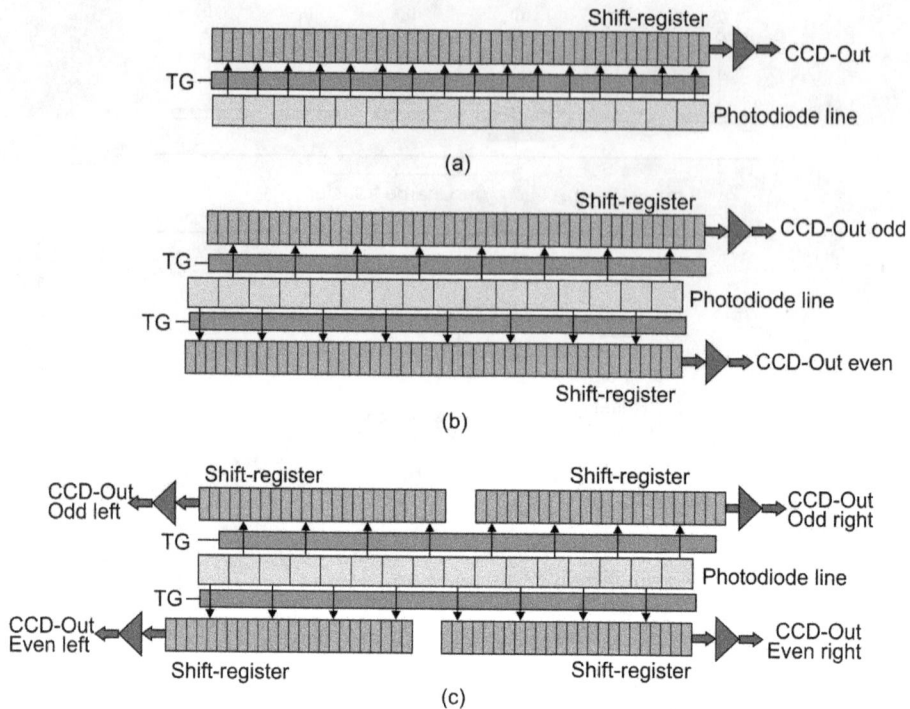

FIGURE 12.34 Linear CCD image sensor: (a) with a single register, (b) with two registers, (c) with four registers.

Linear arrays with different numbers of elements are available, for example, 1024, 2048, 4096. To increase the speed of signal processing, two or even four registers are used (Figure 12.34), which enables faster data transfer and, thus, reduces the time required to refresh the circuit.

12.5.4.1 Full-frame CCD

A diagram of full frame (FF) image sensor architecture is shown in Figure 12.35 [53]. This is the simplest read-out architecture used in CCD instruments. It is composed of an image section, horizontal register and control circuits. In the image section, photon detection and signal charge accumulation are performed. After illumination, the process of a successive row-by-row transfer to the horizontal (read) register follows. First, the charge from the first bottom row is transferred to the horizontal register. From this register, successive charges (pixel by pixel) are transferred to the signal read-out circuit (charge/voltage converter). After reading the content from the last pixel, the next row is sequentially shifted. This process repeats until the charge from the last pixel, the last row, is converted to voltage. Since the imaging section is used for both read-out and charge transport, a mechanical shutter is necessary.

The disadvantage of this architecture is a long reading time, while the advantages are a very low noise level and high sensitivity, as well as a dynamic range of the recorded image, low cost of array fabrication, and high surface fill factor. Transducers of this type are mainly used in scientific research.

12.5.4.2 Frame-transfer CCD

The general structure of frame transfer (FT) image sensor is shown in Figure 12.36. It consists of two sections (areas) – image and memory [54]. In the image section, a photon is detected, and a

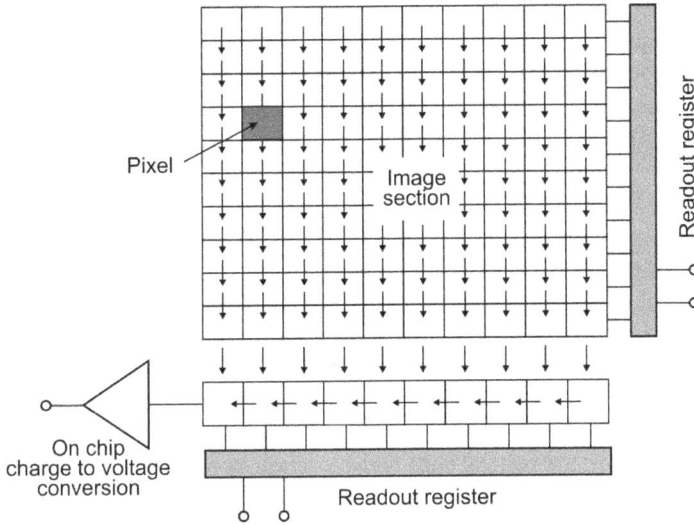

FIGURE 12.35 Pixel layout of the FF CCD.

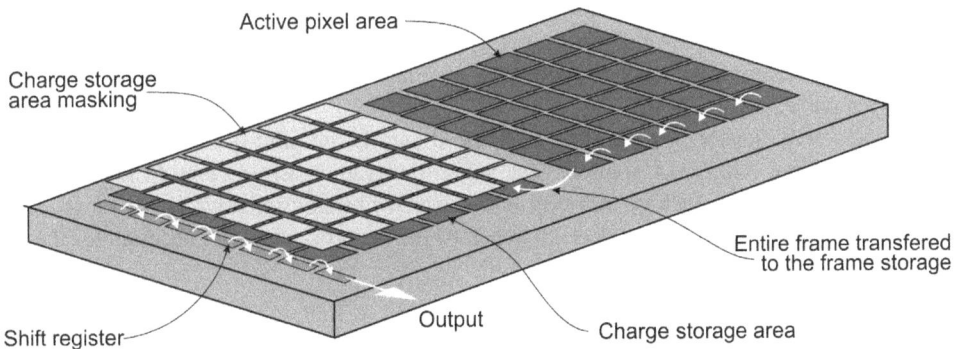

FIGURE 12.36 FT CCD operating principle.

signal charge is accumulated, while in the memory section, a signal charge from the previous image is stored. The picture section contains vertical columns – vertical shift registers. The memory section has the same number of columns and elements as the image section. It is covered with a light, tight aluminium layer. Each register of the image section may be charge-coupled to one corresponding register of the memory section.

During the integration time, the gate electrodes of the CCDs in the image are biased to form a potential well per pixel. Photons incident on the image area generate electron-hole pairs and the electrons are collected in the potential wells. After accumulation of the signal charge, the CCDs in the image and storage areas are driven with the same clock frequency. All the signal charges in the image area are shifted to the storage area by this operation. From this activity, it is commonly referred to as the "frame transfer" converter. The signal charge in the storage area is read out line by line through the horizontal CCD. This type of readout architecture requires small isolation regions between CCD channels, and thus the large fill factor can be achieved.

One disadvantage of the FT-CCD array is the extra real estate for the storage area. In order to reduce smearing of the image during the shifting, the clock frequency for this shifting operation should be as fast as possible. FT CCDs have a much faster read speed than FF CCDs. For example, for a CCD220 chip from e2v (UK), the read-out frequency is of 13.6 MHz, while the frame rate is of 1.3 kHz [55]. The requirement of fast read speed does not occur when a mechanical shutter is used. FT-CCD arrays without the storage area and high resolution have been developed for scientific and industrial applications. Disadvantage of these sensors is a much higher production cost compared to FF CCD converters. They are used in some digital cameras.

12.5.4.3 Interline Transfer CCD

An interline (IL) transfer image sensor is constructed with multiple vertical photosensitive fields connected to vertical CCD shift registers. A diagram of such a sensor is shown in Figure 12.37(a) [54]. Vertical shift registers are shielded from light. They are located between the rows of photosensitive elements. Thus, the read charges move between vertical columns into which the analysed image has been divided. From this property the name was adopted – image converter with an inter-column shift (literally, with an inter-line shift). Such sensors are widely used in commercially available visible range image sensors.

The number of CCDs in the vertical shift registers corresponds to the number of lines present in the TV image field. Time of accumulation of charges under the photosensitive elements is equal to the period of selecting the image. While charges are accumulated in elementary reading cells, vertical CCD registers are isolated from the image section. At the final moment of the integration time, as a result of applying the control pulse to the transfer gate, accumulated charges in elementary reading cells are sent to a potential well of the vertical CCD registers. They are then successively moved line by line to the horizontal register [Figure 12.37(b)]. From this register, point by point, the charge is transferred to the sensor output. Charges transfer to vertical registers occurs during the field blanking pulse.

Advantages of IL sensors are the operation speed and the possibility of electronic adjustment of the exposure time (electronic shutter). The signal integration periods may follow one another directly. However, the presence of registers interleaved with photosensitive elements reduces the active area of such an array. Reduced FF to about 50 per cent, or even less, necessitates the use of microlenses.

12.5.4.4 Frame-interline Transfer CCD

CCD with a frame-interline transfer (FIT) was created as a result of combining the operation concept of FL and IL CCD (Figure 12.38). This type of design solution acts as a very fast electronic shutter and is characterised by a low blurring of the image [56]. The operation of the signal integration and readout from the detector is the same as for the IL CCD. Signal charges, accumulated in the vertical CCD register, are very quickly transferred from the image area to the memory area, allowing

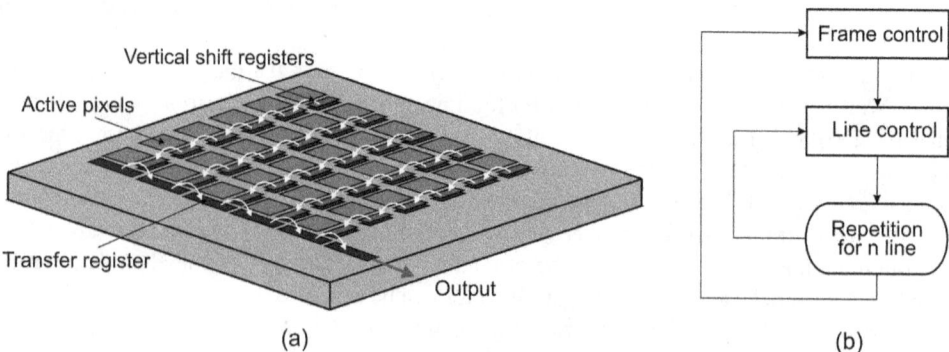

FIGURE 12.37   Interline transfer CCD image sensor: (a) pixel layout, (b) operating principle.

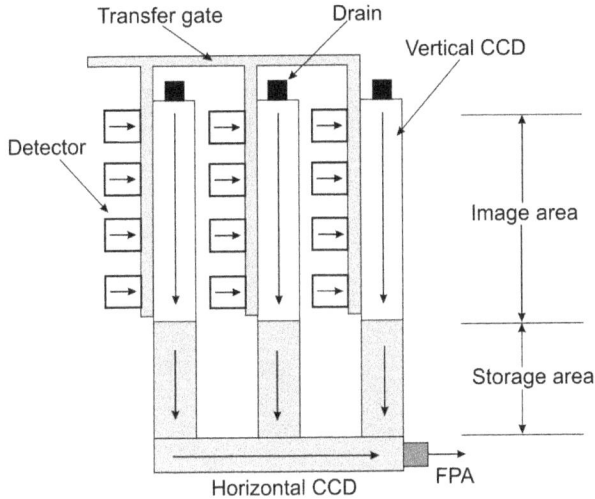

FIGURE 12.38 Frame-interline transfer CCD diagram.

the next frame to accumulate charge. A rapid shift of the signal charge reduces the "blurring" effect caused by carriers generated in the substrate area depth. The operation of reading the signal after this shift is the same as for FT CCD. This structure is preferred in professional cameras.

In the next stage of signal processing in the CCD array, an analogue signal should be converted into a digital signal. In the CCD array, for scientific purposes, 10, 12, 14, and 16 bit analogue-to-digital converters are used. Typically, the number of quantisation levels is smaller than the capacity of the potential well, so there is a certain number of electrons per quantisation level. Suppose we have a 16-bit converter that has 65536 quantisation levels and a potential well capacity of 250000 e-, then we get 3.8e-/quantisation level. Number of electrons per quantisation level is called the conversion factor.

The readout time of photocharges from a CCD array increases as the number of pixels increases. For example, for an array with a resolution of 1024×1024 elements at a signal readout frequency of 100 kHz, it is more than 10 s [57]. This time can be reduced by increasing the signal read-out frequency. However, this causes an increase in current consumption, an increase in power loss and at the same time an increase in the noise of the signal readout circuit. In recent years, an array has been developed that is partitioned (multiport configuration), each partition is connected to a horizontal register and a signal amplifier (Figure 12.39). Thanks to this configuration, it is possible to process data from individual terminals simultaneously, thus increasing the frame rate (number of frames acquired per s). Of course, in this type of solution, the number of output amplifiers increases [57]. Currently, CCD arrays with two, four, and eight terminals are manufactured.

12.5.4.5 Image Sensor Formats

Most sensors are made for camera phones, compact digital cameras, and bridge cameras. Important parameters of visible arrays are the pixel size and its format. Most of these image sensor formats approximate the 3:2 aspect ratio of 35 mm film (see Figure 12.40). The Four Thirds System is a notable exception, with an aspect ratio of 4:3 as seen in most compact digital cameras (see below). The shapes of arrays are typically square or rectangular.

The typical pixel of CCD arrays used in industrial cameras are square-shaped (although there are constructions of a different shape, e.g., rectangular or octagonal) with dimensions in the range of 1.7–14 micrometers [58]. Pixel size and array format are of great importance when selecting optical systems cooperating with it. Arrays of other shapes or sizes are made for special purposes.

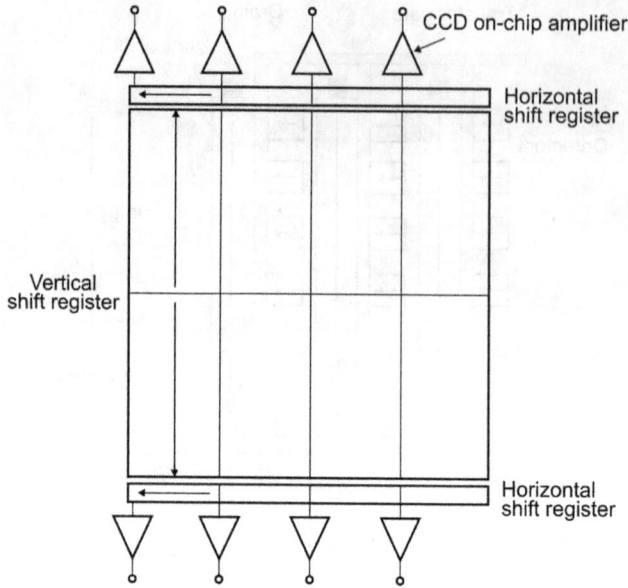

FIGURE 12.39   CCD array with eight terminals.

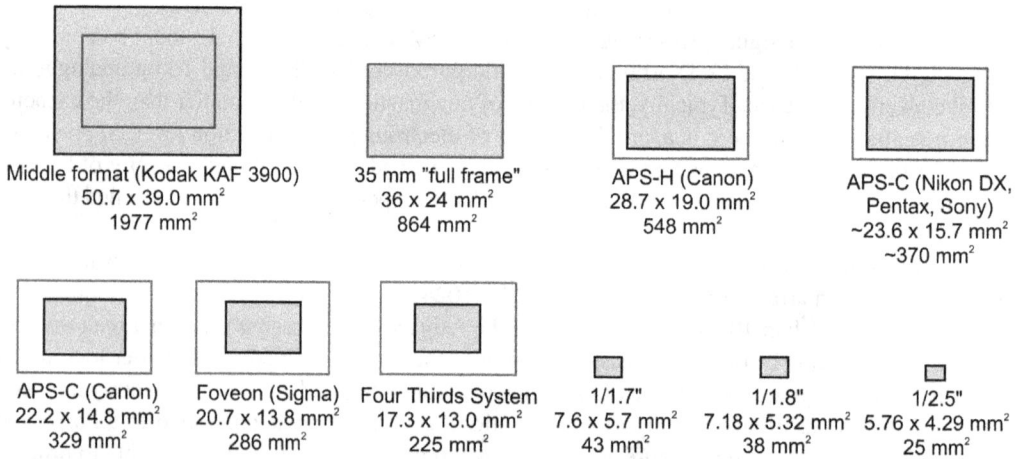

Middle format (Kodak KAF 3900)
50.7 x 39.0 mm²
1977 mm²

35 mm "full frame"
36 x 24 mm²
864 mm²

APS-H (Canon)
28.7 x 19.0 mm²
548 mm²

APS-C (Nikon DX,
Pentax, Sony)
~23.6 x 15.7 mm²
~370 mm²

APS-C (Canon)
22.2 x 14.8 mm²
329 mm²

Foveon (Sigma)
20.7 x 13.8 mm²
286 mm²

Four Thirds System
17.3 x 13.0 mm²
225 mm²

1/1.7"
7.6 x 5.7 mm²
43 mm²

1/1.8"
7.18 x 5.32 mm²
38 mm²

1/2.5"
5.76 x 4.29 mm²
25 mm²

FIGURE 12.40   Examples of CCD array formats. Most of the image sensor formats approximate the 3:2 aspect ratio of 35 mm film.

Table 12.3 presents the main parameters of CCDs from leading manufacturers.

12.6   CMOS DEVICES

An attractive alternative to the CCD readout is coordinative addressing with CMOS switches. In particular, silicon fabrication advances now permit the implementation of CMOS transistor structures that are considerably smaller than the wavelength of visible light and have enabled the practical integration of multiple transistors within a single picture. The configuration of CCD devices requires specialised processing, unlike CMOS imagers that can be built on fabrication lines designed for commercial microprocessors. CMOS have the advantage that existing foundries, intended for

TABLE 12.3
Representative CCD Visible Sensors Offered by Some Major Manufacturers

Manufacturer Model	Number of pixels	Pixel pitch (μm²)	Format (mm²)	Well capacity (e⁻)	Dark current (e/pixel/s)	Dynamic range	Output noise (e⁻ rms)	Output sensitivity (μV/e)
Teledyne e2v CCD47-10	1024×1024	13×13	13.3×13.3	100k	100	50 000:1	2	4.5
Teledyne e2v CCD230-42	2048(H)×2064(V)	15×15	30.7×30.7	150k	0.2		8	2.5
Atmel/Thomson THX7899M	2048×2048	14×14	28.7×28.7	150k	25 pA/cm² @ 25°C	74	13–25	
Kodak KAI 4020	2048×2048	7.4×7.4	16.6(H) ×16(V)	40k	5	60 dB	5	31
Kodak KAF 50100	8176(H)×6132(V)	6×6	49.1(H) ×36.8(V)	40.3	42 pA/cm² (60°C)	70.2	12.5	31
Kodak KAF-6303E	3088(H)×2056(V)	9×9	2765×1848	100k	10 pA/cm² (25°C)	74	15	10
ON Semiconductor KAI-29052	6600(H)×4408(V)	5.5×5.5	36.17×24.11	20k	7 (40°C)	74	10	35
ON Semiconductor KAE–04472	2096(H)×2096(V)	7.4×7.4	5.51(H)×15.51(V)	40k	6	72	10	33
ON Semiconductor KAI-47052	8856(H)×5280(V)	5.5×5.5	48.7(H)×29.0(V)	20k	7	66	10	38
Hamamatsu S10420	1044(H)×22(V)	14×14	14(H)×0.22(V)	60k	50	50000:1	6	6.5
Hamamatsu S11071	2048(H)×64(V)	14×14	28.6(H)×0.89(V)	60k	50	8700:1	23	8
Philips FTF3020-M	3072(H)×2048(V)	12×12	36.864×24.576	500k	20 pA/cm² @ 25°C	72	25	7.5

application specific integrated circuits (ASICs), can be readily used by adapting their design rules. Design rules of 7 nm are currently in production, with pre-production runs of 5 nm design rules. As a result of such fine design rules, more functionality has been designed into the unit cells of multiplexers with smaller unit cells, leading to large array sizes. Figure 12.3 shows the timelines for minimum circuit features and the resulting CCD, IR FPA and CMOS visible imager sizes with respect to the number of imaging pixels. Along the horizontal axis is also a scale depicting the general availability of various MOS and CMOS processes. The ongoing migration to even finer lithography will thus enable the rapid development of CMOS-based imagers having even higher resolution, better image quality, higher levels of integration and lower overall imaging system cost than CCD-based solutions.

CCD sensors have very good dynamic properties, low noise and high sensitivity. Disadvantages of these devices are high current consumption and large size of the systems. Also, the necessity to provide several different supply voltages, necessary for the correct operation of the system, is problematic. Development of digital signal processing technology and reduction of manufacturing costs caused a dynamic development of CMOS sensors. They have the number of advantages. First, progressive miniaturisation makes it possible to create smaller and smaller pixels, resulting in arrays with a very large number of elements. Second, CMOS chips have much lower power consumption than CCDs. Disadvantage of these systems is the noise appearing due to instability of the switching threshold point of transistors connecting pixels to the data bus (capacitive in nature).

CCD and CMOS technologies are compared in Figure 12.24.

12.6.1 Types of Pixels

CMOS chips use passive pixel sensors (PPS), active pixel sensors (APS) and digital pixels (DPS). Table 12.4 shows the schematic diagrams and characteristics of the above pixels.

The term passive pixel should be understood as a system consisting of a detector and a switching transistor. Due to a simpler construction, passive circuits allow for obtaining arrays with a high optical fill factor.

An active pixel consists of detector, preamplifier, and switching transistor. APSs can be equipped with an additional circuitry to control noise in each pixel. This, however, is achieved at the cost of complexity. On the other hand, the image quality improves. Figure 12.41 shows the active pixel structure with a tiny lens system, which serve to focus and concentrate light onto the photodiode surface. Each lenslet is a high-quality optical surface containing refractive elements ranging in size from several hundred to around 10 microns in diameter, depending upon the application. A significant part of the surface is occupied by preamplifier, transistor key and auxiliary elements [59].

A digital pixel consists of detector, analogue-to-digital converter (A/C converter) and memory. Thus, data processing takes place in a given pixel. Placing the amplifier in the active pixel or the A/D converter in the digital pixel causes their dimensions to increase. It also reduces the optical duty cycle factor by up to 50 per cent. The increase of this factor, to about 80 per cent, is achieved by using microlenses.

Different circuits are used to build digital pixels. Figure 12.42 shows a diagram of an elementary DPS cell which is called time-to-first-spike [60]. It is composed of photodiode, reset transistor (key), comparator, control circuit and memory. An important element of this system is the integrating capacity (C_{total}), which consists of photodiode capacitance, comparator input capacitance and mounting capacitance. If the key is on, then this capacitance is charged to the voltage V_{DD}. At the start of the measuring cycle, the key is turned off. The current generated by the photodiode discharges the capacitor, so the potential of the comparator inverting input decreases. If the voltage at the photodiode

TABLE 12.4

Diagrams and Characteristics of Passive, Active and Digital Pixels

Passive pixel (PPS)

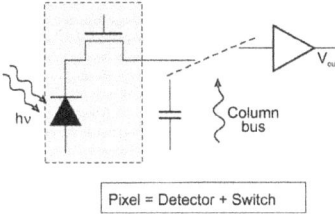

V_{out}

hv

Column bus

Pixel = Detector + Switch

- one transistor (key)
- small pixel area
- high optical fill factor
- high FPN noise
- low signal-to-noise ratio

Active pixel (APS)

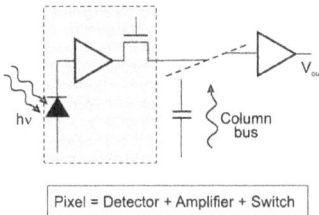

V_{out}

hv

Column bus

Pixel = Detector + Amplifier + Switch

- 1.5–4 transistors per pixel
- larger pixel area
- low optical fill factor
- high signal-to-noise ratio

Digital pixel (DPS)

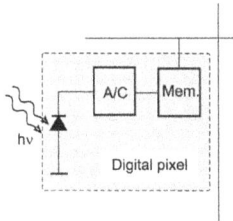

A/C   Mem.

hv

Digital pixel

- 5 transistors per pixel
- big pixels
- low optical fill factor
- no FPN noise

V_{ph} reaches the reference voltage V_{ref} value, a pulse appears at the comparator output. The control circuit, which is triggered by the comparator, stops the capacitance discharge process. Discharge time of this capacitance decreases as the incident radiation intensity increases.

In this method, at the start of processing, simultaneously with the start of a capacitance discharge process, the counter is unlocked and counts pulses delivered to its input from the reference frequency generator. The number of counted pulses, and at the same time the corresponding time value, from the beginning of the integrating capacity discharge cycle to the moment the impulse appears at the comparator output, is stored in a DPS memory.

Figure 12.43 shows a DPS pixel diagram that uses the intensity-to-frequency conversion method. The operation principle of this circuit is similar to that of the circuit discussed above, except that the integrating capacitance is discharged multiple times during the frame duration. The number of capacitance discharge cycles during a frame is directly proportional to the radiation intensity. Each cycle is accompanied by a pulse at the comparator output. These pulses are counted by a counter. In this method, the input current is converted into a pulse train with a frequency proportional to the current value.

Other DPS pixel layout solutions can be found in Reference 61. Discussing them in detail is beyond the scope of this book. Recent reports indicate that work has been undertaken to develop

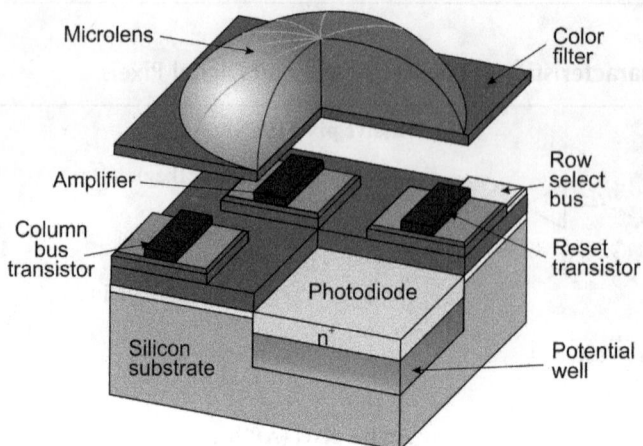

FIGURE 12.41 Active pixel layout.

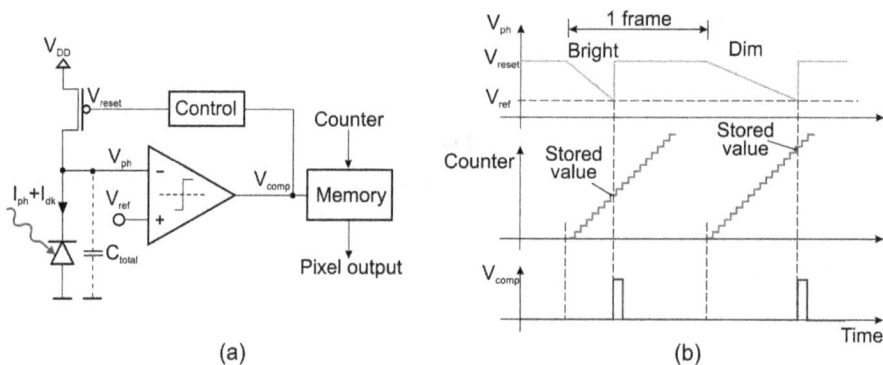

FIGURE 12.42 Digital pixel with irradiance/time converter: (a) diagram, (b) time waveforms at individual points of the system (after Reference 60).

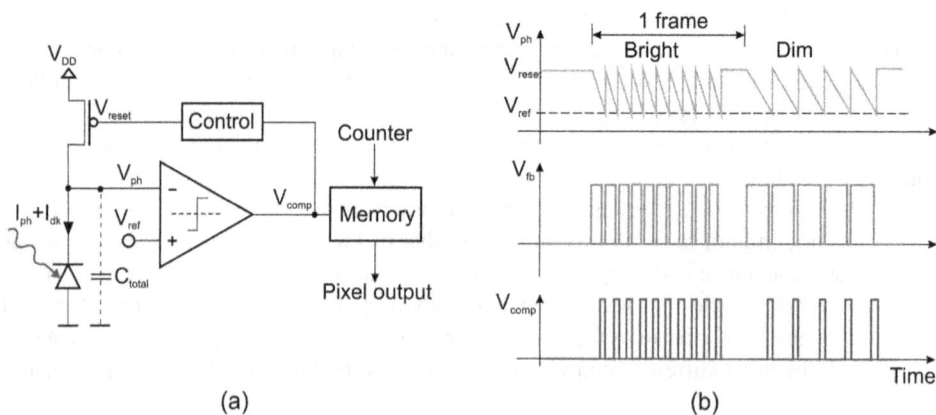

FIGURE 12.43 Digital pixel with intensity-to-frequency converter: (a) diagram, (b) time waveforms at individual points of the system (after Reference 60).

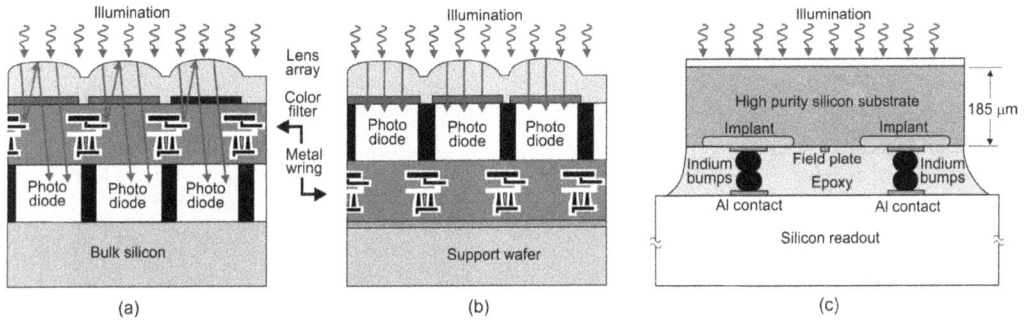

FIGURE 12.44 Cross-section view of different architectures of CMOS imaging sensors: frontside-illuminated (a), backside-illuminated (b), and frontside-illuminated hybrid devices.

a new generation of CMOS sensors [62]. In these digital sensors, all pixels can be read in parallel, which is possible by the association of A/C converter for each pixel.

12.6.2 ARCHITECTURE OF CMOS IMAGING SENSORS

Visible CMOS imaging sensors use two basic architectures:

- Monolithic CMOS (both front side and back side illuminated), for which the photodiodes are included within the silicon readout integrated circuit (ROIC) – see Figure 12.44(a,b); and
- Hybrid CMOS that uses a detector layer for detection of light and collection of photocharge into pixels and a CMOS ROIC for signal amplification and readout – see Figure 12.44(c).

Similar to CCD devices, microlenses have been introduced to the CMOS designs to focus the incoming light onto the photosensitive area of the pixel and to overcome the sensitivity reduction due to a fill factor <100 per cent. However, microlense introduce many design challenges, such as crosstalk. Many of these issues have been solved when CMOS image sensor manufacturers introduced the back-thinning process.

The majority of CMOS imagers are frontside illuminated (FSI). Typical fill factors of FSI sensors range from 30 per cent to 80 per cent. Fabrication of backside illuminated (BSI) sensors is mostly the same as a FSI sensor – photodiodes are laid out first and then the metal layer. After that, the silicon wafer is flipped over, and the excess bulk silicon is ground down until the wafer is only about 10 microns thick [63]. Drawbacks associated with back-thinning of CMOS sensors include lower production yields and higher costs because the thinner silicon wafer makes dies more fragile to produce and more complex to package. Grinding the silicon down allows the wafer to only be as thick as enough to expose the photodiodes. After grinding, the colour filters and microlenses are laid out as with FSI sensors. In this way the device architecture improves the fill factor to nearly 100 per cent.

Impressive progress in the development of hybrid p-i-n Si-CMOS arrays for the large visible and near IR imaging market has been obtained by Raytheon Vision Systems [64]. Arrays as large as 8160×8160 with 8-μm pitch are being produced with > 99.99 per cent operability [65]. The hybrid imagers independently optimise the readout chip and the detector chip with 100 per cent fill factor. One of the key advantages is the use of high resistivity silicon starting material, which results in the ability to fully deplete the intrinsic region of detectors up to 200 μm thick. The deep depleted

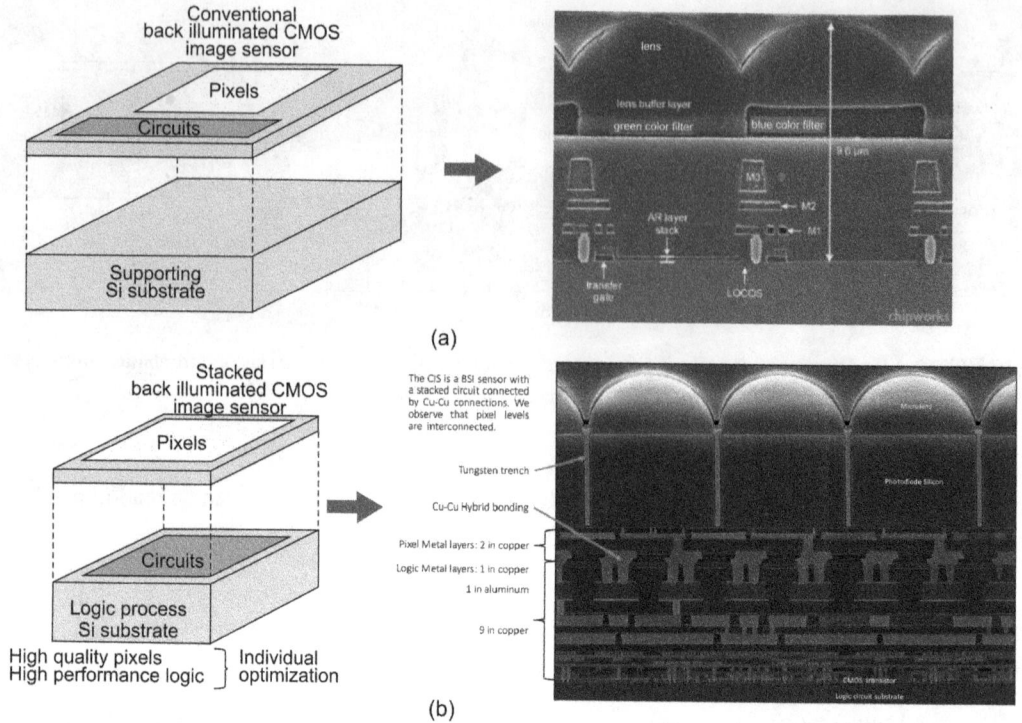

FIGURE 12.45 Digital pixel sensors: (a) conventional chip, layout, (b) 3D-stacked chip generation.

(intrinsic) absorption region is more sensitive to the longer (red) wavelengths of the visible spectrum compared to conventional charge coupled device (CCD) imagers (Figure 7.24).

Basically, the monolithic CMOS chip consists of two layers, the first one containing the pixels, sort of buckets collecting photons, and a second one beneath the first with electronics to read the number of photons accrued by that pixel [see Figure 12.45(b)] [66]. A first command resets the pixel, a second one reads the number of photons captured by the pixel since the reset command. The instant read-out called global shutter, avoids the rolling shutter distortion caused by the time delay as each row of pixels is recorded one after the other. In most existing chips, fast-moving objects become warped as they progress across the frame, because the pixels at the top of the sensor were read earlier than those at the bottom. This can also lead to banding under certain types of artificial lighting.

12.6.3 SIGNAL READOUT CIRCUITS IN CMOS SENSORS

There are ROIC reading systems at the input of image sensors. The most popular circuits include

- self-integrator (SI);
- source follower per detector (SFD);
- capacitor feedback transimpedance amplifiers (CTIA);
- direct injection circuits (DI); and
- MOSFET gate modulation circuits.

They are used in infrared image sensors.

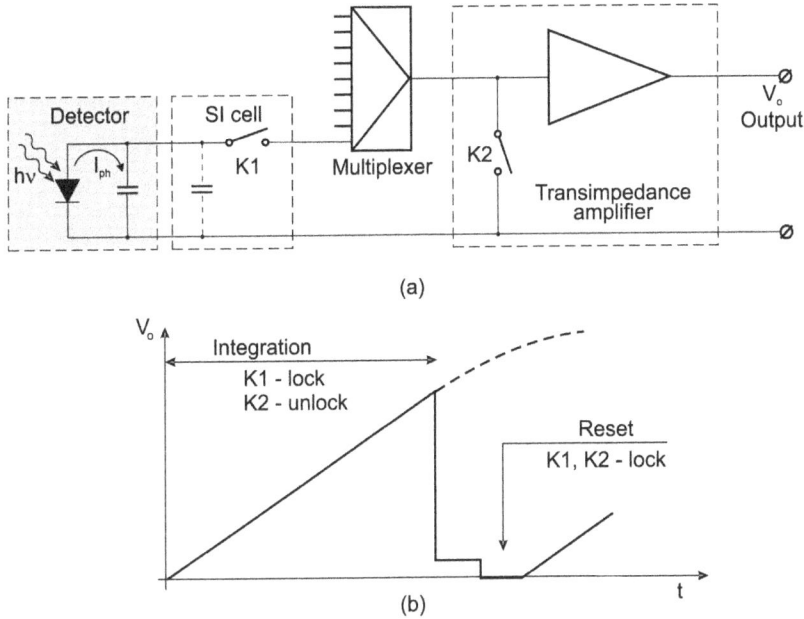

FIGURE 12.46 Self-integrator circuit.

12.6.3.1 SI Circuits

Figure 12.46 shows the basic cell in which a signal integration effect occurs in the input-mode-distributed capacitance. The self-integrator (SI) consists of a detector and a K1 switch made on a MOSFET transistor. A valuable advantage of this solution is that it occupies a very small area. The disadvantage is the lack of signal amplification at the ROIC input. The charge generated by incident photons is stored in the detector capacity and in the capacities of stray connections and the MOSFET switch (K1). Additional capacity can be added, if necessary. After the integration period (time), a signal is transferred by the Z gain transimpedance preamplifier to the circuit output. After the signal is transferred to the sensor output, the capacitance is discharged by the parallel switch K2. In many cases, simply connecting a transimpedance amplifier may be sufficient to discharge the capacitance.

This circuit output voltage, during the integration period, is given by the following equation:

$$V_o = Z \int_0^{t_{int}} I_{ph}(t)\,dt + ZQ_r,\qquad(12.19)$$

where Q_r is the initial charge at the system input, Z is the charge–voltage conversion factor.

The voltage waveform across the sensor capacitances is shown in Figure 12.46(b). If a signal integration time is long, then a non-linear voltage rise will occur, biasing the photodiode in the forward direction. The charge stored in the capacity will then be bypassed by the detector and, as a result, an additional shot noise will occur. For photovoltaic detectors, the voltage at the sensor input terminals will follow the photodiode characteristics. The dynamic range of the SI detector is limited to the level of a reverse voltage present at the detector.

The main source of SI noise is a thermal noise, also called the kTC noise. It is related to fluctuations of the charge stored in the detector capacitance. Changes in the initial charge ΔQ_r cause fluctuations in the detector voltage [Eq. (12.19)].

The RMS value of the SI thermal noise voltage is given by the following equation:

$$V_c^2 = 4kTR_{on} \int_0^\infty \frac{1}{1+\left(2\pi fCR_{on}\right)^2} df = 4kTR_{on}\Delta f, \qquad (12.20)$$

where R_{on} is the resistance of the transistor key in an "on" state. The expression appearing under the integral describes the transfer function of the RC circuit. In turn, the integral from this expression determines the noise bandwidth Δf of the circuit.

For a unipolar RC circuit and white noise, Eq. (12.20) takes the form of

$$V_c = \left[4kTR_{on} \frac{\pi}{2} f_{-3dB} \right]^{1/2}. \qquad (12.21)$$

Thus, the noise equivalent bandwidth Δf appearing in Eq. (12.20) is equivalent to the product of $\pi/2$ and the 3-dB circuit frequency.

The noise voltage can also be defined as the quotient of the noise charge q_c stored in the detector capacitor and the node capacitance (SI cell):

$$V_c = \frac{q_c}{C} = \left(\frac{kT}{C} \right)^{1/2}, \qquad (12.22)$$

where $q_c = (kTC)^{1/2}$.

In practice, the aim is to minimise the stray capacitance at the SI input in order to reduce the kTC noise. In the case when the photon noise dominates, then the maximum permissible input capacitance of the SI system is as follows:

$$C_{max} \le \frac{I_{ph}t_{int}^2}{kT}. \qquad (12.23)$$

The kTC noise is the main source of noise in SI systems. In order to minimise the SI parallel capacity, a smaller capacity detector should be used. Detector capacity is the main component of the SI capacity.

12.6.3.2 SFD Circuits

The source follower per read-out circuit is similar to the SI circuit. Figure 12.47 shows the basic preamplifier cell in which the T2 source follower, T1 reset key and the MOSFET switch T3 are used.

Under the influence of incident radiation, the current generated in the photodiode is integrated into the input node capacitance. This capacitance is equal to the sum of the detector capacitance, the gate capacitance of the source secondary and the junction capacitance. Voltage value on the input node capacitance at the end of the integration period is determined by the following equation:

$$V_t = \frac{I_{det}t_{int}}{C}, \qquad (12.24)$$

where I_{det} is the sum of the photocurrent and the dark current, and C is the input node capacity.

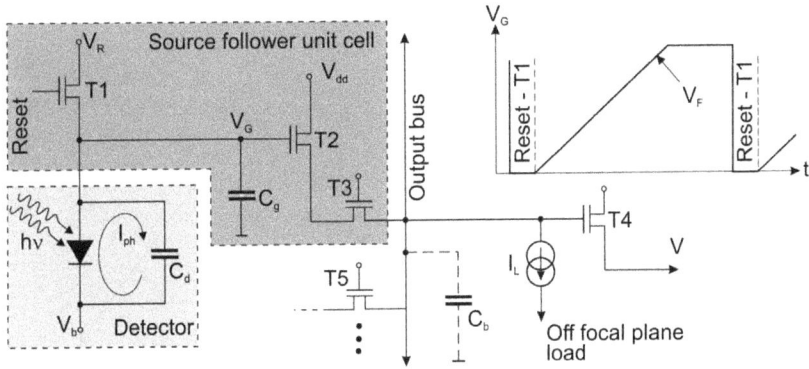

FIGURE 12.47 SFD read-out circuit (after Reference 4).

In an SFD circuit, a voltage increases linearly with an integration time. It is separated by the source MOSFET follower and then switched to the common bus via the T3 transistor. After charging the input mode capacity, the multiplexer reads the resulting voltage, discharges it, and then starts the integration period again. SFD system dynamic range is limited, as to the SI system, by the current-voltage characteristics of the detector. The SFD current load is outside the "reading cell". Thus, the cell only releases power when the output signal is connected to the bus. The source follower current should be large enough to control the multiplexer bus capacity.

SFD circuits are used in those applications where small pixel dimensions are required and where there is a low background level (e.g., in space systems) [67]. In these systems, the charge is accumulated in a sufficiently long time. The integrating capacitance value is mainly determined by the detector capacitance.

In applications where a very high sensitivity is required, the detector capacitance must be small. This makes it possible to obtain a high gain.

The main sources of SFD noise are kTC noise, $1/f$ noise of MOSFETs, and thermal noise of the MOSFET transistor channel resistance.

12.6.3.3 Capacitor Feedback Transimpedance Amplifier

Capacitor feedback transimpedance amplifier (CTIA) is commonly used to amplify electrical signals obtained from infrared radiation detectors [1]. CTIA system circuit ensures high stability of the detector operating conditions, high efficiency of a photocurrent injection, high gain and low noise. Typically, the CTIA circuit performance is better than that of RTIA circuits (with a resistor in a feedback loop). Compared to RTIA circuits, they have a higher upper cut-off frequency and a better *MTF* modulation transfer function. The diagram of the CTIA circuit is shown in Figure 12.48.

The voltage at the CTIA circuit output is as follows:

$$V_o = \frac{K_v I_{det} t_{int}}{C_f (1 + K_u)} = I_{ph} Z_t, \tag{12.25}$$

where Z_t is the CTIA circuit transimpedance. At the end of the cycle, this voltage is sampled and then sent to the output stage. Discharging the capacitor C_f with the bypass switch ends the measurement period and prepares the system for signal detection in the next measurement cycle. Duration of the measurement cycle is equal to the sum of the integration time and the zeroing time. There are also circuits at the CTIA circuit output that reduce drift and correct the reference voltage.

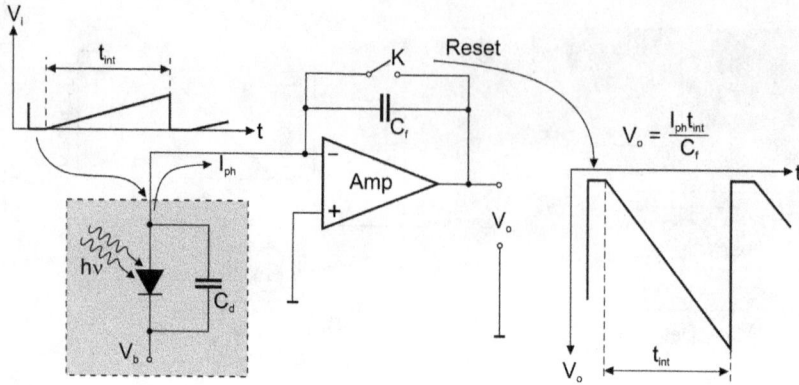

FIGURE 12.48 CTIA circuit.

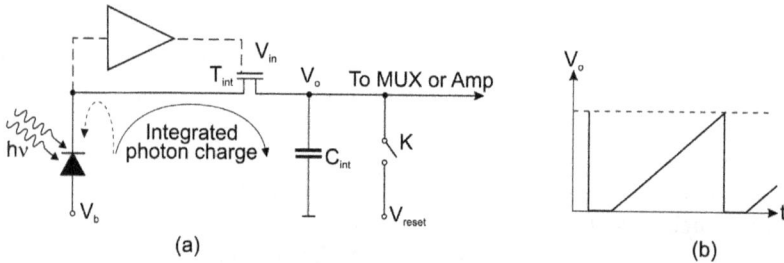

FIGURE 12.49 Charge injection integrator with MOSFET transistor: (a) diagram, (b) voltage waveform at the output of the circuit.

The greatest noise in CTIA is caused by the input transistor of the differential amplifier, which can cause undesirable drift and off-balance voltage. CTIA output noise depends on the gain and noise bandwidth Δf. The gain of the circuit depends on the detector capacity and the capacity in the feedback circuit:

$$\frac{V_{no}}{V_n} \approx \frac{C_f + C_{det}}{C_f}.$$

(12.26)

Most of CTIA circuits are made in the CMOS technology.

12.6.3.4 Injection Circuits

Zero integrators belong to the family of injection circuits. Circuits with charge injection through the active transistor channel or the CCD instrument channel are known. Figure 12.49 shows the zero-crossing integration circuit using a MOSFET.

In this circuit, the signal integration circuit is closed via the channel of the active transistor T_{int}. Charge accumulated in the integration capacitance C_{int} is periodically reset. Since the detector is not directly reset, but the capacitor C_{int} is short-circuited, some residual charge remains in the detector junction capacitance. This charge is integrated in the next measuring cycle causing crosstalk.

The circuit shown in Figure 12.49(a) has been used for many years as an input cell of CCD devices. This configuration takes up a very small area; the second largest after SI systems. This system is designed to detect medium- to high-intensity radiation. Direct injection photocurrent is injected through the source of the transistor bandwidth into the integral capacitance, which is reset to zero at the beginning of the frame. The photocurrent generated in the photodiode causes charging of the capacitor C_{int} during the entire measurement cycle [Figure 12.49(b)]. After the integration period, the capacitor voltage is read out by the multiplexer. The capacitor is then discharged using the switch K.

The gain in DI and CTIA is set using an integrating capacitor, capacitance of which may be very small and does not depend on the detector capacitance. Integrating capacitance can be separated from downstream circuits by a source follower.

If a phase-inverting amplifier with the gain K_v is connected to the DI circuit, we get a feedback-enhanced direct injection (FEDI) system. It reduces the DI circuit input impedance, thereby increasing the injection coefficient and broadening the frequency response [52]. This circuit is also more sensitive compared to the DI circuit.

The dominant noise source of FEDI circuits is the amplifier input noise V_n. The contribution of the voltage noise V_n of the transistor T_{int} is negligible because it is reduced K_v times. Detector noise influence is identical to that of the DI circuit.

12.6.3.5 MOSFET Gate Modulation Circuits

In MOSFET gate modulation circuits, the current generated in the photodiode controls the gate potential, resulting in a change in the drain current. This current charges the integrating capacitor or the potential well of a CCD instrument. For this modulation method, fluctuations of the detector bias voltage occur. To prevent this phenomenon, the detector is biased in a reverse direction. However, this causes an increase in type $1/f$ noise and dark current. In order to reduce crosstalk between consecutive frames, the capacitance C_{int} should be shortened using the analogue switch at the end of the frame. Gate modulation circuits are most often used in photoreceivers operating in conditions of a strong background radiation [67].

Figure 12.50 shows the circuits with the MOSFET transistor gate modulation. Figure 12.50(a) uses the resistor R_L in the photodiode load circuit, while Figure 12.50(b) uses a current mirror (CM) [4]. The photodiode anode voltage depends on the value of the photocurrent, the dark current, the load resistance R_L and the detector bias voltage V_b, and is as follows:

$$V_i = \left(I_{ph} + I_d \right) R_L + V_b. \tag{12.27}$$

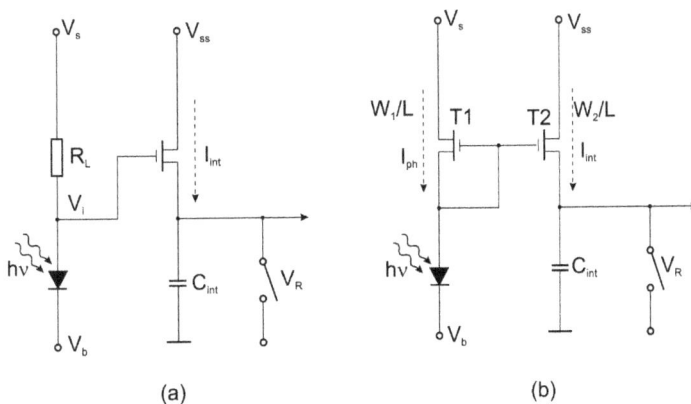

(a)   (b)

FIGURE 12.50 Circuit with gate modulation: (a) with a resistor in the photodiode load circuit, (b) with a current mirror in the photodiode load circuit.

The load resistor should have low noise type $1/f$ and high temperature stability. They are usually made of polycrystalline silicon. This resistor value should be identical for all cells of the detector array.

In gate-modulated circuits, the MOSFET transistor usually operates in the subthreshold (weak inversion) range. The drain current depends on the voltage at the photodiode anode and the K_2 coefficient:

$$I_{drain} = I_{int} K_2 \exp(V_i),$$ (12.28)

where K_2 is the factor dependent on the supply voltage V_s, MOSFET threshold voltage, temperature, and many other factors.

A circuit with modulation of the transistor gate enables a significant reduction of the background radiation influence. When only background radiation falls on the detector, the operating point of this circuit should be chosen so that the drain current is as small as possible. It is possible to select the transistor operating point using the resistor R_L or the detector supply voltage.

Output voltages of individual circuits may differ from each other. This is due to unequal threshold voltages of the MOSFET transistors, the resistance R_L value, or detector resistance.

In the current mirror (CM) preamplifier, the resistor R_L is replaced with a MOSFET [Figure 12.50(b)]. In this circuit, a photocurrent is also a drain current of the first transistor. The way the transistors are connected causes the same gate-source voltage changes. Since these transistors are made in the same technological process, the second transistor drain current will be identical to the photocurrent. In general, the integrator current is a linear function of the detector current (as opposed to the resistor R_L circuit).

In a current mirror preamplifier, it is possible to determine an integration current value. This is done by selecting geometrical dimensions of the transistor pair. Integration current dependence on dimensions of the transistor drain and the detector current is given by the following equation [4]:

$$I_{int} = I_{det} \frac{W_2/L_2}{W_1/L_1},$$ (12.29)

where W and L are the width and length of the MOSFETs drains, respectively.

As already mentioned, CM circuits are used in photoreceivers operating under strong influence of background radiation, with small charge-accumulating capacitances. To reduce the signal integration current, dimensions of the second transistor drain must be reduced in relation to the first transistor dimensions. In this way, a reduction in the integration current value in relation to the photocurrent is achieved. It is also possible to adjust the integration current by selecting the values of voltages supplying both transistors according to the following equation:

$$I_{int} = I_{det} \frac{W_2/L_2}{W_1/L_1} \exp(V_s - V_{ss}).$$ (12.30)

The above analysis is valid assuming that there is 100 per cent efficiency for injecting the detector current into the MOSFET. The injection efficiency depends on the detector resistance and the MOSFET transconductance, which is a photocurrent function.

CM circuits have a high-pattern noise due to unequal transistor threshold voltages or non-uniform injection efficiency. The latter parameter depends largely on the detector resistance. Circuits with a current mirror are characterised by a greater linearity compared to circuits with a resistive load.

Table 12.5 shows a comparison of the most commonly used signal readout systems.

TABLE 12.5
Comparison of the Most Commonly Used Signal Readout Systems

Circuit	Advantages	Disadvantages	Full well capacity [e]	Readout noise [e]	Application
DI	Compact unit cell, stable detector bias at medium to high backgrounds, low impedance detector interface	Unstable detector bias at low current levels	Tens of millions	< 1000	Medium to high photon flux, terrestrial IR systems.
FEDI	Compared with DI, increase in the injection ratio, increase in the frequency response, about a 10-fold decrease in the maximum flux, stable detector bias with average to high backgrounds	Increase in noise caused by use of amplifier, large unit cell, increased power dissipation, bias variation from cell to cell, sometimes compensation of FD-PA system oscillation	Tens of millions	< 1000	Medium and high photon flux, space IR systems
SFD	Used to read the signal from compact unit cell, low power consumption, low noise, high sensitivity	Poor to flux performance, detector bias changes during integration, low dynamic range	100 000	< 15	Low background astronomy (IR and visible detectors)
CTIA	High stability of detector working conditions, high injection efficiency, high gain, high linearity, wide dynamic range, low noise	Complex readout circuit, higher power and noise compared then SFD for low flux, worse performance than DI for high flux	1–10 millions	< 50	Suitable for all backgrounds, space IR and visible detectors

12.6.4 READOUT CIRCUIT ARCHITECTURE FOR CMOS SENSORS

Many CMOS image sensor system solutions are well-known. The most popular include MOS-XY image sensor and MOS sensors with read-out in the horizontal direction.

A diagram of the MOS-XY integrated image sensor is shown in Figure 12.51. The photodiode array is addressed here with an X-Y orthogonal array. MOS transistors act as keys. The photodiode cathode is connected to the source of the MOS key transistor. Its gate is connected to the electrode line (row), and the drain is connected to the array node column. The columns electrodes connect to the busbar via MOS transistors, controlled by the horizontal addressing system.

In a MOS-XY converter, the keying transistors of all nodes of one row of the array are usually activated simultaneously. Photocharges stored in junction capacitors travel to the transistor sources whose sequential opening cause successive photocharges to be released to the busbar. Thus, a line analysis takes place. The busbar end is the output circuit that converts a charge into an output voltage. Advantages of this read-out are a large optical fill factor, high saturation level and compatibility with standard MOS large-scale integrations [56]. The disadvantage of this circuit is a

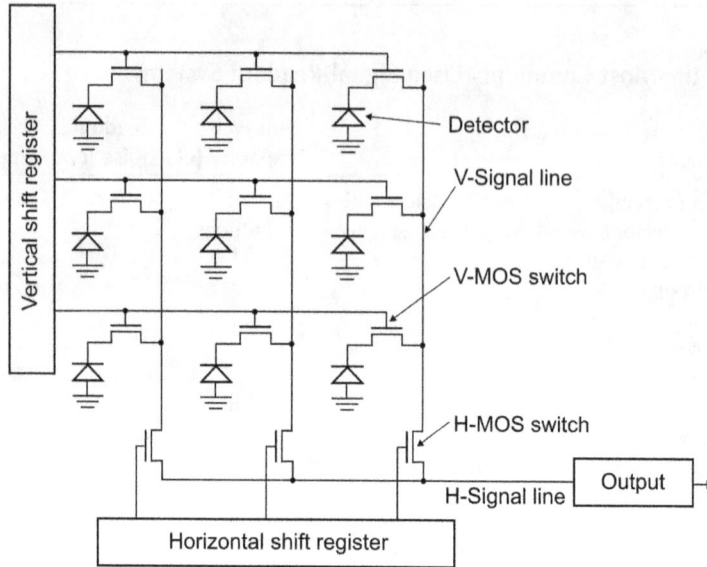

FIGURE 12.51   Diagram of the MOS-XY converter.

large random noise due to a large vertical line capacitance, and a noise resulting from non-uniform horizontal characteristics of the MOSFET transistors. To eliminate this disadvantage, a row-readout MOS converter was developed [68].

12.6.5   CMOS VERSUS CCD

As mentioned in section 12.5, CCDs and CMOS imagers were both invented in the late 1960s and 1970s. In this beginning period CCD became dominant, primarily because they gave far superior images with the fabrication technology available. CMOS image sensors required more uniformity and smaller features than silicon wafer foundries could deliver at the time. To compete with CCD devices, the development of photolithography in the 1990s achieved the expectations of the designers to return to CMOS imagers again. Renewed interest in CMOS was based on lowered power consumption, camera-on-a-chip integration, and lowered fabrication costs from the reuse of mainstream logic and memory device fabrication. The advantages and disadvantages of CCD and CMOS are described in detail in Figure 12.24. Achieving CMOS benefits in practice while simultaneously delivering high image quality has taken far more time, money and process adaptation than original projections suggested. In the mid-1990s CMOS imagers joined CCDs as mainstream, mature technology [69, 70].

The monolithic CMOS devices, where detector array and accompanying readout circuits are fabricated in the same substrate, were developed and commercialised in the mid-1990s. While Sony has been the dominant supplier of CCDs to the imaging and machine markets, this dominance is not evident with CMOS giving more market choice. Key players besides Sony are ON Semiconductor, CMOSIS, eV2 and Teledyne DALSA.

CMOS technology enables system designers to tailor their imaging devices to the needs of their applications. Fairchild Imaging, Andor Technology and PCO CMOS sensors are called Scientific CMOS (sCMOS), since they are designed with a superior combination of features that are able to meet the extreme performance requirements of many scientific applications in biomedical research, astronomy, security and defence. Table 12.6 lists performance characteristics of monolithic CMOS devices that have been designed for scientific applications.

TABLE 12.6
Characteristics of the State-of-the-Art Scientific Monolithic CMOS Devices

Sensor technology	Fairchild sCMOSLTN4625A Back-illuminated	SRI International Back-illuminated	eV2 EV2S16M Back-illuminated
Format	4608×2592	2048×1920	4096×4096
Pixel size (μm)	5.5	10	2.8
Image area (mm)	25.3×14.3		16.22 (diagonal)
Full well capacity (e⁻)	> 40 000	> 220 000	
Dark current (e⁻/pixel/sec)	< 15	< 4	3–5
Read noise (e⁻)	< 5	< 14	< 5
Max. frame rate (fps)	240		16
Power consumption (W)	2		1.6

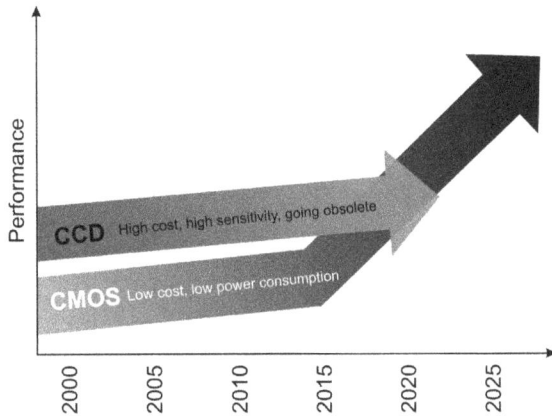

FIGURE 12.52 Development of CMOS imaging sensors.

CMOS technology has been key for meeting the challenges of Moore's Law. Shrinking sensor pixel size, however, poses significant challenges to sensor design. As pixel size gets smaller, the well capacity shrinks, resulting in less dynamic range. The photon collection area also shrinks, causing less sensitivity. Crosstalk, noise, coupling, and non-uniformity become more severe and visible.

In the mid-1980s, APS sensors were invented as a low-cost alternative to the dominant CCD technology. In the early 2000s these sensors were updated to use the new generation CMOS technology – with 3D-stacked DPS sensors. Although early CMOS sensors were only used in low-performance applications, the advent of smart phones pushed manufacturers to rapidly improve their performance (see Figure 12.52). By 2007 CMOS had achieved market parity with CCD sensors, and by 2020 the first sensors capable of surpassing CCD performance appeared. Today, CMOS has matured to the point where it is replacing CCD in all but the most specialised applications. CCD technology and frontside illuminated CMOS APS sensors have passed their maturity stage, and are now in decline, while backside illuminated CMOS APS technology is currently growing. Sales of CCD image sensors on the global market have declined to an unsustainable level due to the ongoing market conversion from CCD towards CMOS image sensors. For this reason, for example, ON Semiconductor has announced to discontinue the production of CCD image sensors.

Figure 12.53(a) shows the pixel sizes of CCD and CMOS arrays during the first twenty years of the twenty-first century. It should be noted that in the initial period smaller pixel sizes in CCD arrays were obtained, while in recent years significant technological advances in the development of CMOS arrays have been achieved, obtaining large array formats and comparable or even smaller pixel sizes [70].

CMOS technology has been the key for meeting the challenges of Moore's Law. Shrinking sensor pixel size, however, poses significant challenges to sensor design. As pixel size gets smaller, the well capacity shrinks resulting in less dynamic range, the sensitivity and gain of charge-voltage conversion increases, while the potential well capacity decreases [see Figure 12.53(b)]. Crosstalk, noise, coupling and non-uniformity become more severe and visible.

The CMOS has overcome CCD technology, particularly in pixel size, critical to mobile applications. Success was defined by the proper timing of leveraging high-volume, low-cost, stable semiconductor processes, pragmatically optimising the size, cost and performance of miniature cameras. The smallest CMOS pixels used in smartphone products today are 0.9-μm sized pixels.

Another problem concerns the phenomenon of light diffraction. The smaller the pixel, the more visible the blurring of the image will be. Thus, we come to a barrier that seems impassable. At

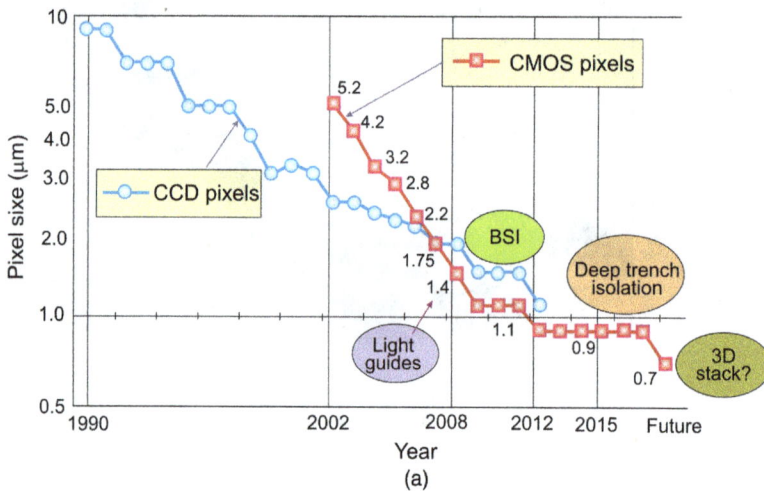

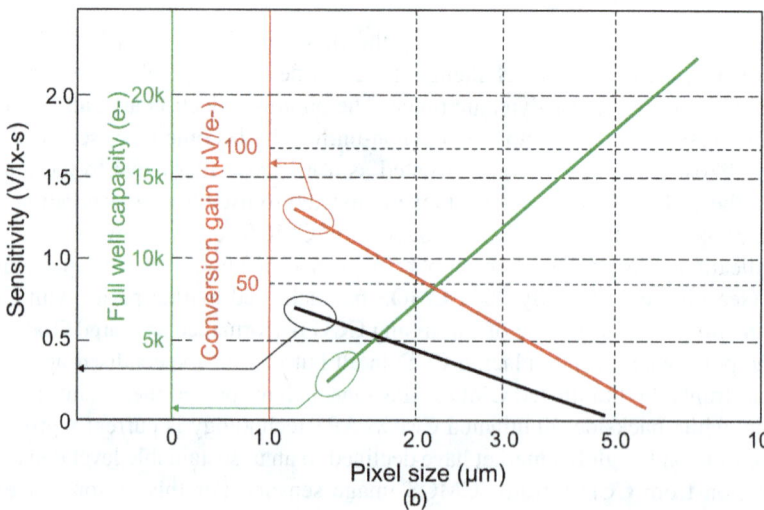

FIGURE 12.53 Changes in pixel sizes in CCD and CMOS arrays: (a) over the years, (b) the impact of pixel sizes on sensitivity, well capacity, and gain.

present, CMOS arrays are beginning to dominate in cameras, for example, single-lens reflex cameras as well as cameras integrated with mobile phones.

Currently, the largest volume of the image sensor market is based on consumer electronics, which prefer high-resolution arrays with small pixel dimensions. Many DPS designs are currently unsuitable for this market segment. However, there are application areas – for example, medicine, security systems, automotive industry and special applications – where the use of arrays with DPS pixels is perfectly justified.

12.7 REPRESENTATIVE FOCAL PLANE ARRAYS

This section concentrates on describing impressive achievements in fabrication focal plane arrays in different spectral ranges from γ-rays to terahertz (THz). Figure 12.54 presents a typical pixel size of electronic image sensors in various imaging bands.

12.7.1 BUTTING VERSUS STITCHING TECHNIQUES

Both *stitching* and *butting* techniques are used in fabrication of large imaging arrays.

Stitching refers to putting various design blocks together during the processing of the semiconductor to make one large, stand-alone imaging array. In most cases stitching is used to make imagers that are larger than the field of view of the lithographic equipment used during the fabrication of the imagers. Readout circuit wafers are processed in standard commercial foundries and can be constrained in size by the die-size limits of the photolithography step and repeat printers. Because of field size limitations in those photography systems, the imager chip sizes must currently be limited to standard lithographic field sizes of less than 32×26 mm for submicron lithography. The stitching photolithographic technique is used to fabricate detector arrays larger than the reticle field of photolithographic steppers. The large array is divided into smaller subblocks. Later, the complete sensor chips are stitched together from the building blocks in the reticle as shown in Figure 12.55. Each block can be photocomposed on the wafer by multiple exposures at appropriate locations. Single

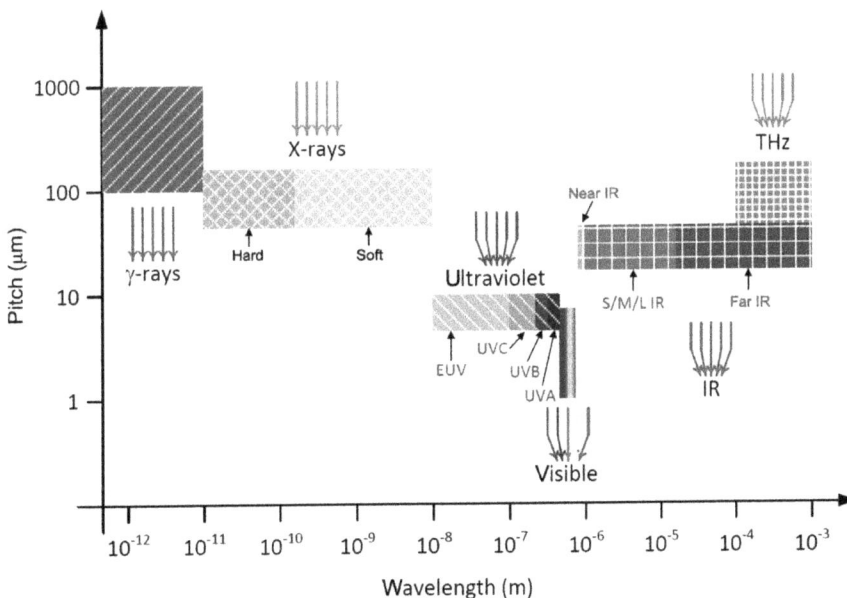

FIGURE 12.54   Variation of typical pixel pitch with imaging band (after Reference 60).

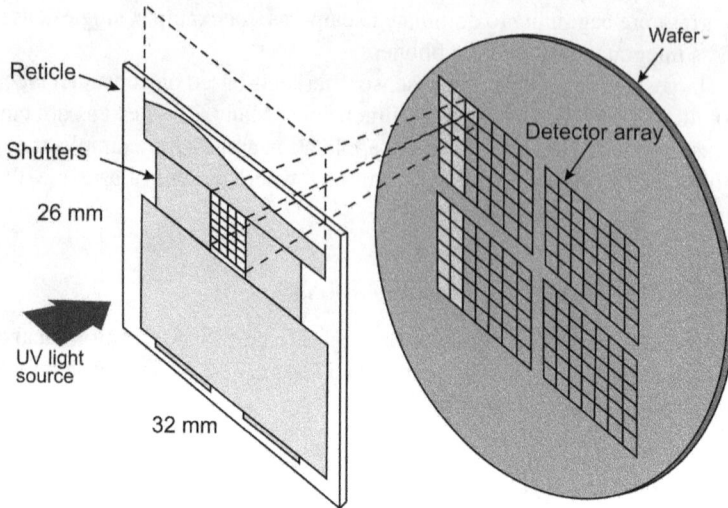

FIGURE 12.55   The photocomposition of a detector array die using array stitching based on photolithographic stepper.

blocks of the detector array are exposed at one time, as the optical system allows shuttering, or selectively exposing only a desired section of the reticle.

Butting refers to tiling closely together separate pieces of semiconductor to come to one large sensitive array. In principle all separate pieces of semiconductor can be operated as a single image sensor. In most cases butting is used to make imagers that are larger than the largest imager a single wafer can hold. Most of the buttable devices are also stitched because stitching is needed to make the largest array possible on a single wafer. If that imager is still not large enough, butting is the only solution. However, not all stitched devices are buttable, because not all stitched devices have a wafer-level size.

Below, butting technique is explained in more detail. Figure 12.56(a) shows a simple draft of an imaging array with a left-driving and a right-driving circuitry, a readout part at the bottom and some extra electronic circuitry at the top. This array is not designed to be butted. To make, for example, two sides buttable, the readout circuitry along two sides needs to be removed in the design, which is shown in Figure 12.56(b). As can be seen in Figure 12.56(c), the total four-sided buttable light sensitive array is four times as large as the size of a single device.

A three-sided buttable architecture is used for medical (mainly CMOS) and astronomy (mainly CCD with shift towards CMOS) applications. Assuming 300 mm wafer sizes, single monolithic sensors of 200×200 mm^2 on a single wafer can be fabricated. Recently, also some attempts to build four-sided buttable CCDs have been realised. In the future, greater use of four-sided buttable designs is expected.

The butting is never perfect; there are always some pixels missing between the two pieces of semiconductor (usually limited to a single line of pixels). Usually, the butted arrays do not use small pixels. Their typical size is several tens of microns.

It should be noted that stitching creates a seamless detector array, as opposed to an assembly of closely butted sub-arrays. The butting technique is commonly used in the fabrication of very large-format sensor arrays. For example, the 1.4 gigapixel (Gpixel) orthogonal transfer array (OTA) CCD imager (spread over an area about 40 cm^2) used in Panoramic Survey Telescope and Rapid Response System (PanSTARRS) is comprised of 64 chips, each of 22 megapixels (Mpixels). Figure 12.57 shows one of the 64 OTA devices. This above 1 gigapixel imager could not be made monolithically, since it exceeds the size of the largest silicon wafers used by the IC industry. Currently silicon wafer sizes do

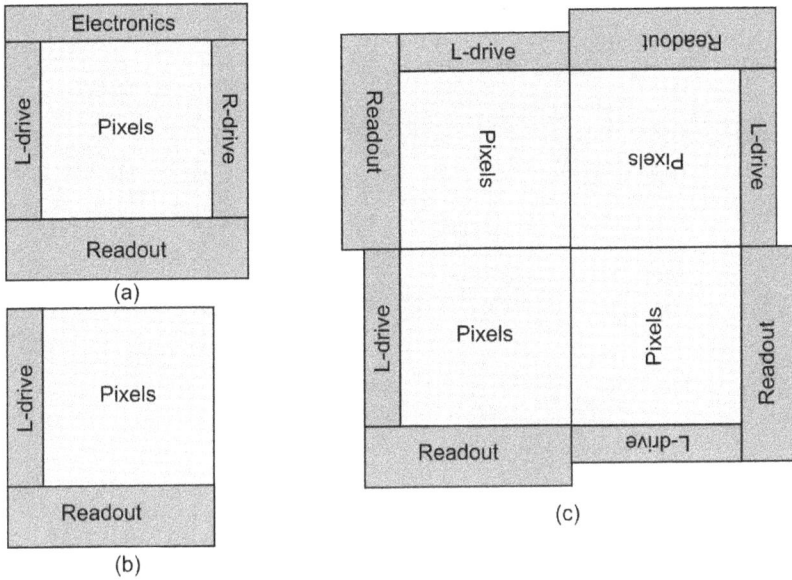

FIGURE 12.56 Four devices butted together (c) based on the device concept of 2-sides buttable imaging array (b). Figure (a) shows a sketch of the floor plan of an image sensor (after Reference 71).

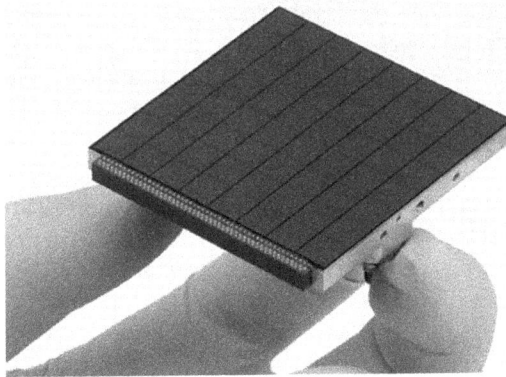

FIGURE 12.57 One of the 64 orthogonal transfer array (OTA) devices used in PanSTARRS camera. The OTA consists of an 8×8 array of 600×600 CCD devices, each of which can be controlled and read out independently (after Reference 72).

not exceed the 300-mm diameter although the silicon-integrated circuit industry is actively exploring a transition to 450 mm diameter wafers. Due to both cost and technological reasons, many imaging chips are made typically using process technologies being run on 200-mm diameter wafers. Gaps between are reduced to as little as a few tens of micrometers, especially for monolithic technologies.

12.7.2 DETECTOR OPERATING TEMPERATURE

Generally, there are two main types of detectors: cooled and uncooled. Cooled detectors require cooling below the ambient temperature. Although uncooled sensors offer significant advantages in

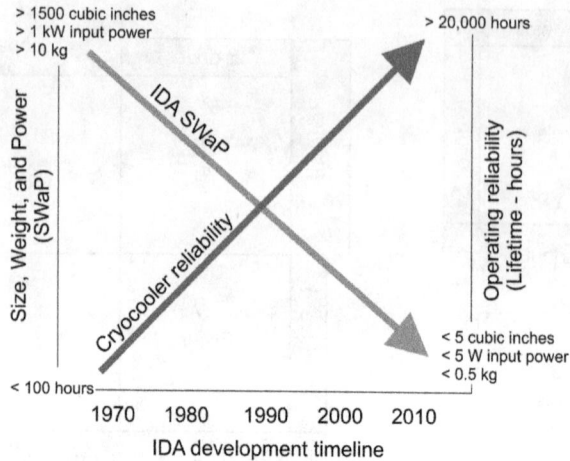

FIGURE 12.58 Evolution of cryocooler and infrared detector packaging.

terms of cost, lifetime, size, weight and power, cooled sensors offer significantly enhanced range, resolution and sensitivity as a result of the lower noise operation.

In the infrared (IR) industry the housing with detector installed is known as an integrated detector assembly (or IDA). When IR sensors began to move out of the laboratory and into tactical application in the 1960s, the first sensors to do so relied on adaptations of laboratory equipment, primarily the refrigerators and vacuum systems. These initial systems were large, heavy and power hungry. As the capability of the systems increased, and the applications extended, the cryogenic and vacuum packaging solutions were better suited for tactical environments – they were lighter and smaller, used less power, required less support and offered high reliability. Figure 12.58 graphically illustrates the trend in size, weight and power (SWaP) consumption and reliability after removing the barriers to IR sensor adoption.

The housing on an IDA is basically a fancy dewar. The detector is located on the base of the inner wall with a window in the base of the outer wall. Cryogenic liquid pour-filled dewars are frequently used for detector cooling in laboratories. They are rather bulky and need to be refilled with liquid nitrogen every few hours. For many applications, especially in the field LN_2, pour-filled dewars are impractical, so many manufacturers are turning to alternative coolers that do not require cryogenic liquids or solids. There are many design considerations and challenges that go into developing an IDA. Figure 12.59 illustrates common elements and features of an IR dewar. Inside the dewar are several additional key components:

- Coldshield – to limit the field of view (FOV) of the detector to the desired optical bundle. The internal features and surfaces of the coldshield stray light coming from outside the desired bundle but coming through the aperture. Typically, coldshields eliminate more than 95 per cent of the stray light.
- Coldfilter – to eliminate the energy outside the region of interest. By cooling the filter, the self-emission of the filter element is minimised. Coldfilters are fabricated from a variety of substrate materials, most commonly silicon, BK7 glass, sapphire, and germanium.

Figure 12.60 is a chart depicting operating temperature and wavelength regions spanned by a variety of available detector technologies. Typical operating temperatures range from 4 K to just below room temperature, depending on the detector technology. Most modern cooled infrared (IR) detectors operate in the temperature range from < 10 K to 150 K, depending on the detector type and

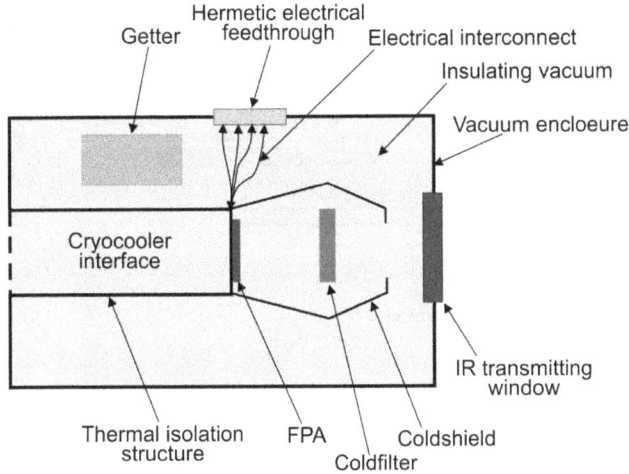

FIGURE 12.59 Components of a dewar.

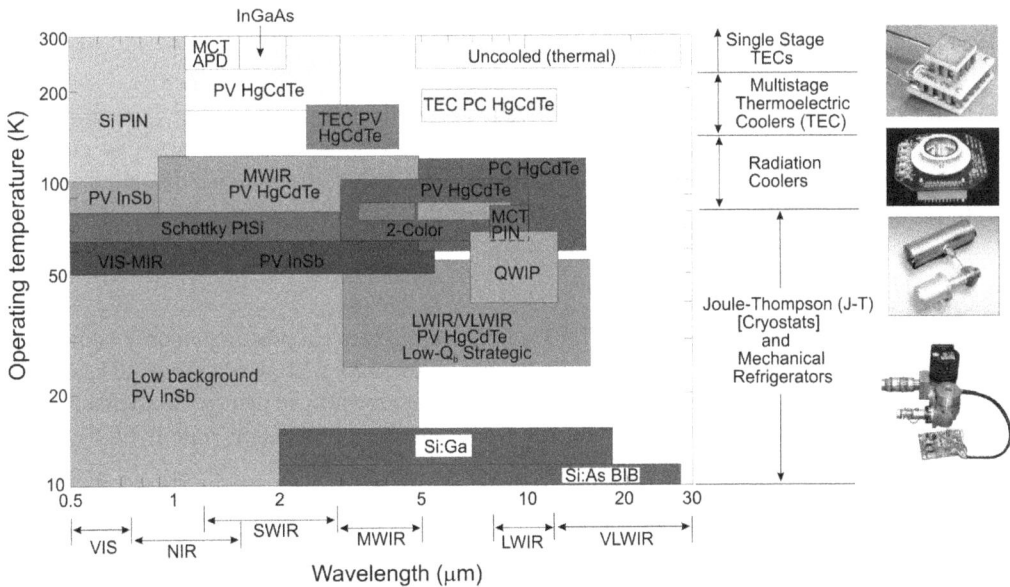

FIGURE 12.60 The operating temperature and wavelength regions spanned by a variety of available IR detector technologies.

performance level. 77 K is a very common temperature because this is relatively easily achievable with liquid nitrogen. Uncooled infrared detectors, despite their name, typically incorporate some degree of temperature control near or slightly below room temperature (~250 K – 300 K) to minimise noise, optimise resolution and maintain stable operating temperature.

The method of cooling varies according to the operating temperature and the system's logistical requirements [73,74]. The two technologies currently available for addressing the cooling requirements of IR and visible detectors are closed-cycle refrigerators and thermoelectric coolers. Closed cycle refrigerators can achieve the cryogenic temperatures required for cooled IR sensors, while thermoelectric coolers are generally the preferred approach to temperature control for

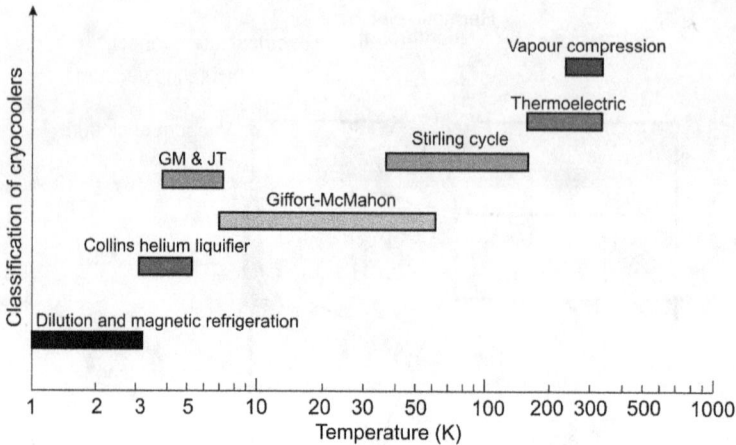

FIGURE 12.61 Temperature ranges for commercial refrigerators (adapted after Reference 73).

uncooled visible and IR sensors. The major difference between the thermoelectric and mechanical cryocoolers is the nature of the working fluid. A thermoelectric cooler is a solid-state device that uses charge carriers (electrons or holes) as a working fluid, whereas mechanical cryocoolers use a gas such as helium as the working fluid.

The selection of a cooler for a specific application depends on cooling capacity, operating temperature, procurement, cost and maintenance and servicing requirements. A survey of currently operating cryogenic systems for commercial, military and space applications are summarised in Figure 12.61.

12.7.3 ULTRAVIOLET AND VISIBLE ARRAYS

As is noted in Chapter 7, the ultraviolet (UV) solid-state imagers are most commonly built with a hybrid structure with typical 320×256 pixels. Recently, first 640×512 pixel hybrid AlGaN arrays with 15-μm pitch have been demonstrated. The wafers were grown by metalorganic chemical vapor deposition of AlGaN epilayers on sapphire substrates and after processing were hybridised with CTIA ROIC (see Figure 12.62).

Today, CMOS image sensors are the dominant imaging device, having overtaken CCDs a decade ago [76]. CMOS devices do not employ pixel-to-pixel charge transfer across the detector area as CCDs do, so they are inherently more radiation tolerant. The megapixel race has pushed manufacturers towards a continuous decrease in pixel size, the image sensor equivalent of Moore's Law. It has been recognised that the smallest pixel available in a specific visible technology lies between 10 and 20 times the minimum feature size of that technology node [77], and their size is in the micron range, with some examples below 1 μm. In general, systems operating at shorter wavelengths are more likely to benefit from small pixel sizes because of the smaller diffraction-limited spot size.

CCD for scientific applications are routinely made with pixel counts exceeding 20 megapixels and the trend to ever-larger single chips will continue. Visible 50 megapixel arrays are now available with digital outputs having ROIC noise levels of less than 10 electrons and offering a sensitivity advantage over consumer products. At present, the largest single-chip CCD arrays exceed 100 megapixels. DALSA has successfully produced a 252 megapixel CCD sensor chip (see Figure 12.63). The active area measures approximately 4×4 inches and 17216×14656 pixels with 5.6 μm size [78].

The record-breaking chips are developed for astronomy applications to assist in the determination of the positions and motions of stars, solar system objects and the establishment of celestial

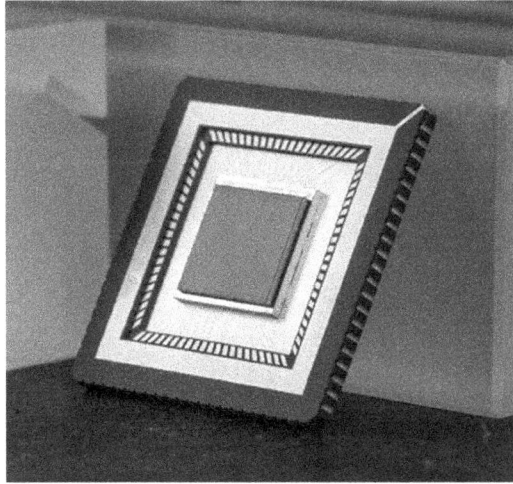

FIGURE 12.62 Solar-blind 640×512/15-μm pitch AlGaN FPAs mounted in 84-pin chip carriers (after Reference 75).

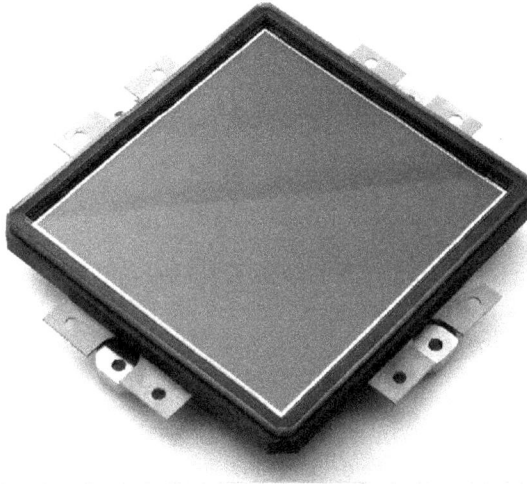

FIGURE 12.63 DALSA 252 megapixel CCD-array with 17216×14656 pixels (96.4×82.1 mm) with 5.6 μm size.

reference frames. The large CCD sensors are now starting to be produced in large quantities to meet the demands of astronomers. In particular, recent development of buttable CCD arrays could be of considerable interest to the photogrammetric and remote-sensing communities.

The development of mosaics of area arrays to produce large-format (above one gigapixel) frame images is an intriguing idea [79]. One of them, the 1.4 gigapixel CCD imager used in PanSTARRS, is comprised of 64 chips, each of 22 megapixels (see Figure 12.57). Another example is a wide area persistent surveillance program such as the Autonomous Real-time Ground Ubiquitous Surveillance – Imaging System (ARGUS-IS) [80, 81], where extremely large mosaics of visible FPAs are used (see Figure 12.64). The 1.8 gigapixel video sensor produces more than 27 gigapixels per second running at a frame rate of 15 Hz. The airborne processing subsystem is modular and scalable providing more than 10 teraops of processing.

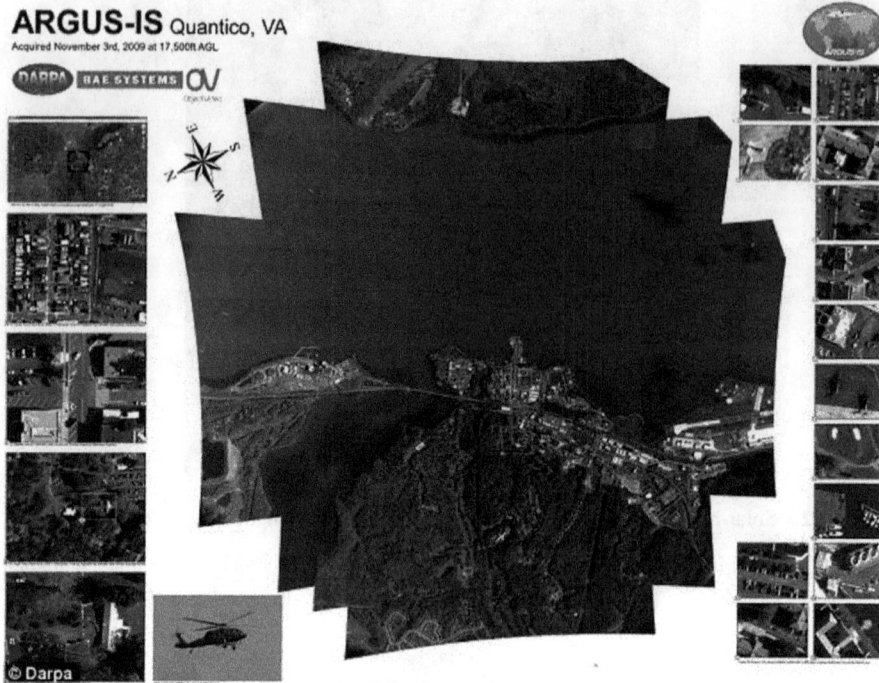

FIGURE 12.64 Sample of ARGUS-IS imagery. Mounted under a YEH-60B helicopter at 17,500 ft. over Quantico, Va., Argus-IS images an area more than 4 km wide and provides multiple 640×480-pixel real-time video windows.

The next milestone in the development of large CCD arrays is the Gaia camera for space missions [82]. Gaia, funded by the European Space Agency (ESA) with EADS Astrium as the prime contractor, is an ambitious space observatory designed to measure the positions of a billion stars with unprecedented accuracy. In order to meet this challenge, Gaia has enlisted the services of e2v Technologies of Chelmsford, in the UK, the world's leading scientific CCD manufacturer. This FPA is populated with 106 back-illuminated devices, each with an active area of 45×59 mm^2 corresponding to 4500×1966 pixels (total number 938 megapixels), each 10×30 µm^2 in size. All of the Gaia CCDs are large-area, full-frame devices. They all have a 4-phase electrode structure in the image section and a 2-phase structure in the readout register, leading to a single, high-performance, two-stage buffered output node. A noise performance better than 10 electrons RMS is expected.

The Gaia spacecraft launched in 2013 is parked at the Earth–Sun L2 Lagrange point, which is a spot 1.5 million kilometres (932,057 miles) behind the Earth, when viewed from the Sun. Gaia operates at a temperature of minus 110°C. This low temperature is maintained by passive thermal control, including the cold radiator on the focal plane assembly and a giant sunshade attached to the top of the spacecraft.

At present, the US Department of Energy's SLAC National Accelerator Laboratory leads in construction of the largest digital camera ever built for astronomy, and will be mounted in 2022 on the 8.4-metre Simonyi Survey Telescope (Chile) [10]. The resolution the Legacy Survey of Space and Time (LSST) camera [see Figure 12.2(a)], as mentioned previously, is high enough that a golf ball can be seen from around 15 miles (24 km) away. This 3.2-gigapixel camera will take a 15-second exposure every 20 seconds, which requires very precise focusing due to the rapid repointing. It will produce data of extremely high quality with minimal downtime and maintenance.

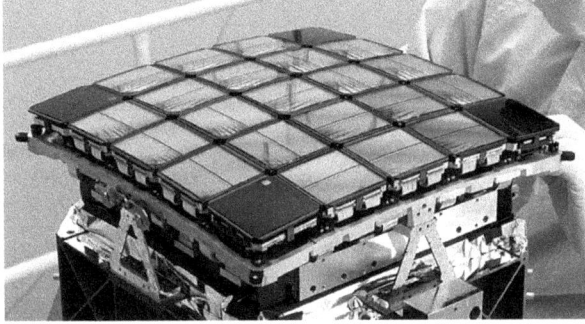

FIGURE 12.65 Image of Kepler focal plane, employing a CCD detector mosaic on a curved spherical substrate.

The emergence of curved detectors potentially will have a very high impact for astronomy [83]. Using curved detectors allows a drastic reduction of the optical systems complexity together with increasing the transmitted flux and reducing the exposure time. In addition, the optics of systems is simplified (less misalignments and instrumental errors) and stabilised (less calibration time, less dependence on the environmental conditions). One example of the impact of curvature in the field is the Kepler FPA, with 95 megapixels, made of 21 large flat format detectors disposed on a highly curved plate (Figure 12.65) [84]. The focal plane consists of an array of 42 CCDs. Each CCD is 2.8×3.0 cm with 1024×1100 pixels. Kepler is a space telescope launched in 2009 and designed to survey a portion of the Milky Way Galaxy in search of exoplanets – planets outside our solar system.

Until recently, CMOS imagers have been at a disadvantage relative to CCDs for readout noise, since the CMOS's readout circuit is inherently higher noise than a CCD amplifier. One reason for higher noise is the capacitance of the sense node of the three transistor CMOS pixel. For a typical pixel size of 5 μm in a 0.25 μm CMOS image sensor process, the sense node capacitance is about 5 fF, corresponding to a responsivity of 32 μV/electron, which limits the lowest readout noise to about 10 electrons. With the development of the four-transistor pixel, monolithic CMOS can achieve the lowest noise levels required by astronomy [17]. The state-of-the-art CMOS pixel architecture utilise up to eight transistor designs by incorporating more electronics in the pixel at the cost of increased noise and reduced fill factor [63].

Tables 12.7 and 12.8 gather characteristics of the standard image sensors manufactured by Teledyne eV [85].

Large visible light detection CCD and CMOS imagers are also fabricated by Fairchild Imaging [86], SRI International [87] and Teledyne Imaging Sensors (TIS). TIS uses both monolithic and hybrid MOS detectors [17, 88]. These highest performance silicon-based image arrays are intended for the astronomical community. Low-noise silicon hybrid arrays H4RG-10 termed HyViSI (Hybrid Visible Silicon Imager), produced in 4k×4k format with 10 μm pixel pitch, achieve high pixel interconnectivity (> 99.99%), low readout noise (< 10 e- rms single CDS), low dark current (< 0.5 e-/pixel/s at 193K), high quantum efficiency (> 90% broadband), and large dynamic range (> 13 bits) [17]. The modular stitching design approach allows fabrication of ROICs ranging from 2k×2k to 16k×16k formats. The chip size of the H4RG-10 is 43.0 mm×45.5 mm, slightly bigger than the 18 μm pixel H2RG (38.8 mm×40.0 mm). Figure 12.66 shows photographs of Teledyne's hybrid silicon p-i-n CMOS sensors. Teledyne's CMOS sensors are fully digital system-on-chip, with all bias generation, clocking, and analogue-to-digital conversion included with the image array.

State-of-the-art scientific CMOS devices with hybrid architecture are available in formats as large as 8k×8k four-side buttable [64, 88–90]. These detectors achieve the same performance as the best deep depletion CCDs.

TABLE 12.7
Standard CCD Image Sensors Fabricated by Teledyne e2V

	Number of pixels	Pixel pitch [μm]	Image size [mm]	Output amplifier type	Maximum readout rate [MHz]	Readout noise [e⁻]	Primary packane type
CCD30-11	256×1024	26×26	6.7×26.7	LS	5	4 (RNB)	20-pin DIL ceramic
CCD42-10	512×2048	13.5×13.5	6.9×27.6	2×VLN	3	2 (RNB)	20-pin DIL ceramic
CCD42-40	2048×2048	13.5×13.5	27.6×27.6	2×VLN	3	2 (RBN)	20-pin DIL ceramic
CCD42-90	4608×2048	13.5×13.5	62.2×27.6	2×VLN	3	2 (RBN)	Invar 3-side buttable +PGA
CCD44-82	4096×2048	15×15	61.4×30.7	2×VLN	2	2 (RBN)	Invar 3-side buttable +PGA
CCD47-10	1024×1024	13×13	13.3×13.3	2×VLN	5	2 (RBN)	24-pin DIL ceramic
CCD55-20	1152×770	22.5×22.5	25.9×17.3	1 VLN+1 LS	7	3 (RNB)	44-pin PGA ceramic
CCD55-30	1152×1252	22.5×22.5	25.9×27.9	1 VLN+1 LS	7	3 (RNB)	44-pin PGA ceramic
CCD62-06	578×385	22×22	12.7×8.5	HSA	12	4 (RNB)	20-pin DIL ceramic
CCD77-00	512×512	24×24	12.3×12.3	2×LS	7	3 (RNB)	24-pin DIL ceramic
CCD303-88	4136×4096	12×12	49.2×49.2	4×VLN	3	3 (RNB)	Invar buttable +2 flex cable
CCD230-42	2064×2048	15×15	30.7×30.7	4×VLN	5	3 (RNB)	78-pin PGA ceramic
CCD230-84	4112×4096	15×15	61.4×61.4	4×VLN	5	3 (RNB)	80-pin PGA ceramic
CCD231-84	4112×4096	15×15	61.4×61.4	4×VLN	3	2 (RNB	SiC buttable + 2 flex cable
CCD231-C6	6160×6144	15×15	92.4×92.2	4×VLN	3	2 (RNB	SiC buttable + 2 flex cable
CCD290-99	9232×9216	10×10	92.4×92.2	16×VLN		2 (RNB)	SiC buttable + 2 flex cable

DIL – dual in line, RNB – at maximum readout rate, LS – large signal scientific amplifier, VLN – very low noise scientific amplifier, HSA – high speed output amplifier

Apart from Teledyne, for over twenty years Raytheon has built hybrid focal planes based on silicon p-i-n photodiodes. The sensor chip assembles (SCAs) can be combined in mosaic configurations to form large composite arrays using 2, 3, and 4 side buttable packages. Recent advancements in latest generation of 8-μm pixels with format up to 8k×8k are presented in References 89 and 90. The current family of devices has very low read-noise ROICs, low detector dark current, operate with a 25 volt bias and deliver 50 per cent mean response operability greater than 99.995 per cent. The detector structure is fully depleted and thickness of active region is changed from 10 to 350 μm, which allows tuning of *MTF* and near-infrared response. Raytheon's latest ROIC deliver 14-bit ADCs, windowing, > 1 Gbit/s outputs, noise flor 5–7 e⁻, and well capacity > 200 ke⁻. Figure 12.67 shows photograph of 8k×8k, 8-μm pixel Si p-i-n based SCA and resulting image.

12.7.4 MICROBOLOMETER ARRAYS

The typical cost of cryogenically cooled imagers of around US$50,000 restricts their installation to critical military applications involving operations in complete darkness. The commercial systems are derived from military systems that are too costly for widespread use. As the volume of production increases, the cost of commercial systems will inevitably decrease. The current market price for a low-cost thermal imager, generally costs around US$1,000. Recently, the first thermal imaging smartphone was launched [91].

TABLE 12.8
Standard CMOS Image Sensors Fabricated by Teledyne e2V

	Number of pixels	Filter	Pixel pitch [µm]	Image size [inches]	Shutter type	Output format	Frame rate [fps]	Maximum readout rate [MHz]	Dynamic range [dB]
Jade 0,5M* – EV76C454	640×860	Mono, Bayer	5.8×5.8	½,9	Global	Parallel 8 bit	60	48	>52
Sapphire 1,3M – EV76C560	1024×1280	Mono, Bayer	5.3×5.3	1/1,8	Global + Rolling	Parallel 10 bit	60 (>100 VGA)	120	62
Sapphire 2M – EV76C570/ 571	1200×1600	Mono, Bayer	4.5×4.5	1/1,8	Global + Rolling	Parallel 10 bit	50–60	120	66
Sapphire WVGA – EV76C541	480×752	Mono, Bayer	4.5×4.5	1/4	Global + Rolling	Parallel 10 bit	125	114	66
Ruby 1,3M – EV76C660	1024×1280	Mono, Bayer	5.3×5.3	1/1,8	Global + Rolling	Parallel 10 bit	60 (>100 at VGA)	120	-
Ruby 1,3M – EV76C661	1024×1280	Mono, Bayer	5.3×5.3	1/1,8	Global + Rolling	Parallel 10 bit	60 (>100 VGA)	120	-
Onyx 1,3M – EV76C664	1024×1280	Mono, Sparse	10×10	1	Global + Rolling	LVDS from 8b to 14b	100 (12bits)	250	58/67/74
Lince 5M181	2048×2560	Mono, Bayer	5×5	1	Global	LVDS from 8b to 12b	250 12bits)	345	58
Lince 5M84	2048×2560	Mono, Bayer	5×5	1	Global	LVDS from 8b to 12b	69 (at 12bits)	88	58

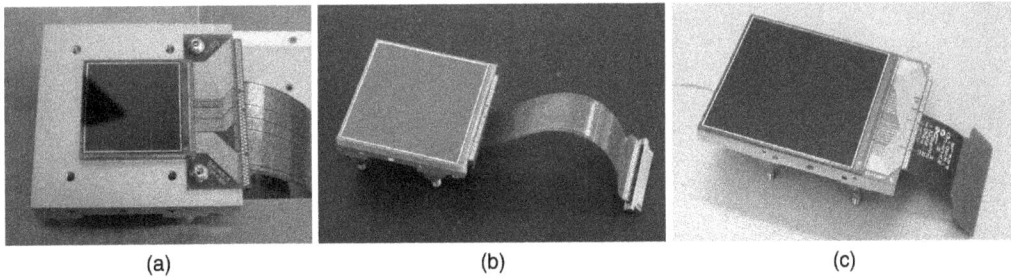

(a) (b) (c)

FIGURE 12.66 Teledyne's hybrid silicon p-i-n CMOS sensors: (a) 1k×1k H1RG-18 HyViSi, (b) 2k×2k H1RG-18 HyViSi, and (c) 4k×4k H4RG-10 (after Reference 17).

It is expected that the thermal-imaging market will reach around US$7.5 billion in value by 2025, at an 8 per cent CAGR (Compound Annual Growth Rate) from 2019 to 2025 [92]. Currently, microbolometer detectors are produced in larger volumes than all other IR array technologies together. Their cost has drastically dropped (about −15% per year). At present, VO_x microbolometer arrays are clearly the most-used technology for uncooled detectors. VO_x is the winner in the battle between different technologies: amorphous silicon, BST and silicon diodes [93].

The key trade-off with respect to uncooled thermal imaging systems is between sensitivity and response time. Thermal conductance, G_{th}, is an extremely important parameter, since *NEDT* is proportional to $G_{th}^{1/2}$, but the response time of the detector is inversely proportional to G_{th}. Therefore,

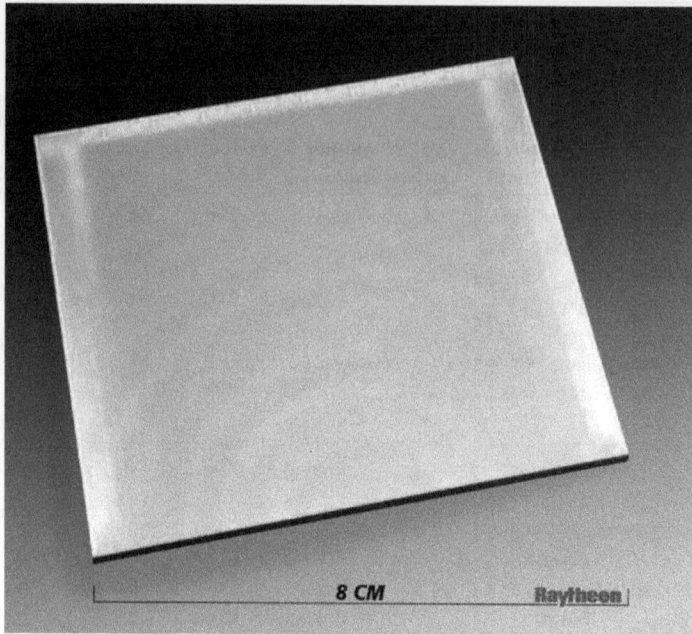

(a)

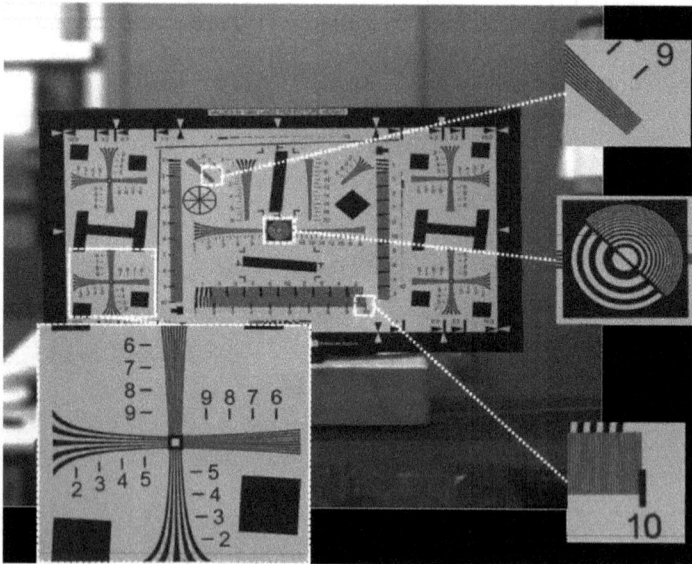

(b)

FIGURE 12.67 Silicon p-i-n SCA: (a) photograph of 8k×8k, 8-μm pixel array and (b) resulting high resolution image (after Reference 90).

a change in thermal conductance due to improvements in material-processing technique improves sensitivity at the expense of time response.

Assuming $f/1$ optics and 100 per cent transmission optics at DC condition, *NEDT* can be estimated as [94]:

$$NEDT = \frac{4G_{th}V_n}{TCR \times FF \times \varepsilon \times R_d \times I_b \times A \times (\Delta P / \Delta T)} \qquad (12.31)$$

This expression includes: the detector noise, V_n, the detector electrical resistance, R_d, the detector bias current, I_b, the thermal coefficient of resistance (TCR), the detector fill factor (FF), the absorption rate, ε and the differential radiation falling on the detector, $\Delta P/\Delta T$ (also called temperature contrast).

Equation (12.31) can be manipulated to include $\tau_{th} = C_{th}/G_{th}$:

$$NEDT = \frac{4C_{th}V_n}{\tau_{th} \times TCR \times FF \times \varepsilon \times R_d \times I_b \times A \times (\Delta P / \Delta T)} \qquad (12.32)$$

If the NEDT is dominated by a noise source that is proportional to G_{th}, which takes place when Johnson and $1/f$ noises are dominant, then the Figure of Merit given by

$$FOM = NEDT \times \tau_{th} = \frac{4C_{th}V_n}{TCR \times FF \times \varepsilon \times R_d \times I_b \times A \times (\Delta P / \Delta T)} \qquad (12.33)$$

can be introduced [95].

Users are interested not only in the sensitivity, but also in their thermal time constants and the FOM described by Eq. (12.33) recognises the trade-off between thermal time constant and sensitivity. Figure 12.68 shows the dependence of NEDT on thermal time constant for three $NEDT \times \tau_{th}$ products. Lynred announced in 2019 a publishing record performance of a 150 mK×msec figure of merit, meaning that the thermal sensitivity was below 50 mK with a thermal time constant below 3 ms.

The demonstrated performance is getting closer to the theoretical limit with the advantages regarding weight, power consumption and cost (SWaP). Because the cost of the optics made of Ge, the standard material, depends approximately on the square of the diameter, reducing the pixel size allows the size and cost of the optics to be reduced. However, the NEDT is inversely proportional to the pixel area, thus, if the pixel size is reducing, improvements in the readout electronics are needed to compensate for this.

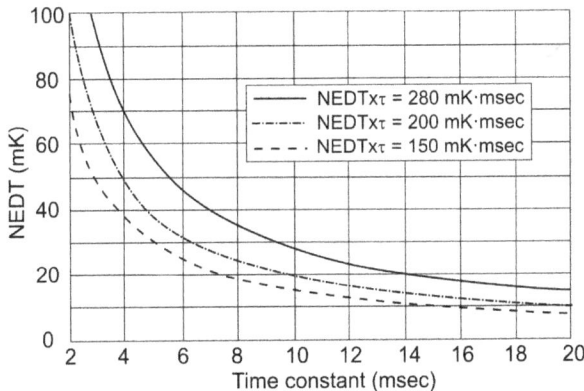

FIGURE 12.68 Calculated microbolometer NEDT and thermal time constant, τ_{th}, for three $NEDT \times \tau_{th}$ products.

The minimum resolvable size of microbolometer pixel, x, is decided by the diffraction limitation. Assuming the Rayleigh criterion, this size is expressed by $x \approx f\theta = 1.22\lambda F$, where θ is the diffraction angle, F is the F-number, and λ is the wavelength focal length of the optical lens. For LWIR detectors with F-number close to 1, the minimum resolvable size is 10–15 μm. Considerations carried out in Reference 95 indicate that resolution still benefits from the oversampling when pixel size is between $0.5\lambda F$ and $1.22\lambda F$. However, in these conditions the resolution quickly saturates as the pixel size decreases [96]. Unlike the photon detectors, where even smaller pixels are preferred to achieve the maximum performance, the CMOS microbolometer arrays are still in the "detector limit" regime, that is, still far from the potential limiting performance. Figure 12.69(b) shows the trends in pixel reduction.

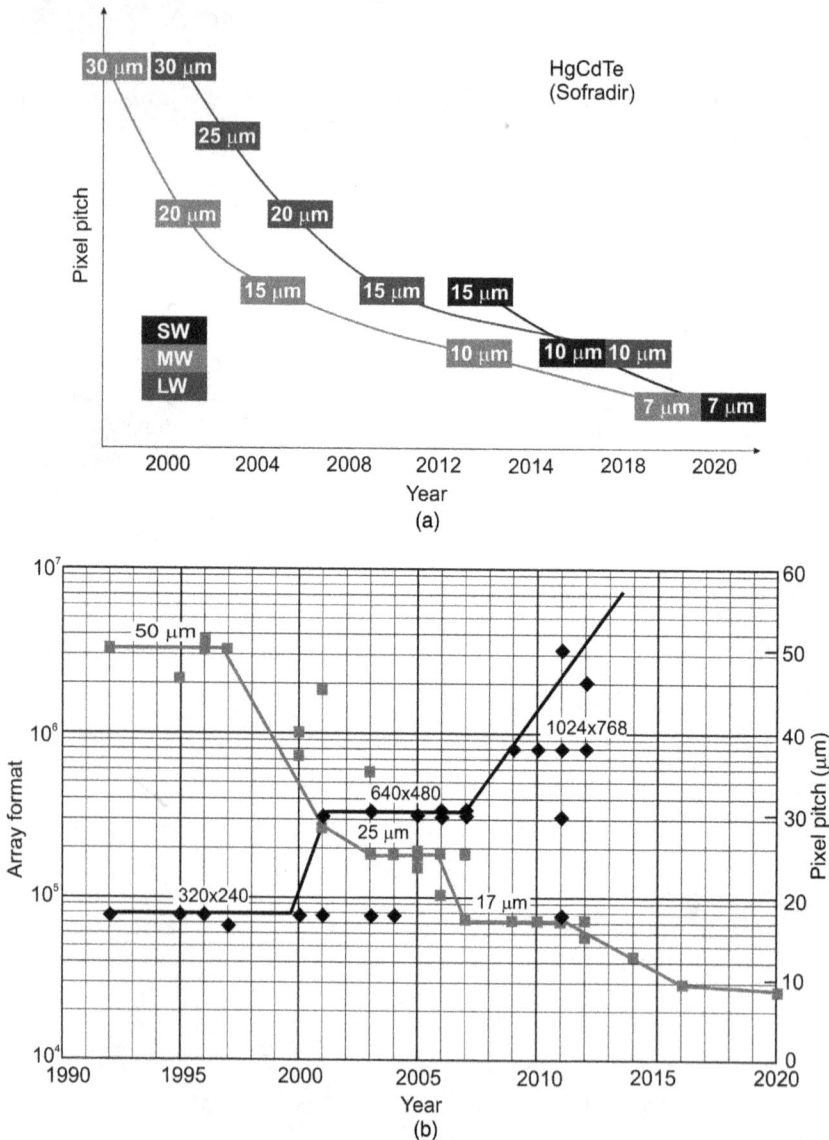

FIGURE 12.69 Pixel pitch for HgCdTe photodiodes fabricated by Sofradir (a) and for silicon microbolometers (b).

The main factor that limits the pixel size reduction in CMOS microbolometer is the responsivity. Smaller pixel results in less IR absorption and low responsivity. To reach smaller pixels for uncooled IR FPA, further improvements in detector technology are necessary, which presents significant challenges in both fabrication process improvements and in pixel design. At the present stage of technology, the detector fill factor and the absorption coefficient are closed to their ideal value and only a little benefit can be expected from the optimisation of these two parameters. More gain can be obtained through improvement of the thermistor material; its TCR and R_d.

At present, the commercially available bolometer arrays are made either from VO_x, amorphous silicon (a-Si), or silicon diodes. Figure 12.70 shows scanning electron microscope (SEM) images of commercial bolometers fabricated by different manufacturers.

The micromachined microbolometers reported to date are classified in two design categories – single and double layer. A single-layer microbolometer, shown schematically in Figure 12.8(d) and (b), is comprised of a transducer element and a leg structure. The pixel design shows a resonant cavity formed by an absorbing layer suspended above a reflecting metal layer. The cavity is used to amplify the absorptance of the incident IR radiation. The microbridge is supported by beams and thermally isolated from the ROIC to increase the sensitivity of the microbolometer.

Figure 12.71 shows example imagery from the DRS 1280×1024, 10-μm pitch uncooled bolometer sensor with $f/1.1$ optics. The image shows unprecedented detail as expected with such a small pixel pitch. Outstanding bolometer performance results in improvements of thermal and spatial resolution and image quality of infrared cameras.

Table 12.9 contains an overview of the main suppliers and specifications for existing products and for bolometer arrays that are in the R&D stage. Most manufacturers of uncooled amorphous silicon (a-Si) and vanadium oxide (VOx) microbolometer FPA products have long been producing imaging devices with 17 μm pixel-pitch arrays. There is general uniformity and compatibility throughout the industry between camera products and optics. As we can see, the similar performance has been described by BAE Systems, DRS, Lynred, L-3, and SCD. The array sizes range from 60×80 up to 1920×1200. Low resolution devices demonstrate very low cost. Some 10/12 μm pixel pitch devices are available in moderate volumes from a small number of manufacturers.

The first thermal camera for smartphone with 156×206 VO_x microbolometer format was introduced in the consumer market by FLIR in 2014. The Seek Thermal camera uses 12-μm pixel design by Raytheon. The camera has a very compact size and is compatible with Android smartphones via its micro-USB connector – see Figure 12.72. Thanks to its strong integration at the die level with wafer-level packaging, this is the world's smallest microbolometer-based thermal imaging camera.

12.7.5 Infrared Photon Detector Arrays

Infrared system performance is highly scenario-dependent and requires the designer to account for numerous different factors when specifying detector performance. It means that a good solution for one application may not be as suitable for a different application. In general, detector material is primary selected based on wavelength of interest, performance criteria and operating temperature (see Figure 12.73). Although efforts have been made over the past 40 years to develop monolithic structures using a variety of infrared photodetector materials (including narrow-gap semiconductors), only a few have matured to a level of practical use. These include Si, PtSi, and more recently PbS, PbSe. Other infrared material systems (InGaAs, InSb, HgCdTe, InAs/GaSb type-II superlattice, GaAs/AlGaAs QWIP, and extrinsic silicon) are used in hybrid configurations. Table 12.10 contains a description of representative IR FPAs that are commercially available as standard products and/or catalogue items from the major manufacturers.

A suitable detector material for near-IR (1.0–1.7-μm) spectral range is Si and InGaAs lattice matched to the InP. Various HgCdTe alloys, in both photovoltaic and photoconductive configurations, cover from 0.7 μm to over 20 μm. InAs/GaSb strained layer superlattices have emerged as an

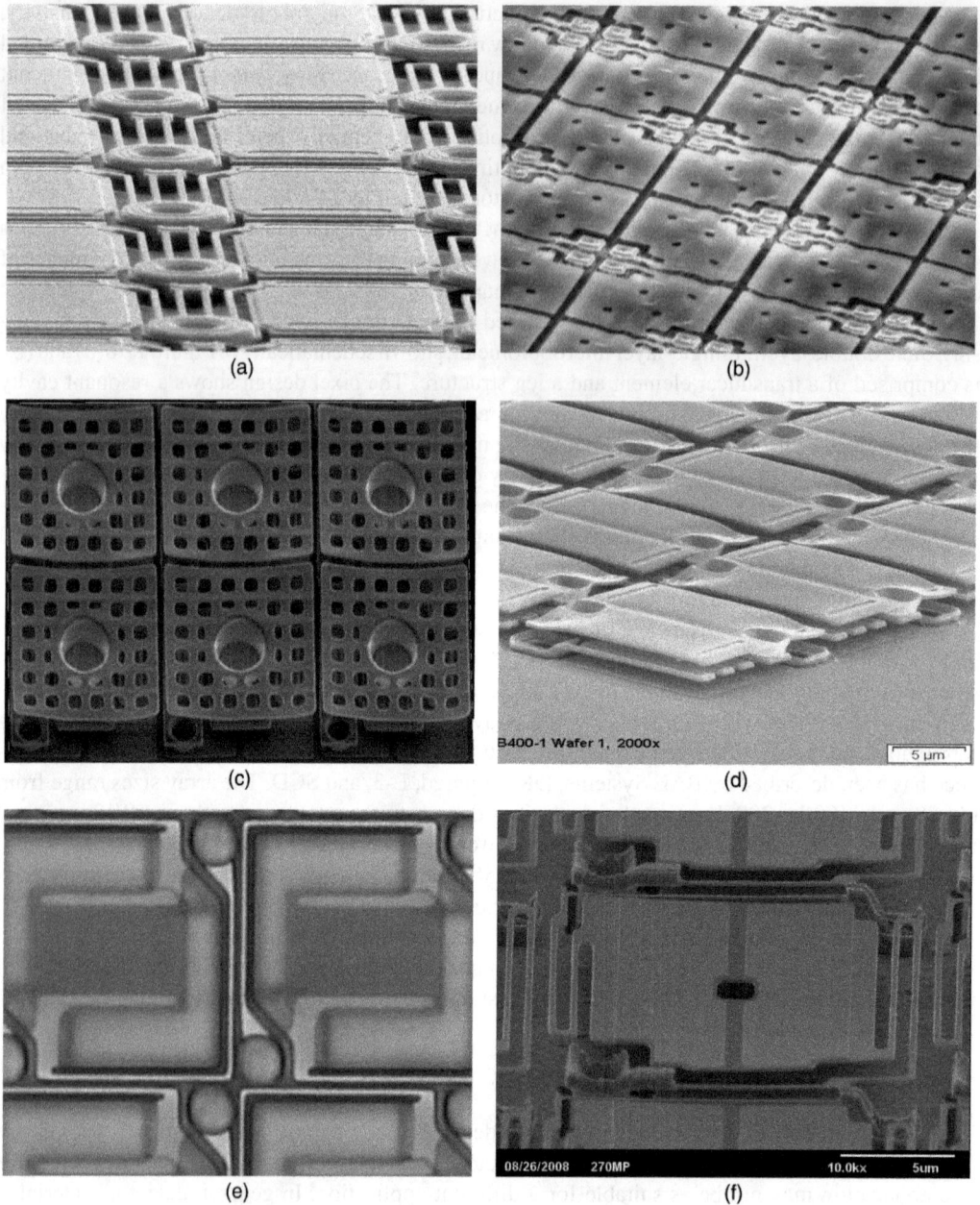

FIGURE 12.70 Commercial bolometer design: (a) VO_x bolometer from BAE, (b) a-Si bolometer from Ulis, (c) VO_x umbrella design bolometer from DRS, (d) VO_x bolometer from Raytheon, (e) VO_x bolometer from SCD, and (f) a-Si/a-SiGe bolometer from L-3 Communications.

alternative to the HgCdTe. Impurity-doped (Sb, As, and Ga) silicon-blocked impurity band (BIB) detectors operating at 10 K have a spectral response cut-off in the range of 16 to 30 μm.

12.7.5.1 InGaAs Arrays

InGaAs ternary alloy is an optimal material choice for SWIR imaging applications due to the ability to operate at room temperature with high quantum efficiency for wavelengths in visible range

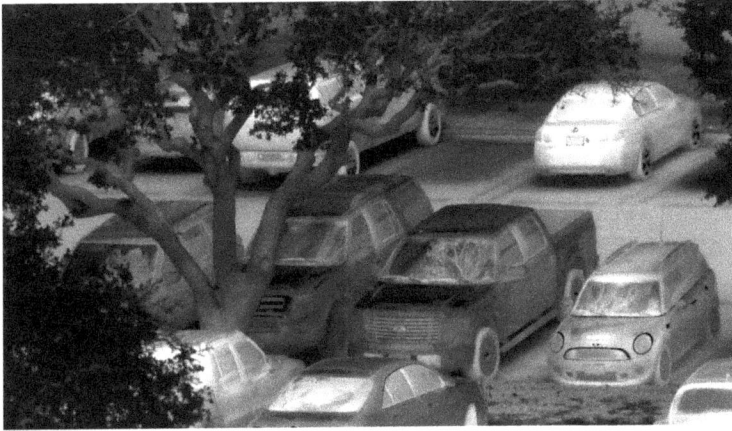

FIGURE 12.71 Image from the DRS 1280×1024, 10-μm pitch uncooled camera running at 30 Hz and operating in 1280×720 format (after Reference 97).

to about 3 μm. These applications span both commercial and industrial opportunities, including semiconductor-wafer inspection, wavefront sensing, astronomy, spectroscopy, machine vision, and military applications (surveillance, active point tracking, and laser radar). The increasing interest in the use of InGaAs detector arrays is driven primarily by potential advantages in detecting objects using target signatures which are dominated by reflection of external sources of illumination as opposed to thermal emission of radiation, which occurs in the longer infrared wavelengths.

Linear array formats of 256, 512, 1024 and 2048 elements have been fabricated for operations in three ranges: 0.9 to 1.7 μm, 1.1. to 2.2 μm, or 1.1 to 2.6 μm, with pixel pitch as small as 12.5 μm [98]. They are available in various sizes, defined by the detector height, pixel pitch, and the number of pixels, and are packaged with 1-, 2- or 3-stage thermoelectric cooling, or without a cooler for externally cooled applications.

The largest and finest pitched imager in $In_{0.53}Ga_{0.47}As$ material system has been demonstrated. Goodrich has presented a high-resolution 1280×1024 InGaAs visible/SWIR imager with 15 μm pixels for day/night imaging [99]. The array with capacitive transimpedance amplification (CTIA) readout unit cells was designated to achieve a noise level of less than 50 electrons, due to its small integration capacitor. The ROIC was readout at 120 frames per second and had a dynamic range of 3000:1 using rolling, nonsnapshot integration. Total measured noise with the detector was 114 electrons using double sampling.

Figure 12.74(a) shows the 1280×1024 1.7 μm InGaAs sensor chip assembly (SCA) for MANTIS (Multispectral Adaptive Networked Tactical Imaging System) program [100]. The detector array is hybridised to an innovative ROIC with unit cell amplifiers designed with a capacitance transimpedance amplifier and a sample/hold circuit. Noise measurements of this SCA at a 30 Hz frame rate are shown in Figure 12.74(b). A fit of noise model assuming domination of kTC and the detector g-r noise implies that the detector R_oA product is $8×10^6$ Ωcm^2 at 280 K and the ROIC contributes approximately 40 electrons of noise. Above 240 K, the detector noise dominates while below 240 K ROIC noise dominates.

In recent years SCD has developed InGaAs/InP product, Cardinal 1280, with 10-μm pitch and 1280×1024 (SXGA) format [101]. The new array is sensitive down to the visible spectrum, with a typical dark current of ~ 0.5 fA at 280K, and a quantum efficiency > 80 per cent at 1550 nm. It also has a low noise imaging mode with 35e- readout noise with internal correlated double sampling.

The standard hybrid technology makes it difficult to fabricate fine-pitch pixel arrays due to the limited scalability of the bump. Sony's research group developed a back-illuminated InGaAs image sensor with 5-μm pitch 1280×1040 format by using Cu-Cu hybridisation connecting different

TABLE 12.9
Representative Commercial Uncooled Infrared Bolometer Arrays

Company	Bolometer type	Array format	Pixel pitch (μm)	Detector NEDT (mK) (f/1, 20–60 Hz)	Time constant (msec)/ Frame rate (Hz)
L-3 (USA)	VO$_x$ bolometer	320×240	37.5	50	
www.l3t.com	a-Si bolometer	160×120 – 640×480	30	50 30–50	
	a-Si/a-SiGe bolometer	320×240 – 1024×768	17		
BAE (USA)	VO$_x$ bolometer	640×480	12	<50	<15 ms
www. fairchildimaging.com	VO$_x$ bolometer	1920×1200	12	<50	
DRS (USA)	VO$_x$ bolometer	320×240	25	<40	≤18 ms/60 Hz
www.leonardodrs. com	VO$_x$ bolometer	320×240	17	<50	60 Hz
	VO$_x$ bolometer	640×480	17	<40	≤14 ms/30 Hz
	VO$_x$ bolometer	1024×768	17	<40	≤14 ms/30 Hz
	VO$_x$ bolometer	640×512	10	<50	60 Hz
	VO$_x$ bolometer	1920×1200	12		60 Hz
Raytheon (USA)	VO$_x$ bolometer	320×240, 640×480	25	30–40 50	
www.raytheon.com/	VO$_x$ bolometer	320×240, 640×480	17		
	VO$_x$ bolometer	1024×480, 2048×1536	17		
Lynred (France)	a-Si bolometer	80×80		<100	100 Hz
www.lynred.com/ products	a-Si bolometer	160×120	17	<60	<10 ms/60 Hz
	a-Si bolometer	320×240	12	<60	<10 ms/60 Hz
	a-Si bolometer	384×288	17	<60	<10 ms/60 Hz
	a-Si bolometer	640×480	17	<50	<12 ms/120 Hz
	a-Si bolometer	1024×768	17	<50	<12 ms/120 Hz
SCD (Israel)	VO$_x$ bolometer	640×480	17	<35	<18
www.scd.co.il	VO$_x$ bolometer	1024×768	17	<35	<14
FLIR Systems (USA)	VO$_x$ bolometer	640×512	12	<60	8 ms/60 Hz
www.flir.com	VO$_x$ bolometer	320×256	12	<50	8 ms/60 Hz
NEC (Japan)	VO$_x$ bolometer	480×360	23.5	25	
www.nec.com	VO$_x$ bolometer	640×480	23.5	<75	
	VO$_x$ bolometer	640×480	12	60	
	VO$_x$ bolometer	320×240	23.5	NEP < 100 pW*	
DALI (China)	a-Si bolometer	640×480	17	<60	5 ms
www.dalithermal. com	a-Si bolometer	384×288	17	<60	5 ms
	a-Si bolometer	160×120	25	<60	5 ms
	a-Si bolometer	640×480	20	50	15 ms

*at 4 THz

materials – InGaAs/InP of photodiode array (PDA) and silicon readout integrated circuit (ROIC). This new process architecture was established for high productivity and pixel-pitch scaling [102]. Figure 12.75(a) shows a schematic diagram of the InGaAs image sensor process. The new process architecture does not increase process damage since the dark current density of the photodiode was at the same level as that obtained for standard hybrid architecture [101–106] – see Figure 12.75(b).

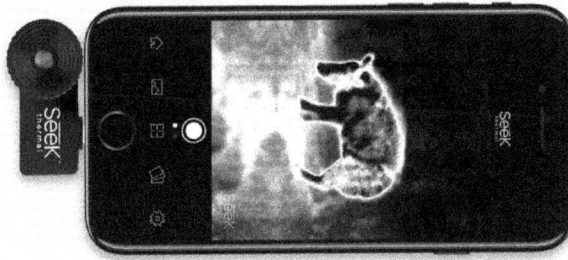

FIGURE 12.72   Smartphone with Seek Thermal camera

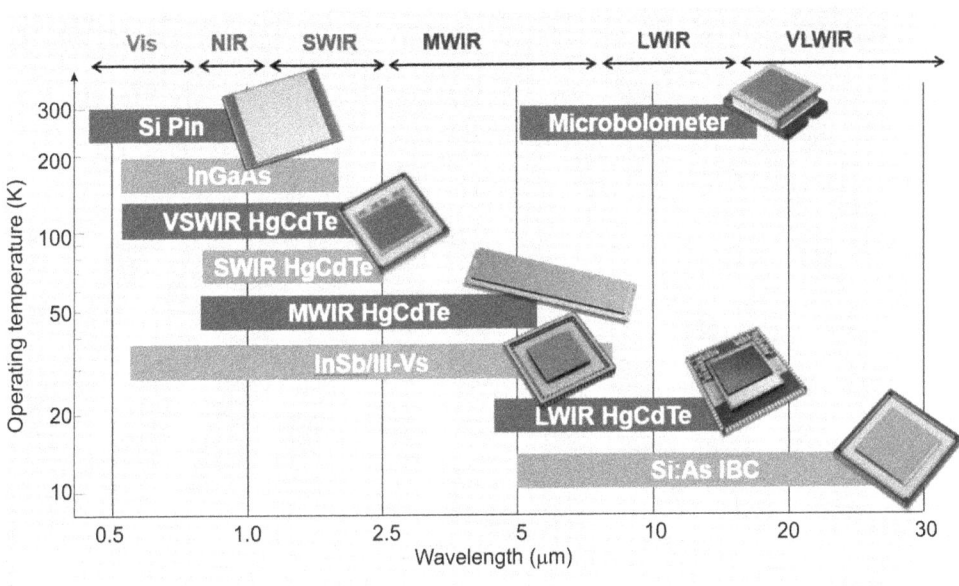

FIGURE 12.73   Detector materials which have the largest interest for infrared detector technology (adapted after Reference 90).

12.7.5.2   InSb Arrays

InSb photodiodes have been available since the late 1950s. They are used in the 1-μm to 5-μm spectral region and must be cooled to approximately 77 K. The applications include infrared homing guidance, threat warning, infrared astronomy, commercial thermal imaging cameras and FLIR (forward looking infrared) systems. One of the most significant recent advances in infrared technology has been the development of large two-dimensional FPAs for use in the staring arrays. Array formats are available with readouts suitable for both high-background $f/2$ operation and for low-background astronomy applications. Linear arrays are rather rarely used.

One of the reasons for selecting InSb for infrared instruments is its broad response, which is shown in Figure 12.76 [107,108]. The internal quantum efficiency is nearly 100 per cent in wide spectral band from 0.4 to 5 μm, which is an advantage of the thinned InSb arrays for this application. The limiting factor in quantum efficiency is the reflection of incident light at the surface, which can be minimised with antireflection coatings.

Large staring InSb focal plane evolution has been driven by astronomy applications. The first InSb array to exceed one million pixels was the ALADDIN array produced in 1993 by Santa

TABLE 12.10
Representative IR Hybrid FPAs Offered by Some Major Manufactures

Manufacturer/Web site	Size/ Architecture	Pixel size (μm)	Detector material	Spectral range (μm)	Oper. temp. (K)	$D^*(\lambda_p)$ (cmHz$^{1/2}$/ W)/*NEDT* (mK)
Sensors	640×512	12.5×12.5	InGaAs	0.7–1.7	300	2.9×10^{13}
Unlimited (USA)	1280×1024	12.5×12.5	InGaAs	0.4–1.7	300	2.9×10^{13}
www.sensorsinc.com						
Raytheon Vision	1024×1024	30×30	InSb	0.6–5.0	50	
Systems	2048×2048	25×25	HgCdTe	0.6–5.0	32	
(USA)	(Orion II)					
www.raytheon.com/	2048×2048	20×20	HgCdTe	0.8–2.5	4–10	
	(Virgo-2k)					
	2048×2048	15×15	HgCdTe/Si	3.0–5.0	78	23
	1024×1024	25×25	Si:As	5–28	6.7	
	2048×1024	25×25	Si:As	5–28		
Teledyne Imaging	4096×4096	10×10	HgCdTe	1.0–1.7	120	
Sensors (USA)	(H4RG)	or 15×15				
www.teledyne-si.com/	4096×4096	10×10	HgCdTe	1.0–2.5	77	
	(H4RG)	or 15×15				
	4096×4096	10×10	HgCdTe	1.0–5.4	37	
	(H4RG)	or 15×15				
	2048×2048	18×18	HgCdTe	1.0–1.7	120	
	(H2RG)					
	2048×2048	18×18	HgCdTe	1.0–2.5	77	
	(H2RG)					
	2048×2048	18×18	HgCdTe	1.0–5.4	37	
	(H2RG)					
Lynred (France)	640×512	15×15	InGaAs	0.9–1.7	300	
www.lynred.com/	320×256	30×30	HgCdTe	7.7–11.7	50–75	<25
products	(Mars)					
	640×512	15×15	HgCdTe	3.7–4.8	90	18
	(Scorpio)					
	640512 (Leo)	15×15	HgCdTe	3.7–4.8	80	20
	1280×720	10×10	HgCdTe	3.7–4.8	120	20
	(Daphnis)					
	1280×1024	15×15	HgCdTe	3.7–4.8	110	20
	(Jupiter)					
	640×512	15×15	HgCdTe	7.7–9.3	90	22
	(Scorpio)					
Selex (Great Brittain)	320×256	24×24	HgCdTe APD	0.8–2.5		
www.	(Saphira)					
leonardocompany.com	640×512	16×16	HgCdTe	3.7–4.95	up to 110	17
	(Hawk MW)					
	640×512	12×12	HgCdTe	3.7–4.95		
	(Hawk MW)					
	1280×720	8×8	HgCdTe	3.7–4.95	110	20
	(SuperHawk)					
	640×512	16×16	HgCdTe	8–10	up to 90	32
	(Hawk LW)					
	640×512	24×24	HgCdTe	MW/LW(dual)	80	28/28
	(CondorII)					

TABLE 12.10 (Continued)
Representative IR Hybrid FPAs Offered by Some Major Manufactures

Manufacturer/Web site	Size/ Architecture	Pixel size (μm)	Detector material	Spectral range (μm)	Oper. temp. (K)	$D^*(\lambda_p)$ (cmHz$^{1/2}$/ W)/NEDT (mK)
IAM	640×512	15×15	HgCdTe	3.4–5.0	95–120	18
www.aim-ir.com	1280×1024	15×15	HgCdTe	3.4–5.0	95–120	25
	640×512	15×15	HgCdTe	7.6–9.0	80	23
SCD	640×512	10×10	InSb	3.6–4.9	77	<25
www.scd.co.il	1280×1024	15×15	InSb	3–5	77	20
	1920×1536	10×10	InSb	1–5.4	150	<25
	1280×1024	15×15	InAsSb nBn	3.6–4.2	77	<28
	640×512	15×15	InAs/GaSb T2SL	7.0–9.3		15
FLIR Systems (USA)	640×512	15×15	InGaAs	0.9–1.7	300	10^{10} ph/ cm^{2}s(NEI)
www.flir.com	1024×1024	18×18	InSb	3–5	80	<25
	640×512	15×15	InAs/GaSb T2SL	7.5–12	80	<40
DRS	1280×760	6×6	HgCdTe	3.4–4.8		<30
Technologies (USA)	640×480	12×12	HgCdTe	3.4–4.8		25
www.leonardodrs.com	2048×2048	18×18	Si:As	5–28	7.8	
	1024×1024	25×25	Si:As	5–28	7.8	
	2048×2048	18×18	Si:Sb	5–40	7.8	

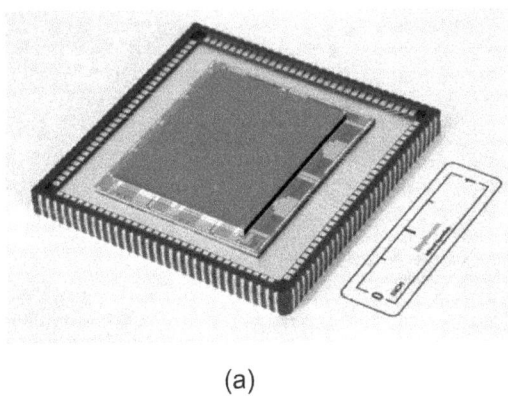

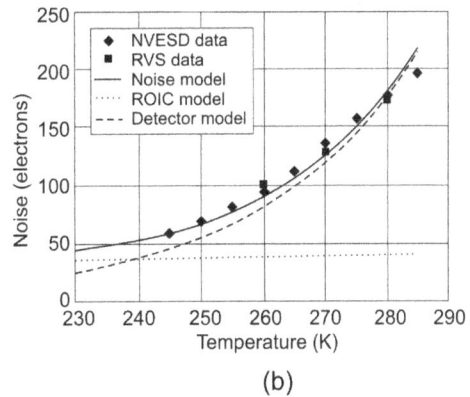

(a)   (b)

FIGURE 12.74 1280×1024 MANTIS InGaAs: (a) sensor chip assembly, and (b) noise at 30 Hz as a function of temperature. The line is a fit of the data to a noise model that includes detector g-r noise and ROIC *kTC* noise (after Reference 100).

Barbara Research Center (SBRC) and demonstrated on a telescope by National Optical Astronomy Observations (NOAO), Tucson, in 1994 [109]. This array had 1024×1024 pixels spaced on 27 μm centres and was divided into four independent quadrants, each containing eight output amplifiers. This solution was chosen due to uncertain yield of large arrays at that time.

The ALADDIN has been upgraded with the larger version, the ORION FPA family. A chronological history of the Raytheon Vision Systems (RVS) astronomical focal plane arrays is shown in Figure 12.77 [108]. The next step in the development of InSb FPAs for astronomy was the 2048×2048

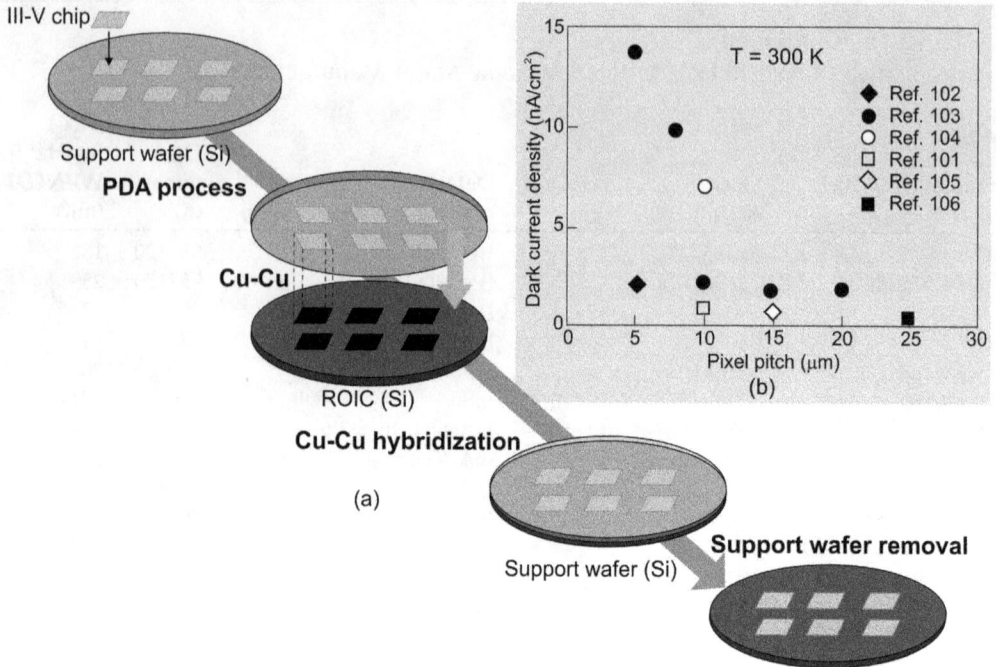

FIGURE 12.75 High-definition InGaAs image sensor: (a) fabrication process of of image sensor, (b) benchmark of InGaAs photodiode dark current measured at room temperature.

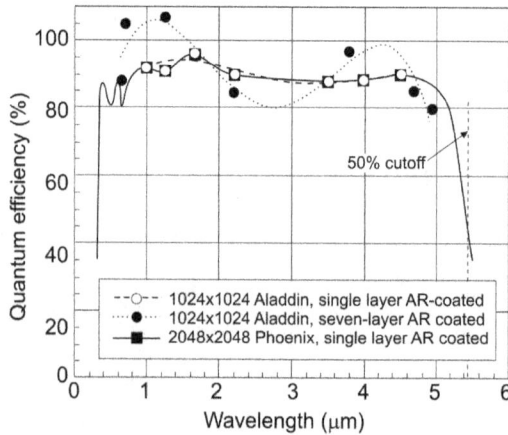

FIGURE 12.76 Quantum efficiency of InSb SCAs as a function of wavelength for a 1024×1024 ALADDIN SCA (single-layer and seven-layer AR-coated) and 2048×2048 PHOENIX SCA (after Reference 108).

ORION SCA. Four ORION SCAs were deployed as a 4096×4096 focal plane in the NOAO near-IR camera [109], currently in operation at the Mayall 4-metre telescope on Kitt Peak, Tucson. This array has 64 outputs, allowing up to a 10 Hz frame rate. Many of the packaging concepts used on the ORION program are shared with the three-sided buttable 2k×2k FPA InSb modules developed by RVS for the James Webb Space Telescope (JWST) mission [110].

PHOENIX SCA is another 2k×2k FPA InSb array that has been fabricated and tested. This detector array is identical to ORION (25-μm pixels), however its readout is optimised for lower

ALADDIN: 1k×1k   ORION: 2k×2k   PHOENIX: 2k×2k

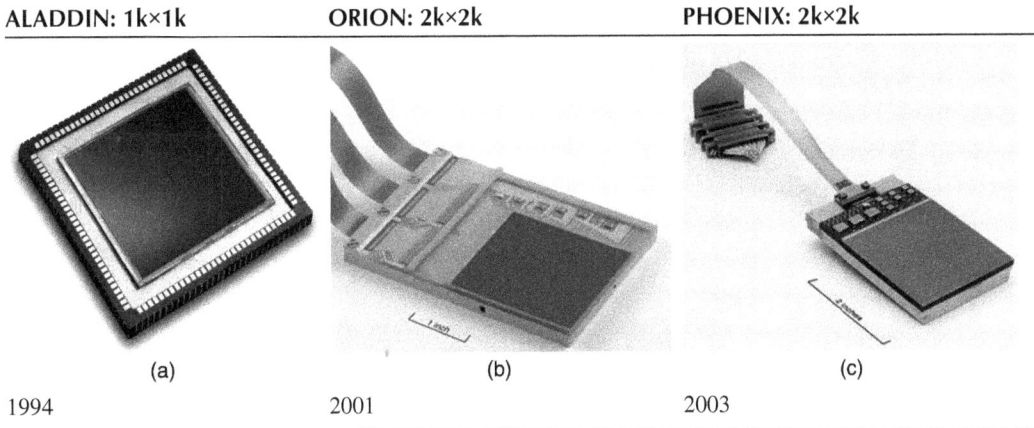

| (a) | (b) | (c) |
| 1994 | 2001 | 2003 |

FIGURE 12.77   Timeline and history development of the InSb RVS astronomy arrays (after Reference 108).

frames rates and lower power dissipation. With only four outputs, the full frame read time is typically ten seconds. The smaller number of outputs allows a smaller module package that is three-sided buttable [107]. Three-sided buttable modules allow the possibility to realise a large detection area.

Different formats of InSb FPAs also have found many high background applications, including missile systems, interceptor systems and commercial imaging camera systems. With an increasing need for higher resolution, several manufacturers have developed megapixel detectors. L-3 Cincinnati Electronics is the manufacturer of large-format/wide-area surveillance sensors with 16.7 megapixels and an ultra-wide field-of-view. This imaging engine is capable of detecting and identifying features that small-format sensors would miss. It is currently in use by United States assets in overseas combat zones. Table 12.11 presents typical performance specifications for this InSb sensor.

12.7.5.3   HgCdTe Arrays

HgCdTe photodiodes are available to cover the spectral range from 1 to 20 µm. Spectral cut-off can be tailored by adjusting the HgCdTe alloy composition. Most applications are concentrated in the SWIR (1–3 µm), MWIR (3–5 µm) and LWIR (8–12 µm). Also, development work on improving performance of very LWIR (VLWIR) photodiodes in the 13–18 µm region for important Earth-monitoring applications are undertaken.

A number of architectures are used in the development of IR HgCdTe FPAs. The best results have been obtained using hybrid architecture. Higher-density detector configuration leads to higher image resolution as well as greater system sensitivity. Pixel sizes ranging from as small as 5 µm square have been demonstrated [111]. While the size of individual arrays continues to grow, the very large FPAs required for many space missions by mosaicking a large number of individual arrays [112]. An example of a large mosaic developed by Teledyne Imaging Sensors (TIS) is shown in Figure 12.78. The mosaic consists of four 2RG arrays, each 2048×2048 format and 18-µm pixel pitch.

Sapphire buffered with CdZnTe became a standard substrate for SWIR and MWIR devices. LWIR devices are typically based on CdZnTe substrates. Efforts to extend the performance of HgCdTe into the LWIR range has been also pursued using MOVPE-grown HgCdTe on GaAs and GaAs/Si substrates in the United Kingdom [113]. The next approach to reach production is connected with silicon-based alternative substrates, such as CdZnTe/Si. Significant advantages of HgCdTe/Si are evident and available in large area wafers, and because the coupling of the Si substrates with Si

TABLE 12.11
Performance Characteristics of Sensors with Large Format InSb Arrays

	L-3 Cincinnati Electronics (Large-Format/Wide-Area Surveillance Sensors)	SCD (Blackbird IDCA)
View of integrated detector		
Format	4096×4096	1920×1536
Pixel Size	15×15 μm²	10×10 μm²
FPA power consumption	2/5 W	400 mW
Cooler power steady state	< 55 W	20 W
Weight	~ 15 lb.	700 gr
NEDT	Dependent upon integration time	< 24 mK

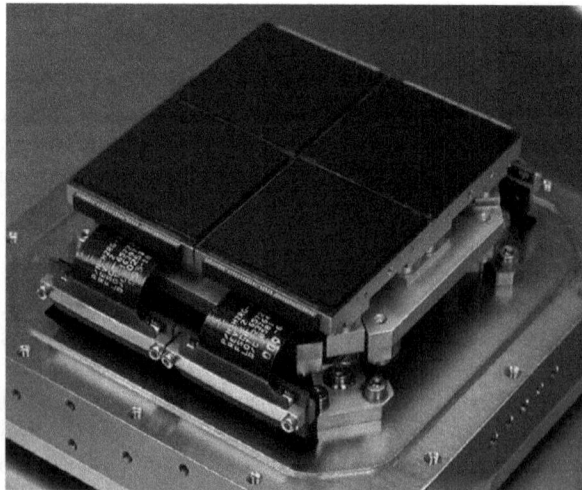

FIGURE 12.78 Packaging of mosaic four Hawaii-2RG arrays fabricated by Teledyne Imaging Sensors for used in astronomy observations.

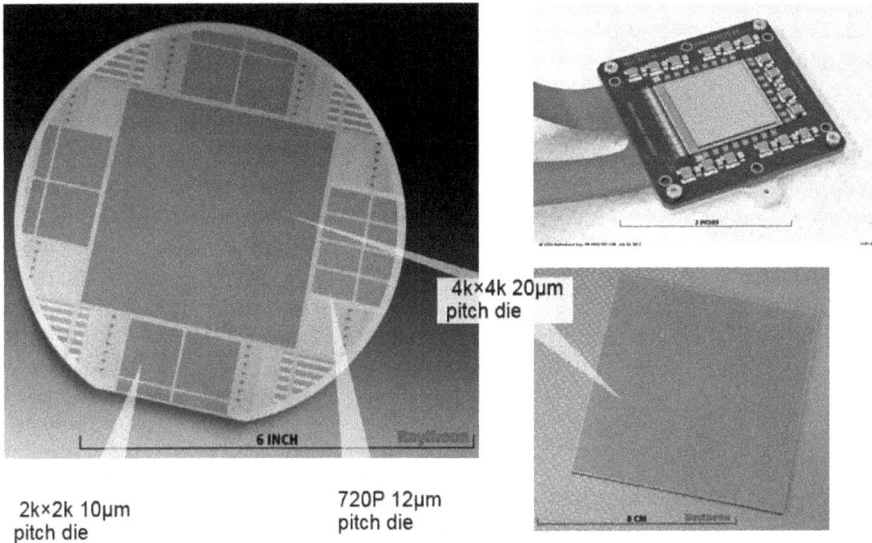

FIGURE 12.79   6-inch diameter HgCdTe/Si detector fabricated using MBE (after Reference 90).

TABLE 12.12
MWIR HgCdTe Focal Plane Arrays

Company	Lynred (Daphnis)	Leonardo (HexaBlu 1280)	AIM (HiPIR-1280M)
Array size	1280×720	1280×960	1280×1024
Pixel pitch	10×10 μm²	6×6 μm²	15×15 μm²
Spectral response	3.7–4.8 μm	3.4–4.8 μm	3.4–5 μm
Operating temperature	up to 120 K	80 to 100 K	95 to 120 K
Max charge capacity	4.2×10⁶ e⁻	4.8×10⁶ e⁻	6×10⁶ e⁻
Pixel output rate	up to 20 MHz		up to 10 MHz
Frame rate	up to 85 Hz full frame rate	60 Hz	50 Hz
NEDT	< 20 mK	< 30 mK	25 mK
Operability	> 99.8%	> 99.5%	> 99.3%

readout circuitry in an FPA structure allows fabrication of very large arrays exhibiting long-term thermal cycle reliability [114]. Figure 12.79 shows 6-inch diameter HgCdTe/Si detector wafer, a 4k×4k format 20-μm pixel array composed of FPA operabilities greater than 99.9 per cent. This is equivalent-size array for an 8k×8k 10-μm pixel format. This technology readiness provides affordable large-format arrays for current and future IR applications.

SWIR, MWIR and LWIR electronically scanned HgCdTe arrays with CMOS multiplexer are commercially available from several manufactures. Table 12.10 presents the worldwide situation in the industry while Tables 12.12 and 12.13 list typical performance specifications for larger MWIR, and LWIR staring arrays fabricated by Sofradir, Leonardo (formerly Selex) and AIM. Most manufactures produce their own multiplexer designs because these often have to be tailored to the applications.

HgCdTe ternary alloy is also used for fabrication of two-colour devices. Multicolour detector capabilities are highly desirable for advanced infrared (IR) imaging systems, since they provide enhanced target discrimination and identification combined with lower false-alarm rates. By

TABLE 12.13
LWIR HgCdTe Focal Plane Arrays

Parameter	Lynred (Scorpio)	Leonardo (Eagle)	AIM (HiPIR-1280L)
Array size	640×512	1280×720	1280×1024
Pixel pitch	$15 \times 15 \ \mu m^2$	$12 \times 12 \ \mu m^2$	$15 \times 15 \ \mu m^2$
Spectral response	7.7–9.3 μm at 80 K	8–10 μm	7.6–9 μm
Operating temperature	up to 90 K	up to 90 K	70 K
Max charge capacity	$1.36 \times 10^7 \ e^-$	$1.8 \times 10^7 \ e^-$	$6 \times 10^6 \ e^-$
Pixel output rate	up to 8 MHz	up to 10 MHz	up to 10 MHz
Frame rate	up to 210 Hz full frame rate		50 Hz
NEDT	22 mK	19 mK	30 mK
Operability	> 99.8%	> 99.8%	> 99.0%

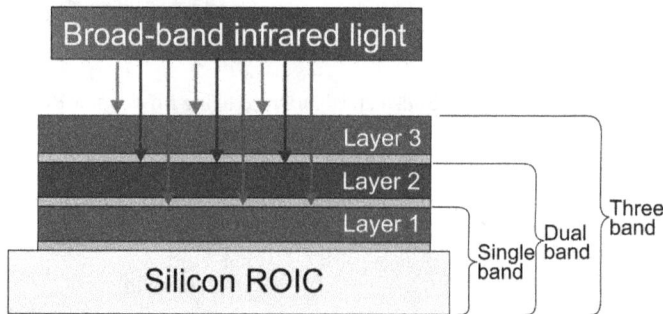

FIGURE 12.80 Structure of a three-colour detector pixel. Infrared flux from the first band is absorbed in Layer 3, while longer wavelength flux is transmitted through the next layers. The thin barriers separate the absorbing bands.

providing this new dimension of contrast, multiband detection also offers advanced colour processing algorithms to further improve sensitivity above that of single-colour devices. Multispectral IR FPAs are highly beneficial for a variety of applications such as missile warning and guidance, precision strike, airborne surveillance, target detection, recognition, acquisition and tracking, thermal imaging, navigational aids and night vision, and so on [115].

The unit cell of integrated multicolour FPAs consists of several collocated detectors, each sensitive to a different spectral band (see Figure 12.80). Radiation is incident on the shorter band detector, with the longer wave radiation passing through to the next detector. Each layer absorbs radiation up to its cut-off, and hence is transparent to the longer wavelengths, which are then collected in subsequent layers. In the case of HgCdTe, this device architecture is realised by placing a longer wavelength HgCdTe photodiode optically behind a shorter wavelength photodiode.

Figure 12.81 illustrates examples of the spectral response from different two-colour HgCdTe photodiodes [116]. Note that there is minimal crosstalk between the bands, since the short wavelength detector absorbs nearly 100 per cent of the shorter wavelengths. The separate photodiodes in a two-colour detector perform exactly like single-colour detectors in terms of achievable performance variation ($R_o A$ product and dark current) with the wavelength at a given temperature [117].

Raytheon Vision Systems has developed two-colour, large-format infrared FPAs to support the U.S. Army's third-generation FLIR systems in both 640×480) and "high definition" 1280×720 formats with 20×20 μm unit cells (see Figure 12.82(a) [118]. The megapixel arrays are implemented in 3rd Gen eLRAS3 FLIR systems [see Figure 12.82(b)]. The ROICs share a common chip architecture

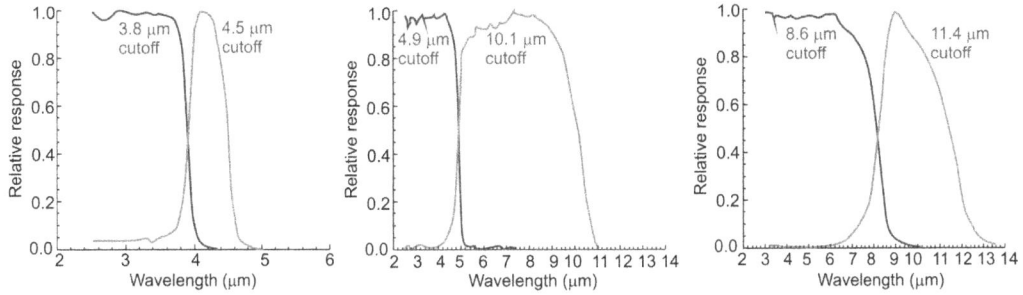

FIGURE 12.81 Spectral response curves for two-colour HgCdTe detectors in various dual-band combinations of MWIR and LWIR spectral bands (after Reference 116).

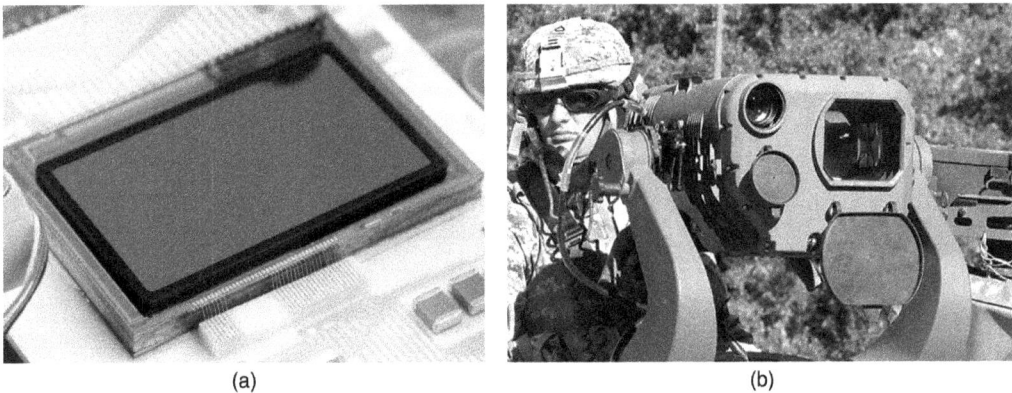

FIGURE 12.82 Dual-band megapixel MW/LW HgCdTe FPAs: (a) RVS 1280×720 format HgCdTe FPAs mounted on dewar platforms (after Reference 118), 3rd Gen eLRAS3 FLIR system with implemented MW/LW two-colour array.

and incorporate identical unit cell circuit designs and layouts; both FPAs can operate in either dual-band or single-band modes. High-quality MWIR/LWIR 1280×720 FPAs with cut-offs ranging out to 11 μm at 78K have demonstrated excellent sensitivity and pixel operabilities exceeding 99.9 per cent in the MW band and greater than 98 per cent in the LW band. Median 300 K *NEDT* values at *f*/3.5 of approximately 20 mK for the MW and 25 mK for the LW have been measured for dual-band operation at 60 Hz frame rate with integration times corresponding to roughly 40 per cent (MW) and 60 per cent (LW) of full well charge capacities. Typical integration times were about 3 ms and 0.1 ms for MW and LW spectral bands, respectively. As shown in Figure 12.83 [117, 118], excellent high resolution IR camera imaging with *f*/2.8 FOV broadband refractive optics at 60 Hz frame rate has been achieved.

12.7.5.4 Lead Salt Arrays

Lead salts were among the first polycrystalline thin-film materials sensitive to the IR radiation used for military applications. Early research works on the materials as infrared detectors were carried out during the 1930s, and the first useful devices were processed by Germans, Americans and British during and just after World War II. Modern lead salt detector arrays contain more than a thousand elements on a single substrate. Operability exceeding 99 per cent is readily achieved for these arrays.

A considerable breakthrough in developing low-cost PbS and PbSe detectors for threat-warning systems was achieved by Northrop Grumman [120, 121]. The focal planes on these detectors are

(a)

(b)

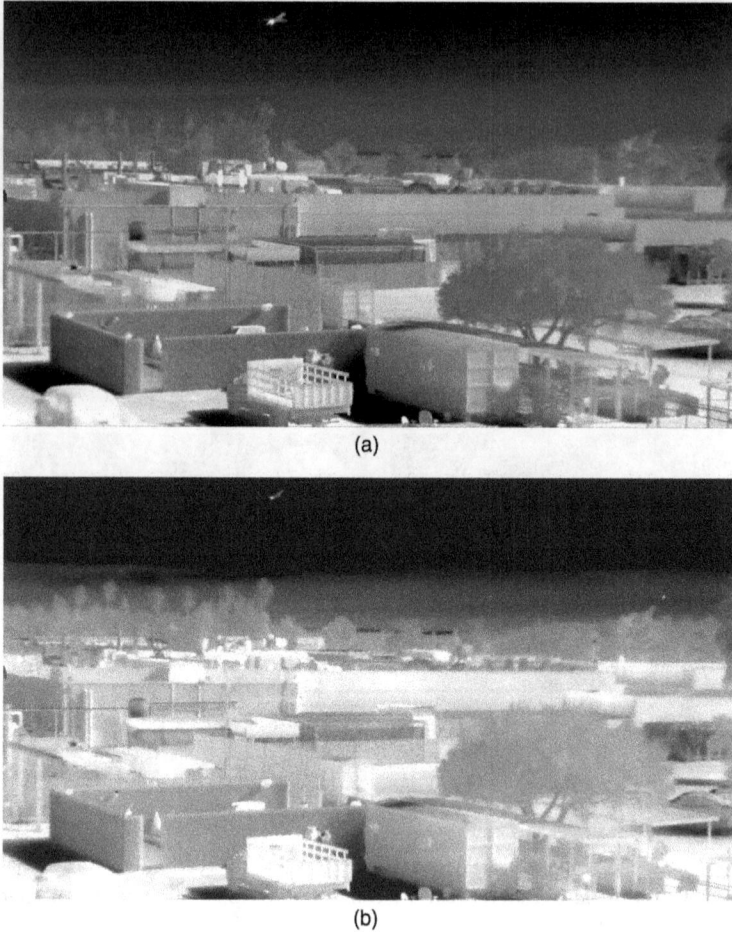

FIGURE 12.83 A still camera image taken at 78 K with $f/2.8$ FOV and 60 Hz frame rate using two-colour 20 μm unit-cell MWIR/LWIR 1280×720 HgCdTe hybrid FPA: (a) MWIR and (b) LWIR (after Reference 119).

PbSe-deposited on silicon readouts. The remarkable aspect of these MWIR detectors is that they are cooled (non-cryogenically) with two thermoelectric coolers. The arrays are 320×240 pixels with 60-μm pixels and 99.6 reproducibility. Sensitivities are now 30 mK with an $f/1$ optic and a 2.5-ms integration time, operating at 230 K (see Table 12.14). These arrays with unique properties (high speed, mid-wave non-cryocooled) can be produced at low cost compared with conventional hybridised, single-crystal IRFPAs. Figure 12.84 exhibits broadband IR across the entire PbSe sensitivity range. The sensor was placed on a rooftop 40 metres in elevation at mid-day under sunny conditions facing a parking lot whose furthest features are at a slant range of 1 km.

12.7.5.5 QWIP Arrays

Various types of MWIR and LWIR high resolution hybrid QWIPs are offered for different applications (FLIR, IRST, reconnaissance, surveillance, airborne camera etc.). The arrays can be assembled in various long vacuum-life dewar and cooler configuration in order to meet the different mechanical and cooling needs of the systems.

The performance figures of merit of state-of-the-art QWIP and HgCdTe FPAs are similar because the main limitations come from the readout circuits. Performance is, however, achieved with very

TABLE 12.14
Specifications for 320×240 Lead Salt Focal Plane Arrays

	Monolithic 320×240 PbS [120]	Monolithic 320×240 PbSe [121]
Pixel size (μm)	30×30	60×60
Detectivity (cmHz$^{1/2}$/W)/NEI*	8×10^{10} (ambient); 3×10^{11} (220 K)	$NEI = 0.07$ μW/cm^2
NEDT (mK)		30 (f/1 optics) (230K)
Type of signal processor	CMOS	CMOS
Time constant (ms)	0.2 (ambient); 1 (220 K)	
Integration options	Snapshot	
Number of output lines	2	
Frame rate (Hz)	60	400
Integration period	Full frame time	
Mux dynamic range (dB)	69	
Active heat dissipation (mW)	200 max	
Operability (%)	> 99	> 99.6
Mux transimpedance (MΩ)	100	
Detector bias (V)	0–6 (user adjustable)	

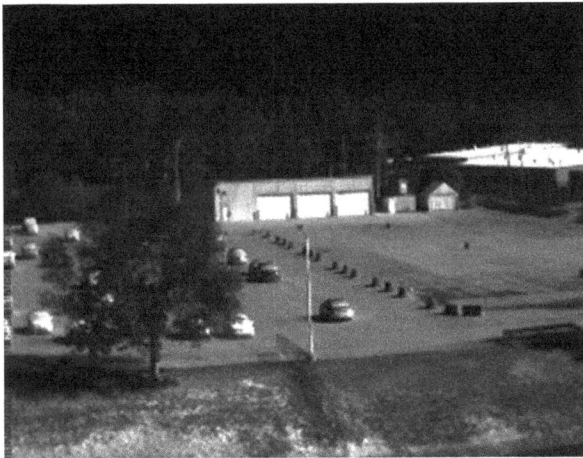

FIGURE 12.84   Image frame data collected on a rooftop, viewing parking lot of Northrop Grumman Rolling Meadows Campus. f/1 lens was broad band with no spectral filter. NEDT performance was measured to be 30 mK with 99.6 per cent pixel operability at 230 K operating temperature (after Reference 121).

different integration times. The very short integration time of LWIR HgCdTe devices (typically below 300 μs) is very useful to freeze a scene with rapidly moving objects. Due to excellent homogeneity and low photoelectrical gain, QWIP devices achieve an even better NEDT [19]; due to low quantum efficiency, however, the integration time must be 10–100 times longer, and typically is between 5 and 20 ms. The choice of the best technology is therefore driven by the specific needs of a system. QWIPs are adequate for any application requiring frame rates no higher than 30 or 60 Hz. The examples are several hundreds of Catherine cameras manufactured by the Thales Research Technology [122] – the cameras contain Vega and Sirius FPAs hybridised and integrated in sensor chip assembly by Sofradir [123] (see Table 12.15). Also, a wide set of QWIP configurations is offered by Lockheed Martin Corporation (see Table 12.15).

TABLE 12.15
Performance of LWIR QWIP Arrays

Parameter	Sofradir (Catherine camera) [123]	Lockheed Martin (ImagIR camera) [124]
Array size	640×512	1024×1024
Pixel pitch	20×20 μm^2	19.5×19.5 μm^2
Spectral response	$\lambda_p = 8.5\pm0.1$ μm, $\Delta\lambda = 1$ μm @ 50%	8.5–9.1 μm
Operating temperature	70–73 K	73 K
Integration type	Snapshot	Snapshot
Max charge capacity	1.04×10^7 e$^-$	8.1×10^6 e$^-$
Frame rate	up to 120 Hz full frame rate	up to 200 Hz full frame rate
NEDT	31 mK (300 K, f/2) 7 ms integration time	< 35 mK
Operability	> 99.9%	> 99.95%
Nonuniformity	< 5%	

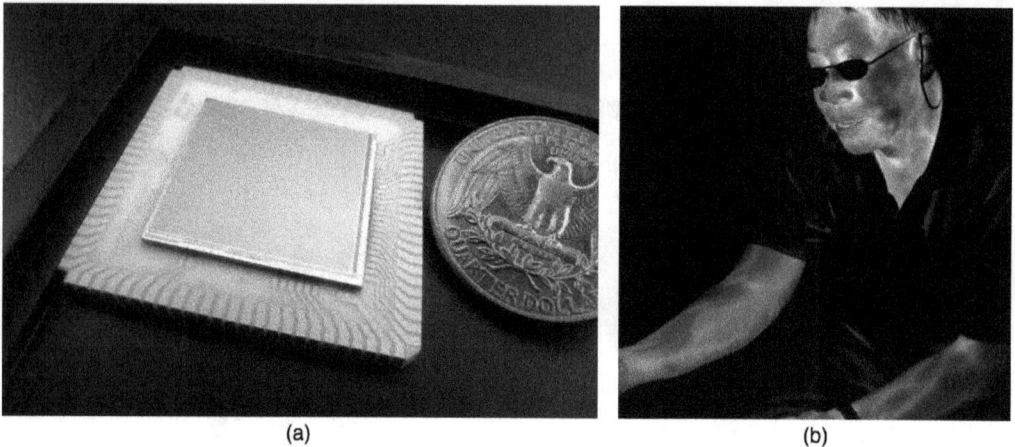

(a)   (b)

FIGURE 12.85 Megapixel QWIP array: (a) picture a 1024×1024 pixel QWIP FPA mounted on a 84-pin lead less chip carrier, (b) one frame of MWIR (5.1 μm) video taken at a frame rate of 10 Hz at temperature 90 K using a ROIC capacitor having a charge capacity of 8×10^6 electrons (after Reference 125).

One magapixel hybrid MWIR and LWIR QWIP with 18 μm pixel size has been demonstrated (see Figure 12.85) with excellent imaging performance using transitions from bound to extended states and from bound to miniband states. Gunapala *et al.* [125] have demonstrated the MWIR detector arrays with a *NEDT* of 17 mK at 95 K operating temperature, *f*/2.5 optics and a 300 K background, and the LWIR detector array with a *NEDT* of 13 mK at 70 K operating temperature, the same optical and background conditions as the MWIR detector array. This technology can be readily extended to a 2k×2k array. Figure 12.85(b) shows frames of video images taken with 5.1 μm cut-off 1024×1024 pixel camera.

QWIPs are ideal detectors for the fabrication of pixel co-registered simultaneously readable two-colour IR FPAs because a QWIP absorbs IR radiation only in a narrow spectral band and is transparent outside of that absorption band [126]. Thus it provides zero spectral crosstalk when two spectral bands are more than a few microns apart. Individual pixels in a multiband QWIP detector array are fabricated using a process similar to that used for their single-band counterparts, except for the via holes that need to be added to electrically connect with the silicon ROIC.

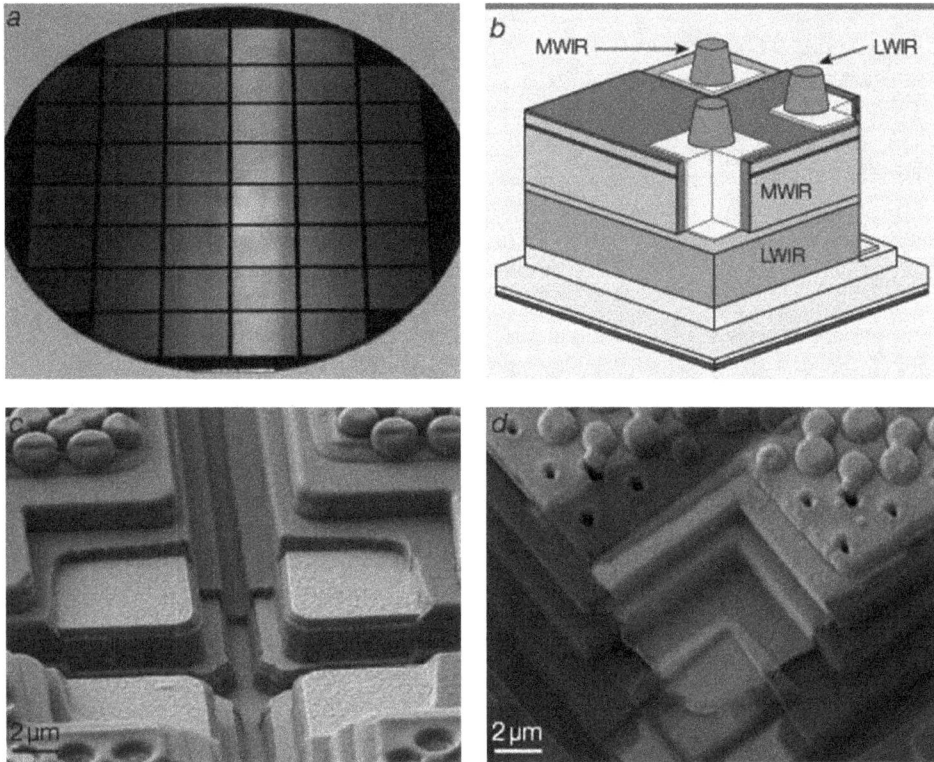

FIGURE 12.86 Two-colour MWIR/LWIR QWIP FPA: (a) 48 FPAs processed on a 4-inch GaAs wafer, (b) 3D view of pixel structure, (c) electrical connections to the common contact, and (d) the pixel connections are brought to the top of each pixel using the gold via connections (after Reference 127).

Figure 12.86 provides insight into dual-band QWIP processing technology developed at Jet Propulsion Laboratory (JPL) [127], based on four-inch wafers to fabricate 320×256 MWIR/LWIR dual-band QWIP devices with pixels collocated and simultaneously readable. As shown in Figure 12.86(b), the carriers emitted from each multiquantum well (MQW) region are collected separately using three contacts. The middle contact layer [see Figure 12.86(c)] is used as the detector common. The electrical connections to the detector common and the LWIR connection are brought to the top of each pixel using via connections. Electrical connections to the common contact and the LWIR pixel connection are brought to the top of each pixel using the gold via connections visible in the figure. This elaborate processing technology could lead to 2-D imaging arrays that can detect separate bands on a single pixel.

The research group from JPL has implemented a MWIR/LWIR pixel co-registered simultaneously readable 1024×1024 dual-band device structure [128, 129]. The pitch of the detector array was 30 μm and the actual MWIR and LWIR pixel sizes were 28×28 μm². The experimentally measured *NEDT* values were 27 and 40 mK for MWIR and LWIR, respectively.

12.7.5.6 Barrier and Type-II Superlattice Arrays

Hitherto, two material systems are used in fabricating both MWIR and LWIR FPAs: HgCdTe ternary alloy and III-V structures based on type-II superlattices (T2SLs). The position of the second class of materials has increased due to implementation of novel structures like barrier detectors, for example, nBn structures (see section 8.5). Recently, Rogalski *et al.* critically analysed the performance of both classes of photodetectors [130]. Results from their paper are as follows:

- III-V materials have inherently short Shockley-Read lifetimes below 1μs, and require barrier architecture to operate at reasonable temperatures, and as such are diffusion-current limited. This applies both to the simple alloy and the T2SL versions.
- HgCdTe alloys have long Shockley-Read lifetimes > 100 μs depending on the cut-off wavelength. They can thus operate with either architecture and may be diffusion or depletion current limited.
- III-Vs offer similar performance to HgCdTe at an equivalent cut-off wavelength, but with a sizeable penalty in operating temperature due to the inherent difference in Shockley-Read lifetimes.

An important advantage of T2SLs is the high quality, high uniformity and stable nature of the material. In general, III-V semiconductors are more robust than their II-VI counterparts due to stronger, less ionic chemical bonding. As a result, III-V-based FPAs excel in operability, spatial uniformity, temporal stability, scalability, producibility and affordability – the so-called "ibility" advantages [131]. Moreover, the status of III-Vs materials can be strengthened since Hg-containing devices can potentially lead to health and environmental concerns, so evaluation of alternative materials is required.

The nBn sensor design is self-passivating, decreasing leakage current and associated noise while improving reliability and manufacturability. Because of its simple design (see Table 8.2), the array technology is a major advance in the state of the art for large infrared FPAs.

The first commercially nBn InAsSb arrays sensor developed by Lockheed Martin Santa Barbara Focalplane operate at 145 to 175 K temperatures. In IRCameras' implementation of Santa Barbara Focalplane's MWIR nBn sensor, a 1280×1024 format, a 12-μm-pixel-pitch detector is packaged in a 1.4-in.-diameter dewar with an overall dewar housing length of about 3.8 in., including the cooler. With a long life, 25,000 h cryocooler consuming about 2.5 W and electronics adding another 2.5 W, the total camera core power draw is only about 5 W total. A high spatial resolution image acquired with nBn sensor running at 160 K was presented in Reference 132. Also, SCD has developed advanced InAsSb (MWIR [133]) and T2SL (LWIR [134]) barrier detectors enable diffusion limited dark currents comparable with HgCdTe "Rule 07" and high quantum efficiency – above 50 per cent. Table 12.16 presents typical performance specifications.

The most spectacular results of the Vital Infrared Sensor Technology Acceleration (VISTA) US government program were presented during the 2017 SPIE Defense and Security Conference in Anaheim (*Proc. SPIE* 10177). This program was devoted to innovative approaches for infrared FPA technology to enhance infrared sensor capabilities. The feasibility of a small pixel had been demonstrated (5–10-μm pitch) T2SL FPA technology as an attractive alternative to HgCdTe

---

TABLE 12.16
InSb-based FPA Manufactured by SCD SemiConductors (after Reference 135)

Parameter	Value	
	InAsSb HOT nBn	pB_pp T2SL
Spectral range	3.6 – 4.2 μm	9.3 μm (filter)
Array format	1280×1024	640×512
Pixel pitch	10 μm	15 μm
Well capacity	2 Me⁻	6 Me⁻
Maximum frame rate	90 Hz	360 Hz
Power consumption	< 2.5 W	
NEDT	< 25 mK	15 mK
Weight	~ 750 gr.	

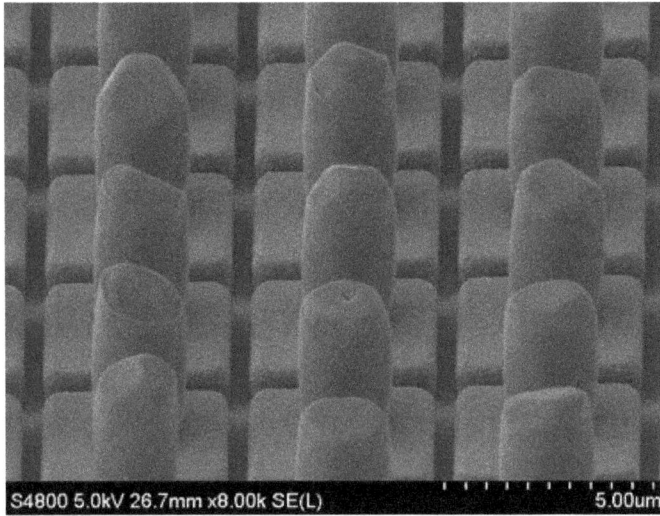

FIGURE 12.87   An SEM photo of fabricated 5-μm pixels using a high-aspect ratio dry etch process resulting > 80 per cent physical fill factor (after Reference 136).

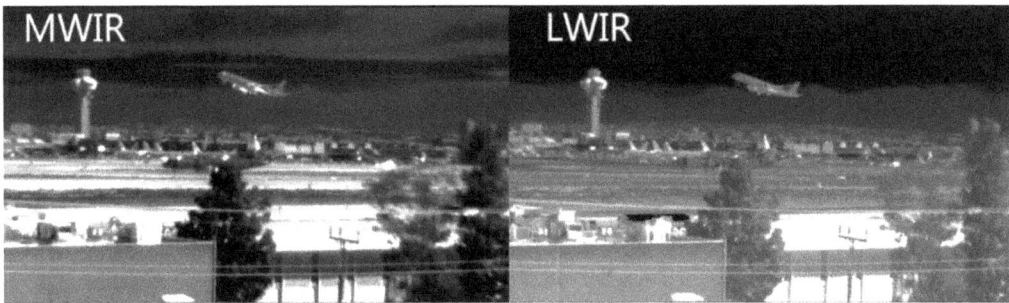

FIGURE 12.88   Pictures acquired with a dual band 1280×720, 12-μm pitch, T2SL MW/LW FPA. The image was captured at 80K and f/4 optics (after Reference 137).

technology, mainly due to lower cost, ease of scalability to larger formats (e.g. 8k×8k/10-μm), and better uniformity. Infrared FPAs with 2k×2k/10-μm and 2k×1k/5-μm formats have been demonstrated by developing high-aspect ratio dry etching for mesa delineation (fill factor > 80%; see Figure 12.87), proper device passivation by dielectric layer and high-aspect ratio indium bump schemes (operability > 99.9%). Resulting MWIR hybrids operating at 150 K show low dark current with low turn-on bias, low *NEDT* (< 20 mK at 150 K using *f*/2.3 optics), and high operability for both 5 μm and 10 μm pixels.

The VISTA program focuses also on large-format dual-band MWIR/LWIR sensing applications. Excellent manufacturability and high uniformity of T2SLs superlattices also have been demonstrated for HD-format (1280×720, 12-μm pitch) T2SL dual-band MWIR/LWIR FPAs grown on GaSb substrates – see Figure 12.88 [137]. The reliability test was carried out by cycling the array's temperature from 70 K to 290 K over 2,000 times. No degradation in either the sensitivity or the operability of the MWIR and LWIR bands was observed, confirming the stability of hybridisation and post-process. The rapid maturation of this technology makes it a strong candidate for deployment in future dual band MW/LW systems.

TABLE 12.17
Comparison of LWIR Existing State-of-the-Art Device Systems for LWIR Detectors

	Bolometer	HgCdTe	QWIP	Type-II SLs
Maturity level	TRL 9	TRL 9	TRL 9	TRL 6-7
Status	Material of choice for application requiring medium to low performance	Material of choice for application requiring high performance	Commercial	Research and development
Operating temp.	Un-cooled	Cooled	Cooled	Cooled
Manufacturability	Excellent	Poor	Excellent	Very good
Cost	Low	High	Medium	Medium
Prospect for large format	Excellent	Very good	Excellent	Excellent
Availability of large substrate	Excellent	Poor	Excellent	Very good
Military system examples	Weapon sight, night vision goggles, missile seekers, small UAV sensors, unattended ground sensors	Missile intercept, tactical ground and air born imaging, hyper spectral, missile seeker, missile tracking, space based sensing	Being evaluated for some military applications and astronomy sensing	Being developed in university and evaluated industry research environment
Limitations	Low sensitivity and long time constants	Performance susceptible to manufacturing variations. Difficult to extend to > 14-μm cut-off	Narrow bandwith and low sensitivity	Requires a significant investment and fundamental material breakthrough to mature
Advantages	Low cost and requires no active cooling, leverages standard Si manufacturing equipment	Near theoretical performance, will remain material of choice for minimum of the next several years	Low cost applications. Leverages commercial manufacturing processes. Very uniform material	Theoretically better then HgCdTe, leverages commercial III-V fabrication techniques

Note: TRL – technology readiness level.

Next, we follow after Reference 80 in order to compare different detector technologies existing on the global market. Table 12.17 provides a snapshot of the current state of development of LWIR detectors fabricated from different material systems. Note that TRL means technology readiness level. The highest level of TRL (ideal maturity) achieves a value of 10. The highest level of maturity (TRL = 9) is credited to microbolometers, HgCdTe photodiodes and QWPs. A little less, TRL = 6/7, for T2SLs. The type-II $A^{III}B^{V}$ superlattice structures have great potential for LWIR spectral range application with performance comparable to HgCdTe for the same cut-off wavelength. Strong progress toward mature superlattice and barrier detector technologies, including their commercialisation, has been observed in the last decade.

PROBLEMS

Example 12.1

Consider a three-phase Si-CCD with 5 μm cell size, with an acceptor doping level $N_a = 10^{14}$ cm^{-3}, and a dark current per pixel $I_d = 0.01$ pA. What is the clock driving voltage required? What is the saturation level and the dynamic range? What is the signal for a 100 lux illumination on the CCD?

Example 12.2

Usually, the performance of MWIR and LWIR focal plane arrays (FPAs) is limited by the readout circuits (by storage capacity of the ROIC). The current generated in a biased photon detector is integrated onto a capacitive node with a carrier well capacity of N_w. Find the relation of charge-handling capacity with *NEDT* for target of 300 K for MW and LW bands, respectively.

Example 12.3

If the *NEDT* of a system were measured to be 0.25 K, and the scan rate were then slowed by a factor of 2, what would the new *NEDT* be?

Example 12.4

Consider a satellite in space located 200 km from a spherical source of 1-m diameter that radiates as a blackbody of 2000 K against a background of cold black space (see figure below). The electro-optical system of satellite has parameters given in the table.

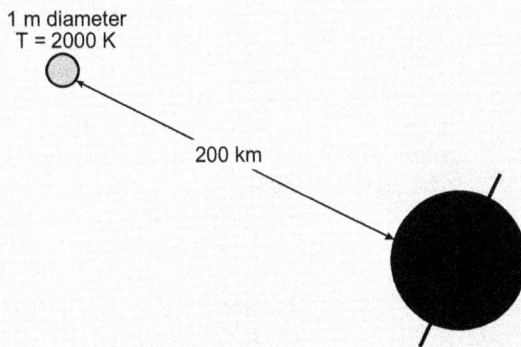

Source: Satellite configuration

Estimate:
- the detector noise-equivalency power (*NEP*);
- whether the source represents a point source for satellite configuration;
- the noise equivalent irradiance of the system;
- the signal-to-noise ratio.

Example 12.5

Derive the noise equivalent difference temperature (*NEDT*) for the thermal imaging system shown in Figure 12.12. On the graph shown in this figure, A_s and A_d are, respectively, the surfaces of the object and the detector, r is the distance of the object to the lens (system optics), A_{ap} and D are the surface and the diameter of the lens (aperture, entrance-pupil). The detector is placed in focal plane of the system in the distance $\approx f$ to the entrance pupil. The optic's system is opened to $F/\#$ (i.e., $F = f/D$ with $A_{ap} = \pi D^2/4$).

Satellite Parameters

Primary mirror diameter, D_o	0.2 m
f/# of optics	*f*/3
Detector area, A_d	1 cm^2
Detector detectivity, D^*	10^{10} Jones
Wavelength band	8–12 μm
Electrical bandwidth, Δf	1 Hz

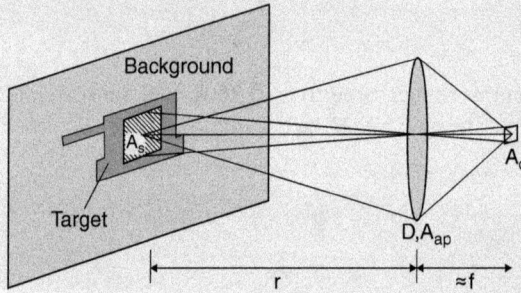

REFERENCES

1. G.H. Rieke, *Detection of Light: From Ultraviolet to the Submillimeter*, Cambridge University Press, Cambridge, 2003.
2. J.D. Vincent, S.E. Hodges, J. Vampola, M. Stegall, and G. Pierce, *Fundamentals of Infrared and Visible Detector Operation and Testing*, Wiley, Hoboken, NJ, 2016.
3. E.L. Dereniak and G.D. Boreman, *Infrared Detectors and Systems,* John Wiley, New York, 1996.
4. J.L. Vampola, "Readout electronics for infrared sensors", in *The Infrared and Electro-Optical Systems Handbook*, Vol. 3, pp. 287–342, edited by W.D. Rogatto, SPIE Press, Bellingham, 1993.
5. W.S. Boyle and G.E. Smith, "Charge coupled semiconductor device", *Bell. Syst. Techn. Jour.* 49, 72–74 (1970).
6. G.F. Amelio, M.F. Tompsett, and G.E. Smith, "Experimental verification of the charge coupled device concept", *IEEE Trans. Electron Devices* ED-18, 986–992 (1970).
7. *CCD Imaging Databook*, Loral Fairchild Imaging Sensors, 1991.
8. *CCD Image Sensors and Cameras*, DALSA, 1991.
9. http://image-sensors-world.blogspot.com/2012/09/teledyne-dalsa-announces-60mp-medium.html.
10. N. Lavars, "World's largest camera sensor snaps first ever 3,200-megapixel photo", https://newatlas.com/photography/worlds-largest-camera-first-3200-megapixel-photo/.
11. P. Jerram and J. Beletic, "Teledyne's high performance infrared detectors for space missions", *Proc. SPIE* 11180, 111803D-2 (2018).

12. P. Norton, "Detector focal plane array technology", in *Encyclopedia of Optical Engineering*, pp. 320–348, ed. R. Driggers, Marcel Dekker, New York, 2003.

13. L. Beiser and R.B. Johnson, "Scanners", *Handbook of Optics*. Vol. I, Chapter 30, 3rd edition; ed. M. Bass, McGraw Hill, 2010.

14. V.P. Ponomarenko and A.M. Filachev, "Linear and matrix IR detectors at RD&P center Orion", *Proc. SPIE* 4369, 25–42 (2001).

15. www.hamamatsu.com/sp/hpe/HamamatsuNews/HamaNews_0113.pdf.

16. A. Rogalski, "Infrared detectors at the beginning of the next millennium", *Opto-Electron. Rev.* 9(2), 173–187 (2001).

17. Y. Bai, J. Bajaj, J.W. Beletic, and M.C. Farris, "Teledyne imaging sensors: silicon CMOS imaging technologies for X-ray, UV, visible and near infrared", *Proc. SPIE* 7021, 702102 (2008).

18. A. Rogalski, A. Bielecki, and J. Mikołajczyk, "Detection of optical radiation", in *Handbook of Optoelectronics*, Vol. 1, pp. 65–123, edited by J.P. Dakin and R.G.W. Brown, CRC Press, Boca Raton, 2018.

19. A. Rogalski, *Infrared and Terahertz Detectors*, CRC Press, Boca Raton, 2019.

20. *Prescient & Strategic Intelligence*, www.psmarketresearch.com/market-analysis/image-sensors-market.

21. M. Kimata, "My life in IRFPA R&D", *Proc. SPIE* 10177, 1017727-1-11 (2017).

22. R. Thorn, "High density infrared detector arrays", U.S. Patent No. 4, 039, 833, 1977.

23. I.M. Baker and R.A. Ballingall, "Photovoltaic CdHgTe-silicon hybrid focal planes", *Proc. SPIE* 510, 121–129 (1984).

24. I.M. Baker, "Photovoltaic IR detectors", in *Narrow-Gap II-VI Compounds for Optoelectronic and Electromagnetic Applications*, pp. 450–473, ed. P. Capper, Chapman & Hall, London, 1997.

25. A. Turner, T. Teherani, J. Ehmke, C. Pettitt, P. Conlon, J. Beck, K. McCormack, L. Colombo, T. Lahutsky, T. Murphy, and R.L. Williams "Producibility of VIP scanning focal plane arrays", *Proc. SPIE* 2228, 237–248 (1994).

26. M.A. Kinch, "HDVIP FPA technology at DRS", *Proc. SPIE* 4369, 566–578 (2001).

27. *Handbook of 3D Integration, Technology and Applications of 3D Integrated Circuits*, 2nd edition; edited by P. Garrou, C. Bower, and P. Ramm, Wiley-VCH, Weinheim, 2008.

28. J.M. Lloyd, *Thermal Imaging Systems,* Plenum Press, New York, 1975.

29. A. Redjimi, D. Knežević, K. Savić, N. Jovanović, M. Simović, and D. Vasiljević, "Noise equivalent temperature difference model for thermal imagers, calculation and analysis", *Sci. Tech. Rev.* 64(2), 42–49 (2014).

30. www.dxomark.com/itext/measurements-and-protocols/MTF.jpg.

31. ASTM E1213-97, *Standard Test Method for Minimum Resolvable Temperature Difference for Thermal Imaging Systems*, 2009.

32. K. Chrzanowski, *Testing Thermal Imagers. Practical guide*, Military University of Technology, Warsaw, 2010, www.inframet.com/Literature/Testing%20thermal%20imagers.pdf.

33. A. Daniels, *Field Guide to Infrared Systems, Detectors, and FPAs*, 3rd edition, SPIE Press, Bellingham, 2018.

34. J. Johnson, "Analysis of image forming systems," in *Image Intensifier Symposium*, AD 220160, Warfare Electrical Engineering Department, U.S. Army Research and Development Laboratories, Ft. Belvoir, Virginia, pp. 244–273, 1958.

35. U. Adomeit, "Infrared detection, recognition and identification of handheld objects", *Proc. SPIE* 8541, 85410O-1-9 (2012).

36. J.L. Miller, "Future sensor system needs for staring arrays", *Infrared Phys. & Technol.* 54, 164–169 (2011).

37. A. Rogalski, J. Antoszewski, and L. Faraone, "Third-generation infrared photodetector arrays," *J. Appl. Phys.* 105, 091101–44 (2009).

38. J. Chouinard, *The Fundamentals of Camera and Image Sensor Technology,* www.visiononline.org/userassets/aiauploads/file/cvp_the-fundamentals-of-camera-and-image-sensor-technology_jon-chouinard.pdf.

39. www.pco.de/fileadmin/fileadmin/user_upload/pco-product_sheets/PCO_scmos_ebook.pdf.

40. http://hamamatsu.magnet.fsu.edu/articles/ccdsatandblooming.html.

41. Kodak CCD Primer, KCP-001, *Charge-Coupled Device Image Sensors*. Eastman Kodak Company – Microelectronics Technology Division, Rochester, NY, 2010, www1.phys.vt.edu/~jhs/phys3154/KodakCCDPrimer.pdf.

42. O. Djazovski, "Focal plane arrays for optical payloads", in *Optical Payloads for Space Missions*, pp. 793–837, edited by S. N. Qian, Wiley, Chichester, 2016.

43. J.H. Giles, T.D. Ridder, R.H. Williams, D.A. Jones, and M.B. Denton, "Selecting a CCD camera", *Anal. Chem. News & Features* 70(19), 663A-668A (1998).

44. https://keyassets.timeincuk.net/inspirewp/live/wp-content/uploads/sites/13/2014/12/Bayer-filter.jpg.

45. *High Performance Silicon Imaging. Fundamentals and Applications of CMOS and CCD Sensors*, 2nd edition, edited by D. Durini, Elsevier, Duxford, 2020.

46. https://encyclopedia2.thefreedictionary.com/Super+CCD.

47. "X-3: New single-chip colour CCD technology," *New Technology*, 20–24, March/April 2002.

48. R.F. Lyon and P. Hubel, "Eyeing the camera: Into the next century", *IS&T/SID Tenth Color Imaging Conference*, 349–355, 2001.

49. *Introduction to Charge-Coupled Devices*, www.ysctech.com/digital-microscope-CCD-camera-info.html.

50. M.H. White, D.L. Lampe, F.C. Blaha, and I.A. Mack, "Characterization of surface channel CCD image arrays at low light levels", *IEEE J. Solid-State Circuits* SC-9(1), 1–13 (1974).

51. E.R. Fossum and B. Pain, "Infrared readout electronics for space science sensors: State of the art and future directions", *Proc. SPIE* 2020, 262–285 (1993).

52. G.F. Amelio, "Impact of large CCD image sensing arrays", *Proc. CCD 74 Int. Conf.* 6, paper 1/3 (1974).

53. *CCD Architecture*, https://andor.oxinst.com/learning/view/article/ccd-sensor-architectures.

54. *CCD Sensor Types*, www.stemmer-imaging.com/en/knowledge-base/ccd/.

55. https://i0.wp.com/img.directindustry.com/pdf/repository_di/191249/e2v-ccd220-back-illuminated-l3vision-sensor-electron-multiplying-adaptive-optics-ccd-732427_1b.jpg?resize=720%2C1017.

56. M. Kimata and N. Tubouchi, "Charge transfer devices", in *Infrared Photon Detectors*, pp. 94–144, edited by A. Rogalski, SPIE Optical Engineering Press, Bellingham, WA, 1995.

57. *Hamamatsu Catalogue. Chapter 4. Image Sensors*, www.scribd.com/document/343028020/e05-Handbook-Image-Sensors

58. www.vision-doctor.com/en/camera-technology-basics/sensor-and-pixel-sizes.html.

59. *Introduction to CMOS Image Sensors*, www.olympus-lifescience.com/es/microscope-resource/primer/digitalimaging/ cmosimagesensors/.

60. O. Skorka and D. Joseph D, "CMOS digital pixel sensors: technology and applications", *Proc. SPIE* 9060, 90600G1–14 G14 (2014).

61. M. El-Desouki, M.J. Deen, Q. Fang, L. Liu, Tse F, and D. Armstrong, "CMOS image sensors for high speed applications", *Sensors* 9, 430–444 (2009).

62. *CMOS Sensors*, www.stemmer-imaging.com/en-se/knowledge-base/cmos/.

63. J. Ohta, *Smart CMOS Sensors and Applications*, 2nd edition, CRC Press, Boca Raton, 2019.

64. S. Kilcoyne, N. Malone, B. Kean, J. Cantrell, J. Fierro, L. Meier, S. DeWalt, C. Hewitt, J. Wyles, J. Drab, G. Grama, G. Paloczi, J. Vampola, and K. Brown, "Advancements in large-format Si PIN hybrid focal plane technology", *Proc. SPIE* 9219, 921906-1-11 (2014).

65. J. Drab, "Multilevel wafer stacking for 3D circuit integration", *Raytheon Technology Today*, Issue 1, 30–31, 2015.

66. V. Suntharalingam, R. Berger, S. Clark, J. Knecht, A. Messier, K. Newcomb, D. Rathman, R. Slattery, A. Soares, C. Stevenson, K. Warner, D. Young, L.P. Ang, B. Mansoorian, and D. Shaver, "A four-side tileable back illuminated, three-dimensionally integrated megapixel cmos image sensor", MIT Lincoln Laboratory, 2009.

67. L.J. Kozlowski, S.A. Cabelli, D.E. Cooper, and K. Vural, "Low background infrared hybrid focal plane array characterization", *Proc. SPIE* 1946 , 199–213 (1993).

68. D.J. Sauer, F.L. Hsueh, F.V. Shallcross, G.M. Meray, and T.S. Villani, "A 640×480 element PtSi IR sensor with low-noise MOS-X-Y addressable multiplexer", *Proc. SPIE* 1308, 81–87 (1990).

69. J. Nakamura, *Image Sensors and Signal Processing for Digital Still Camera*, CRC Press, Boca Raton, 2006.

70. D. Durini, *High Performance Silicon Imaging. Fundamentals and Applications of CMOS and CCD Sensors*, 2nd edition, Duxford, 2020.

71. *Butting versus Stitching*, https://harvestimaging.com/blog/?p=1568.

72. J.L. Tonry, B.E. Burke, S. Isani, P.M. Onaka, and M.J. Cooper, "Results from the Pan-STARRS Orthogonal Transfer Array (OTA)", *Proc. SPIE* 7021, 702105 (2008).

73. A.R. Jha, *Cryogenic Technology and Applications*, Elsevier, Oxford, 2006.

74. P.T. Blotter and J.C. Batty, "Thermal and mechanical design of cryogenic cooling systems," in *The Infrared and Electro-Optical Systems Handbook*, Vol. 3, 343433, edited by W.D. Rogatto, Infrared Information Analysis Center, Ann Arbor, MI, and SPIE Press, Bellingham, 1993.

75. R. Rehm, R. Driad, L. Kirste, S. Leone, T. Passow, F. Rutz, L. Watschke, and A. Zibold, "Toward AlGaN focal plane arrays for solar-blind ultraviolet detection", *Phys. Status Solidi A* 217, 1900769 (2020).

76. *Image Sensor, Market Review and Forecast 2009*, Strategies Unlimited, PennWell, September (2009).

77. E.R. Fossum, "CMOS image sensors: electronic camera-on-a-chip", *IEEE Trans. Electron. Dev.* 44, 1689–1698 (1997).

78. K. Jacobson, "Recent developments of digital cameras and space imagery", www.ipi.uni-hannover.de/fileadmin/ipi/publications/2011_GISOSTRAVA_KJ.pdf.

79. G. Patrie, "Gigapixel frame images: Part II. Is the holy grail of airborne digital frame imaging in sight?", *GeoInformatics*, 24–29, March 2006.

80. *Seeing Photons: Progress and Limits of Visible and Infared Sensor Arrays*, Committee on Developments in Detector Technologies; National Research Council, 2010, www.nap.edu/catalog/12896.html

81. B. Leininger, J. Edwards, J. Antoniades, D. Chester, D. Haas, E. Liu, M. Stevens, C. Gershfield, M. Braun, J.D. Targove, S. Weind, P. Brewere, D.G. Madden, K.H. Shafique, "Autonomous Real-time Ground Ubiquitous Surveillance – Imaging System (ARGUS-IS)," *Proc. SPIE* 6981, 69810H-1–11 (2008).

82. "Billion pixel Gaia camera starts to take shape", https://sci.esa.int/web/gaia/-/48901-billion-pixel-gaia-camera-starts-to-take-shape.

83. O. Iwert and B. Delabrea, "The challenge of highly curved monolithic imaging detectors", *Proc. SPIE* 7742, 774227 (2010).

84. E.W. Dunham, J.C. Geary, R.H. Philbrick, C. Stewart, and D. Koch, "The Kepler mission's focal plane", *Proc. SPIE* 4854, 558–566 (2003).

85. *Standard CMOS and CCD Image Sensors*, www.teledyne-e2v.com/content/uploads/2017/07/29884_Teledyne-E2V_CMOS-and-CCD-Sensors_v5_1_aw_web.pdf.

86. www.fairchildimaging.com/products/.

87. *Advanced Imaging System*, www.sri.com/advanced-imaging-systems/.

88. Y. Bai, W. Tennant, S. Anglin, A. Wong, M. Farris, M. Xu, E. Holland, D. Cooper, J. Hosack, K. Ho, T. Sprafke, R. Kopp, B. Starr, R. Blank and J. W. Beletic, "4K×4K format, 10 μm pixel pitch H4RG-10 hybrid CMOS silicon visible focal plane array for space astronomy", *Proc. SPIE* 8453, 84530M-1-18, 2012.

89. B.W. Kean, S. Kilcoyne, N.R. Malone, G. Wilberger, R. Troup, S. Miller, K.C. Brown, J. Vampola, "Advancements in large-format Si PIN hybrid focal plane technology", *Proc. SPIE* 8511, 851111-1-10, 2012.

90. B. Starr, L. Mears, C. Fulk, J. Getty, E. Beuville, R. Boe, C. Tracy, E. Corrales, S. Kilcoyne, J. Vampola, J. Drab, R. Peralta, C. Doyle, "RVS large format arrays for astronomy", *Proc. SPIE* 9915, 99152X-1-14, 2016.

91. *The World's First Thermal Imaging Smartphone*, www.flir.com/home/news/details/?ID=74197.

92. *Thermal Imager Industry: The Chinese Triumph*, www.yole.fr/ThermalImaging_MarketUpdate_GuidBolometer.aspx.

93. *Uncooled Detectors for Thermal Imaging Cameras*, www.flirmedia.com/MMC/CVS/Appl_Stories/AS_0015_EN.pdf.

94. F. Niklaus, C. Jansson, A. Decharat, J.-E. Källhammer, H. Pettersson, and G. Stemme, "Low to medium vacuum atmosphere: performance model and tradeoffs", *Proc. SPIE* 6542, 1M-1–12 (2007).

95. M. Kohin and N. Butler, "Performance limits of uncooled VO$_x$ microbolometer focal-plane arrays", *Proc. SPIE* 5406, 447–453 (2004).

96. A. Rogalski, P. Martyniuk, and M. Kopytko, "Challenges of small-pixel infrared detectors: A review", *Rep. Prog. Phys.* 79, 046501 (2016).

97. G.D. Skidmore, "Uncooled 10 μm FPA development at DRS", *Proc. SPIE* 9819, 98191O-1-8 (2016).

98. http://xenics.com/en/products/cameras; www.sensorsinc.com/products/linescan-cameras/.

99. M.D. Enriguez, M.A. Blessinger, J.V. Groppe, T.M. Sudol, J. Battaglia, J. Passe, M. Stern, and B.M. Onat, "Performance of high resolution visible-InGaAs imager for day/night vision", *Proc. SPIE* 6940, 69400O (2008).

100. A. Hoffman, T. Sessler, J. Rosbeck, D. Acton, and M. Ettenberg, "Megapixel InGaAs arrays for low background applications", *Proc. SPIE* 5783, 32–38 (2005).

101. R. Fraenkel, E. Berkowicz, L. Bykov, R. Dobromislin, R. Elishkov, A. Giladi, I. Grimberg, I. Hirsh, E. Ilan, C. Jacobson, I. Kogan, P. Kondrashov, I. Nevo, I. Pivnik, and S. Vasserman, "High definition 10 μm pitch InGaAs detector with asynchronous laser pulse detection mode", *Proc. SPIE* 9819, 1–8 (2016).

102. S. Manda, R. Matsumoto, S. Saito, S. Maruyama, H. Minari, T. Hirano, T. Takachi, N. Fujii, Y. Yamamoto, Y. Zaizen, T. Hirano, and H. Iwamoto, "High-definition visible-SWIR InGaAs image sensor using Cu-Cu bonding of III-V to silicon wafer", *2019 IEEE International Electron Devices Meeting (IEDM)*, 390–393 (2019).

103. H. Yuan, M. Meixell, J. Zhang, P. Bey, J. Kimchi, and L.C. Kilmer, "Low dark current small pixel large format InGaAs 2D photodetector array development at Teledyne Judson Technologies", *Proc. SPIE* 8353, 835309 (2012).

104. A. Rouvié, J. Coussement, O. Huet, JP. Truffer, M. Pozzi, E.H. Oubensaid, S. Hamard, V. Chaffraix, and E. Costard, "InGaAs focal plane array developments and perspectives", *Proc. SPIE* 9451, 945105-1-8 (2015).

105. R. Fraenkel, E. Berkowicz, L. Bikov, R. Elishkov, A. Giladi, I. Hirsh, E. Ilan, C. Jakobson, P. Kondrashov, E. Louzon, I. Nevo, I. Pivnik, A. Tuito, and S. Vasserman, "Development of low SWaP and low noise InGaAs detectors", *Proc. SPIE* 10177, 1017703 (2017).

106. J.A. Trezza, N. Masaun, and M. Ettenberg, "Analytic modeling and explanation of ultra-low noise in dense SWIR detector arrays", *Proc. SPIE* 8012, 80121Y (2011).

107. A. W. Hoffman, E. Corrales, P. J. Love, J. Rosbeck, M. Merrill, A. Fowler, and C. McMurtry, "2K×2K InSb for astronomy", *Proc. SPIE* 5499, 59–67 (2004).

108. E. Beuville, D. Acton, E. Corrales, J. Drab, A. Levy, M. Merrill, R. Peralta, and W. Ritchie, "High performance large infrared and visible astronomy arrays for low background applications: instruments performance data and future developments at Raytheon", *Proc. SPIE* 6660, 66600B (2007).

109. A.M. Fowler, D. Bass, J. Heynssens, I. Gatley, F.J. Vrba, H.D. Ables, A. Hoffman, M. Smith, and J. Woolaway, "Next generation in InSb arrays: ALADDIN, the 1024×1024 InSb focal plane array readout evaluation results", *Proc. SPIE* 2268, 340–45 (1994).

110. A. M. Fowler, K. M. Merrill, W. Ball, A. Henden, F. Vrba, and C. McCreight, "Orion: A 1–5 micron focal plane for the 21st century", in *Scientific Detectors for Astronomy: The Beginning of a New Era*, edited by P. Amico, 51–58, Kluwer, Dordrecht, 2004.

111. J.M. Armstrong, M.R. Skokan, M.A. Kinch, and J.D. Luttmer, "NDVIP five micron pitch HgCdTe focal plane arrays", *Proc. SPIE* 9070, 907933 (2014).

112. J.W. Beletic, R. Blank, D. Gulbransen, D. Lee, M. Loose, E.C. Piquette, T. Sprafke, W.E. Tennant, M. Zandian, and J. Zino, "Teledyne Imaging Sensors: Infrared imaging technologies for astronomy & civil space", *Proc. SPIE* 7021, 70210H (2008).

113. C.D. Maxey, J.C. Fitzmaurice, H.W. Lau, L.G. Hipwood, C.S. Shaw, C.L. Jones, and P. Capper, "Current status of large-area MOVPE growth of HgCdTe device structures for infrared focal plane arrays", *J. Electronic Materials* 35, 1275–1282 (2006).

114. J.M. Peterson, J.A. Franklin, M. Readdy, S.M. Johnson, E. Smith, W.A. Radford, and I. Kasai, "High-quality large-area MBE HgCdTe/Si", *J. Electronic Materials* 36, 1283–1286 (2006).

115. P. Norton, J. Campbell, S. Horn, and D. Reago, "Third-generation infrared imagers", *Proc. SPIE* 4130, 226–236 (2000).

116. P.R. Norton, "Status of infrared detectors", *Proc. SPIE* 3379, 102–114 (1998).

117. E.P.G. Smith, L.T. Pham, G.M. Venzor, E.M. Norton, M.D. Newton, P.M. Goetz, V.K. Randall, A.M. Gallagher, G.K. Pierce, E.A. Patten, R.A. Coussa, K. Kosai, W.A. Radford, L.M. Giegerich, J.M. Edwards, S.M. Johnson, S.T. Baur, J.A. Roth, B. Nosho, T.J. de Lyon, J.E. Jensen, and R.E. Longshore, "HgCdTe focal plane arrays for dual-color mid- and long-wavelength infrared detection", *J. Electronic Materials* 33, 509–516 (2004).

118. D.F. King, J.S. Graham, A.M. Kennedy, R.N. Mullins, J.C. McQuitty, W.A. Radford, T.J. Kostrzewa, E.A. Patten, T.F. McEwan, J.G. Vodicka, and J.J. Wootan, "3rd-generation MW/LWIR sensor engine for advanced tactical systems", *Proc. SPIE* 6940, 69402R (2008).

119. D.F. King, W.A. Radford, E.A. Patten, R.W. Graham, T.F. McEwan, J.G. Vodicka, R.F. Bornfreund, P.M. Goetz, G.M. Venzor, and S.M. Johnson, "3rd-generation 1280×720 FPA development status at Raytheon Vision Systems", *Proc. SPIE* 6206, 62060W (2006).

120. T. Beystrum, R. Himoto, N. Jacksen, and M. Sutton, "Low cost Pb salt FPAs", *Proc. SPIE* 5406, 287–294 (2004).

121. K. Green, S.-S. Yoo, and Ch. Kauffman, "Lead salt TE-cooled imaging sensor development", *Proc. SPIE* 9070, 9070-1-7 (2014).

122. J. Wallace, "Photonics products: MWIR and LWIR detectors: QWIPs capture LWIR images at low cost", *Laser Focus World*, July 10, 2015.

123. E. Costard and Ph. Bois, "THALES long wave QWIP thermal imagers", *Infrared Phys. Technol.* 50, 260–269 (2007).

124. www.termografia.com/PDF/imag_ir.pdf.

125. S.D. Gunapala, S.V. Bandara, J.K. Liu, C.J. Hill, B. Rafol, J.M. Mumolo, J.T. Trinh, M.Z. Tidrow, and P.D. LeVan, "1024×1024 pixel mid-wavelength and long-wavelength infrared QWIP focal plane arrays for imaging applications", *Semicond. Sci. Technol.* 20, 473–480 (2005).

126. S.D. Gunapala, S.V. Bandara, J.K. Liu, J.M. Mumolo, C.J. Hill, S.B. Rafol, D. Salazar, J. Woollaway, P.D. LeVan, and M.Z. Tidrow, "Towards dualband megapixel QWIP focal plane arrays", *Infared Phys. Technol.* 50, 217–226 (2007).

127. S. Gunapala, "Megapixel QWIPs deliver multi-color performance", *Compd. Semicond.* 10, 25–28, October 2005.

128. A. Soibel, S. D. Gunapala, S. V. Bandara, J. K. Liu, J. M. Mumolo, D. Z. Ting, C. J. Hill, and J. Nguyen, "Large format multicolor QWIP focal plane arrays", *Proc. SPIE* 7298, 729806 (2009).

129. S. Gunapala, S.V. Bandara, J.K. Liu, J.M. Mumolo, D.Z. Ting, C.J. Hill, J. Nguyen, B. Simolon, J. Woolaway, S.C. Wang, W. Li, P.D. LeVan, and M.Z. Tidrow, "Demonstration of megapixel dual-band QWIP focal plane array", *IEEE J. Quantum. Electron.* 46, 285–293 (2010).

130. A. Rogalski, P. Martyniuk, and M. Kopytko, "Type-II superlattice photodetectors versus HgCdTe photodiodes", *Prog. Quantum Electron.* 68, 100228 (2019).

131. P.Y. Delaunay, B.Z. Nosho, A.R. Gurga, S. Terterian, and R.D. Rajavel, "Advances in III-V based dual-band MWIR/LWIR FPAs at HRL", *Proc. SPIE* 10177, 101770T-1-12 (2017).

132. A. Adams and E. Rittenberg, "HOT IR sensors improve IR camera size, weight, and power", *Laser Focus World*, January 2014, 83–87.

133. P.C. Klipstein, E. Avnon, Y. Benny, E. Berkowicz, Y. Cohen, R. Dobromislin, R. Fraenkel, G. Gershon, A. Glozman, E. Hojman, E. Ilan, Y. Karni, O. Klin, Y. Kodriano, L. Krasovitsky, L. Langof, I. Lukomsky, I. Nevo, M. Nitzani, I. Pivnik, N. Rappaport, O. Rosenberg, I. Shtrichman, L. Shkedy, N. Snapi, R. Talmor, R. Tessler, E. Weiss and A. Tuito, "Development and production of array barrier detectors at SCD", *J. Electronic Materials* 46(9), 5386–5393 (2017).

134. https://scdusa-ir.com/products/.

135. P.C. Klipstein, E. Avnon, D. Azulai, Y. Benny, R. Fraenkel, A. Glozman, E. Hojman, O. Klin, L. Krasovitsky, L. Langof, I. Lukomsky, M. Nitzani, I. Shtrichman, N. Rappaport, N. Snapi, E. Weiss and A. Tuito, "Type II superlattice technology for LWIR detectors", *Proc. SPIE* 9819, 9819-20 (2016).

136. H. Sharifi, M. Roebuck, S. Terterian, J. Jenkins, B. Tu, W. Strong, T.J. De Lyon, and R.D. Rajavel, J. Caulfield, and J.P. Curzan, "Advances in III-V bulk and superlattice-based high operating temperature MWIR detector technology", *Proc. SPIE* 10177, 101770U-1-6 (2017).

137. P.Y. Delaunay, B.Z. Nosho, A.R. Gurga, S. Terterian, and R.D. Rajavel, "Advances in III-V based dual-band MWIR/LWIR FPAs at HRL", *Proc. SPIE* 10177, 101770T-1-12 (2017).

Index

For Product Safety Concerns and Information please contact our EU
representative GPSR@taylorandfrancis.com
Taylor & Francis Verlag GmbH, Kaufingerstraße 24, 80331 München, Germany

www.ingramcontent.com/pod-product-compliance
Lightning Source LLC
Chambersburg PA
CBHW060951210326
41598CB00031B/4785

9 781032 069227